Fundamentals of
Molecular
Diagnostics

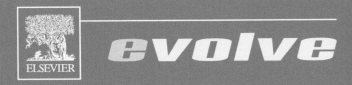

ELSEVIER

evolve

⁘ *To access your Instructor Resources, visit:*

http://evolve.elsevier.com/Bruns/molecular

Evolve® Student Resources for *Bruns: Fundamentals of Molecular Diagnostics offers the following features*

Instructor Resources

- **Web Links**
  Links to places of interest on the web specifically for molecular diagnostics.

- **Content Updates**
  Find out the latest information on relevant issues in the field.

Fundamentals of
Molecular
Diagnostics

David E. Bruns, M.D.
Professor of Pathology
University of Virginia Medical School;
Director of Clinical Chemistry and Associate Director of
    Molecular Diagnostics
University of Virginia Health System
Charlottesville, Virginia;
Editor, *Clinical Chemistry*
Washington, DC

Edward R. Ashwood, M.D.
Professor of Pathology
University of Utah School of Medicine
Chief Medical Officer/Laboratory Director
ARUP Laboratories
Salt Lake City, Utah

Carl A. Burtis, Ph.D.
Senior Technical Specialist
Health Services Division
Oak Ridge National Laboratory
Oak Ridge, Tennessee;
Clinical Professor of Pathology
University of Utah School of Medicine
Salt Lake City, Utah

Consulting Editor
Barbara G. Sawyer, Ph.D., M.T.(A.S.C.P.),
    C.L.S.(N.C.A.), C.L.Sp.(M.B.)
Professor
Department of Laboratory Sciences and Primary Care
School of Allied Health Sciences
Texas Tech University Health Sciences Center
Lubbock, Texas

SAUNDERS

ELSEVIER

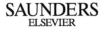

11830 Westline Industrial Drive
St. Louis, Missouri 63146

FUNDAMENTALS OF MOLECULAR DIAGNOSTICS   ISBN: 978-1-4160-3737-8
Copyright © 2007 by Saunders, an imprint of Elsevier Inc.

Library of Congress Control Number: 2007921086

Publishing Director: Andrew Allen
Executive Editor: Loren Wilson
Senior Developmental Editor: Ellen Wurm
Publishing Services Manager: Pat Joiner
Senior Project Manager: Rachel E. Dowell
Design Direction: Margaret Reid
Cover Designer: Jyotika Shroff

To our students, children, and grandchildren,
who teach us and are our future

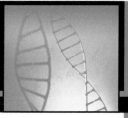
Edward R. Ashwood, M.D.
Professor of Pathology
University of Utah School of Medicine
Chief Medical Officer/Laboratory Director
ARUP Laboratories
Salt Lake City, Utah

Patrick M. M. Bossuyt, Ph.D.
Professor of Clinical Epidemiology
Chair of the Department of Clinical Epidemiology,
　　Biostatistics, & Bioinformatics
Academic Medical Center
University of Amsterdam
Amsterdam, The Netherlands
Introduction to Evidence-Based Molecular Diagnostics

David E. Bruns, M.D.
Professor of Pathology
University of Virginia Medical School;
Director of Clinical Chemistry and Associate Director of
　　Molecular Diagnostics
University of Virginia Health System
Charlottesville, Virginia;
Editor, *Clinical Chemistry*
Washington, DC
Introduction to Evidence-Based Molecular Diagnostics and
　　Reference Information

Carl A. Burtis, Ph.D.
Senior Technical Specialist
Health Services Division
Oak Ridge National Laboratory
Oak Ridge, Tennessee;
Clinical Professor of Pathology
University of Utah School of Medicine
Salt Lake City, Utah

Angela M. Caliendo, M.D., Ph.D.
Professor and Vice Chair
Pathology and Laboratory Medicine
Emory University School of Medicine;
Director, Emory Medical Laboratories
Emory University Hospital
Atlanta, Georgia
*Molecular Methods in Diagnosis and Monitoring of Infectious
　　Diseases*

Rossa W.K. Chiu, M.B.B.S., Ph.D., F.H.K.A.M.
　　(Pathology), F.R.C.P.A.
Associate Professor
Department of Chemical Pathology
The Chinese University of Hong Kong;
Honorary Senior Medical Officer
Department of Chemical Pathology
Prince of Wales Hospital
Hong Kong SAR
China
Principles of Molecular Biology and Nucleic Acid Isolation

Kojo S. J. Elenitoba-Johnson, M.D.
Associate Professor of Pathology
Director, Division of Translational Pathology
Director, Molecular Genetic Pathology Program
University of Michigan Medical School
Ann Arbor, Michigan
Molecular Genetics in Diagnosis of Human Cancers

Andrea Ferreira-Gonzalez, Ph.D.
Professor of Pathology
Virginia Commonwealth University;
Director Molecular Diagnostics Laboratory
Virginia Commonwealth University Medical Center
Richmond, Virginia
*Molecular Methods in Diagnosis and Monitoring of Infectious
　　Diseases*

Amy R. Groszbach, C.L.Sp.(M.B.)
Education Specialist II
Molecular Genetics Laboratory;
Instructor of Laboratory Medicine
Mayo Clinic College of Medicine
Mayo Clinic
Rochester, Minnesota
Specimen Collection and Processing

Sultan Habeebu, M.D., Ph.D.
Molecular Genetic Pathology Fellow
Department of Pathology
Baylor College of Medicine and Texas Children's Hospital
Houston, Texas
*Molecular Methods in Diagnosis and Monitoring of Infectious
　　Diseases*

Doris M. Haverstick, Ph.D.
Associate Professor of Pathology
University of Virginia
Charlottesville, Virginia
Specimen Collection and Processing

Malek Kamoun, M.D., Ph.D.
Professor, Department of Pathology and Laboratory Medicine
University of Pennsylvania
Philadelphia, Pennsylvania
Identity Assessment

Anthony A. Killeen, M.D., Ph.D.
Associate Professor
Director of Clinical Pathology
Department of Laboratory Medicine and Pathology
University of Minnesota
Minneapolis, Minnesota
Design and Operation of a Molecular Diagnostics Laboratory

Noriko Kusukawa, Ph.D.
Adjunct Associate Professor of Pathology
University of Utah School of Medicine;
Assistant Vice President
ARUP Laboratories
Salt Lake City, Utah
Genomes and Nucleic Acid Alterations and *Nucleic Acid Techniques*

Yuk Ming Dennis Lo, M.A., D.M., D.Phil., F.R.C.P., M.R.C.P., F.R.C.Path.
Dr. Li Ka Shing Professor of Medicine and Professor of Chemical Pathology
Department of Chemical Pathology
The Chinese University of Hong Kong;
Honorary Consultant Chemical Pathologist
Prince of Wales Hospital
Shatin, New Territories
Hong Kong SAR
China
Principles of Molecular Biology and *Nucleic Acid Isolation*

Elaine Lyon, Ph.D., F.A.C.M.G.
Assistant Professor (Clinical) of Pathology
Director of Molecular Genetics
University of Utah School of Medicine
Salt Lake City, Utah
Design and Operation of a Molecular Diagnostics Laboratory

Gwendolyn A. McMillin, Ph.D.
Assistant Professor of Pathology
University of Utah School of Medicine;
Medical Director of Clinical Toxicology, Drug Abuse Testing, Trace Elements
Co-Medical Director of Pharmacogenomics
ARUP Laboratories
Salt Lake City, Utah
Pharmacogenetics

Christopher P. Price, Ph.D., F.R.C.Path.
Visiting Professor in Clinical Biochemistry
University of Oxford
Oxford, United Kingdom
Introduction to Evidence-Based Molecular Diagnostics

James Versalovic, M.D., Ph.D.
Assistant Professor of Pathology
Baylor College of Medicine;
Director, Division of Molecular Pathology
Department of Pathology
Texas Children's Hospital
Houston, Texas
Molecular Methods in Diagnosis and Monitoring of Infectious Diseases

Cindy L. Vnencak-Jones, Ph.D.
Associate Professor of Pathology and Pediatrics
Vanderbilt University School of Medicine;
Director, Molecular Genetics Laboratory
Vanderbilt University Medical Center
Nashville, Tennessee
Inherited Diseases

Victor W. Weedn, M.D., J.D.
Visiting Professor
Forensic Science and Law Program
Bayer School of Natural and Environmental Sciences
School of Law
Duquesne University
Pittsburgh, Pennsylvania
Identity Assessment

Peter Wilding, Ph.D., F.R.C.Path.
Professor Emeritus
Department of Pathology and Laboratory Medicine
University of Pennsylvania Medical Center
Philadelphia, Pennsylvania
Miniaturization: DNA Chips and Devices

Thomas M. Williams, M.D.
Professor of Pathology
University of New Mexico;
Director, Genetics and Cytometry Division
TriCore Reference Laboratories
Albuquerque, New Mexico
Identity Assessment

Carl T. Wittwer, M.D., Ph.D.
Professor of Pathology
University of Utah Medical School
Salt Lake City, Utah
Genomes and Nucleic Acid Alterations and *Nucleic Acid Techniques*

Reviewers

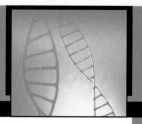

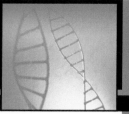

Foreword

In the late 1990s, a small number of clinical laboratories, primarily based in university hospitals, established new laboratory sections where emerging nucleic acid–based technologies were adapted for diagnostic purposes. In the ensuing 15 years, we have witnessed the development and growth of these early efforts into the discipline of molecular diagnostics. Today the majority of university hospital laboratories, reference laboratories, and many large private hospital laboratories offer sophisticated menus in molecular diagnostic testing. Further, we are beginning to see the dissemination of molecular diagnostics into community laboratory settings through technological innovation. Molecular diagnostics has become an essential component in the laboratory evaluation of a diversity of human disease conditions, both inborn and acquired. As a participant in the growth of molecular diagnostics, I have often reflected on the pressing need for textbooks that offer current and comprehensive information on molecular diagnostics. This need has made itself most apparent when teaching molecular diagnostics to medical technologists, technologists in training, medical students, and pathology residents and fellows. In this context, I am particularly enthused to introduce the first edition of *Fundamentals of Molecular Diagnostics*, edited by Drs. David E. Bruns, Edward R. Ashwood, and Carl A. Burtis.

The editors have assembled an outstanding group of authors who are recognized experts in their respective areas of molecular diagnostics. With an orientation towards serving as a textbook for a course in molecular diagnostics, the text appropriately begins with chapters on basic principles of molecular biology and nucleic acid chemistry, followed by an in-depth description of the genomic alterations interrogated in molecular diagnostic assays. The next section of the text focuses on techniques, instrumentation, and operational principles for a molecular diagnostics laboratory, and admirably describes the core elements needed for establishing a molecular diagnostics laboratory. Extensive discussion is devoted to specimen collection and processing, nucleic acid purification and amplification, and detection techniques. The polymerase chain reaction, which has become the dominant analytical technique in molecular diagnostics, is presented in a state-of-the-art manner. The inclusion of a chapter on evidence-based molecular diagnostics adds an important perspective beyond the technical.

The third section of the text focuses on applications. The chapter on inherited disorders provides an in-depth introduction to the complexity of genetic testing from single nucleotide alterations to full gene analysis to imprinting and mitochondrial genetics. The concept of genetic predisposition is exemplified by discussion of inherited breast cancer and familial colon cancer. A chapter on identity assessment provides the reader with an understanding of how variations in the human genome are used for tissue typing in organ transplantation, assessment of bone marrow engraftment, parentage testing, and forensics. Molecular diagnostics has tremendously impacted the field of infectious diseases, becoming integral in the diagnosis and monitoring of several key infectious diseases, including human immunodeficiency virus (HIV) and hepatitis C virus. The impact of molecular diagnostics on these major pathogens and others is reflected in the chapter on infectious diseases. Notably, the role of molecular diagnosis in the emerging field of bioterrorism is also addressed. Reflecting the current and comprehensive nature of the text, a chapter is devoted to pharmacogenetics, the study of genetic variation and how it impacts drug metabolism. The final chapter concludes with an extensive review of genomic alterations that contribute to the development and progression of malignancies and that are assessed for diagnostic, therapeutic, and monitoring purposes.

In addition to the in-depth text discussions, each chapter is highlighted by illustrations that describe and reinforce concepts and show examples of diagnostic results. Each chapter begins with a set of Key Words and Definitions that serve as guides for the most critical concepts. Throughout the text, example questions are provided, and an additional, unique feature is a focus on ethical issues raised by molecular diagnostic testing that are presented in case scenarios accompanied by points for discussion.

It has been a rewarding, intellectual adventure to be a participant in the growth of molecular diagnostics and it is gratifying to see how fully the field has developed. This growth is amply reflected in *Fundamentals of Molecular Diagnostics*, and I look forward to using this new text as a reference and in my teaching.

Karl V. Voelkerding, M.D.

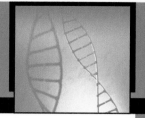

Preface

Molecular diagnostics is the youngest and fastest growing field of laboratory science. Most areas of medicine depend most heavily on 19th and 20th century technologies such as microscopes, stethoscopes, and Lina Hesse's agar for growing of bacteria. By contrast, the exciting scientific and technological advances that make molecular diagnostics possible occurred in our lifetimes. The application of these technologies to medical diagnostics comes at an equally exciting time in medicine in which evidence-based medicine is teaching us better ways to study and use tests in making diagnoses and in selecting and guiding therapy. Not surprisingly, molecular diagnostics is growing rapidly, and writing a book about it requires the collaboration of experts.

BACKGROUND

This new book on molecular diagnostics had its origins when we were updating the *Tietz Textbook of Clinical Chemistry and Molecular Diagnostics*. We quickly realized that the coverage of molecular diagnostics needed to expand beyond the single short chapter on nucleic acids to become a new section of the textbook. Fortunately, each of the leading experts whom we invited to prepare a new chapter on a selected aspect of molecular diagnostics agreed to do so, and each of them produced an excellent manuscript, often with one or more expert co-authors. The new chapters were published in the Fourth Edition of the *Tietz Textbook*.

The present work builds on the *Tietz Textbook* chapters to capture the *fundamentals* of molecular diagnostics; it does not aim to provide *details* of the field or extensive reference lists found in larger reference books. The book was prepared with the needs of students in mind, including medical technologists and pathology residents and others with diverse backgrounds. Special effort has been taken to make the text understandable without prior knowledge of the field.

In preparing this book, we benefited not only from the collaboration of outstanding authors but also from the expert help of Barbara G. Sawyer, Ph.D., M.T.(A.S.C.P.), C.L.S.(N.C.A.), C.L.Sp.(M.B.). Professor Sawyer teaches molecular diagnostics, among other topics, to Medical Technology and Medical Laboratory Technician students. Professor Sawyer served as a consulting editor on this book as she did for the Fifth and Sixth Editions of *Tietz Fundamentals of Clinical Chemistry*. The parallels of this book with the companion *Tietz Fundamentals of Clinical Chemistry* will be apparent to the many readers who are familiar with that book.

FEATURES

This book contains educational features that are not present in the chapters published in the *Tietz Textbook of Clinical Chemistry and Molecular Diagnostics*. These include:

- **learning objectives** for each chapter
- a list of **key words and their definitions** at the beginning of each chapter
- Advanced Concepts (AC) sections (found in shaded boxes) that go beyond material found in introductory courses and provide enrichment, challenges, or background
- separate discussions (found in blue-shaded boxes) of **ethical issues** in nearly every chapter
- a **glossary** of technical terms
- a section of **reference information** that will make the book useful for later reference
- a short list of **self-study questions** (written by the expert authors) at the end of each chapter

We trust that these will prove as useful as similar features for users of *Tietz Fundamentals of Clinical Chemistry*.

ANCILLARIES

The **Evolve Web site** for *Fundamentals of Molecular Diagnostics* offers instructors additional educational material including an instructor's manual and a 250-question test bank.

We trust that these will prove as useful as similar features have for users of *Tietz Fundamentals of Clinical Chemistry*.

We are grateful for the opportunity to prepare this book for students of molecular diagnostics. We have enjoyed working with our team of dedicated authors who have invested untold hours in preparing clearly written chapters that are authoritative and up-to-date. We have also benefited from working with the staff of Elsevier, including Loren Wilson, Ellen Wurm, and Rachel E. Dowell. Their professionalism and sound advice are cheerfully acknowledged. Ellen Wurm even joined our weekly conference calls throughout the years of planning, writing, editing, and producing this book and its predecessor.

Molecular diagnostics is changing lives each day, and the impact of the field on society will expand greatly as even more powerful molecular tests are introduced. We hope that the short ethics sections, each only a few paragraphs long and set off from the body of the text, will not only provide a brief respite from the reading of challenging technical information, but will encourage students, whether technologists, physicians, or doctoral scientists, to reflect on the critical roles they play in this exciting adventure that we call molecular diagnostics.

David E. Bruns
Edward R. Ashwood
Carl A. Burtis

Contents

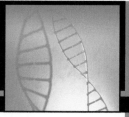

Fundamentals of
Molecular
Diagnostics

SECTION I

PRINCIPLES

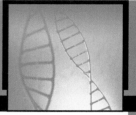

Chapter 1

Principles of Molecular Biology

Y.M. Dennis Lo, M.A., D.M., D. Phil., F.R.C.P., F.R.C. Path.
Rossa W.K. Chiu, M.B.B.S., Ph.D., F.R.C.P.A., FHKAM (Pathology)

OBJECTIVES

1. Define the genetic code and state the central dogma.
2. Compare genotyping and phenotyping.
3. Discuss the differences between DNA and RNA, including physical and chemical structure, physiological function, and utility in clinical diagnostic testing.
4. Compare and contrast the chemical makeup of purines and pyrimidines.
5. Describe the structure of a eukaryotic chromosome.
6. Describe the physical structure and chemical composition of chromatin and its appearance during cell cycle stages.
7. Differentiate centromeres and telomeres and state the function of each.
8. List the processes involved in DNA replication, RNA transcription, and mRNA translation.
9. State the physiological function of DNA and RNA polymerases.
10. State the importance of epigenetics, particularly DNA methylation, in gene function.
11. Describe the structure of mitochondrial DNA; compare this with nuclear DNA and pseudogenes.
12. State the clinical utility of assays for circulating nucleic acids.
13. Describe the human genome and the Human Genome Project.

KEY WORDS AND DEFINITIONS

Allele: A copy of a gene; alleles may demonstrate sequence variations that determine variations in the functional characteristics of a translated protein.

Autosome: A nonsex chromosome; there are 22 pairs of autosomes in the human genome.

Base Pair: A purine and a pyrimidine nucleotide bound by hydrogen bonds; in DNA base pairing, adenine binds to thymine and guanine pairs with cytosine, and in RNA base pairing, adenine binds to uracil.

Centromere: A primary constriction in a chromosome; centromeres play an important role in directing the movement of chromosomes between daughter cells during cell division.

Chromatin: Nuclear DNA and its associated structural proteins; chromatin is arranged and organized in a hierarchical fashion in which the degree of its condensation increases with higher levels of structural organization.

Chromosome: A highly ordered structure of a single double-stranded DNA (dsDNA) molecule, compacted many times with the aid of structural DNA-binding proteins.

Codon: A three-nucleotide sequence that "codes" for an amino acid during translation; there are 64 possible codons in nuclear DNA.

DNA: Deoxyribonucleic Acid: A molecule that carries genetic information and is a double-stranded polymer of nucleotides.

DNA-Binding Proteins: Proteins that recognize and bind to specific DNA sequences. Some of such proteins are involved in the regulation of DNA transcription.

DNA Methylation: The addition of a methyl group to the fifth carbon position of cytosine residues in CpG dinucleotides; this epigenetic process is implicated in growth and development of organisms.

Epigenetics: Processes that alter gene function or its interpretation by mechanisms other than those that rely on DNA sequence change; these processes include DNA methylation, genomic imprinting, histone modification, chromatin remodeling, and others.

Euchromatin: Genomic regions that are rich in genes and are in general less compactly organized during interphase.

Exon: The coding region of a gene that will be expressed as protein following translation.

Exonuclease: A nuclease that releases one nucleotide at a time (serially) beginning at one end of a nucleic acid; exonuclease activity excises incorrectly paired nucleotides during replication.

Gene: A unit of DNA that specifies production of proteins and RNA molecules required for cellular function.

Genetic Code: The complete list of nucleotide codons and the amino acids or actions they "code" for.

Genome: The complete set of chromosomes; the total complement of hereditary information; the human genome contains two copies, termed alleles, of each autosomal gene.

Genotype: The primary nucleotide sequences of the two gene alleles.

Heterochromatin: Genomic regions that are gene poor or span transcriptionally silent genes and are more densely packed during interphase.

Heteroplasmy: The presence of more than one population of mitochondrial DNA sequences in a cell consequent to the accumulation of sequence variations.

Histone: A structural protein involved in the three-dimensional organization of nuclear DNA.

Homoplasmy: The presence of a homogeneous population of mitochondrial genomes in a cell.

Human Genome Project: A project undertaken by the International Human Genome Sequencing Consortium to decipher the three billion base pairs in the human genome; the project was completed in 2003.

Intron: A noncoding region of a gene, locked between exons, that will not be translated into protein.

MicroRNAs: Short noncoding RNA molecules around 22 nucleotides in length that play a role in regulation of gene expression by interfering with effective translation of mRNA to proteins.

Mitochondrial DNA: The circular DNA within a mitochondrial organelle that codes for polypeptides involved in the oxidative phosphorylation pathway; this DNA is typically transmitted across generations by maternal inheritance.

Nucleases: Enzymes that catalyze the hydrolysis of nucleic acid by cleaving chains of nucleotides into smaller units.

Nucleic Acid: A polymer made of nucleotide monomers (a sugar moiety, a phosphoric acid, and purine or pyrimidine bases); examples are deoxyribonucleic acid (DNA) and ribonucleic acid (RNA).

Nucleosome: A unit of chromatin consisting of nucleosome core particles (146 base pairs of dsDNA) and linker DNA wound around an octamer of histone proteins.

Nucleotide: A unit of DNA or RNA, consisting of one chemical base (purine or pyrimidine) plus a phosphate molecule and a sugar molecule (deoxyribose or ribose).

Phenotype: The observable characteristics of an organism; includes visible features (eye color, height), and chemical and behavioral characteristics; reflects interaction of genes and environment.

Polymerase: Enzymes involved in DNA replication and transcription; DNA polymerase III reads a parent DNA template and attaches nucleotides to a growing daughter strand according to the base-pairing rules of dsDNA; RNA polymerase II binds to a promoter region of a DNA strand to initiate transcription.

Promoter: A regulatory region of DNA that serves to bind RNA polymerase II that in turns binds other substances that will lead to initiation of transcription; promoters control the rate and timing of a protein's production.

Purine: A base containing two carbon-nitrogen rings; adenine and guanine are purines.

Pyrimidine: A base containing one carbon-nitrogen ring; cytosine, thymine, and uracil are pyrimidines.

Replication: The faithful reproduction of the DNA content from parent to daughter cells during cell division.

RNA: Ribonucleic Acid: A biological substance similar to DNA with the exceptions of being single stranded, containing ribose as the sugar moiety, having an extra hydroxyl group, and containing uracil instead of thymine; there are different functional types of RNA including messenger (coding) RNA (mRNA), ribosomal RNA (rRNA), transfer RNA (tRNA), and other small noncoding RNAs, such as microRNA.

Telomere: The DNA sequences at the end of a chromosome; telomeres contain repetitive nucleotide sequences that protect the ends of chromosomes from recombination with other chromosomes.

Transcription: The process of transferring sequence information from the gene regions of DNA to an RNA message.

Translation: The process whereby an mRNA sequence forms an amino acid sequence with the help of tRNA and eventual enzymatic peptide bond formation between amino acids to synthesize polypeptides; translation occurs on cytoplasmic ribosomes.

Molecular diagnostics represents one of the most rapidly developing areas in many diagnostic disciplines, including clinical chemistry, clinical hematology, clinical immunology, clinical microbiology, and tissue pathology. Advances in the field have been made possible by our improved understanding of molecular biology and genetics and of their relationships with human diseases and the development of powerful technologies for the analysis of **nucleic acids.** The chapters in this book attempt to provide an overview of the important advances in molecular diagnostics. The fundamental concepts in molecular biology are reviewed in this chapter. Molecular diagnostic techniques and operational requirements are discussed in Chapters 3 to 8. The subsequent chapters focus on key applications of molecular diagnostics, specifically inherited diseases (Chapter 9), identity (Chapter 10), infectious diseases (Chapter 11), pharmacogenetics (Chapter 12), and the assessment of malignancies (Chapter 13).

LANDMARK DEVELOPMENTS IN GENETICS AND MOLECULAR DIAGNOSTICS

Amazing developments in biotechnology took place in the late twentieth century. For example, we witnessed the decoding of the human **genome,** cloning of organisms, and progress in stem cell research and gene therapy. Many of these advances would not have been possible without the many earlier landmark discoveries that unveiled the mysteries of genetics and paved the way for modern molecular diagnostics.[9] Genetics began modestly when Mendel experimented with garden peas. His findings, published in 1866 and suggesting the concepts of **alleles** and **genes** as discrete units of heredity, essentially captured the most fundamental concepts in inheritance. In 1910

Morgan revealed that the units of heredity are contained within **chromosomes,** but it was Avery in 1944 who confirmed through studies on bacteria that it was **deoxyribonucleic acid (DNA)** that carried the genetic information. Franklin and Wilkins studied DNA by x-ray crystallography, which subsequently led to the unraveling of the double-helical structure of DNA by Watson and Crick in 1953. In the 1960s Smith demonstrated that DNA can be cleaved by restriction enzymes, which Arber had discovered earlier and that facilitated the subsequent development of recombinant DNA technologies. Nathans furthered the work on restriction enzymes and was the first to construct a genetic map. In 1975 the Southern blot was invented, which allowed the detection of specific DNA sequences. Soon after, in 1977, DNA-sequencing methodologies were developed, and the first complete DNA sequence of an organism, a bacteriophage, was published. Prenatal genetic diagnosis of sickle cell disease was first shown to be feasible by Kan and Chang in 1981. In 1985 Mullis and co-workers developed the **polymerase** chain reaction (PCR), which provided a rapid way to make many copies of a DNA molecule (see Chapter 5). DNA microarrays, which allow the simultaneous interrogation of gene transcripts, became a reality in 1996. Remarkably the draft human genome sequence was released in 2001 and completed in 2003.

This is a brief account of a fraction of the many great discoveries that shaped modern genetics and molecular diagnostics. Whereas the explosive accumulation of genetic knowledge has translated into escalating clinical demands for molecular diagnostics, improved molecular diagnostic techniques have reciprocally led to the discovery of new genetic knowledge. An understanding of the fundamental aspects of molecular biology, as outlined in this chapter, is required for the effective implementation and interpretation of molecular diagnostics. The chapter begins with an overview of the essential principles of molecular biology followed by a more in-depth discussion of the key aspects, starting with the Watson and Crick model of DNA, through to the end discussion of the greatest biotechnological achievement of mankind in our time, the **Human Genome Project.**

THE ESSENTIALS

Genes are the basic units of inheritance corresponding to defined segments of DNA that encode for a protein or **ribonucleic acid (RNA)** product with biological functions. DNA is a biological substance that carries genetic information and is a polymer of **nucleotides** or bases. Genetic information is faithfully reproduced from parent to daughter cells during cell division through the process of DNA **replication.** When genes are expressed ("switched on"), the DNA sequence is transcribed into RNA. RNA molecules are polymers of ribonucleotides and exist in a number of functional forms, such as messenger RNA (mRNA), ribosomal RNA (rRNA), and transfer RNA (tRNA). mRNA is the product of a transcribed nucleotide sequence and is in turn translated into a protein, which is a polymer of amino acids. Each amino acid is encoded by a triplet nucleotide code, termed a **codon.** The human **genetic code** comprises 64 codons encoding for the 21 amino acids and 3 stop codons. The mRNA codons are read by the anticodon regions of tRNA molecules, which are small RNAs that bring the corresponding amino acid to the growing polypeptide chain. The polypeptide chain is synthesized by ribosomes, which are macromolecular complexes containing rRNA. Recently, it has been recognized that certain other RNA molecules that do not encode for a protein product, termed noncoding RNAs, have specialized biological functions. An example of such noncoding RNA is **microRNA.**[1]

Most human cells contain two full complements of the human genome, which is organized and packaged into 23 pairs of chromosomes. A chromosome is a highly ordered structure of a single DNA molecule with specialized structural features, namely a **centromere** and two **telomeres.** Every individual inherits one complement of the human genome from his or her father and one set from the mother. Thus the human genome contains two copies of each **autosome.** Although a gene sequence encodes for a specific protein with defined functions, alleles of genes may demonstrate sequence variations that in turn determine the variations in the functional characteristics of the protein between individuals. The primary nucleotide sequences of the two gene alleles form the **genotype,** and the expressed function or biological effect of the gene product is termed the **phenotype.** Thus one could study a human disease or trait at the genetic level through the determination of the allelic sequence of a gene (i.e., genotyping) or at the protein level through assessments of the protein function (i.e., phenotyping). Examples of phenotyping include the investigation of enzyme concentrations or activities, ABO blood groups, and electrophoretic mobility of hemoglobin variants. The choice of genotyping or phenotyping for making a diagnosis depends on the specific diagnostic application.

NUCLEIC ACID STRUCTURE AND ORGANIZATION

There is an intimate relationship between nucleic acid structure and function. The physiological function of nucleic acid is facilitated by its "strategically designed" structure. Although an alteration in the structure of nucleic acids would lead to an altered function, an altered function, on the other hand, may be seen as an altered structure. Thus a discussion of nucleic acid structure is pertinent to further discussions on nucleic acid function.

Molecular Compositions and Structures of DNA and RNA

The physicochemical properties and function of nucleic acids are largely governed by the compositions and structures of DNA and RNA. A single molecule of DNA is a polymer consisting of a backbone of invariant composition and of side groups arranged in a variable sequence (Figures 1-1, 1-2). The polymer is synthesized from monomers of nucleotides composed of the sugar deoxyribose, a phosphate residue, and a purine or pyrimidine base (Figure 1-1). The **purines** are adenine (A) and guanine (G) and contain two carbon-nitrogen rings (Figure 1-1). The **pyrimidines** are cytosine (C) and thymine (T) and contain one carbon-nitrogen ring (Figure 1-1). The four nucleotide building blocks of DNA are abbreviated dATP (deoxyadenine-triphosphate), dGTP (deoxyguanine-triphosphate), dCTP (deoxycytosine-triphosphate), and dTTP (deoxythymine-triphosphate), respectively. Nucleotides are joined by phosphodiester bonds that link the 5′-phosphate group of one to the 3′-hydroxyl group of the next (Figure 1-1). There are no 3′-3′ or 5′-5′ linkages; thus the sugar and phosphate moieties make up the nonspecific portions of the molecule

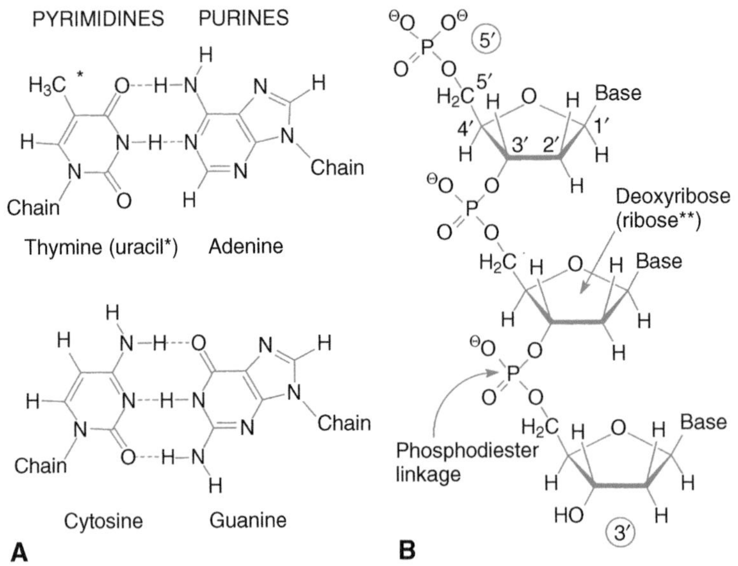

Figure 1-1

A, Purine and pyrimidine bases and the formation of complementary base pairs. Dashed lines indicate the formation of hydrogen bonds. (In RNA, thymine is replaced by uracil, which differs from thymine only in its lack of the methyl group.) **B,** A ssDNA chain. Repeating nucleotide units are linked by phosphodiester bonds that join the 5' carbon of one sugar to the 3' carbon of the next. Each nucleotide monomer consists of a sugar moiety, a phosphate residue, and a base. (In RNA, the sugar is ribose, which adds a 2'-hydroxyl to deoxyribose.)

(Modified from Piper MA, Unger ER. Nucleic acid probes: a primer for pathologists, Chicago: ASCP Press, 1989.)

(Figure 1-2). The sequence of the bases varies from molecule to molecule and uniquely identifies each DNA polymer, which, as discussed later, determines the identity and function of the protein or RNA products that the DNA encodes.

Although the purines and pyrimidines are of different compositions and sizes, when in the proper orientation, adenine forms hydrogen bonds with thymine, and guanine forms hydrogen bonds with cytosine to form flat ("planar") structures of similar dimensions (Figure 1-2). The hydrogen bonding between the two bases leads to the formation of a **base pair.** This and the fact that the base portion of each nucleotide is hydrophobic contribute to the energetically favorable secondary structure of DNA: a right-handed, double-stranded helix, the Watson and Crick structure (Figure 1-2). The planar base pairs stack in the inside of the helix, 10 bases per turn, whereas the hydrophilic sugar-phosphate backbone forms noncovalent bonds with surrounding water molecules. For the two DNA polymers to form the proper hydrogen bonds between the bases, two requirements must be fulfilled: (1) the polymers must run in opposite directions (antiparallel) as defined by the free hydroxyl groups at each end (3'-5' vs. 5'-3'), and (2) the sequences of each molecule must be such that A:T and G:C hydrogen bonds are always formed by the process of base pairing. Two DNA strands that meet these requirements are called complementary. Owing to base pairing and the double-helical conformation, dsDNA is an exceptionally stable molecule. Retention of the base pairs in the inner portion of the helix prevents disruption by water molecules. The helical conformation places each monomer in an identical orientation within the molecule and forms the same secondary bonds as every other monomer. This secondary bonding contributes to the overall stability. Because the base pairs are of similar size, the helix retains a constant angle of rotation and prevents distortion (Figure 1-2). All of these features dictate that all dsDNA molecules, regardless of base sequence, retain the same shape and size within a pH range of approximately 4 to 9. Outside these limits, the base pair bonds are disrupted, and the helix unwinds.

RNA is chemically very similar to DNA, but differs in important ways. The sugar unit is ribose, which has an added hydroxyl group at the 2' position, and the methylated pyrimidine uracil (U) (Figure 1-1) replaces thymine. RNA exists in various functional forms, but typically as a single-stranded polymer that is much shorter than DNA and has an irregular three-dimensional structure. Research from recent years has revealed that RNA conformations are not random structures, and the folding mechanism of RNA molecules is complex.[8] The folding produces a secondary structure that can be depicted in a two-dimensional drawing. The secondary structure adopted by an RNA molecule is to a large extent related to its nucleotide sequence. The secondary structure for particular RNA sequences can be as reproducible as the secondary structure of a protein. It is now known that RNA molecules can further interact to form complex tertiary structures (three-dimensional, like a sculpture). Formation of these structures involves other chemical interactions within the RNA molecule and is intimately related to novel functions of RNA, such as the catalytic activity of ribozymes.[8]

Chromosome Structure

DNA molecules are extremely long and in the eukaryotic cell are maintained in orderly and compact three-dimensional structures. Each diploid human cell (that is, cells with two sets

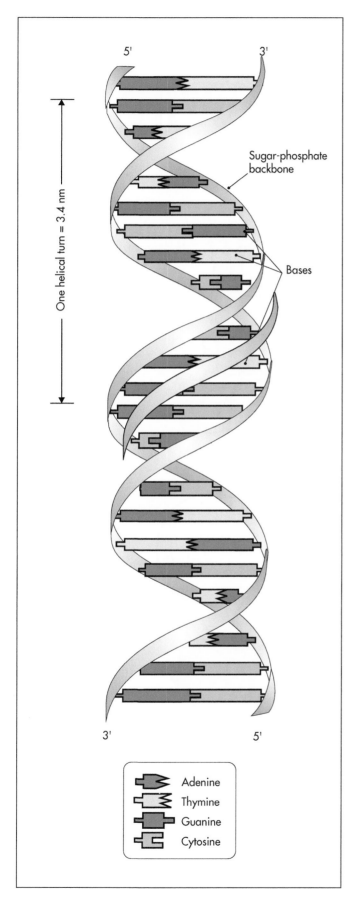

of chromosomes) contains two full complements of the human genome, each copy consisting of approximately 3.2 billion nucleotides. This vast amount of genetic material is organized into 23 chromosome pairs, with one member of each pair being of maternal origin and the other of paternal origin. The two chromosomes of each pair are similar (homologous) and, except for the sex chromosomes (X and Y), contain the same genes arranged in the same sequence. Each chromosome is a highly ordered structure of a single dsDNA molecule, compacted many times with the aid of structural **DNA-binding proteins** (Figure 1-3). The chromosomes are in their most compact state and appear as fingerlike structures during cell division (specifically in the stage called metaphase). A primary constriction, the centromere, is also notable on each chromosome (Figure 1-3). The ends of the chromosomes are termed the telomeres (Figure 1-3). Both the centromeres and telomeres have specialized functions to be discussed below. The nonsex chromosomes, the autosomes, in the human genome are numbered in the order of decreasing size. The chromosomal arrangement of human DNA not only allows the packaging of the vast human genome into the limited physical dimensions of the cell nucleus, but also governs one of the mendelian laws of inheritance on independent assortment whereby genes located on different chromosomes recombine at random from one generation to the next. In addition, as will be discussed later, the structural organization of the human genome is intimately related to the control of DNA transcription, replication, recombination, and repair.[11,16]

Nuclear DNA in conjunction with its associated structural proteins, including **histone** and nonhistone proteins, is known as **chromatin.** Chromatin is arranged and organized in a hierarchical fashion in which the degree of condensation increases with higher levels of structural organization.[11] The **nucleosome** represents the most basic level of chromatin organization and is present as repeated units along the full length of each chromosome (Figure 1-3).[16] Each nucleosome unit consists of a nucleosome core particle and 20 to 80 base pairs of linker DNA, which spans between adjacent nucleosomes. A nucleosome core particle involves 146 base pairs of dsDNA tightly wound around an octamer of histone proteins, two each of four histone proteins, namely H2A, H2B, H3, and H4. The linker DNA segments are associated with the linker histone H1. Nucleosomes are further packed in successive levels of complexity[11] and ultimately can be seen as discrete chromosomes during cell division (Figure 1-3). Integrity of the nucleosomal structure is crucial to the maintenance of the higher-order arrangements of chromatin.

Chromatin condensation is a dynamic process that changes in a coordinated fashion in association with the cell cycle (i.e., during the ordered set of changes that lead to cell growth and division of cells to produce two daughter cells). In general chromatin is much less condensed during interphase of the cell cycle, at which time DNA is replicated. However, the extent of

Figure 1-2
The DNA double helix, with sugar-phosphate backbone and pairing of the bases in the core forming planar structures.
(From Jorde LB, Carey JC, Bamshad MJ et al, editors. Medical genetics, 3rd ed. St Louis: Mosby, 2006.)

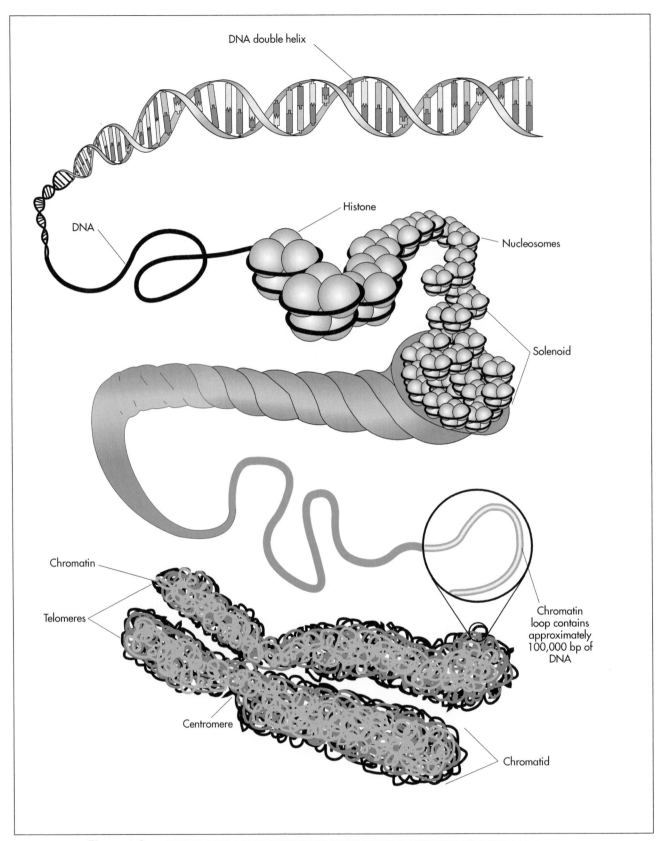

Figure 1-3

Structural organization of human chromosomal DNA. dsDNA is wound around histones to form nucleosomes. Nuclear DNA in conjunction with its associated structural proteins is known as chromatin. Chromatin in its most compact state forms chromosomes. The primary constriction of a chromosome is the centromere, and the chromosome's ends are the telomeres.
(From Jorde LB, Carey JC, Bamshad MJ, editors. Medical genetics, 3rd ed. St Louis: Mosby, 2006.)

chromatin condensation during interphase varies among regions of the genome. Genomic regions that are rich in genes are in general less compactly organized and are termed **euchromatin.** Regions that are gene poor or span over transcriptionally silent genes (i.e., genes that are not being transcribed) are more densely packed and are called **heterochromatin.** Our understanding of the biological role of heterochromatin and the mechanisms that govern its formation and assembly has improved in recent years. Heterochromatin is important for the maintenance of specialized chromatin structures, X-chromosome inactivation in females, maintenance of genome stability by stabilizing repetitive DNA sequences, and regulation of gene expression.[10] Eukaryotic chromosomes contain two specialized regions of heterochromatin, namely the centromere and the telomeres. The former plays an important role in directing the movement of chromosomes between daughter cells during cell division, and the latter contains repetitive nucleotide sequences that protect the ends of chromosomes from recombination with other chromosomes. The number of telomeric repeats in somatic cells decreases with age, but is maintained in germ cells and malignant cells by the enzyme telomerase. It has been appreciated in recent years that telomeres and telomerase play important roles in the pathological conditions of human diseases.[2] Besides the large centromeric or telomeric blocks of heterochromatin, smaller domains of heterochromatin are scattered throughout the genome and are associated with the control of gene expression. The assembly of heterochromatin starts at the most basic level of chromatin organization, the nucleosomes, and involves **DNA methylation,** histone modifications, noncoding RNAs, and sequence-specific DNA-binding proteins.[10] The functional implications of the structural organization of chromatin will be discussed further later in the chapter.

NUCLEIC ACID PHYSIOLOGY AND FUNCTIONAL REGULATION

Nucleic acids form the repository for hereditary information and provide the means of translating that information into the cellular machinery of life. Gene expression refers to the process of transforming the genetic blueprint into functional products that participate in various biological processes of a cell. The process of gene expression is governed by the central dogma. The central dogma specifies that biological information is transferred from DNA to RNA to protein (Figure 1-4). The faithful reproduction of the DNA content from parent to daughter cells during cell division is termed **replication.** A gene is expressed through the **transcription** of its DNA sequence into RNA. A polypeptide is then synthesized through **translation** of the RNA base sequence into the corresponding amino acid sequence.

Replication

Each time a cell divides, the entire DNA content of that cell must be faithfully duplicated so that the total complement of hereditary information (the human genome) is retained in each daughter cell. This process is called replication. Owing to the laws of base pairing (which state that adenine pairs only with thymine and guanine only with cytosine), the sequence of a single strand of DNA dictates the sequence of its complementary strand. In replication, each of the two parent strands of a dsDNA molecule serves as the template for the synthesis of a daughter strand (Figure 1-5). The process is called semiconser-

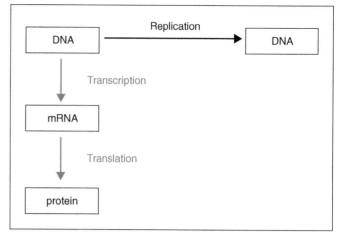

Figure 1-4
The central dogma.

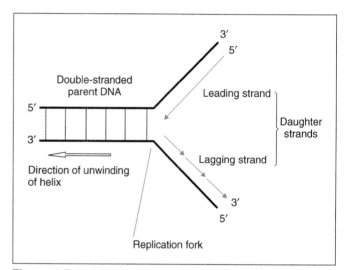

Figure 1-5
DNA replication. dsDNA is separated at the replication fork. The leading strand is synthesized continuously, whereas the lagging strand is synthesized discontinuously, but joined later by DNA ligase.

vative because the duplicated dsDNA molecules produced in this manner are each composed of one parent (conserved) strand and one daughter strand. For replication to occur, the original double-stranded helix must be separated, which is an energetically unfavorable event. This is accomplished with a combination of DNA-specific proteins and enzymes, and synthesis of both daughter strands proceeds as the parent strands separate. Replication is initiated at multiple sites (origins of replication) during this process, but each origin of replication is used only once during a single cell cycle.

Daughter strands are synthesized by DNA polymerase III, an enzyme that reads the parent template and attaches nucleotides to the growing daughter strand according to the base-pairing rules of dsDNA. DNA polymerase III begins synthesis at the replication fork (Figure 1-5), the point of strand separation, with a short RNA primer that base pairs to the parent template. Later this primer is excised and replaced with DNA by the DNA repair enzyme, DNA polymerase I. Because DNA polymerase III synthesizes DNA only in the 5'-3' direction, one daughter strand, the leading strand, is synthesized continuously, whereas the other, the lagging strand, must be synthesized discontinuously (i.e., in short segments) (Figure 1-5). The fragments on the discontinuous strand are then joined by the DNA ligase enzyme. Many other proteins are involved in unwinding and stabilizing the parent strands for synthesis, in protecting single-stranded regions, in recognizing initiation sites, and in synthesizing the RNA primer. In addition to synthetic capabilities, the DNA polymerases possess a special **onuclease** or "proofreading" function. When an incorrect nucleotide is added to the growing polymer, a conformational change brings the chain in contact with the **exonuclease** portion of the enzyme, which cuts out ("excises") the incorrect nucleotide. This helps maintain the integrity of the original DNA sequence.

Transcription

The information in DNA is arranged in units specifying production of proteins and RNA molecules required for cellular function. These units, called genes, include coding regions specifying the amino acid sequence of a protein and the regulatory regions, called **promoters,** controlling the rate and timing of that protein's production (Figure 1-6). The coding region of a gene is divided into segments, called **exons,** interspersed with noncoding regions termed **introns** (Figure 1-6). The number and size of introns and exons differ among genes. The production of proteins is mediated by RNA molecules that carry the information for specific proteins from the DNA in the nucleus to the cytoplasm, where the proteins are synthesized. These are mRNAs. The process of transferring the sequence information from DNA to the RNA message is called transcription.

Like replication, transcription requires separation of the duplex DNA strands and uses a polymerase to copy the template DNA strand. For transcription the polymerase is RNA polymerase II, which binds to sequences in the promoter. Promoters occur approximately 100 bases "upstream" (i.e., at the 5' end) from the initiation site of transcription where the first

ribonucleotide unit is paired with the template. (In RNA, thymine is replaced by uracil, which pairs with adenine.) Promoters are usually rich in thymine and adenine in repeating patterns and have been referred to as TATA boxes. Initiation of transcription requires many protein cofactors to bind to RNA polymerase to form the active initiation complex. Other regions of DNA, known as enhancers, may interact with the initiation complex to stimulate or repress transcription.

The end of transcription (or "chain termination") occurs in response to specific sequences. The RNA transcript quickly detaches from the template DNA because restoration of the DNA-DNA duplex is energetically more favorable than retaining the DNA-RNA hybrid or a segment of single-stranded DNA (ssDNA). The end product is a complementary sequence of ribonucleotides called pre-mRNA that contains the information necessary for protein synthesis (Figure 1-6). Additional modifications are required, however, before the mRNA can be exported to the cytoplasm where protein synthesis takes place. The 5' end of the pre-mRNA molecule is modified by the addition of 7-methyl guanosine residues to form a structure called a cap (Figure 1-6). The 3' end is modified by the addition of multiple adenine bases, called the poly A tail (Figure 1-6). Both the cap and tail are necessary for translation of mRNA into protein, and they protect the mRNA molecule from degradation by exonucleases. Excision or splicing of the noncoding introns is carried out by a molecular complex termed a spliceosome. These complexes are composed of multiple small nuclear ribonucleoprotein particles (snRNPs). Spliceosomes mediate the cleavage and ligation of RNA at specific recognition sequences, termed the splicing donor and acceptor sequences. After the introns are removed, the exons are juxtaposed to each other, forming a mature mRNA molecule (Figure 1-6) that is transported into the cytoplasm where protein synthesis takes place.

Translation

Translation is the process whereby the mRNA sequence directs the amino acid sequence during protein synthesis. Twenty-one amino acids are involved in protein synthesis, and each is speci-

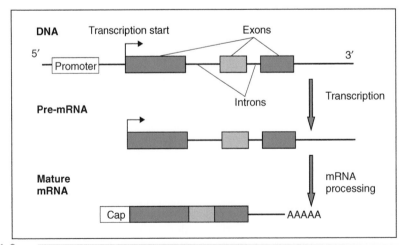

Figure 1-6

DNA transcription and mRNA processing. A gene that encodes for a protein contains a promoter region with a variable number of introns and exons. Transcription commences at the transcription start site. Pre-mRNA is processed by capping, polyadenylation, and intron splicing and becomes a mature mRNA.

fied by a three-nucleotide sequence known as a codon (Table 1-1). Because there are 64 possible codons, most amino acids are specified by more than one codon. In addition, two codons do not code for amino acids, but signal termination of protein synthesis (stop codons), and one codon, UGA, codes for either a stop or for the amino acid selenocysteine, depending on the adjacent sequences or RNA-binding proteins. The full menu of codon sequences forms the *genetic code*, which is shown in Table 1-1. Translation takes place on ribosomes, which are ribonucleoprotein complexes that function as protein synthesis factories. A ribosome binds to the initiation site on mRNA to form an initiation complex. During synthesis, codons are "read" by tRNA, short RNA molecules that have a sequence complementary to an amino acid codon (anticodon) and are bound to the amino acid molecule specified by the codon. As synthesis proceeds, the appropriate tRNA anticodon base pairs with the next mRNA codon. An enzyme on the ribosome then catalyzes the formation of a peptide bond between the amino acid bound to the tRNA and the growing protein chain. The previous tRNA is released, and the next tRNA is added. The ribosome moves along the mRNA until a stop codon is reached and synthesis is complete. The ribosome and the protein product are then dissociated from the mRNA. More than one ribosome can move along an mRNA molecule at a time, forming a polyribosome.

Genetics and Epigenetics

Genetic and **epigenetic** phenomena are intimately related. In general, genetic events are related to the sequence information of DNA and thus include the consequences of the transmission of a particular DNA sequence (e.g., the inheritance of DNA mutations or polymorphisms) or the acquisition of DNA sequence variations (e.g., the accumulation of somatic mutations in aging or cancer development). These abnormalities are discussed in some of the subsequent chapters. On the other hand, there have been inconsistent views regarding the definition of epigenetics. In most circumstances, epigenetics encompasses processes that alter gene function or its interpretation by mechanisms other than those that rely on DNA sequence change. Practically, epigenetics has evolved to include the study of DNA methylation, genomic imprinting, histone modification, chromatin remodeling, and other processes. Most of these processes add another dimension to gene expression control.

DNA methylation is the most widely studied epigenetic phenomenon. DNA methylation refers to the addition of a methyl group to the fifth carbon position of cytosine residues in CpG dinucleotides, also termed CpG sites. Not all CpG sites in the human genome are methylated. The genomic locations and distribution of methylated CpG sites are referred to as the methylation profile of a particular cell or tissue. Approximately 80% of all CpG dinucleotides in the human genome are methylated, and these mainly include isolated CpG dinucleotides and clusters, termed CpG islands, in nonpromoter DNA repeat elements (Figure 1-7).[13] These patterns of methylation are faithfully reproduced during DNA replication by maintenance DNA methyltransferases (DNMT1) so that the methylation pattern is inherited by daughter cells at cell division. In addition, DNA methylation is involved in the regulation of growth and development of organisms. The methylation profile varies between different stages of development and different tissues in the growing organism. The process starts after embryo fertilization when the genome becomes almost fully demethylated (except imprinted loci, see discussion later in this chapter) to pave the way for the establishment of developmentally related patterns of DNA methylation by de novo DNA methyltransferases (DNMT3a and DNMT3b). Genomic imprinting and gene dosage compensation of X-linked genes in females, termed X-inactivation or lyonization, are special epigenetic processes also mediated by DNA methylation. Genomic imprinting is an epigenetic phenomenon whereby the genetic function of alleles at certain genetic loci is determined by whether a particular allele is originally inherited from the father or mother. The human insulin-like growth factor-2 H19 (IGF2-H19) locus on chromosome 15 is an example of an imprinted locus. Inheriting

TABLE 1-1	The Genetic Code (Translation of mRNA to Amino Acids During Protein Synthesis)			
NUCLEOTIDE POSITION IN THE CODON				
		3RD			
1st	**2nd**	**U**	**C**	**A**	**G**
U	U	Phenylalanine	Phenylalanine	Leucine	Leucine
	C	Serine	Serine	Serine	Serine
	A	Tyrosine	Tyrosine	Stop	Stop
	G	Cysteine	Cysteine	Selenocysteine*	Tryptophan
C	U	Leucine	Leucine	Leucine	Leucine
	C	Proline	Proline	Proline	Proline
	A	Histidine	Histidine	Glutamine	Glutamine
	G	Arginine	Arginine	Arginine	Arginine
A	U	Isoleucine	Isoleucine	Isoleucine	Methionine
	C	Threonine	Threonine	Threonine	Threonine
	A	Asparagine	Asparagine	Lysine	Lysine
	G	Serine	Serine	Arginine	Arginine
G	U	Valine	Valine	Valine	Valine
	C	Alanine	Alanine	Alanine	Alanine
	A	Aspartic acid	Aspartic acid	Glutamic acid	Glutamic acid
	G	Glycine	Glycine	Glycine	Glycine

*The codon UGA can code for either selenocysteine or stop.

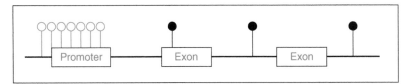

Figure 1-7
Normal DNA methylation pattern in the human genome. Sites of CpG dinucleotides are indicated by circles. CpG islands in association with gene promoters are generally unmethylated, whereas isolated CpG dinucleotides are methylated. Open circles: unmethylated; filled circles: methylated.

both gene alleles solely from either the father or mother, instead of inheriting one each of the paternal and maternal alleles as in the usual circumstance, results in significantly different clinical outcomes, namely Prader-Willi and Angelman syndromes, respectively (see Chapter 9). This observation suggests that the two alleles at the locus impart different functions depending on whether they are of maternal or paternal origin. The paternal or maternal origins of the respective alleles are marked by differential methylation patterns of the imprinted gene locus from the time of germ cell development.

Besides its role in growth and development, DNA methylation is a well-recognized epigenetic mechanism to mediate gene silencing.[13] With the exception of CpG islands within DNA repeat elements, other CpG islands, particularly those found in promoter regions of active genes, are unmethylated in the homeostatic state (Figure 1-7). If, on the contrary, the promoter CpG islands become hypermethylated, the genes would become transcriptionally silenced. Aberrant hypermethylation of gene promoters, particularly those of tumor suppressor genes and genes involved in DNA repair, is a well-known phenomenon in tumor development.[13] The methylation of gene promoters has been shown to hinder the association of methylation-sensitive transcription factors, thus preventing gene activation. In addition, hypermethylated sites attract the binding of methyl-CpG binding proteins, such as methyl-CpG binding protein 2 (MECP2) and methyl-CpG binding domain proteins (MBD1 and MBD2), which further block the association of a number of transcription factors and thus block transcription.[13] More importantly, it is now appreciated that these methyl-CpG binding proteins have the ability to recruit histone deacetylases, a phenomenon that leads to deacetylation of histones and that ultimately represses transcription.

As discussed, histones are an integral part of nucleosomes, the basic repeating structural unit of chromatin. The histone proteins can be modified posttranslationally by processes that include acetylation, methylation, phosphorylation, and ubiquitination.[16] Acetylation of certain lysines of histones H3 and H4 by histone acetyltransferases decreases histone-DNA interaction and improves the accessibility of DNA to transcriptional activation. On the contrary, histone deacetylation by histone deacetylases promotes the formation of compact nucleosomes, leading to repression of transcription. Histone deacetylation is a key component in the assembly of heterochromatin, the transcriptionally inactive chromatin.[10]

Besides the histone modifications, nucleosomes can be remodeled by ATP-dependent processes, including octamer sliding, DNA looping, and histone substitution.[16] Octamer sliding allows the relocation of histone octamers to adjacent DNA segments. DNA looping refers to the mechanism whereby the DNA segment originally wrapped around the nucleosome could be unlooped. Histone substitution allows the replacement of octamer subunits with variant histones. Consequently, nucleosomes are dynamic structures that can be remodeled according to the transcriptional demands of the cell. Furthermore, energy-dependent processes also exist that facilitate the remodeling of higher-order chromatin structures with implications for genetic events, such as DNA transcription, replication, repair, and recombination. In summary, gene function is moderated by an interrelated web of epigenetic mechanisms. The interdependency between the control of gene function or expression and the structural organization of chromatin can be appreciated from the dual structural and functional effects of CpG methylation, histone modification, heterochromatin formation, and nucleosomal and chromatin remodeling.

BEYOND THE NUCLEAR GENOME

Up to this point, we have focused our attention on the nuclear genome. In fact the cell also has a separate genome in the mitochondria, and nucleic acids are found even outside the cell.

The Mitochondrial Genome

The mitochondrial genome is the other important genetic component of eukaryotic cells. The human mitochondrial genome is a circular piece of DNA and is 16,500 bases (16.5 kb) in length.[23] **Mitochondrial DNA** is transmitted between generations by maternal inheritance, with the mitochondria coming from the oocytes and not (usually) from sperm. Multiple copies of mitochondrial DNA are present within each mitochondrion, and each cell contains a variable number of mitochondria depending on the energy requirements of the particular cell type. Thus certain cell types may contain up to several thousand copies of mitochondrial DNA. This greater abundance, compared with that of nuclear DNA, makes mitochondrial DNA attractive for certain testing applications in which sample DNA is limited (e.g., crime scene investigations, pathogen detection, and paleontology). Mitochondrial DNA is double stranded for most of its length except at the replication and transcription control region (the D-loop). Unlike the nuclear genome, the mitochondrial genome is not packaged into nucleosomal units. Instead, it has a unique structural organization, which researchers have just begun to unravel. It encodes for 13 polypeptides, all involved in the oxidative phosphorylation pathway; two rRNAs; and all of the 22 tRNAs required for mitochondrial protein synthesis. Several other proteins are also required for normal mitochondrial function and are encoded by nuclear genes.

The mutation rate of mitochondrial DNA is 10 to 20 times higher than that of nuclear DNA. This high rate has been viewed as a result of the poor fidelity of mitochondrial DNA polymerase. Inherited germ-line mutations in the mitochondrial genome generally lead to neurodegenerative and/or myopathic diseases, such as MELAS (myopathy, encephalopathy, lactic acidosis, and strokelike episodes) and Leber's hereditary optic neuropathy. Somatic mutations, on the other hand, are associated with aging and cancer development.[23] Consequent to the accumulation of sequence variations, more than one population of mitochondrial DNA sequences may be present in a cell. This state is termed **heteroplasmy** as opposed to **homoplasmy** in which the cell contains a homogeneous population of mitochondrial genomes. When performing genetic analysis for mitochondrial DNA, a note of caution is warranted on the potential problems related to the presence of nuclear pseudogenes, which are DNA segments in the nuclear genome with significant similarity (homology) to the mitochondrial genome.[24] The close resemblance of the nuclear and mitochondrial DNA segments may result in the false-positive detection of mitochondrial DNA sequences,[24] and thus the specificity of PCR systems for mitochondrial DNA detection needs to be carefully evaluated. Disorders associated with mitochondrial DNA and tests for the disorders are discussed in Chapter 9.

Circulating Nucleic Acids

Besides being confined within cellular boundaries, nucleic acid molecules are also present in the blood circulation. In the 1940s intriguing data appeared that pointed to the existence of cell-free DNA and RNA in human plasma.[3] Apart from studies in the field of virology, the study of nucleic acids in the circulation was largely neglected until the 1990s when it was realized that specific nucleic acid sequences were released in association with certain pathological or physiological processes. The field has since grown rapidly because it represented a new means to performing molecular diagnostics. More specifically, nucleic acid sequences derived from tumors, the unborn fetus, transplant donors, and traumatized tissues have been found in the plasma of cancer patients, pregnant women, transplant recipients, and patients suffering acute pathologies, respectively. Thus the potential for developing clinical applications of molecular diagnostics is vast.

Cancer DNA in Plasma

In 1994 two groups simultaneously reported the presence of tumor-associated oncogene mutations in DNA in the plasma and serum of cancer patients.[12] These reports were rapidly followed by the detection of other cancer-associated molecular changes[12] in DNA found in plasma and serum, including microsatellite alterations, oncogene amplifications, epigenetic changes, mitochondrial mutations, and viral nucleic acids. The detection and quantification of circulating tumor-derived DNA in plasma and serum have been shown to allow the detection, monitoring, and prognostication of a variety of cancers.[12] The mechanism through which DNA is released into the plasma and serum has generally been thought to be because of cell death,[5] probably through a combination of two types of cell death, apoptosis and necrosis. Consistent with this view, circulating DNA in cancer patients has been shown to consist mainly of short DNA fragments.[3] The functional implication

of circulating tumor DNA remains unclear, although provocative hypotheses have been proposed regarding the possibility that such DNA may mediate "genometastasis."

Fetal DNA in Maternal Plasma

The presence of tumor-derived DNA in the plasma of cancer patients has inspired researchers to look for other types of circulating nucleic acids. In particular, the similarity between the placenta and a malignant neoplasm has led to the discovery of cell-free fetal DNA in the plasma and serum of pregnant women.[3,18] Fetal DNA has been shown to be present in the plasma of almost all pregnant women, from the early first trimester onward, and to be present in increasing concentrations as gestation progresses. Following delivery, fetal DNA is cleared rapidly from maternal plasma, with half removed in about 16 minutes. The discovery of cell-free fetal DNA in maternal plasma and serum has opened up new possibilities for noninvasive prenatal diagnosis.[3] Fetal DNA is readily detectable in maternal plasma, but its concentration is lower than the concentration of the mother's own DNA. Thus most workers in the field have attempted to detect unique genetic markers that the fetus has inherited from the father (e.g., Y chromosomal markers for a male fetus or an altered gene that is present in the father but not in the mother). This technology has now been used for the noninvasive prenatal diagnosis of a number of conditions, including sex-linked disorders, RhD status, congenital adrenal hyperplasia, achondroplasia, and β-thalassemia.[3] Fetal RhD status determination in RhD-negative women has been adopted as a routine service by several laboratories. In addition to the qualitative mutation analyses of fetal DNA in maternal plasma, quantitative aberrations have also been reported in a number of pregnancy-associated disorders, including preeclampsia, preterm labor, trisomy, hyperemesis gravidarum, and invasive placentation.[3] These data have generally been produced by the measurement of fetal-derived Y chromosomal DNA sequences in the plasma or serum of women carrying male fetuses. However, classes of markers have been developed that do not depend on fetal gender or polymorphisms; these include circulating fetal RNA and epigenetic sequences. Hence, fetal nucleic acid measurement for prenatal screening might become a realistic possibility.

Other Applications of Circulating DNA

Apart from oncology and fetomaternal medicine, plasma DNA also has other applications in molecular diagnostics. In a situation analogous to the presence of a fetus in a pregnant woman, DNA derived from a transplanted organ has also been detected in the plasma of the transplant recipient.[20] It has been hypothesized that a measurement of graft-derived DNA concentration might provide a noninvasive method for monitoring graft rejection, analogous to the situation of urine DNA measurement following kidney transplantation.[25] In addition, the association between plasma DNA and cell death has also prompted investigators to measure circulating DNA concentrations in various conditions associated with tissue injury, including trauma, myocardial infarction, and stroke.[4]

Plasma RNA

The detection of cell-free DNA in plasma has prompted investigators to determine if cell-free RNA may also be present in the plasma.[19] The first cell-free RNAs detected in the circulation were tumor-derived RNAs, including tumor-associated viral RNA and a tissue-specific mRNA transcript, in the plasma and serum of cancer patients. Since then a number of RNA targets, including telomerase components and multiple epithelial mRNA transcripts, have been detected in the plasma and serum of patients suffering from a variety of cancers. One apparent paradox in the detection of RNA in plasma is the well-known lability of RNA.[19] Indeed, if purified RNA is added to plasma, the RNA molecules are largely degraded within seconds. However, when endogenous plasma RNA is studied, the RNA molecules are remarkably stable, with concentrations remaining unchanged for extended periods at room temperature. The stability of endogenous plasma RNA has recently been shown to be related to the fact that such RNA molecules appear to be associated with particulate matter.[19] One possible nature of such particulate matter is apoptotic bodies (i.e., small pieces of cells that died by apoptosis).

Fetal RNA has been found in the plasma of pregnant women.[3] Recently the placenta has been shown to be a major organ responsible for the release of fetal RNA into maternal plasma. Thus placental mRNA transcripts, such as those for (1) human placental lactogen, (2) the beta subunit of human chorionic gonadotropin, and (3) corticotropin releasing hormone, have been detected in maternal plasma. Through the use of expression microarray analysis, literally hundreds of new fetal RNA markers potentially suitable for study in maternal plasma could be developed. The quantitative analysis of placental mRNA in maternal plasma has the potential to be used in the monitoring of pregnancy-associated disorders, such as preeclampsia. Apart from cancer and pregnancy, circulating RNA has also been detected in patients with acute trauma.[4] It is expected that further clinical applications will be forthcoming during the next few years.

THE HUMAN GENOME PROJECT

The Human Genome Project is the biggest biological project ever undertaken by mankind. Apart from its ambitious goal of deciphering the 3 billion base pairs that make up the human genetic code, it also represents a model for the planning, organization, and execution of large-scale biological projects.[6] The first serious discussion of the feasibility of such a project can be traced back to the mid 1980s. In 1988 a special committee of the U.S. National Research Council of the U.S. National Academy of Sciences formulated a 15-year human genome project, costing about $200 million a year. The latter part of the project was marked by a highly publicized race between a publicly funded group of investigators and a private effort. The public effort, undertaken by the International Human Genome Sequencing Consortium, consisted of investigators from 20 centers located in six countries: the United States, the United Kingdom, Japan, China, France, and Germany. The completion of a draft sequence was announced June 26, 2000, and it was published in two landmark papers, one from the public team and one from the private team, in February 2001.[17,22] The final sequence was accomplished in April 2003, with 99.99% sequencing accuracy, with no gaps.

The human genome consists of 3.2 Gb (3,200,000,000 base pairs) of DNA. Among these sequences, some 2.95 Gb consists of weakly staining, potentially gene-rich euchromatic regions. Only about 1.1% to 1.4% is sequence that encodes proteins. More than half of the DNA consists of various types of repeated sequences. The number of genes in the human genome has been estimated to be between 26,000 and 31,000. These estimates provide an interesting comparison with the 6000 genes estimated for a yeast cell, 13,000 for a fruit fly, 18,000 for a worm, and 26,000 for a plant. With the basic sequence decoded, the project that awaits biologists is the even more difficult task of elucidating the biological functions of these stretches of DNA.

An understanding of our genetic heritage has the potential of providing a quantum leap in the understanding of the biology of life. It will also greatly enhance the ability to elucidate the molecular basis of diseases.[15] Developments in the genome project have also given us enhanced ability to develop tests for the molecular diagnosis of numerous diseases. In the longer term, these developments also provide new targets for the pharmaceutical industry. On the other hand, the vast amount of biological reference data that has been generated and the development of high-throughput analytical tools, such as microarrays and tandem mass spectrometry, have led to the emergence of various disciplines of systems biology. Systems biology refers to the large-scale analysis of the total complement of genetic sequences, gene expression profiles, protein expression patterns, or protein interactions within a cell or tissue; these disciplines are termed, respectively, genomics, transcriptomics, proteomics and metabolomics. These developments have the potential to revolutionize the way molecular diagnostics will be conducted in the future.

Apart from its scientific merits, it is important to realize the enormous nonscientific implications of the Human Genome Project. It was visionary for the early proponents of the Human Genome Project to set aside part of the budget of the project to study the social, legal, and ethical implications of this project (Ethics Box 1-1).[5] The most commonly expressed fear by the public is that genetic information may be used in ways that could harm people.[7]

The Human Genome Project can be regarded as a foundation on which future large-scale biological projects can be built.[6] One important extension of our knowledge of the human genome is a detailed understanding of the heritable variation in the human genome. One class of such variations is the single nucleotide polymorphism (SNP). A landmark public project, the International HapMap Project, has provided detailed information about the patterns of linkage disequilibrium of SNPs and SNP haplotypes across the human genome.[21] Another large-scale project is the Encyclopedia of DNA Elements (ENCODE) Project (http://www.genome.gov/ENCODE/), which aims to identify all of the functional elements in the human genome. Mankind's understanding of life is likely to be expanded in a synergistic manner by related efforts, such as proteomics and the Human Epigenome Project,[14] which aims to elucidate potentially all of the methylation sites across the human genome and in multiple tissue types. The twenty-first century will likely be the century when a key biological revolution will take place.

ETHICS Box 1-1   Social and Ethical Implications of the Human Genome Project

Although we celebrate the many positive outcomes of the Human Genome Project (HGP), we must consider its social and ethical implications. Court cases about genetic information[6] highlight the far-reaching effects of the HGP. Problems emerge when the moral and social framework has not been clearly defined regarding how, when, why, and to whom genetic testing should be applied. Prominent issues can be broadly divided into three categories that involve how genetic information should be obtained, interpreted, and disseminated.

A. OBTAINING GENETIC INFORMATION

Before genetic testing is undertaken, counseling of the tested individual should be conducted. The content of the discussion forms the basis for the individual to make informed choices about consent to the testing, the form of testing, and the ensuing actions related to the outcome of the testing. The use of genetic counseling implies that the individual has the autonomy to make decisions regarding the testing. However, uncertainties arise when in the process of the work-up of a hereditary disease, a key family member refuses testing. Similarly, do individuals have the right to refuse testing for a genetic trait that may make them a hazard to the public in certain occupations? How about mandatory testing as part of a public health initiative? There are also concerns regarding the testing of fetuses and minors.

B. INTERPRETATION OF GENETIC INFORMATION

The interpretation of the test results often determines later actions. Often, however, the results cannot be interpreted with absolute certainty, and definitive medical advice cannot be given because the understanding of molecular biology is far from complete. The inheritance of a genetic predisposition may not definitely translate to the eventual manifestation of a disease. First, the penetrance (i.e., the chance of expression) of the trait may not be absolute. Even with the expression of the disease, disease severity may be variable between individuals. Furthermore, for complex diseases, each susceptibility locus may contribute only modestly to the predisposition to the disease. On the other hand, negative results of testing of one genetic locus may not be interpreted as absolute evidence of freedom of risk because different mutations or different genes may lead to the same disease manifestations.

The principles of disease screening require that preventive measures and/or therapeutic strategies are available to prevent or delay the progression of diseases for which testing is undertaken.[5] How can one ensure that adequate resources are available for the delivery of such measures in an equitable manner? Moreover, currently untreatable diseases and other information can be identified "unintentionally" during testing. For example, it is not uncommon for nonpaternity to be revealed during familial testing for a hereditary disease. How should such "extra" information be handled?

C. DISSEMINATION OF GENETIC INFORMATION

Genetic testing generates information regarding the current or future health status and possibly the biological limitations of an individual. Such information may have implications beyond those affecting the individual himself or herself. Information regarding the inheritance of a genetic mutation can have implications for family members, and certain disease traits may make a person unsuitable for certain jobs. Should such information be made available to the parties concerned? The most debated fear is for one to use genetic information in a discriminatory fashion, such as determining the insurability of an individual. As a result, the Genetic Information Nondiscrimination Act was passed by the U.S. Senate that prohibits the act of using genetic information to deny an individual an insurance policy or employment.[7] However, how insurance premiums should be determined in light of the available genetic information remain unresolved.

The previous discussion provides more questions than answers. Resolution of these questions will require active debate involving individuals from all walks of life. Legislative measures will be needed to draw the limits or boundaries of how the healthcare professions should obtain, interpret, disseminate, and use genetic information. There is no doubt that the information and tools made available by the HGP are changing the practice of laboratory medicine.

REFERENCES

1. Alvarez-Garcia I, Miska EA. MicroRNA functions in animal development and human disease. Development 2005;132:4653-62.
2. Blasco MA. Telomeres and human disease: ageing, cancer and beyond. Nat Rev Genet 2005;6:611-22.
3. Chiu RWK, Lo YMD. The biology and diagnostic applications of fetal DNA and RNA in maternal plasma. Curr Top Dev Biol 2004;61:81-111.
4. Chiu RWK, Rainer TH, Lo YMD. Circulating nucleic acid analysis: diagnostic applications for acute pathologies. Acta Neurochir Suppl 2005;95:471-4.
5. Clayton EW. Ethical, legal, and social implications of genomic medicine. N Engl J Med 2003;349:562-9.
6. Collins FS, Morgan M, Patrinos A. The human genome project: lessons from large-scale biology. Science 2003;300:286-90.
7. Collins FS, Watson JD. Genetic discrimination: time to act. Science 2003;302:745.
8. Conn GL, Draper DE. RNA structure. Curr Opin Struct Biol 1998;8:278-85.
9. Garwin L, Lincoln T. A century of Nature: twenty-one discoveries that changed science and the world. Chicago: The University of Chicago Press, 2003.
10. Grewal SI, Moazed D. Heterochromatin and epigenetic control of gene expression. Science 2003;301:798-802.
11. Horn PJ, Peterson CL. Molecular biology. chromatin higher order folding—wrapping up transcription. Science 2002;297:1824-7.
12. Johnson PJ. A framework for the molecular classification of circulating tumor markers. Ann N Y Acad Sci 2001;945:8-21.
13. Jones PA, Baylin SB. The fundamental role of epigenetic events in cancer. Nat Rev Genet 2002;3:415-28.
14. Jones PA, Martienssen R. A blueprint for a human epigenome project: the AACR human epigenome workshop. Cancer Res 2005;65:11241-6.
15. Kerem B, Rommens JM, Buchanan JA, Markiewicz D, Cox TK, Chakravarti A, et al. Identification of the cystic fibrosis gene: genetic analysis. Science 1989;245:1073-80.
16. Khorasanizadeh S. The nucleosome: from genomic organization to genomic regulation. Cell 2004;116:259-72.
17. Lander ES, Linton LM, Birren B, Nusbaum C, Zody MC, Baldwin J, et al. Initial sequencing and analysis of the human genome. Nature 2001;409:860-921.
18. Lo YMD, Corbetta N, Chamberlain PF, Rai V, Sargent IL, Redman CW, et al. Presence of fetal DNA in maternal plasma and serum. Lancet 1997;350:485-7.
19. Lo YMD, Chiu RWK. The biology and diagnostic applications of plasma RNA. Ann N Y Acad Sci 2004;1022:135-9.
20. Lo YMD, Tein MSC, Pang CCP, Yeung CK, Tong KL, Hjelm NM. Presence of donor-specific DNA in plasma of kidney and liver-transplant recipients. Lancet 1998;351:1329-30.
21. The International HapMap Consortium. A haplotype map of the human genome. Nature 2005;437:1299-1320.
22. Venter JC, Adams MD, Myers EW, Li PW, Mural RJ, Sutton GG, et al. The sequence of the human genome. Science 2001;291:1304-51.
23. Wallace DC. Mitochondrial disease in man and mouse. Science 1999;283:1482-8.
24. Wallace DC, Stugard C, Murdock D, Schurr T, Brown MD. Ancient mtDNA sequences in the human nuclear genome: a potential source of

errors in identifying pathogenic mutations. Proc Natl Acad Sci U S A 1997;94:14900-5.

25. Zhang J, Tong KL, Li PK, Chan AY, Yeung CK, Pang CC, et al. Presence of donor-and recipient-derived DNA in cell-free urine samples of renal transplantation recipients: urinary DNA chimerism. Clin Chem 1999;45:1741-6.

REVIEW QUESTIONS

1. With regard to mitochondrial DNA,
   A. the sequence is identical from individual to individual.
   B. the sequence is identical within a single nuclear family.
   C. meiotic recombination is an important mechanism for generating interindividual variation.
   D. it is a nucleic acid molecule of approximately 16.5 kb.
   E. it is an ssDNA molecule.

2. Fetal DNA in maternal plasma
   A. represents more than 50% of the DNA that is present in maternal plasma.
   B. can be used to detect a mitochondrial DNA mutation that the fetus has inherited from the mother.
   C. is useful for determining the RhD status of a fetus carried by an RhD-positive pregnant woman.
   D. can be used to determine if a fetus has inherited an X-linked mutation from the mother.
   E. is useful for the prenatal investigation of hemophilia A.

3. The human genome
   A. consists of a single DNA molecule of 3.2 Gb in length.
   B. is protein coding for 95% of its length.
   C. is 10 times larger than the human mitochondrial DNA genome.
   D. codes for more than 20,000 genes.
   E. is exactly identical in all cells within a human body.

4. The dsDNA structure
   A. is formed by two DNA polymers with the phosphate groups stacked in the center and the bases forming the backbone.
   B. involves base pairing between adenine and uracil, and cytosine and guanine.
   C. involves the pairing of complementary DNA strands.
   D. is unwound during DNA replication, but limited to one site at a time.
   E. is in the form of a left-handed helix.

5. Chromatin
   A. is most condensed during the interphase of the cell cycle when DNA replication takes place.
   B. refers to the genetic material found within mitochondria.
   C. refers to a complex involving nuclear DNA and ribosomal proteins.
   D. can be further classified as euchromatin or heterochromatin depending on its compactness.
   E. in its most basic structural form consists of a segment of DNA wound around a hexamer of histone proteins.

6. DNA methylation
   A. is a process that involves nucleotide sequence changes.
   B. may affect the transcription rate of a gene.
   C. is involved in the inactivation of the X chromosome in males.
   D. is seen in all CpG dinucleotides in the human genome.
   E. describes the addition of a methyl group to the fifth carbon position of guanine residues in CpG dinucleotides.

7. RNA molecules
   A. are single stranded in nature and appear as a helical structure.
   B. function only as intermediates for protein production.
   C. adopt random structures.
   D. contain methylated cytosines, which is a distinguishing feature from DNA.
   E. may have catalytic activity like a (protein) enzyme.

8. DNA replication
   A. describes the process of transferring the sequence information in DNA to RNA.
   B. results in daughter cells that are haploid in nature.
   C. involves the base pairing of an RNA primer to the template DNA strand.
   D. involves DNA synthesis in the 3′ to 5′ direction.
   E. is mediated by DNA polymerase II.

9. DNA transcription
   A. is mediated by RNA polymerase II.
   B. takes place in ribosomes.
   C. occurs more readily within heterochromatin.
   D. may be followed by mRNA processing, which involves the splicing of exons.
   E. is activated through the binding of transcription factors to the replication fork.

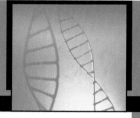

Chapter 2

Genomes and Nucleic Acid Alterations

Carl T. Wittwer, M.D., Ph.D.
Noriko Kusukawa, Ph.D.

OBJECTIVES

1. Describe the human genome, including size, composition, designation of specific genetic components, and genetic content.
2. Identify what constitutes a polymorphism.
3. Characterize a single nucleotide polymorphism; state the different forms of an SNP and its role in disease.
4. State the role of amplified genes in disease; give an example of a disease caused by amplified genes.
5. Compare and contrast bacterial and viral genomes with the human genome.
6. State the differences between nucleases, endonucleases, ligases, and polymerases, including physiological roles and possible use in genetics testing.
7. Given a specific restriction endonuclease, describe what DNA sequence it recognizes and what type of "end" is produced.

KEY WORDS AND DEFINITIONS

Alteration: A variation or change in DNA sequence. It may be benign or may cause disease.
Aneuploidy: An abnormal amount of DNA, usually used in reference to an abnormal number of chromosomes.
Deletion: A DNA sequence that is missing in one sample compared with another. Deletions may be as small as one nucleotide or as large as an entire chromosome.
Endonuclease: An enzyme that hydrolyzes an internal phosphodiester bond, splitting a nucleic acid into two or more parts.
Exonuclease: An enzyme that removes terminal nucleotides from a polynucleotide.
Haplotype: The association of specific alleles at multiple loci on one chromosome strand.
Indel: A sequence variant arising from both an insertion and a deletion.

Insertion: An extra DNA sequence that is present in one sample compared with a reference sequence.
Intergenic: DNA sequence between genes.
Ligase: An enzyme that covalently joins two DNA strands.
Microsatellites: Short segments of DNA (1 to 13 bases long) that are repeated end to end, also known as short tandem repeats (STRs).
Minisatellites: Repeated segments of DNA that are 14 to 500 bases long, also known as variable number of tandem repeats (VNTRs).
Missense: A nucleotide substitution that codes for a different amino acid. Although these sequence changes are commonly referred to as missense "mutations," this is strictly a misnomer because they may be benign and cause no disease.
Mutation: Usually refers to a sequence alteration that causes disease. However, in some contexts, refers to any sequence variant. This chapter describes disease-causing sequence alterations.
Nonsense: A nucleotide substitution that results in a stop codon, prematurely terminating the protein.
Nuclease: An enzyme that degrades nucleic acid.
Oligonucleotide: A short single-stranded polymer of nucleic acid.
Polymerase: An enzyme that sequentially adds nucleotides onto a growing polynucleotide, usually requiring a primer and a template.
Pseudogene: A genetic element that does not result in a functional gene product, usually because of accumulated sequence changes.
Restriction Endonuclease: An endonuclease, usually from bacteria, that cuts nucleic acid in a sequence-specific manner.
Reverse Transcriptase: A polymerase that catalyzes synthesis of DNA from an RNA template.
Short Tandem Repeats (STRs): Short segments of DNA (1 to 13 bases long) that are repeated end to end, also known as microsatellites.
Single Nucleotide Polymorphism (SNP): A single nucleotide variant that occurs in the population at a frequency of at least 1%. SNPs may be benign or may cause disease.
Transposon: A mobile genetic element that can delete and insert itself variably into the genome.

Variable Number of Tandem Repeats (VNTRs): Repeated segments of DNA that are 14 to 500 bases long, also known as minisatellites.

Molecular diagnostics focuses on medically important sequence variations within a background of complex genomic structure. This chapter reviews the organization of human, bacterial, and viral genomes and the spectrum of variations in nucleic acids that are of medical concern. Then, the enzymes that allow processing of nucleic acids into forms that are amenable to analytical interrogation are described.

GENOMES AND NUCLEIC ACID ALTERATIONS

Basic molecular biology and nucleic acid chemistry was introduced in Chapter 1. In what follows, the structures of human, bacterial, and viral genomes are reviewed. Nucleic acid alterations of medical interest are introduced, emphasizing concepts relevant to molecular diagnostic techniques.

Human Genome

Each human cell contains two copies of a 3.2-billion-member sequence code of nucleic acids on 46 chromosomes. Box 2-1 lists statistics for the human genome and the types of variations found that are important in clinical diagnostics.

Three quarters of human DNA is **intergenic** or between genes. More than 60% of this intergenic sequence consists of "parasitic" DNA regions of transposable elements 100 to 11,000 bases in length. Between 2 million and 3 million of these elements are present in each copy of the genome. They contribute to genetic recombination and chromosome structure and provide an evolutionary record of sequence variation and selection.

Intergenic DNA also carries most of the simple sequence repeats (SSRs) present in the genome. These repeats are known as **microsatellites** or **short tandem repeats (STRs)** when the repeat unit is 1 to 13 bases and **minisatellites** or **variable number of tandem repeats (VNTRs)** when the repeat unit is 14 to 500 bases. SSRs are critical markers in genetic linkage studies and in forensic or medical identity testing. They are formed by slippage during replication and are highly polymorphic between individuals. The most common SSRs are dinucleotide repeats, such as ACACAC and ATAT. On average approximately one SSR occurs every 2000 bases.

One quarter of the human genome consists of genes. There are about 30,000 genes in the human genome. The average gene covers 27,000 bases, but only about 1300 of these bases code for amino acid sequences. These coding regions, or exons, are interspersed throughout the gene. On average there are about nine exons per gene. The noncoding areas between exons are known as introns. Within a gene, 95% of the sequence is covered by introns, whereas only 5% consists of coding sequences within exons. Coding sequences make up only 1.1% to 1.4% of the total genome.

Sequence Variation Within the Human Genome

If the DNA of any two individuals is compared, there is on average one difference every 1250 bases (i.e., approximately 99.9% of the sequence is identical between randomly chosen copies of the genome). Any sequence change (compared with a reference sequence) is called a sequence variant or **alteration.**

BOX 2-1

The Human Genome and Its Sequence Variation

THE HUMAN GENOME: 3.2 BILLION BASE PAIRS, 23 CHROMOSOME PAIRS (47-245 MILLION BASE PAIRS PER CHROMOSOME)

Genes (25%)		Intergenic Sequences (75%)	
24%	Intron sequences	45%	Parasitic (**transposon-**derived repeats)
1.1%-1.4%	Exon sequences	5%	Segmental duplications
		3%	Simple sequence repeats (SSRs, STRs)
		22%	Other

Number of genes: ~30,000
Average gene:
27,000 base pairs
9 exons
1340 bases of coding sequence
446 amino acids

SEQUENCE ALTERATIONS: 99.9% IDENTITY (1 DIFFERENCE EVERY 1250 BASES BETWEEN RANDOMLY SELECTED HAPLOID GENOMES)

Single Nucleotide Polymorphisms (SNPs): identified every 100-300 bases

97%	Noncoding
3%	Within exons

Disease-Causing Variants

70%	SNPs
49%	Missense (amino acid substitution)
11%	Nonsense (termination)
9%	Splicing
<1%	Regulatory
23%	Small insertions and/or deletions
7%	Gross lesions (large insertions and/or deletions, repeats, rearrangements, complex alterations)

EPIGENETIC ALTERATIONS
Variable initiation
Alternative splicing
Methylation (regulation)
Histone phosphorylation, methylation, acetylation

Data compiled from the human gene mutation database[2] and Lander et al.[1]

If a sequence variant or alteration is present in at least 1% of a population it is a polymorphism. Many sequence variants, alterations, and polymorphisms in the genome do not affect human health and are benign or silent. For example, **single nucleotide polymorphisms (SNPs)** and SSRs found in the intergenic sequence are rarely associated with disease. Similarly, most of the SNPs in introns, except for splicing and regulatory variants, are not known to affect gene function. In addition, some of the SNPs within exons are silent alterations that do not code for a change in amino acid sequence because of the redundancy in the genetic code. Still other SNPs in exons code for amino acid changes that do not affect protein function. Even such silent SNPs may nonetheless be of considerable medical interest as genetic markers.

The most common sequence variations are single base changes, also known as **single nucleotide polymorphisms** or SNPs. Millions of SNPs have been described, and many new SNPs continue to be reported. Some SNPs are common in the population, with allele frequencies of 0.1 to 0.5 (i.e., present in 10 to 50 of every 100 copies studied), though other single base changes are very rare. Although an SNP has been identified every 100 to 300 bases, many of these are not found frequently in the population. The vast majority of SNPs (97%) occur in noncoding regions; only 3% of SNPs are associated with exons.

Sequence Variations That Cause Human Disease

Sequence alterations that are known to cause disease are often called **mutations,** although the more cumbersome, "disease-causing variant," is more precise. About 70% of known disease-causing variants are SNPs. Most of the remaining disease-causing variants (23%) are small **insertions** or **deletions.** The remainder (7%) are more complex sequence changes, including (1) large insertions or deletions, (2) copy number changes, (3) repeat expansions, (4) translocations, and (5) rearrangements (see Box 2-1).

Single Nucleotide Polymorphisms

Most SNPs that cause disease are **missense** and result in an amino acid substitution, whereas significantly fewer are **nonsense** variants that result in a termination codon and premature polypeptide chain termination. Approximately 9% of disease-causing variants are SNPs that affect splicing sites and result in altered concatenation of coding sequences. Finally, less than 1% of known disease-causing variants are SNPs that affect the regulatory efficiency of transcription by altering promoter and/or enhancer regions in introns or the stability of the RNA transcript.

Insertions, Deletions, Rearrangements, and Short Tandem Repeats

The small insertion and/or deletion variants account for about 23% of the nucleic acid sequence alterations that cause disease. An insertion refers to the presence of extra bases, whereas deletion implies the absence of certain bases in comparison with a reference sequence. Insertions and deletions often cause a shift of the codon reading frame, resulting in altered amino acid sequence downstream of the variation—commonly followed by chain termination from a nonsense codon. An **indel** implies both an insertion and a deletion at the same locus (e.g., replacement of TG with AGGTC).

The remaining 7% of variants that cause disease are mostly larger lesions, including (1) duplications or deletions of entire exons or genes, (2) chromosomal translocations, (3) SSR expansions (e.g., increased number of trinucleotide repeat), (4) gene rearrangements (e.g., B- and T-cell gene rearrangements), and (5) complex polymorphic loci related to health and disease (e.g., HLA).

Haplotypes

Often, sequence variants are inherited together in a contiguous block, or **haplotype.** A schematic representation of haplotypes (and alleles) and an explanation are given in Figure 2-1 and its legend.

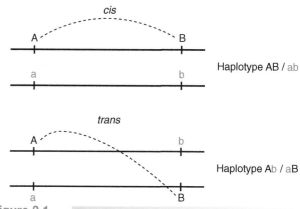

Figure 2-1

Schematic diagram of haplotypes. Two polymorphic sites reside on each of two chromosomes. One site carries either allele "A" or allele "a." The other site is either "B" or "b." The possible *haplotypes* are: AB/ab, in which allele A and allele B are on the same chromosome (in which case A and B are said to be in *cis*), or Ab/aB, in which allele A and B are on different chromosomes (and are referred to as being in *trans*).

Disease associations may depend not on any particular sequence variant but on the overall effect of several linked alleles that define the haplotype. For example, enzyme function depends on the haplotype that defines the amino acid sequence in the protein. When the haplotype linkage of alleles is strong (e.g., in the example in Figure 2-1, when allele A is always found with allele B on the same chromosome), genotype determination at a single locus may identify the haplotype (and disease association) with high confidence. However, methods for determining the *cis* and/or *trans* phase of alleles at distant loci are necessary when the haplotype linkage is weak and also when the disease association and/or haplotype linkage is first being established. Haplotypes may be defined by the phases of many polymorphic loci.

Alterations in Mitochondrial DNA

Most human genetic material is present in two copies, with the exception of the unpaired sex chromosome in males and mitochondrial DNA. The presence of only a single copy of genes on the X and Y chromosome in males leads to well-known sex-linked disorders. In contrast, the 16,500 bp mitochondrial genome is present in more than 1000 copies per cell, constituting about 0.3% of human DNA. Allele fractions may vary over a wide range when all mitochondria in a cell are considered. That is, sequence variations in mitochondrial DNA are *heteroplasmic*, meaning that the ratio of wild-type to variant alleles within a cell can vary almost continuously, sometimes resulting in a wide range of symptoms even when only one sequence variant is involved.

Numerical Gene Alterations and Cellular DNA Content

Sometimes genes or even chromosomes are present in more than two copies. If extra copies of genes lose their function, they are known as **pseudogenes.** It is important to distinguish pseudogenes from functional genes because sequence variations in pseudogenes are seldom of clinical importance. Some very important genes are present in many copies so that overall protein expression is not affected if a chance variation occurs in one copy. Most genes, however, are present in only two copies and the normal gene dosage is two. When these genes, such as *HER-2-neu,* are present in more than two functional copies, the genes are said to be amplified. As a result, more mRNA transcripts and protein are usually made, resulting in cellular abnormalities and possible progression to cancer. Many cancers and some genetic disorders are correlated with abnormal (increased or decreased) chromosome numbers or **aneuploidy.** The specific chromosomal alterations can be determined by cytogenetics, or the overall DNA content can be determined by flow cytometry.

Human Epigenetic Alterations

In addition to the sequence alterations considered above, epigenetic alterations, including alternative splicing and methylation, affect gene expression. (See the section "Genetics and Epigenetics" in Chapter 1 for descriptions and discussion.) Even though the number of genes may be limited to 30,000, variable transcription initiation and exon splicing are estimated to produce about 90,000 mRNA transcripts and protein products.

Methylation of cytosine to form 5-methylcytosine occurs frequently; about 70% of CpG dinucleotides in the human genome are methylated. Although not inherited, interest in this "5th base" has increased recently as correlations with cancer have been reported. CpG islands are about 1000 bases in length and are often found near the 5′ end of genes. These regions consist of clusters of CG dinucleotides that are usually not methylated in normal cells. However, CpG methylation correlates with condensed chromatin structure and promoter inactivation; an important example occurs in tumor-suppressor genes.

As described in Chapter 1, DNA is associated with proteins in nucleosomes. Gene expression can be altered by histone phosphorylation, acetylation, and methylation. Our understanding of epigenetic alterations and their relation to disease is rapidly developing.

Bacterial Genomes and Sequence Variants

Bacterial genomes are considerably less complex than human or other eukaryotic genomes. Common bacteria have only one chromosome, usually a circular DNA double helix of 4 million to 5 million base pairs, about 1000 times less than the amount of DNA in a human cell. About 90% of the DNA in bacteria codes for protein. There are no introns, but there are multiple small intergenic regions of repetitive sequences that are dispersed throughout the genome. The common bacterium *Escherichia coli* contains about 4300 genes.

In addition to the large circular chromosome that carries essential genes, bacteria also carry accessory genes in smaller circles of double-stranded DNA (dsDNA) known as plasmids. Plasmids range in size from 1000 to more than 1 million base pairs. Plasmids are important in molecular diagnostics because they often encode pathogenic factors and antibiotic resistance.

The bacterial repertoire of DNA can be altered by: (1) gain or loss of plasmids; (2) single-base changes, small insertions, and deletions as in eukaryotic genomes; and (3) larger segmental rearrangements, including inversions, deletions, and duplications. Some genes, such as those for ribosomal RNA, are present in many copies and have been used to identify different species of bacteria. In addition, the intergenic repetitive sequences serve as multiple targets for **oligonucleotide** probes, enabling the generation of unique DNA profiles or fingerprints for individual bacterial strains.

Viral Genomes and Sequence Variants

Viral genomes are considerably less complex than bacterial genomes. Common viruses that infect humans vary in size from about 5000 to 250,000 bases, or 20 to 1000 times less than the amount of nucleic acid in *E. coli.* Because viruses use the host's cellular machinery, they do not need as many genes. Small viruses may encode only several genes, but the larger viruses can encode hundreds. The viral genome consists of either DNA or RNA, and the nucleic acid may be single stranded or double stranded, linear, or circular with one or multiple fragments and/or copies per viral particle. As in bacteria, there are no introns. In fact, in some viruses the exons overlap with different reading frames coding different products from the same nucleic acid sequence. Noncoding regions are usually present at the terminal ends of linear genomes. Repeat segments are often found as terminal or internal repeats and may be inverted.

Sequence alterations in viruses are common. Areas of high sequence variation may be interspersed between conserved domains. Higher frequencies of variation have been correlated with lower polymerase fidelity and may allow escape from antibody recognition and from antiviral drugs. Common sequence variants in viruses include single base changes, insertions, and deletions. Sequence diversity within a viral species may be so great that consensus sequences for molecular typing are difficult to find.

NUCLEIC ACID ENZYMES

Nucleic acid enzymes are critical tools for the techniques used in molecular diagnostics. Common enzymes that act on nucleic acids include those that synthesize longer polymers and those that degrade nucleic acid into shorter fragments. These enzymes are critical for DNA replication and for transcription and must be present in all cells that replicate. In addition to general-function enzymes, a variety of unique enzymes, found in bacteria and viruses, act on specific nucleic acid sequences. Many of these enzymes have been purified and synthesized in vitro, sometimes "engineered" with alterations that improve their performance or stability (e.g., at high temperatures needed to dissociate dsDNA in laboratory tests). Our ability to manipulate nucleic acids in vitro with these enzymes has made modern molecular biology possible. Enzymes are also used extensively in nucleic acid diagnostics, including sample preparation, probe labeling, signal generation, and amplification of targets and probes.

Nucleases are enzymes that hydrolyze one or more phosphodiester bonds in nucleic acid polymers. Nucleases may require a free hydroxyl end (**exonucleases**), with specificity for the 3′ or 5′ end, or may act only on internal bonds (**endonucleases**). For example, some probe techniques are based on 5′-exonuclease activity that cleaves nucleic acids between two fluorescent labels. Nucleases can be DNA or RNA specific and may act on only double- or single-stranded polymers. For example, DNAse I digests dsDNA, and S1 nuclease acts only on single-stranded DNA (ssDNA). DNAse I can be used to specifically degrade DNA in nucleic acid mixtures when only RNA is of interest. RNAses are very stable enzymes that are common laboratory contaminants.

Restriction endonucleases are found in bacteria; these enzymes prevent replication of foreign DNA. Their action is sequence specific, requiring recognition sequences of usually 4 to 10 nucleotides on a dsDNA molecule. At each location where this sequence is found, the enzyme cuts both strands in a reproducible manner, resulting in either staggered or blunt-end cuts. For example, *EcoRI* is a restriction enzyme from *E. coli* that recognizes the 6-base sequence GAATTC and cuts between the G and the A on both strands, producing a staggered cut:

5′ . . . G/AATTC . . . 3′
3′ . . . CTTAA/G . . . 5′

Note that "blunt-end" cuts would be produced if the enzyme hydrolyzed the bond between A and T.

Restriction enzymes are used for digesting large fragments of DNA into smaller pieces and for preparing DNA from different sources to be joined together in cloning procedures. Nicking enzymes are restriction enzymes that cut only one strand of double-stranded nucleic acid.

Ligases catalyze the formation of phosphodiester linkages between two nucleic acid chains. DNA ligases are not sequence specific and require the presence of a complementary template. In contrast, RNA ligases used in mRNA processing do not require a template, but are sensitive to sequence.

Polymerases catalyze the synthesis of complementary nucleic acid polymers using a parent strand as a template. In vitro these enzymes can extend an oligonucleotide primer that is annealed to a template strand. Extension requires that the 3′OH of the extending end is free and that nucleotide triphosphates (NTPs) are present. Extension stops if you run out of template or NTPs or if no 3′OH groups are available at the extending end. Thermostable polymerases, such as *Thermus aquaticus* (*Taq*) DNA polymerase, are essential reagents for the automation of many nucleic acid amplification procedures because of their stability at high temperatures that are used in the procedures.

Reverse transcriptase is found in retroviruses and catalyzes the synthesis of DNA from either an RNA or a DNA template. Retroviruses have RNA genomes, and reverse transcriptase activity is required as part of their replication. In vitro reverse transcriptase is used to make complementary DNA (*cDNA*) copies of RNA in samples and may be used for cloning, probe preparation, and nucleic acid assays.

REFERENCES

1. Lander ES, Linton LM, Birren B, Nusbaum C, Zody MC, Baldwin J, et al. Initial sequencing and analysis of the human genome. Nature 2001;409:860-921.
2. Stenson PD, Ball EV, Mort M, Phillips AD, Shiel JA, Thomas NS, et al. Human gene mutation database (HGMD): 2003 update. Hum Mutat 2003;21:577-81.

REVIEW QUESTIONS

1. About what percentage of bases in the human genome code for proteins?
   A. 1%
   B. 5%
   C. 10%
   D. 20%
   E. 50%

2. Approximately how many genes are in the human genome?
   A. 3000
   B. 10,000
   C. 30,000
   D. 100,000
   E. 300,000

3. How many pairs of chromosomes are in normal diploid human cells?
   A. 23
   B. 32
   C. 16
   D. 48
   E. 1

4. What percentage of the genetic sequence is identical between two people?
   A. 50%
   B. 75%
   C. 90%
   D. 99%
   E. 99.9%

5. Which of the following statements about polymerases is false?
   A. Polymerases catalyze the synthesis of nucleic acid sequences.
   B. Polymerases require a parent nucleic acid strand as a template.
   C. DNA polymerase from *Thermus aquaticus* (*Taq*) is thermostable (i.e., it is stable at high temperature).
   D. Polymerases are important as reagents in molecular diagnostics.
   E. None of the above

SECTION II

TECHNIQUES AND INSTRUMENTATION

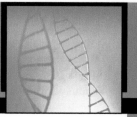

Chapter **3**

Specimen Collection and Processing

Doris M. Haverstick, Ph.D.
Amy R. Groszbach, C.L.Sp.(M.B.)

OUTLINE

Specimen Collection
    Blood
    Urine
    Feces
    Cerebrospinal Fluid
    Synovial Fluid
    Amniotic Fluid
    Chorionic Villus Sampling
    Pleural, Pericardial, and Ascitic Fluids
    Buccal Cells
    Solid Tissue
    Hair and Nails
Handling of Specimens for Analysis
    Maintenance of Specimen Identification
    Preservation of Specimens in Transit
    Separation and Storage of Specimens
    Transport of Specimens
Ethical Issues

OBJECTIVES

1. State the differences between plasma, serum, and whole blood.
2. Clarify the mechanisms of ethylenediaminetetraacetic acid (EDTA) and heparin anticoagulants; explain why heparin is an inappropriate anticoagulant for amplification procedures.
3. Identify specific additives with specific stopper color and list the correct order of draw using an evacuated tube system.
4. Define hemolysis and state how it interferes with molecular diagnostic testing.
5. Demonstrate correct patient identification and specimen labeling procedures.
6. Compare various body fluids and their utility in molecular diagnostic testing.
7. Describe appropriate specimen preparation for transport to a distant site.
8. Summarize specimen storage requirements for specific specimens including whole blood, plasma, isolated cells, and extracted DNA.

KEY WORDS AND DEFINITIONS

Amniocentesis: Removal of amniotic fluid from the amniotic sac, normally through the mother's abdomen.
Anticoagulant: Any substance that prevents blood clotting.
Arthrocentesis: Withdrawal of joint fluid.
Buccal Cells: Epithelial cells from the inside of the mouth (cheek).
Formalin-Fixed, Paraffin-Embedded (FFPE) Tissue: Tissue that has been permanently fixed with formalin and then embedded in paraffin before the preparation of microscopy slides.
Hemolysis: Disruption of the membranes of blood cells causing release of hemoglobin and other components of the cells.
Lymphostasis: Blockade of the normal flow of lymph.
Optimal Cutting Temperature (OCT) Compound: A water-soluble compound composed of polyvinyl alcohol and polyethylene glycol that surrounds but does not infiltrate tissue.
Phlebotomist: One who practices phlebotomy; the individual who withdraws blood from a patient.
Phlebotomy: The puncture of a vein to collect blood.
Plasma: The fluid portion of the blood in which the cells are suspended. Differs from serum in that it contains fibrinogen and related proteins that are removed when blood clots to produce serum.
Preanalytical Variables: Factors that affect specimens before analytical testing begins.
Sample: Part of a whole. A plasma **sample** is obtained from a blood specimen. A portion of a urine specimen that is taken for testing is a **sample** of the urine specimen. A blood specimen is also a **sample** of all the blood of the person being tested, and a liver biopsy is a **sample** of the patient's liver tissue; see also **specimen.**
Serum: The clear liquid that separates from blood on clotting.
Skin Puncture: Collection of capillary blood usually from a pediatric patient by making a thin cut in the skin, often the heel of the foot.
Specimen: Tissue, fluid or other material taken for testing; contrast with **sample.**
Venipuncture: The process of obtaining a blood specimen from a vein.

Venous Occlusion: Temporary blockage of return blood flow to the heart through the application of pressure, usually using a tourniquet.

This chapter provides a review of the **preanalytical variables** involved in the (1) collection, (2) processing, and (3) storage of common types of **specimens** and **samples** used for diagnostic testing. There will be particular emphasis on aspects of these activities that affect molecular diagnostic tests and their interpretation to facilitate integration of requests for specialized testing with more routine analyses. As with routine testing, many errors can occur during the collection, processing, and transport of biological specimens for molecular diagnostic analysis. Such errors are considered preanalytical errors and are known to contribute to delayed and suboptimal patient care. Minimizing these errors through careful adherence to the concepts below and any individual institutional policies will result in more reliable information for use in quality patient care by healthcare professionals.

SPECIMEN COLLECTION

Examples of biological materials that are analyzed in clinical laboratories include (1) whole blood, (2) **serum,** (3) **plasma,** (4) urine, (5) feces, (6) saliva, (7) spinal, synovial, amniotic, pleural, pericardial, and ascitic fluids, and (8) various types of tissue. All these specimens also are used for molecular diagnostic testing. Specimens with nucleated cells yield genomic DNA to detect genetic alterations in the patient. Specimens devoid of patient cells are useful in detection of infectious agents, often by quantification of agent-specific RNA. The Clinical and Laboratory Standards Institute (CLSI, formerly known as the National Committee for Clinical Laboratory Standards or NCCLS) has published several procedures for collecting many of the most common specimen types under standardized conditions,[3-6] including one publication devoted exclusively to specimens for use in molecular diagnostics.[7]

Blood

Blood for analysis may be obtained from veins, arteries, or capillaries. Venous blood is usually the specimen of choice, and **venipuncture** is the method for obtaining this specimen. In young children and for many point-of-care tests, **skin puncture** is frequently used to obtain what is mostly capillary blood. The process of collecting the blood is known as **phlebotomy** (from *phleb*, which means vein, and *tome*, to cut or incise) and should always be performed by a trained **phlebotomist.**

Venipuncture

In the clinical laboratory, venipuncture is defined as all of the steps involved in obtaining an appropriate and identified blood specimen from a patient's vein.[3]

Preliminary Steps

Before any specimen is collected, the phlebotomist must confirm the identity of the patient. Two or three items of identification should be used (e.g., name, medical record number, date of birth, social security number, or address if the patient is an outpatient). In specialized situations, such as paternity testing or other tests of medico-legal importance, establishment of a chain of custody for the specimen may require additional patient identification, such as a photograph, either provided as part of the identification process or taken to confirm the identity of the patient.

Identification must be an active process. Where possible, the patient should state his or her name, and the phlebotomist should verify information on the patient's wrist band if the patient is hospitalized. If the patient is an outpatient, the phlebotomist should ask the patient to state his or her name and confirm the information on the test requisition form with identifying information provided by the patient. In the case of pediatric patients, the parent or guardian should be present and provide active identification of the child. In many institutions, at this point in the process the patient should also be asked about latex allergies. If present and if latex gloves or a latex tourniquet may be used, the phlebotomist should secure an alternative tourniquet and put on gloves that are latex free. Finally, for some tests for genetic diseases, the performing laboratory may request a signed consent form from the patient and this should be completed at this time if not provided by the requesting physician.

Before collection of a specimen, a phlebotomist should be properly dressed in personal protective equipment (PPE), such as an impervious gown and gloves, applied immediately before approaching the patient to adhere to standard precautions against potentially infectious material and to limit the spread of infectious disease from one patient to another.[8] If the phlebotomist is to collect a specimen from a patient in isolation in a hospital, the phlebotomist must put on a clean gown and gloves and a face mask and goggles before entering the patient's room. The face mask limits the spread of potentially infectious droplets, and the goggles limit the possible entry of infectious material into the eye. The extent of the precautions required will vary with the nature of a patient's illness and the institution's policies and bloodborne pathogen plan to which a phlebotomist must adhere. If airborne precautions are indicated, the phlebotomist must wear an N95 TB respirator.

The patient should be comfortable: seated or supine (if sitting is not feasible) and should have been in this position for as long as possible before the specimen is drawn. For an outpatient, it is generally recommended that the patient be seated before the completion of the identification process to maximize their relaxation. At no time should venipuncture be performed on a standing patient. Either of the patient's arms should be extended in a straight line from the shoulder to the wrist. An arm with an inserted intravenous line should be avoided, as should an arm with extensive scarring or a hematoma at the intended collection site. If a woman has had a mastectomy, arm veins on that side of the body should not be used because the surgery may have caused **lymphostasis** (blockade of normal lymph node drainage), affecting the blood composition. If a woman has had double mastectomies, blood should be drawn from the arm of the side on which the first procedure was done. If the surgery was done within 6 months on both sides, a vein on the back of the hand or at the ankle should be used.

Before performing a venipuncture, the phlebotomist should estimate the volume of blood to be drawn and select the appropriate number and types of tubes for the blood, plasma, or serum tests requested. In many settings, this will be facilitated by computer-generated collection recommendations and should be designed to collect the minimum amount necessary for testing. The sections below on "Collection with Evacuated Blood Tubes" and "Order of Draw for Multiple Collections" discuss the types of tubes and recommended order of draw for multiple specimens in more detail. In addition to tubes, an appropriate needle must also be selected. The most commonly used sizes are 19 to 22 gauge. The larger the gauge number is, the smaller the bore. The usual choice for an adult with normal veins is 20 gauge; if veins tend to collapse easily, a size 21 is preferred. For volumes of blood from 30 to 50 mL, an 18-gauge needle may be required to ensure adequate blood flow. A needle is typically 1.5 inches (3.7 cm) long, but 1-inch (2.5-cm) needles, usually attached to a winged or butterfly collection set, are also used. All needles must be sterile, sharp, and without barbs.

Location

The median cubital vein in the antecubital fossa, or crook of the elbow, is the preferred site for collecting venous blood in adults because the vein is both large and close to the surface of the skin.[15] Veins on the back of the hand or at the ankle may be used, although these are less desirable and should be avoided in people with diabetes or other individuals with poor circulation. In the inpatient setting, it is appropriate to collect blood through a cannula that is being inserted for long-term fluid infusions at the time of first insertion to avoid the need for a second stick. In severely ill individuals or those requiring many intravenous injections, an alternative blood-drawing site should be chosen. Selection of a vein for puncture is facilitated by palpation. An arm containing a cannula or arteriovenous fistula should not be used without consent of the patient's physician. If fluid is being infused intravenously into a limb, the fluid should be shut off for 3 minutes before a specimen is obtained and a suitable note made in the patient's chart and on the result report form. Specimens obtained from the opposite arm or below the infusion site in the same arm may be satisfactory for most tests, although not for some chemistry tests.[16]

Preparation of Site

The area around the intended puncture site should be cleaned with whatever cleanser is approved for use by the institution. Three commonly used materials are a prepackaged alcohol swab, a gauze pad saturated with 70% isopropanol, and a benzalkonium chloride solution (Zephiran chloride solution, 1:750). Cleaning of the puncture site should be done with a circular motion and from the site outward. The skin should be allowed to dry in the air. No alcohol or cleanser should remain on the skin because traces may cause **hemolysis** and invalidate test results. Once the skin has been cleaned, it should not be touched until after the venipuncture has been completed.

Venous Occlusion

After the skin is cleaned, either a blood pressure cuff or a tourniquet is applied 4 to 6 inches (10 to 15 cm) above the intended puncture site (distance for adults). This obstructs the return of venous blood to the heart and distends the veins (**venous occlusion**). When a blood pressure cuff is used as a tourniquet, it is usually inflated to approximately 60 mm Hg (8.0 kPa). Tourniquets are typically made from precut soft rubber strips or from Velcro. It is rarely necessary to leave a

tourniquet in place for longer than 1 minute, but even within this short time the composition of blood changes. Although the changes that occur in 1 minute are slight, marked changes have been observed after 3 minutes for many chemistry analytes.[16] There are no known changes affecting molecular diagnostics.

Timing

For most current molecular diagnostic tests, the time of day is unlikely to contribute to altered or invalid test results. However, the time at which a specimen is obtained is important for those blood constituents that undergo marked diurnal variation (e. g., corticosteroids and iron) and for those used to monitor drug therapy.

Order of Draw for Multiple Blood Specimens

In general, blood for molecular testing is not affected by the physiological changes associated with application of a tourniquet.[13,16] The composition of blood drawn first (i.e., the blood closest to the tourniquet) is most representative of the composition of circulating blood and should therefore be used for those analytes, such as calcium, that are pertinent to critical medical decisions. Blood drawn later shows a greater effect from venous stasis, and recommended order of draw (see below) has been developed with these changes in mind.[13,16]

In a few patients, backflow from blood tubes into veins occurs owing to a decrease in venous pressure. The dangerous consequences of this occurrence may be prevented if only sterile tubes are used for collection of blood. Backflow is minimized if the arm is held downward and blood is kept from contact with the stopper during the collection procedure. To minimize problems if backflow should occur and to optimize the quality of specimens—especially to prevent cross contamination with **anticoagulants**—blood should be collected into tubes in the order outlined in Table 3-1. This table also provides the recommended number of inversions for each tube type because it is critical that complete mixing of any additive with the blood collected be accomplished as quickly as possible.

The selection of which tube type is to be used for molecular diagnostic testing will depend in large measure on whether the testing is for genomic DNA of the patient (yellow ACD tube or white K ethylenetriaminetetraacetic acid (EDTA) with gel tube) or RNA or DNA from an infectious agent (lavender K or Na EDTA). In general, blood collected for molecular testing that requires amplification should never be drawn into a heparin-containing tube. A more complete discussion of the choice of anticoagulants for molecular testing is presented below.

Collection with Evacuated Blood Tubes

Evacuated blood tubes are usually considered to be less expensive and more convenient and easier to use than syringes and thus are the collection device of choice in many institutions. Evacuated blood tubes may be made of soda-lime or borosilicate glass or plastic (polyethylene terephthalate). Because of the decreased likelihood of breakage and subsequent exposure to infectious materials, many laboratories have converted from glass tubes to plastic tubes. There are several types of evacuated tubes used for venipuncture collection.[9] They vary by the type of additive added and volume of the tube. The different types of additives are identified by the color of the stopper used

TABLE 3-1	Recommended Order of Draw for Multiple Specimen Collection	
Stopper Color	**Contents**	**Number of Inversions**
Yellow	Sterile media for blood culture	8
Royal blue	No additive	0
Clear	Nonadditive; discard tube if no royal blue used	0
Light blue	Sodium citrate	3-4
Gold/red	Serum separator tube	5
Red/red, orange/ yellow, royal blue	Serum tube, with or without clot activator, with or without gel	5
Green	Heparin tube with or without gel	8
Tan (glass)	Sodium heparin	8
Royal blue	Sodium heparin, sodium EDTA	8
Lavender, pearl white, pink/pink, tan (plastic)	EDTA tubes, with or without gel	8
Gray	Glycolytic inhibitor	8
Yellow (glass)	ACD for molecular studies and cell culture	8

Modified from information in Clinical and Laboratory Standards Institute/ NCCLS. Evacuated tubes and additives for blood specimen collection: CLSI-approved standard H1-A5, 5th ed. Wayne, PA: Clinical and Laboratory Standards Institute, 2003 and So you're going to collect a blood specimen: an introduction to phlebotomy, 11th ed. FL Kiechle, Ed. Northfield, Il: College of American Pathologists, 2005.

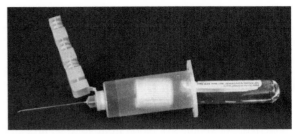

Figure 3-1
Assembled venipuncture set.
(From Flynn JC. Procedures in phlebotomy, 3rd ed. St Louis: Saunders, 2005.)

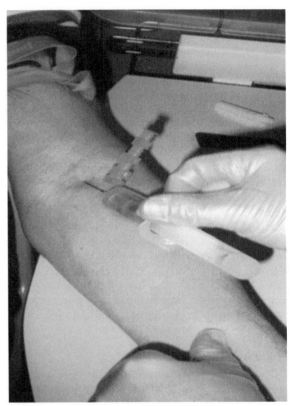

Figure 3-2
Venipuncture. (Courtesy Mayo Clinic, Rochester, Minn.) (See Color Plate 1.)

(Table 3-2). Additional tubes, not listed, are sold for special applications, such as RNA isolation. These less common tubes must be validated by each laboratory before use.

Blood collected into a tube containing one additive should never be transferred into other tubes, because the first additive may interfere with tests for which a different additive is specified. Additionally, transfer of the additive from one tube to another should be minimized (or adverse effects reduced) through a strict adherence to recommendations for order of tube use (Table 3-1).

A typical system for collecting blood in evacuated tubes is shown in Figure 3-1.[11] This is an example of a commonly used single-use device that incorporates a cover that is designed to be placed over the needle when collection of the blood is complete, thereby reducing the risk of a puncture of the phlebotomist by the now-contaminated needle. A needle or winged (butterfly) set is screwed into the collection tube holder, and the tube is then gently inserted into this holder. The tube should be gently tapped to dislodge any additive from the stopper before the needle is inserted into a vein; this prevents aspiration of the additive into the patient's vein.

After the skin is cleaned, the needle should be guided gently into the patient's vein (Figure 3-2); once the needle is in place, the tube should be pressed forward into the holder to puncture the stopper and release the vacuum. When blood begins to flow into the tube, the tourniquet should be released without moving the needle. The tube is filled until the vacuum is exhausted. It is critically important that the evacuated tube be filled completely. Many additives are provided in the tube based on a "full" collection; deviation or short draws can be a source of preanalytical errors because they can significantly affect test results. Once the tube is filled completely, it can then be withdrawn from the holder, mixed gently by inversion, and replaced by another tube, if this is necessary. Other tubes may be filled using the same technique with the holder in place. When several tubes are required from a single blood collection, a shutoff valve—consisting of rubber tubing that slides over the needle opening—is used to prevent spillage of blood during exchange of tubes.

Blood Collection with Syringe

Syringes are customarily used for patients with difficult veins. If a syringe is used, the needle is placed firmly over the nozzle of the syringe, and the cover of the needle is removed. If the syringe has an eccentric nozzle, the needle should be arranged

TABLE 3-2	Coding of Stopper Color to Indicate Additive in Evacuated Blood Tube		
Tube Type	**Additive**	**Stopper Color**	**Alternative**
Gel separation tubes	Polymer gel/silica activator	Red/black	Gold
	Polymer gel/silica activator/lithium heparin	Green/gray	Light gray
Serum tubes (nonadditive)	Silicone-coated interior	Red	Red
	Uncoated interior	Red	Pink
Serum tubes (with additives)	Thrombin (dry additive)	Gray/yellow	Orange
	Particulate clot activator	Yellow/red	Red
	Thrombin (dry additive)	Light blue	Light blue
Whole blood/plasma tubes	K_2 EDTA (dry additive)	Lavender	Lavender
	K_3 EDTA (liquid additive)	Lavender	Lavender
	Na_2 EDTA (dry additive)	Lavender	Lavender
	Citrate, trisodium (coagulation)	Light blue	Light blue
	Citrate, trisodium (erythrocyte sedimentation rate)	Black	Black
	Sodium fluoride (antiglycolic agent)	Gray	Light/gray
	Heparin, lithium (dry or liquid additive)	Green	Green
	Potassium oxalate/sodium fluoride	Light gray	Light gray
	Lithium heparin/iodoacetate	Light gray	Light gray
Specialty tubes (microbiology)			
Blood culture	Sodium polyanethol sulfonate (SPS)	Light yellow	Light yellow
Specialty tubes (chemistry)			
Lead	Heparin, potassium (liquid additive)	Tan	Tan
Trace elements	Heparin, sodium (dry additive)	Royal blue	Royal blue
Stat chemistry	Silicone-coated interior (serum tube)	Royal blue	Royal blue
	Thrombin	Gray/yellow	Orange
Specialty tubes (molecular diagnostics)			
Plasma	K_2EDTA (dry additive)/polymer gel/silica activator	Opalescent white	Opalescent white
	ACD solution A (Na_3 citrate, 22.0 g/L; citric acid, 8.0 g/L; dextrose, 24.5 g/L)	Bright yellow	Bright yellow
	ACD solution B (Na_3 citrate, 13.2 g/L; citric acid, 4.8 g/L; dextrose, 14.7 g/L)	Bright yellow	Bright yellow
Mononuclear cell preparation tube	Sodium citrate with density gradient polymer fluid	Blue/black	Blue/black
	Sodium heparin with density gradient polymer fluid	Green/red	Green/red

Modified from information In Clinical and Laboratory Standards Institute. Evacuated tubes and additives for blood specimen collection: CLSI-approved standard H1-A5, 5th ed. Wayne, Pa: Clinical and Laboratory Standards Institute, 2003 and in the Becton Dickinson Web page (http://www.bd.com/).

with the nozzle downward but the bevel of the needle upward. The syringe and needle should be aligned with the vein to be entered and the needle pushed into the vein at an angle to the skin of approximately 15°. When the initial resistance of the vein wall is overcome as it is pierced, forward pressure on the syringe is eased, and the blood is withdrawn by gently pulling back the plunger of the syringe. Should a second syringe be necessary, a gauze pad may be placed under the hub of the needle to absorb the spill; the first syringe is then quickly disconnected and the second put in place to continue the draw. After removal of the needle from the syringe, drawn blood should be quickly transferred by gentle ejection into tubes prepared for its receipt. The tubes should then be capped and gently mixed.

Vigorous withdrawal of blood into a syringe during collection or forceful transfer from the syringe to the receiving vessel may cause hemolysis of blood. Hemolysis is usually less when blood is drawn through a small-bore needle than when a larger-bore needle is used.

Completion of Collection

When blood collection is complete and the needle withdrawn, the patient should be instructed to hold a dry gauze pad over the puncture site, with the arm raised to lessen the likelihood of leakage of blood. The pad may then be held in place by a bandage or by a nonadhesive strap (which avoids pulling hairs on the arm when it is removed); these are removed after 15 minutes. With a collection device, such as shown in Figure 3-1, the needle is covered, and the needle and tube holder are immediately discarded into a sharps container. In the event that a winged (butterfly) set was used, the wings are pushed forward to cover the needle, or with newer equipment available, a button is pressed, releasing a spring that retracts the needle. If a syringe was used, the needle and syringe (still attached) should then be discarded in a hazardous waste receptacle.

All tubes should then be labeled per institutional policy. Most institutions have a written procedure prohibiting the advance labeling of tubes because this is seen as providing the potential for mislabeling, one of the most common sources of preanalytical error. Gloves should be discarded in a hazardous waste receptacle if visibly contaminated or in noncontaminated trash if not visibly contaminated. Depending upon institutional policy, hands should be washed with soap and water, or an alcohol-based hand cleanser should be used before applying new gloves and proceeding to the next patient.

Venipuncture in Children

The techniques for venipuncture in children and adults are similar. However, children are likely to make unexpected movements, and assistance in holding them still is often desirable. Either a syringe or evacuated blood tube system may be used to collect specimens. A syringe should be either the tuberculin type or a 3-mL–capacity syringe, except when a large volume of blood is required for analysis. A 21- to 23-gauge needle or 20- to 23-gauge butterfly needle with attached tubing is appropriate to collect specimens. In general, in the pediatric population, alternative collection through skin puncture is often used.

Skin Puncture

Skin puncture is an open collection technique in which the skin is punctured by a lancet and a small volume of blood collected into a microdevice. Skin puncture blood is more like arterial blood than venous blood. In practice it is used in situations in which (1) sample volume is limited (e.g., pediatric applications), (2) repeated venipunctures have resulted in severe vein damage, or (3) patients may have been burned or bandaged, and veins are therefore unavailable for venipuncture. This technique is also commonly used when the sample is to be applied directly to a testing device in a point-of-care testing situation or to filter paper. It is most often performed on the (1) tip of a finger, (2) earlobe, and (3) heel or big toe of infants. For example, in an infant younger than 1 year, the lateral or medial plantar surface of the foot should be used for skin puncture; suitable areas are illustrated in Figure 3-3.[1] In older children, the plantar surface of the big toe may also be used, although blood collection should be avoided on ambulatory patients from anywhere on the foot. The complete procedure for collecting blood from infants using skin puncture is described in a CLSI document.[4]

To collect a blood specimen by skin puncture, the phlebotomist first thoroughly cleans the skin with a gauze pad saturated with an approved cleaning solution as outlined above for venipuncture. If an alcohol swab is used, the alcohol must be allowed to evaporate from the skin so that hemolysis does not occur. When the skin is dry, it is quickly punctured by a sharp stab with a lancet. The depth of the incision should be less than 2.5 mm to prevent contact with bone. To minimize the

possibility of infection, a different site should be selected for each puncture. The finger should be held in such a way that gravity assists the collection of blood on the fingertip and the lancet held to make the incision as close to perpendicular to the fingernail as possible.[15] Massage of the finger to stimulate blood flow should be avoided because it causes the outflow of debris and tissue fluid, which does not have the same composition as plasma. To improve circulation of the blood, the finger (or the heel in the case of heelsticks) may be warmed by application of a warm, wet washcloth or a specialized device, such as a heel warmer, for 3 minutes before applying the lancet. The first drop of blood is wiped off, and subsequent drops are transferred to the appropriate collection tube by gentle contact. Filling should be done rapidly to prevent clotting, and introduction of air bubbles should be prevented.

Blood is collected into capillary blood tubes by capillary action. A variety of collection tubes is commercially available (Figure 3-4). Containers are commercially available that contain different anticoagulants, such as sodium and ammonium heparin, and some are available in brown glass for collection of light-sensitive analytes, such as bilirubin (see section below on anticoagulants). As with evacuated blood tubes, to prevent the possibility of breakage and spread of infection, capillary devices are frequently plastic or coated with plastic. A disadvantage of some of the collection devices shown in Figure 3-4 is that blood tends to pool in the mouth of the tube and must be flicked down the tube creating a risk of hemolysis. Drop-by-drop collection should be avoided because it increases hemolysis. The correct order of filling of these devices is the same as for evacuated blood tubes (Table 3-1).

Capillary tubes are alternative containers for plasma or whole blood for molecular testing. However, the yield of genomic DNA is generally limited. For pediatric patients particularly, **buccal cells** (see below) serve as a better specimen type. Kits for isolation of DNA from capillary tubes exist; individual laboratories will need to determine the best method for their use.

For the collection of blood specimens on filter paper for molecular genetic testing and neonatal screening, the skin is cleaned and punctured as described previously. The first drop of blood should be wiped away. Then the filter paper is gently

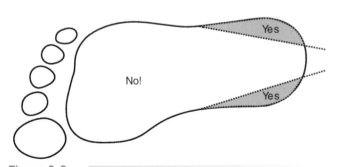

Figure 3-3
Acceptable sites for skin puncture to collect blood from an infant's foot.
(Modified from Blumenfeld TA, Turi GK, Blanc WA. Recommended site and depth of newborn heel punctures based on anatomical measurements and histopathology. Reprinted with permission from Elsevier [Lancet 1979:1:230-3].)

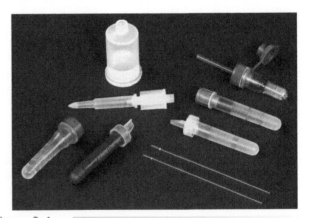

Figure 3-4
Microcollection tubes.
(From Flynn JC. Procedures in phlebotomy, 3rd ed. St Louis: Saunders, 2005.)

touched against a large drop of blood that is allowed to soak into the paper to fill the marked circle. Only a single application per circle should be made. The paper is examined to verify that there has been complete penetration of the paper. The procedure is repeated to fill all the circles. Avoid milking or squeezing of the finger or foot because this procedure contributes tissue fluids. The filter papers should be air-dried (generally 2 to 3 hours to prevent mold or bacterial overgrowth) before storage in a properly labeled paper envelope. Blood should never be transferred onto filter paper after it has been collected in capillary tubes because partial clotting may have occurred, compromising the quality of the specimen.

Arterial Puncture
There is rarely a need for arterial puncture for molecular diagnostic testing; however, such specimens are acceptable when collected into an appropriate container. Arterial punctures require considerable skill and are usually performed only by physicians or specially trained technicians or nurses. The preferred sites of arterial puncture are, in order, the (1) radial artery at the wrist, (2) brachial artery in the elbow, and (3) femoral artery in the groin. Because leakage of blood from the femoral artery tends to be greater, especially in the elderly, sites in the arm are most often used. The proper technique for arterial puncture is described in a CLSI document.[5]

Anticoagulants and Preservatives for Blood
Serum is defined as the watery portion of blood after coagulation has occurred and is the specimen of choice for many assay systems for chemistry testing. However, for molecular diagnostics, anticoagulated whole blood or plasma is more likely to be the specimen of choice. A number of anticoagulants are available, including heparin, EDTA, acid citrate dextrose (ACD), sodium fluoride, citrate, oxalate, and iodoacetate.

Heparin
Heparin is the most widely used anticoagulant for chemistry and hematology testing, but is unacceptable for most tests performed using polymerase chain reaction (PCR) due to inhibition of the polymerase enzyme by this large molecule. Heparin is a mucoitin polysulfuric acid and is available as sodium, potassium, lithium, and ammonium salts, all of which can adequately prevent coagulation. Heparin also has the disadvantages of high cost and a more temporary action of anticoagulation than chemical means, such as those discussed below. In some special circumstances, a heparin tube can be shared with a molecular diagnostic laboratory if a nonheparinized tube is not available. The molecular laboratory can extract DNA from heparinized samples, but may experience reduced amplification as a result of the enzyme inhibition mentioned above. Chapters 4 and 5 discuss mechanisms for extracting DNA and overcoming inhibition.

Ethylenediaminetetraacetic Acid
EDTA is a chelating agent of divalent cations such as Ca^{2+} and Mg^{2+} that is particularly useful for hematological examinations and isolation of genomic DNA because it preserves the cellular components of blood. It is used as the disodium, dipotassium, or tripotassium salt, the last two being more soluble. It is commonly used as the anticoagulant in collection of specimens for qualitative and quantitative human immunodeficiency virus

(HIV), hepatitis C, and cytomrgalovirus (CMV) determinations by molecular techniques. It is effective at a final concentration of 1 to 2 g/L of blood. Higher concentrations hypertonically shrink the red cells. EDTA prevents coagulation by binding calcium, which is essential for the clotting mechanism. Blood collection tubes are prepared by adding a 0.1% solution of an EDTA salt followed by evaporation of water at room temperature. Newer advances using EDTA include the inclusion of a gel barrier to separate plasma from cells (white tubes, Table 3-2). In blue/black tubes (see Table 3-2), incorporation of a density gradient allows recovery of nucleated cells after centrifugation, thus increasing the yield of DNA.

Acid Citrate Dextrose
As indicated above, the collection of specimens into EDTA is often used for isolation of genomic DNA from the patient. However, additional and complementary diagnostic tests, such as cytogenetic testing, may be requested at the same time. For this reason, samples for molecular diagnostics are often collected into ACD anticoagulant so as to preserve both the form and function of the cellular components. There are two ACD tube designations, ACD A and ACD B. These differ by the concentration of the additives only (Table 3-2). Both enhance the vitality and recovery of the white blood cells for several days after collection of the specimen thus being suitable for both molecular diagnostic testing and cytogenetic testing.

Solution A is for an 8.5-mL blood draw (10 mL total volume), whereas solution B is for either a 3-mL or a 6-mL blood draw (7 mL total volume). The amount of extracted DNA required for the specific test(s) requested will determine the size of tube necessary for specimen collection.

Additional Anticoagulants
Blood collected in the following anticoagulants may be used for both pathogen and genomic nucleic acid isolation. However, when testing is performed using FDA (Food and Drug Administration)-approved test systems, validation of the sample type may be required. Such validation is also required for newer "maximum nucleic acid" collection tubes containing proprietary buffer solutions.

Sodium fluoride is a weak anticoagulant, but is often added as a preservative for blood glucose. As a preservative, together with another anticoagulant, such as potassium oxalate, it is effective at a concentration of approximately 2 g/L of blood; when used alone for anticoagulation, a three to five times greater concentration is required. It exerts its preservative action by inhibiting the enzyme systems involved in glycolysis. Sodium iodoacetate at a concentration of 2 g/L is an effective antiglycolytic agent and a substitute for sodium fluoride. Because it has no effect on urease, it was used historically when glucose and urea tests were performed on a single specimen.

Sodium citrate solution (not to be confused with the ACD solution described above), at a concentration of 34 to 38 g/L in a ratio of 1 part to 9 parts of blood, is widely used for coagulation studies because the effect is easily reversible by addition of Ca^{2+}. Because citrate binds calcium, it is clearly unsuitable as an anticoagulant for specimens for measurement of this element.

Sodium, potassium, ammonium, and lithium oxalates inhibit blood coagulation by forming rather insoluble complexes with calcium ions. Potassium oxalate ($K_2C_2O_4 \cdot H_2O$), at a concentration of approximately 1 to 2 g/L of blood, is the most widely used oxalate. At concentrations of greater than 3 g oxalate per liter, hemolysis is likely to occur.

Collection of Blood from Intravenous or Arterial Lines

When blood is collected from a central venous catheter or arterial line, it is necessary to ensure that the composition of the specimen is not affected by the fluid that is infused into the patient. The fluid is shut off using the stopcock on the catheter, and 10 mL of blood is aspirated through the stopcock and discarded before the specimen for analysis is withdrawn. This is particularly important for molecular diagnostics because the stopcock is often heavily saturated with heparin to prevent clotting.

In theory, blood may be collected from the veins of an arm below an intravenous line without interference from the fluid being infused because retrograde blood flow does not occur in the veins, and the fluid that is infused must first circulate through the heart and return to the tissue before it reaches the sampling site.

Hemolysis

Hemolysis is defined as the disruption of the red cell membrane and results in the release of hemoglobin. Serum shows visual evidence of hemolysis when the hemoglobin concentration exceeds 200 mg/L. Slight hemolysis has little effect on most test values. However, a notable effect may be observed on those constituents that are present at a higher concentration in erythrocytes than in plasma.[13,16]

In molecular diagnostic testing, it is possible for the hemoglobin to interfere with the amplification reaction, particularly when RT-PCR is the first step in the analysis of RNA. In some situations, the isolation of nucleic acid is sufficiently selective that free hemoglobin from the ruptured cells is removed and will not cause a problem. However, with hemolyzed blood, alternative or additional extraction methods are usually needed to ensure that the greatest amplification of DNA is achieved. To determine the extent of contamination with hemoglobin, the (optical) absorbance of a sample is read on a spectrophotometer to measure the amount of protein present in the sample. DNA absorbs light at a 260 nm wavelength, whereas proteins absorb at either 230 nm or 280 nm wavelength. Chapter 5 discusses this issue in more detail.

Urine

Currently, urine is an uncommon specimen type in the molecular diagnostic laboratory for genomic testing, although some laboratories use urine samples for bladder cancer screening and monitoring of therapy of bladder cancer. However, urine is frequently used for molecular testing for infectious agents, such as *Chlamydia*, a common sexually transmitted organism, or BK virus, associated with potential rejection and/or failure of transplanted kidneys. Since most requests are for a specific organism, an untimed or random urine specimen collected into a sterile container with no preservative is usually acceptable. A clean, early morning specimen is usually the most concentrated specimen and thus is preferred. Bacterial examination either using molecular techniques or microscopically of the first 10 mL of urine voided is most appropriate to detect urethritis, whereas the midstream specimen is best for investigating

bladder disorders including detection of genomic abnormalities of bladder cells associated with neoplasia.

Catheter specimens are used for microbiological examination in critically ill patients or in those with urinary tract obstruction, but should not normally be obtained just for examination of chemical constituents. The suprapubic tap specimen is a useful alternative because the tap is unlikely to cause infection. After appropriate cleaning of the skin over the full bladder, a 22-gauge spinal needle is passed through a small wheal made by a local anesthetic. The bladder is penetrated, and the urine withdrawn into the syringe.

Even though tests in the clinical laboratory are not usually affected by lack of sterile collection procedures, the patient's genitalia should be cleaned before each voiding to minimize the transfer of surface bacteria to the urine. Details of collection of urine specimens are contained in a CLSI guideline.[6] Timed urine collections[16] are rarely indicated for molecular diagnostic testing.

Collection of Urine from Children

To obtain a sterile urine specimen for culture from an infant, a suprapubic tap is performed. The collection of specimens from older children is done as in adults, using assistance from a parent when this is necessary.

Urine Preservatives

For molecular testing, chemical preservation of urine is not routinely used and is generally not recommended. The most common preservatives used, however, and the recommended volumes per timed collection are listed in Table 3-3. Preservatives have different roles, but are usually added to reduce bacterial action or chemical decomposition or to solubilize constituents that might otherwise precipitate out of solution. Another application is to decrease atmospheric oxidation of unstable compounds. Some specimens should not have any preservatives added because of the possibility of interference with analytical methods. Since urine is an uncommon specimen type for molecular testing, little has been published on the effects, if any, of these preservatives on amplification techniques. Therefore it is the responsibility of each laboratory to identify acceptable specimens for each molecular test performed on urine particularly.

When a urine collection is complete, the specimen should be delivered without delay to the clinical laboratory. For a

TABLE 3-3	Commonly Used Urine Preservatives
Preservative	**Concentrations/Volumes**
HCl	6 mol/L; 30 mL per 24 hour collection
Acetic acid	50%; 25 mL per 24 hour collection
Na_2CO_3	5 g per 24 hour collection
HNO_3	6 mol/L; 15 mL per 24 hour collection
Boric acid	10 g per 24 hour collection
Toluene	30 mL per 24 hour collection
Thymol	10% in isopropanol; 10 mL per 24 hour collection

Adapted from information provided in Clinical and Laboratory Standards Institute. Routine urinalysis and collection, transportation, and preservation of urine specimens: CLSI-approved guideline GP16-A2, 2nd ed. Wayne, Pa: Clinical and Laboratory Standards Institute, 2001.

timed specimen,[16] the volume should be measured by using graduated cylinders or by weighing the container and urine when preweighed or uniform containers are used. The mass in grams may be reported as if it were the volume in milliliters.

Before a specimen is transferred into small containers for each of the ordered tests, it must be thoroughly mixed to ensure homogeneity because the specific gravity, volume, and composition of the urine may all vary throughout the collection period. For molecular diagnostic testing of urine, it is often necessary to concentrate the specimen by centrifugation and resuspension of the sediment pellet in a small volume of the supernatant urine or a suitable buffer for extraction to optimize the yield of nucleic acids. For this reason, aliquoting directly into a plastic centrifuge tube is generally recommended. Any small container into which an aliquot is transferred should not be a plastic bottle if toluene or another organic compound has been used as a preservative; metal-free containers must be used for trace metal analyses.

Feces

Although currently most tests for infectious agents in feces are made through immunological identification of specific antigens associated with individual bacterial agents, increasingly direct molecular identification of pathogens is being used. Most requests for fecal testing will be made in the presentation of diarrhea, often liquid or bloody. The presence of heme in a fecal specimen will be associated with the same problems of inhibition of particularly RT-PCR discussed above with the hemolyzed venipuncture specimen. Additional preparative work may be necessary to remove any heme present.

Testing of the patient's own DNA in stool is uncommon, but recent developments in the diagnosis of colon cancer may change that. DNA isolated from fecal samples is representative of the genetic composition of the colonic mucosa at the time of stool collection. The differential and quantitative analysis of stool DNA integrity has been proposed as a sensitive and specific biomarker useful for the detection of colorectal cancer.[2]

Usually, no preservative is added to the feces, but the container should be kept refrigerated throughout the collection period, and care should be taken to prevent contamination from urine.

Cerebrospinal Fluid

The most common use of spinal fluid in molecular diagnostics is for the rapid identification of an infectious agent. Spinal fluid is normally obtained from the lumbar region, although a physician may occasionally request analysis of fluid obtained during surgery from the cervical region or from a cistern or ventricle of the brain. Spinal fluid is examined when there is a question as to the presence of a cerebrovascular accident, meningitis, demyelinating disease, or meningeal involvement in malignant disease. In general, spinal fluid is cell poor unless there is an infection or malignancy present.

Lumbar punctures should always be performed by a physician, who will collect 3 to 4 mL of fluid into each of multiple tubes. Up to 20 mL of spinal fluid can be safely removed from an adult, although this amount is not usually required. The collection tubes, generally screw-top plastic or glass, should be sterile, especially if microbiological tests are required. Because the initial specimen may be contaminated by tissue debris or

skin bacteria, the first tube should be used for chemical or serological tests, the second for microbiological tests including molecular diagnostics, and the third for microscopic and cytological examination. The same procedure is used for infants and children, but the volume of fluid withdrawn should be the minimum for the requested tests.

Synovial Fluid

The most common use of synovial (joint) fluid in molecular diagnostics is to assess the presence of infectious microorganisms that lead to complications of great severity. Examples of organisms that the laboratory may test for include the presence of *Borrelia burgdorferi,* the causative agent in Lyme disease; *Staphylococcus aureus* for the presence of a staph infection; and aerobic gram-negative bacilli for the presence of *Salmonella, Pasteurella,* or *Pseudomonas,* which can lead to the loss of limbs if left untreated.

The technique of obtaining synovial fluid for examination is called **arthrocentesis.** Synovial fluid is withdrawn from joints to aid characterization of the type of arthritis and to differentiate noninflammatory effusions (leakage into the cavity) from inflammatory fluids. Normally, only a very small amount of fluid is present in any joint, but this volume is usually very much increased in the presence of inflammatory conditions. Arthrocentesis should be performed by a physician using sterile procedures, and the technique must be modified from joint to joint depending on the anatomical location and size of the joint. The physician should establish priorities for the tests to be performed in case the available volume is insufficient for all tests. Sterile plain tubes should be used for molecular diagnostics, for culture, and for glucose and protein measurements; an EDTA tube is necessary for a total leukocyte, differential, and erythrocyte count. Microscopic slides are prepared for staining with Gram or other stains indicated and for gross visual inspection.

Amniotic Fluid

Collection of amniotic fluid, **amniocentesis,** is performed by a physician (1) for prenatal diagnosis of congenital disorders, (2) to assess fetal maturity, or (3) to look for Rh isoimmunization or intrauterine infection. Virtually any molecular diagnostic assay can be applied to the DNA from an amniotic fluid specimen. Some of the more common molecular diagnostic assays include tests for sickle cell anemia, Tay-Sachs disease, and thalassemia.

The gestational timing for sample collection is dependent upon the clinical question. Although ultrasound is not essential, amniocentesis is best performed with its assistance to aid localization of the placenta and to determine the presentation of the fetus. The best sites for obtaining amniotic fluid are behind the neck of the fetus, below its head, or from other unoccupied areas of the amniotic cavity.

The skin is cleaned and anesthetized as for other similar procedures, and 10 mL of fluid is aspirated into a syringe connected to the spinal needle that is typically used. Sterile containers, such as polypropylene test tubes or urine cups, are used to transport the fluid to the laboratory. There are few complications from amniocentesis. Occasionally a bloody tap is made, but normally the fluid is clear and yellow. The blood may come from the uterine wall, the placenta, or even the fetus. Determination of fetal hemoglobin can be used to help ascertain the source if it is important to do so.

For prenatal determination of genetic disorders, the cellular content of the amniocentesis sample may not provide sufficient nucleic acid for analysis. For cytogenetic studies and to obtain more DNA the fluid is usually cultured under highly specialized conditions to expand the number of cells. If culture will be required, amniotic fluid specimens should be transferred into a T-25 tissue culture flask. During transport the specimen should be kept at a cool temperature, but not allowed to freeze. The amniotic fluid, normally clear and yellow, is then distributed into one or more flasks, and growth (expansion of the number of cells) is facilitated by incubation with specialized culture medium. Nine to 12 days of culturing is used to obtain a sufficient number of cells for DNA extraction. The cells are gently removed from the surface of the flask through the use of the enzyme trypsin, mixed, and placed into a collection tube. The sample is then ready for DNA extraction.

Chorionic Villus Sampling

Chorionic villus sampling (CVS) allows for earlier diagnosis than amniotic fluid analysis. With CVS, testing can be performed at a gestation period of 10 to 12 weeks, whereas with amniotic fluid, testing cannot be performed until week 15 to 20 of gestation. CVS is the technique of inserting a catheter or needle into the placenta and removing some of the chorionic villi, vascular projections from the chorion. This tissue has the same chromosomal and genetic makeup as the fetus and can be used to test for disorders that may be present in the fetus. When sampling chorionic villus, ultrasound is performed to assess the placenta and its position. The sample of the placenta is obtained either through the vagina or through the abdomen depending upon the location of the placenta. The specimen is examined under a microscope by a physician at the time of collection to determine the quality, quantity, and integrity of the chorionic villi. Once received by the laboratory, specimen quality is further assessed by examining the specimen for branching, budding, and veining. The specimen is then placed in culture medium and allowed to grow for up to 3 weeks. Once the cells are fully confluent, they are treated as with cells from amniotic fluid (above) for DNA extraction.

Maternal cell contamination testing is used to definitively assess the source of isolated cells in both an amniotic fluid sample and CVS. Such confirmation of the source of the sample is strongly recommended for any prenatal diagnostic testing and may be required as a quality monitor in some laboratories.

Pleural, Pericardial, and Ascitic Fluids

The primary use of these fluids in the molecular diagnostic laboratory is for infectious agent identification and for the detection of cancer cells. Some of the types of organisms found in these fluids include the fungi of Candida, Sporothrix, and Cryptococcus species; Mycobacterium tuberculosis that causes tuberculosis; and Streptococcus pneumoniae that causes pneumonia. Gastrointestinal cancers have also been detected by the presence of free cells in the pleural fluid.[14]

The pleural, pericardial, and peritoneal cavities normally contain a small amount of serous fluid that lubricates the opposing parietal and visceral membrane surfaces. Inflammation or infections affecting the cavities cause fluid to accumulate. The fluid may be removed to determine if it is an effusion or an exudate, a distinction made possible by protein or enzyme analysis. The collection procedure is called paracentesis. When specifically applied to the pleural cavity, the procedure is a thoracentesis; if applied to the pericardial cavity, a pericardiocentesis. Paracentesis should be performed only by skilled and experienced physicians. Pericardiocentesis has now been largely supplanted by echocardiography.

Paracentesis is rarely associated with complications. Occasionally, blood-stained fluid is obtained because of a puncture of a small blood vessel. If adhesions are present between the intestine and abdominal wall, a part of the intestine could be perforated by a peritoneal tap. With a thoracentesis, pneumothorax and bronchopleural fistulas are potential complications.

Buccal Cells

Collection of buccal cells (cells of the oral cavity of epithelial origin) has been identified as providing an excellent source of genomic DNA. Collection of buccal cells is often viewed as less invasive than collection of blood. It is particularly useful for collecting cells with the patient's genomic DNA when the patient has had blood transfusions and thus has blood with another person's (or persons') DNA. Similarly, it is useful after bone marrow transplantation when the circulating blood cells are derived wholly or partially from the donor of the bone marrow. Two methods are used commonly to collect buccal cells: rinsing with mouthwash and the use of swabs.

Rinsing of the oral cavity generally provides a higher yield of cells than does use of swabs. For these collections, the patient is provided with a small amount of mouthwash and instructed to rinse well for a minimum of 60 seconds and then return the mouthwash to a collection tube. There is no harm in doing this longer than 60 seconds, but shortening the time may decrease the yield of buccal cells. Mouthwash solutions high in phenol and ethanol are destructive to the recovered cells and should be avoided. It is necessary for each laboratory to validate a list of acceptable solutions.

Although more commonly used for collection of specimens for microbiological testing, swabs also are used to collect buccal cells for molecular genetics testing. A sterile Dacron or rayon swab with a plastic shaft is preferred because calcium alginate swabs or swabs with wooden sticks may contain substances that inhibit PCR-based testing. After collection the swab should be stored in an air-tight plastic container or immersed in liquid, such as phosphate-buffered saline (PBS) or viral transport medium. In general, the yield of cells and nucleic acid is lower with swabs than with rinsing.

Solid Tissue

Until recently the solid tissue most often analyzed in the clinical laboratory was malignant tissue from the breast for estrogen and progesterone receptors. During surgery at least 0.5 to 1 g of tissue is removed and trimmed of fat and nontumor material. The tissue is quickly frozen, within 20 minutes, preferably in liquid nitrogen or in a mixture of dry ice and alcohol. A histological section should always be examined at the time of analysis of the specimen to confirm that the specimen is indeed malignant tissue.

More recently, somatic gene analyses, such as T-cell receptor rearrangement and clonal expansion, are providing important information for clinicians. For these studies, the molecular diagnostic laboratory often receives material that has been

formalin-fixed, paraffin embedded (FFPE) tissue. In general, neutral buffered formalin, containing no heavy metals, will not interfere with amplification reactions. However, the recovery of nucleic acids is greatly decreased if the tissue has been over-fixed. DNA can still be extracted from tissue embedded in paraffin, but the DNA will be degraded to low molecular weight fragments. In most cases, segments of DNA will amplify in a PCR reaction, but Southern blot methodologies will not work well because most require high molecular weight DNA.

Tissue structure can be retained without permanent fixation by freezing specimens in an **optimal cutting temperature compound (OCT).** OCT is a mixture of polyvinyl alcohol and polyethylene glycol that surrounds but does not infiltrate the tissue. The sample is then frozen at ~−80 °C, and sections are prepared for review by a pathologist. OCT is fully water soluble and should be completely removed from a tissue specimen before it is used as a source of DNA. In general, higher molecular weight DNA can be extracted from OCT-fixed tissues than from FFPE samples.

Hair and Nails

The use of hair or nail in molecular diagnostics is limited to forensic analysis (genomic DNA identification) at this time. Hair and fingernails or toenails have been used for trace metal and drug analyses. However, collection procedures have been poorly standardized, and quantitative measurements are better obtained on blood or urine.

HANDLING OF SPECIMENS FOR ANALYSIS

Maintenance of Specimen Identification

Valid test results require a (1) representative, (2) properly collected, and (3) properly preserved specimen. Proper identification of the specimen must be maintained at each step of the testing process. Every specimen container must be adequately labeled even if the specimen must be placed in ice or if the container is so small that a label cannot be placed along the tube, as might happen with a capillary blood tube. Direct labeling of a capillary blood tube by folding the label like a flag around the tube is preferred. For small volumes of urine submitted in a screw-cap urine cup and any specimen submitted in a screw-cap test tube or cup, the label should be placed on the cup or tube directly, not on the cap. The minimum information on a label should include a patient's name, location, identifying number, and the date and time of collection. All labels should conform to the laboratory's stated requirements to facilitate proper processing of specimens. No specific labeling should be attached to specimens from patients with infectious diseases to suggest that these specimens should be handled with special care. All specimens should be treated as if they are potentially infectious.

Preservation of Specimens in Transit

Specimens must be properly treated both during transport to the laboratory and from the time the serum, cells, etc. have been separated until analysis can begin. For some tests, specimens must be kept at 4 °C from the time the blood is drawn until the specimens are analyzed; others require remaining at or near room temperature. In the case of blood fluids for molecular diagnostics, freezing of the specimen before isolation of the specific component to be analyzed should be avoided. By contrast, if the specimen is a section of solid tissue, freezing is the method of choice. After isolation of the component of the specimen to be analyzed (such as isolation of plasma from blood), delays in analysis may contribute to preanalytical errors.

For all test constituents that are thermally labile, serum and plasma should be separated from cells in a refrigerated centrifuge, although this is rarely necessary for molecular diagnostic testing.

For the molecular diagnostic laboratory, the largest challenge is the recovery of RNA from transported specimens. Depending on the tissue source, RNA yields will vary, primarily because of the amount of RNA present at the time of collection. Specimens from liver, spleen, or heart have large amounts of RNA, but specimens from skin, muscle, and bone have lower RNA content. Tissue samples should be frozen immediately. On the other hand, a blood specimen should never be frozen before separation of the cellular elements because of hemolysis and released heme that may interfere with subsequent amplification processes. For tissue samples, it is critical to choose the disruption method best suited for the specific type of tissue. Thorough cellular disruption is critical for high RNA quality and yield. RNA that is trapped in intact cells is often removed with cellular debris by centrifugation.[12]

Although transport of specimens from the patient to the clinical laboratory is often done by messenger, pneumatic tube systems have been used to move the specimens more rapidly over long distances within the hospital. Hemolysis may occur in these systems unless the tubes are completely filled and movement of the blood tubes inside the specimen carrier is prevented. The pneumatic tube system should be designed to eliminate sharp curves and sudden stops of the specimen carriers because these factors are responsible for much of the hemolysis that may occur. With many systems, however, the plasma hemoglobin concentration may be increased and the amount of hemolysis may contribute to poor nucleic acid recovery and/or amplification. In special cases, such as in a patient undergoing chemotherapy whose cells are fragile, samples should be centrifuged before being placed in the pneumatic tube system or identified as "messenger delivery only."

For specimens that are collected in a remote facility with infrequent transport by courier to a central laboratory, proper specimen processing must be done in the remote facility so that appropriately separated and preserved components are delivered to the laboratory. This necessitates that the remote facility has ready access to all commonly used preservatives and wet ice.

Separation and Storage of Specimens

Plasma or serum should be separated from cells as soon as possible and certainly within 2 hours. Premature separation of serum, however, may permit continued formation of fibrin, which can clog sampling devices in testing equipment. If it is impossible to centrifuge a blood specimen within 2 hours, the specimen should be held at room temperature rather than at 4 °C to decrease hemolysis. For most plasma samples used for molecular diagnostics, the plasma should be removed from the primary tube promptly after centrifugation and held at −20 °C in a freezer capable of maintaining this temperature. Frost-free freezers should be avoided because they have a wide temperature swing during the freeze-thaw cycle.

Cryopreservation of white blood cells and DNA is one method to store and maintain samples for extended periods of time. Whole blood specimens can be centrifuged, and the white cells can be removed and cryopreserved at −20 °C until these cells are required for DNA extraction. For even longer periods of storage, isolated DNA can be stored at −70 °C. The extracted DNA should not be exposed to repetitive cycles of freezing and thawing since this can lead to the shearing of the DNA. After completely thawing these extracted DNA samples, it is important to fully mix the sample to ensure a homogeneous specimen.

Specimen tubes should be centrifuged with stoppers in place. Closure reduces evaporation that occurs rapidly in a warm centrifuge with the air currents set up by centrifugation. Stoppers also prevent aerosolization of infectious particles. Specimen tubes containing volatiles, such as ethanol, must be stoppered while they are spun. Centrifuging specimens with the stopper in place also maintains anaerobic conditions that are important in the measurement of carbon dioxide and free calcium.

Transport of Specimens

Although the discussion below uses the specific example of referral laboratory testing by another laboratory, many of the issues, such as regulations related to shipping, are also relevant to a laboratory that receives specimens from outlying clinics via a (laboratory owned and/or operated) courier service.

Before a referral laboratory is used for any tests, the quality of its work should be verified by the referring laboratory. Guidelines for selection and evaluation of a referral laboratory have been published.[10] For laboratories accredited by the College of American Pathologists (CAP), it is a requirement that the referring laboratory validate that the referral lab is CLIA certified by obtaining a copy of the CLIA certificate before the shipping of specimens. For molecular diagnostic testing, this is of particular importance because often the latest genetic test being requested by a physician has not yet moved from research interest status to patient care status and may not be available in a CLIA-certified laboratory.

Specimen type and quantity and specimen handling requirements of the referral laboratory must be observed, and test results reported by a referral laboratory must be identified as such when they are filed in a patient's chart. The director of a referring laboratory has the responsibility to ensure that specimens will be adequately transported to the referral laboratory. Also, the director should determine the benefits of different services and should keep in mind that the fastest service is usually the most expensive. The director should also know that specimens should not be sent to a referral laboratory at the end of the week because more delays in transit occur during weekends than during the working week, and deterioration of specimens is more likely.

It should be assumed that transport from a referring laboratory to a referral laboratory may take as long as 72 hours. Under optimal conditions, a referring laboratory should retain enough specimen for retesting should an unanticipated problem arise during shipment. The tube used for holding a specimen (primary container) should be so constructed that the contents do not escape if the container is exposed to extremes of heat, cold, or sunlight. Reduced pressure of 0.50 atmosphere (50 kPa) may be encountered during air transport, together with vibration, and

specimens should be protected by a suitable container from these adverse conditions. Variability of temperature is a significant factor in causing instability of test constituents.

Polypropylene and polyethylene containers are usually suitable for specimen transport. Glass should be avoided because of its tendency to break. Polystyrene is also unsuitable because it may crack when frozen. The containers must be leak proof and should have a Teflon-lined screw cap that does not loosen under the variety of temperatures to which the container may be exposed. The materials of both stopper and container must be inert and must not have any effect on the concentration of the analyte.

In situations in which sample delivery for molecular analysis will be delayed, extracted nucleic acid, usually DNA only, can be transported in a buffer solution or water or it can be dried down and shipped as a loose powder. With either method, the DNA should be transported at ambient temperatures and not be exposed to extremely high temperatures for an extended period of time because the DNA will begin to degrade, and testing may be compromised.

The shipping or secondary container used to hold one or more specimen tubes or bottles must be constructed to prevent the tubes from banging against each other. Corrugated, fiberboard, or Styrofoam boxes designed to fit around a single specimen tube are commonly used. A padded shipping envelope provides adequate protection for shipping single specimens. When specimens are shipped as drops of blood on filter paper (e.g., for neonatal screening), the paper should be enclosed in a paper envelope to ensure that the sample remains dry. The initial paper envelope can be placed in a shipping envelope and transported to the testing facility; rapid shipping is rarely required for dried blood on paper.

For transport of frozen or refrigerated specimens, a Styrofoam container should be used. The container walls should be 1 inch (2.5 cm) thick to provide effective insulation. The container should be vented to prevent buildup of carbon dioxide under pressure and a possible explosion. Solid carbon dioxide (dry ice) is the most convenient refrigerant material for keeping specimens frozen, and temperatures as low as −70 °C can be achieved. The amount of dry ice required in a container depends on the size of the container, the efficiency of its insulation, and the time for which the specimens must be kept frozen. One piece of solid dry ice (about 3 inches × 4 inches × 1 inch) in a container with 1-inch Styrofoam walls and a volume of 125 cubic inches (2000 cm^3) will maintain a single specimen frozen for 48 hours.

Various laws and regulations apply to the shipment of biological specimens.[7,8,10] Although they theoretically apply only to etiological agents (known infectious agents), all specimens should be transported as if the same regulations applied. Airlines have rigid regulations covering the transport of specimens. Airlines deem dry ice a hazardous material; therefore the transport of most clinical laboratory specimens is affected by the regulations, and those that package the specimens should be trained in the appropriate regulations, such as the U.S. Air International Transport Association (IATA).

The various modes of transport of specimens influence the shipping time and cost, and each laboratory will need to make its own assessment as to adequate service. The objective is to ensure that the properly collected, processed, and identified specimen arrives at the testing facility in time and under the

ETHICS Box 3-1

ETHICAL SITUATION A

Patient A, pregnant with her first child, comes to the laboratory with physician orders for an HIV viral load test as follow-up to her positive HIV antibody test. The patient is upset because she feels she has no risk factors for HIV and cannot understand how she could be HIV-antibody positive, even though she understands that HIV testing is part of the standard prenatal work-up. You, too, are surprised because you remember drawing the prenatal panel on this woman. If anyone would be positive, you would have suspected Patient B, the woman who was seen in the infectious disease clinic that same day.

The more you think about the initial day of draw, you remember that you had had a minor car accident on your way to work that morning and had been pretty upset. You realize that there is a very strong possibility that you could have mislabeled the tubes.

DILEMMA

You are already under probation for a performance issue and realize that if the positive HIV test result on Patient A is wrong, that will be determined when the viral load test is performed. Do you self-report and run the risk of losing your job or figure that you do not need to say anything because you are not sure the samples were switched and anyway, the "correct" results on Patient A will come out eventually?

POINTS FOR DISCUSSION

○ Although it is true that the positive (false or not) HIV test will be confirmed for Patient A, what about Patient B?

○ Do you look into the computer to check her results, hoping maybe they were both positive?

○ But what about your institutional policies on HIPAA and checking patient results?

○ What about the other tests that were run on Patient A as part of the prenatal work-up? Were any of these other tests likely to be performed on blood from the same tube that you suspect was mislabeled?

○ What are the obligations of every member of the healthcare team in patient care?

ETHICAL SITUATION B

A sample for a specific assay (assay A) was analyzed in a molecular diagnostic laboratory and was found to have a positive and unusual result. The supervisor of the laboratory asked that the technologist in the sample preparation area extract DNA from any cells remaining on that specimen. The supervisor plans to use a part of the original specimen as a control for assay X. The patient's specimen did not originally have testing for assay X ordered on it so no one in the laboratory knows the result of this specimen for assay X. Realizing that the laboratory cannot perform a test on the patient's blood that was not ordered by the physician, the supervisor will make the name anonymous.

Question: Is it ethical for the supervisor to perform test X on this sample when this test was not ordered on it originally? What happens if the patient produces a positive result that could have serious implications?

Discussion: The supervisor should not perform an assay that was not ordered on the specimen. Even if the sample is nameless, the laboratory has a responsibility to report all positive results. If test X was not ordered originally and a positive result is found on this patient, the laboratory has an obligation to call the client and disclose the result of this additional testing. If the supervisor needs a control specimen for assay X, the supervisor should anonymously identify a sample that has been analyzed with assay X.

---

correct storage conditions so that the analytical phase can then proceed.

ETHICAL ISSUES

Medical technologists and phlebotomists face special ethical issues related to molecular diagnostic testing. These may occur during specimen collection or later. Two such scenarios are described in Ethics Box 3-1 to stimulate thought and reflection.

The presence of ethical professionals in the clinical laboratory has been important in medicine ever since the advent of the clinical laboratory, and the advent of progressively more powerful tools in the laboratory has made their presence ever more important. We recommend discussion and understanding of the types of issues in the Ethics Box 3-1.

REFERENCES

1. Blumenfeld TA, Turi GK, Blanc WA. Recommended site and depth of newborn heel skin punctures based on anatomic measurements and histopathology. Lancet 1979;1:230-3.
2. Boynton KA, Summerhayes IC, Ahlquist DA, Shuber AP. DNA integrity as a potential marker for stool-based detection of colorectal cancer. Clin Chem 2003;49:2112-3.
3. Clinical and Laboratory Standards Institute. Procedures for the collection of diagnostic blood specimens by venipuncture: CLSI-approved standard H3-A5, 5th ed. Wayne, Pa: Clinical and Laboratory Standards Institute, 2003.
4. Clinical and Laboratory Standards Institute/NCCLS. Procedures and devices for the collection of capillary blood specimens: CLSI/NCCLS approved standard H4-A5, 5th ed. Wayne, Pa: Clinical and Laboratory Standards Institute, 2004.
5. Clinical and Laboratory Standards Institute/NCCLS. Procedures for the collection of arterial specimen: CLSI/NCCLS approved standard H11-A4, 4th ed. Wayne, Pa: Clinical and Laboratory Standards Institute, 2004.
6. Clinical and Laboratory Standards Institute/NCCLS. Routine urinalysis and collection, transportation, and preservation of urine specimens: CLSI/NCCLS approved guideline GP16-A2, 2nd ed. Wayne, Pa: Clinical and Laboratory Standards Institute, 2001.
7. Clinical and Laboratory Standards Institute/NCCLS. Collection, transport, preparation, and storage of specimens for molecular methods. CLSI/NCCLS approved guideline MM12-A, 1st ed. Wayne, Pa: Clinical and Laboratory Standards Institute, 2006.
8. Clinical and Laboratory Standards Institute/NCCLS. Protection of laboratory workers from occupationally acquired infections: CLSI/NCCLS approved guideline M29-A3, 3rd ed. Wayne, Pa: Clinical and Laboratory Standards Institute, 2005.
9. Clinical and Laboratory Standards Institute/NCCLS. Evacuated tubes and additives for blood specimen collection: CLSI/NCCLS approved standard H1-A5, 5th ed. Wayne, Pa: Clinical and Laboratory Standards Institute, 2003.
10. Clinical and Laboratory Standards Institute/NCCLS. Selecting and evaluating a referral laboratory: CLSI/NCCLS approved guideline GP9-A. Wayne, Pa, Clinical and Laboratory Standards Institute, 1998.
11. Flynn JC. Procedures in phlebotomy, 3rd ed. St Louis: Saunders, 2005.
12. Groszbach A. Nucleic acid preparation, 4th Annual University of Connecticut Molecular Review Symposium, 26th Annual Meeting of the Association of Genetic Technologists, Minneapolis, Mn, May 30, 2001.
13. Ladenson JH. Nonanalytical sources of variation in clinical chemistry results. In: Gradwohl's clinical laboratory methods and diagnosis, 8th ed. Sonnenwirth AC, Jarett L, Eds. St Louis: CV Mosby Co, 1980.
14. Natsugoe S, Tokuda K, Matsumoto M. Molecular detection of free cancer cells in pleural lavage fluid from esophageal cancer patients. Int J Mol Med 2003;12:771-5.

15. So you're going to collect a blood specimen: an introduction to phlebotomy, 11th ed. Kiechle FL, Ed. Northfield, Il: College of American Pathologists. 2005.
16. Young DS, Bermes EW, Haverstick DM. Specimen collection and processing. In: Tietz textbook of clinical chemistry and molecular diagnostics, 4th ed. Burtis CA, Ashwood ER, Bruns DE, Eds. St Louis: Elsevier Saunders, 2006:41-58.

REVIEW QUESTIONS

1. Which of the following is not a patient identifier?
    A. Patient name
    B. Date of birth
    C. Social security number
    D. Medical record number
    E. Name of patient's parents

2. Which anticoagulant is not recommended for blood samples that will be used in a molecular diagnostic laboratory?
    A. Heparin
    B. ACD
    C. EDTA
    D. Potassium oxalate
    E. Sodium citrate

3. A hemolyzed sample of blood arrives in a molecular diagnostic laboratory for genetic testing. How should the hemolyzed sample be handled?
    A. Reject the sample.
    B. Ask for a redraw.
    C. Extract the sample with standard extraction procedures.
    D. Extract the sample with alternative or additional extraction procedures.
    E. Digest the entire specimen and extract the DNA according to standard extraction procedures.

4. DNA was extracted from a hemolyzed blood sample. The technologist wants to know if the isolated DNA is contaminated with hemoglobin. Which instrument will be used to provide that information?
    A. Fluorometer
    B. Spectrophotometer
    C. Electrophoresis apparatus (agarose gel)
    D. Thermocycler
    E. LightCycler

5. A blood specimen for genetic testing arrives in the molecular diagnostic laboratory with a different name on the blood tube from that on the test requisition. How should the laboratory handle the situation?
    A. Contact the ordering physician, explain the situation, and ask for a redraw.
    B. Have a genetic counselor ask the client for more patient information.

    C. Have the laboratory call the client and ask for clarification.
    D. Have the laboratory call the client's physician for more information on the client.
    E. Do nothing and extract the sample.

6. Genomic DNA analysis is requested on a specimen received in the hospital laboratory at 1600 on a Friday afternoon and collected at 0900 in a remote location. The referral laboratory that will analyze the specimen requires receipt of the specimen within 96 hours of collection. Routine specimen transport indicates that the specimen will arrive at the testing facility at 2100 Tuesday. Which of the following is(are) acceptable?
    A. Reject the specimen with no further action.
    B. Alter the collection time to indicate a 9 PM (2100) collection rather than 9 AM (0900) collection time.
    C. Contact the requesting physician and request a new specimen or the addition of an order for DNA extraction to provide stable DNA that will allow analysis of the specimen.
    D. Set up the test in your own laboratory.
    E. Find a different laboratory that does not have such a stringent requirement.

7. The correct order of draw if multiple tests are requested is the following:
    A. EDTA plasma, lithium plasma, serum (gel barrier), serum (no gel), ACD.
    B. Serum (no gel), serum (gel barrier), lithium plasma, EDTA plasma, ACD.
    C. ACD, lithium plasma, serum (gel barrier), serum (no gel), EDTA plasma.
    D. Serum (no gel), lithium plasma, EDTA plasma, serum (gel barrier), ACD.
    E. ACD, serum (no gel), serum (gel barrier), lithium plasma, EDTA plasma.

8. Which of the following are considered preanalytical errors?
    A. Incorrect patient name, short-draw tube, and hemolysis
    B. Incorrect patient medical record number, switched tubes during extraction of nucleic acid, and hemolysis
    C. Specimen stored at 4 °C rather than at required room temperature, RT-PCR Master Mix solution had Mg^{2+} rather than Mn^{2+} added, and hemolysis
    D. Incorrect ICD-9 code on requisition, incorrect patient medical record number, and hemolysis
    E. Wrong tube type drawn, wrong test ordered by physician, and hemolysis

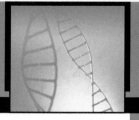

Chapter 4

Nucleic Acid Isolation

Y.M. Dennis Lo, M.A., D.M., D. Phil., F.R.C.P., F.R.C. Path.
Rossa W.K. Chiu, M.B.B.S., Ph.D., F.R.C.P.A., FHKAM (Pathology)

OBJECTIVES

1. List five types of specimens from which DNA and RNA can be isolated; state the requirement a specimen must have before DNA can be extracted from it.
2. Compare liquid- and solid-phase DNA extraction.
3. State the purpose of RNA extraction and isolation.
4. List the steps involved in DNA and RNA extraction.
5. Describe the assessment of isolated nucleic acids using ultraviolet (UV) spectrophotometry and gel electrophoresis.
6. Calculate the purity of isolated RNA or DNA given absorbance values.
7. Describe three automated techniques for isolation of nucleic acids.
8. State the problems involved with isolation of circulating nucleic acids.
9. Discuss the technical issues concerned with maximizing isolation of circulating nucleic acids.
10. Explain the fact that a higher quantity of DNA can be isolated from a serum sample than from a plasma sample.

KEY WORDS AND DEFINITIONS

Absorbance: The measurement of radiant energy absorbed by a solution (or a substance in a solution); this measurement is related to the concentration of a substance, such as DNA or RNA, in that solution.
DNase: A nuclease that specifically degrades DNA.
Extraction: The technique of removing a substance (in this case, DNA or RNA) from surrounding material.
Isolation: The separation of a substance from its surrounding material.
RNase: A ubiquitous nuclease that specifically degrades RNA.

Throughput: A term that describes analytical productivity; a process with high throughput is one in which a large number of samples are analyzed per hour or other appropriate time period.

Many of the key advances in understanding of DNA and RNA have been achieved by study of purified nucleic acids. In the molecular diagnostic laboratory, some tests can be performed directly on samples of biological fluids, but techniques for *isolation* of nucleic acids often are critical. Nucleic acid **isolation** refers to the process of separating DNA or RNA from its surrounding material. Nucleic acid **extraction** is the technique of removing DNA or RNA from surrounding material. The process of nucleic acid isolation involves the extraction procedures and other procedural steps, such as blood centrifugation or tissue grinding.

DNA ISOLATION

Extraction of DNA and/or RNA is usually a key preliminary step to subsequent molecular analysis. Many protocols have been developed over the years. In selecting the most appropriate protocol for one's laboratory, some of the issues worth considering include the (1) specimen type and its available volume, (2) required yield, (3) purity and size of the isolated nucleic acids, (4) ease of operation, (5) **throughput,** and (6) cost and (7) whether the protocol involves the use of hazardous reagents and (8) whether it is amenable to automation. With the advent of the polymerase chain reaction (PCR), molecular analyses could be performed on a variety of specimens, including (1) whole blood, (2) plasma, (3) serum, (4) tissue biopsies, (5) cultured cells, (6) buccal swabs, (7) cerebrospinal fluid, (8) amniotic fluid, (9) paraffin-embedded tissues, and (10) others. Although various commercial protocols are available for DNA extraction, most protocols can be classified into one of a few categories that involve either liquid- or solid-phase extraction. In general, solid-phase extraction methods are more commonly used because of the (1) relative ease of operation, (2) ability to process large batches of specimens, (3) high reproducibility, and (4) adaptability to automation. However, solution-based methods are still favored when large quantities of DNA or large sample volumes are involved.

Because the phosphate esters of the nucleic acid backbone are strong acids and exist as anions at neutral pH, DNA is soluble in water up to about 10 g/L of solution, and it is precipitated by the addition of alcohol. Alcohol precipitation has therefore been used in many nucleic acid extraction protocols, both liquid- and solid-phase protocols. In general, most DNA extraction protocols involve an initial step of cell lysis whereby both the cellular and nuclear membrane envelopes are disrupted. Cellular proteins are then removed by salt precipitation or degraded enzymatically. An additional step of **RNase** digestion is optional. The genomic DNA that remains in solution is then precipitated by the addition of alcohol. The DNA precipitate is isolated and rehydrated. The resultant DNA extract is then stored until subsequent analysis. For the solution-based protocols, cellular debris and protein are usually separated from the soluble DNA fraction by solvent extraction through the use of solvents with different solubility constants. The well-known phenol-chloroform protocols are based on this principle. After the DNA is precipitated by alcohol, the DNA pellet is isolated by manual removal of the excess alcohol solution. Careful attention to this step is required to prevent the inadvertent removal of the DNA pellet, which is quite fine or loose in some instances. Before rehydration of the DNA pellet, it is air-dried to remove the remaining drops of alcohol. Because of the number of manual steps involved, the sample throughput of these solution-based methods is limited. Another disadvantage is that both phenol and chloroform are hazardous chemicals.

On the other hand, solid-phase extraction methods are more robust and are generally based on the principle of DNA adsorption onto silica in the presence of chaotropic salts, such as guanidine thiocyanate and alcohol. The silica is typically coated onto membrane filters or magnetic particles. Silica-impregnated filters that are housed in plastic columns are the most commonly adopted format. DNA binds reversibly with silica depending on the ionic strength of the environment.[19] After cell lysis and protein digestion, DNA is precipitated by the addition of alcohol. The solution is then allowed to pass through the silica-impregnated filter, which binds and purifies the DNA from other debris present in the alcohol solution. Either centrifugation or vacuum manifolds are typically used for the filtration step. The bound DNA is usually washed and subsequently eluted using nuclease-free water or low ionic strength buffers. Similarly, methods based on the use of silica-coated magnetic particles allow the isolation and purification of alcohol-precipitated DNA from other debris. The precipitated DNA binds to the fine magnetic particles by silica adsorption. The solution is then placed under a magnetic field whereby the DNA molecules on the magnetic beads are retained. The magnetic beads are subsequently removed from the purified DNA before the final elution step by changing the ionic strength of the solution to promote disassociation of the DNA from silica. Both the filter column and magnetic particle methods are applicable to various scales of operation. Isolated columns have been used for the extraction of a small number of specimens. The 96-well plate formats are available from some commercial providers and allow the processing of specimens at medium throughput. Moreover, the protocols can be further adapted for use on automated platforms for large-scale processing (see discussion below).[11,13]

RNA ISOLATION

RNA analysis and therefore RNA extraction are required for studies on gene expression. RNA molecules are generally less stable than DNA because, unlike DNA, RNA is not protected by a stable double-helical conformation and, in addition, RNA is subject to alkaline hydrolysis via the 2′-hydroxyl group of its ribose moiety. Although both DNA and RNA are degraded enzymatically by DNA- and RNA-specific nucleases (**DNase** and **RNase**, respectively), RNases are nearly ubiquitous, making it much more difficult to work with native RNA molecules in the laboratory. Thus certain issues warrant special attention when one undertakes operations on RNA, including its extraction.[8] Because of the inherent instability of RNA, clinical specimens intended for RNA analysis should be (1) processed promptly in the fresh state; (2) preserved by the immediate addition of preservation agents, such as RNA*later*™ (Ambion, Austin, Tex.), or (3) snap frozen by liquid nitrogen. The number of freeze-thaw cycles should be minimized for both the specimens and solutions of extracted RNA. Utmost care is needed to prevent RNase contamination. This care includes the use of RNase-free reagents, RNase-free plastic ware, and the cleaning or decontamination of the working surfaces and equipment with RNase-free detergents or chemicals. Water treated with diethylpyrocarbonate (DEPC) for the inactivation of RNase is widely used. As the DNA sequence of eukaryotic genes differs from their mRNA counterparts only by the presence of introns, there exists a possibility in which both DNA and RNA segments are coamplified in specimens contaminated with DNA. Therefore care must be taken to prevent DNA contamination. Alternatively, DNA digestion by DNase I treatment is commonly incorporated as an additional step during the process of RNA purification.[5]

The underlying principles for RNA extraction are essentially identical to those of DNA isolation and purification. Both solution-based and solid-phase extraction protocols are available. Similarly, RNA molecules are (1) first released by lysis of cells; (2) isolated and purified from the protein and lipid debris, either by phenol-chloroform extraction or reversible binding to silica; and (3) precipitated by use of alcohol. However, the composition of lysis buffers typically includes phenol (e.g., Trizol reagent from Invitrogen, Carlsbad, Calif.), sodium dodecyl sulfate, or guanidinium salts because these buffers not only lyse cells directly, but also inhibit RNase effectively.[7] The successful isolation of high quality RNA is thus dependent to some extent on the degree of cellular exposure to these denaturants. Therefore tissue specimens need to be ground to a fine powder form before lysis. To prevent RNA degradation during grinding, the procedure should be performed on either snap-frozen tissues or specimens preserved with RNA stabilizing agents.[8] The above procedures are relevant to the isolation of total RNA, which comprises mRNAs, rRNAs, small nuclear RNAs, and tRNAs. Protocols have been developed for the isolation of mRNA that are based on the capture of the poly-adenylated tails on the 3′ ends of mRNA by hybridization to cellulose-bound oligo(dT) molecules.[8]

ASSESSMENT OF NUCLEIC ACID YIELD AND QUALITY

Nucleic acid molecules absorb UV light maximally at a wavelength of 260 nm owing almost entirely to the constituent bases. Thus DNA or RNA yield can be quantified by spectrophotometric measurement of the **absorbance** at 260 nm, with higher absorbance values indicating higher yield. For example, a solution containing 50 mg/L of pure double-stranded DNA has an absorbance of 1.0 at 260 nm. Alternatively, isolated nucleic acids can be subjected to agarose gel electrophoresis and their yield quantified by densitometric measurements whereby brighter electrophoretic bands indicate higher yield. Spectrophotometric and densitometric methods are also used for the assessment of the quality of the extraction of DNA and RNA. Purity is evaluated by assessing the ratio of the spectrophotometric absorbances at 260 nm and 280 nm (A260/A280), the latter reflecting the presence of the aromatic amino acids in the contaminating proteins. Values greater than 1.8 indicate minimal contamination with proteins. The sizes of the isolated genomic DNA can be estimated by gel electrophoresis. Good quality DNA extractions are generally associated with higher molecular weight fragments (Figure 4-1). Similarly, total RNA integrity can be assessed by estimating the size distribution of the extracted RNA and the appearances of the 18S and 28S rRNA peaks (Figure 4-2). Total RNA preparations of high quality generally have a 28S/18S ratio greater than 2.0. With RNase degradation, the RNA size distribution is shifted toward the smaller fragments with a reduction in the 28S/18S rRNA ratio (Figure 4-2). Similarly, high quality mRNA preparations isolated by oligo(dT)-cellulose should display broad size ranges.

In assessing the yield and quality of DNA and/or RNA extracts, electrophoretic methods provide better precision and more information regarding quality, for instance, the size distribution of the isolated DNA or RNA. Modern improvements in instrumentation have led to the development of spectrophotometric and electrophoretic systems, which require the input of only microvolumes of extracted DNA and/or RNA for assessment. One spectrophotometer for this purpose uses only 1 μL of sample (ND-1000 Spectrophotometer, Nanodrop Technologies Wilmington, Del.). Automated analyzers that use prefabricated chips with microfluidic channels and are designed for the electrophoresis of microvolumes of DNA and RNA have also become available.[17] One such example is the Agilent 2100 bioanalyzer (Agilent Technologies, Palo Alto, Calif.). These systems allow the sensitive and precise quantification of nucleic acids while requiring minute amounts of sample input, leaving the bulk of the precious DNA and/or RNA sample for molecular analysis.

AUTOMATED NUCLEIC ACID ISOLATION

Many molecular diagnostic protocols that were originally developed by research laboratories have now been adopted by clinical laboratories. With this shift, additional protocol requirements need to be considered. Among these requirements, the clinical laboratory needs to (1) improve analytical throughput, (2) minimize the need for manual handling, (3) ensure consistent and reliable assay performance, and (4) comply with regulatory or accreditation specifications. Automation of the molecular diagnostic procedures is thus often considered. This consideration is particularly relevant to the process of nucleic acid isolation because it involves many manual steps. Many commercial systems address the automation of this process. In general, the automated nucleic acid isolation systems are based on the solid-phase extraction principles discussed above. For example, the MagNA Pure instruments from Roche Diagnostics (Basel, Switzerland)[13] adopt the use of silica-coated magnetic bead separation. The BioRobot Universal system (Qiagen, Hilden, Germany), on the other hand, is based on the use of silica-impregnated filter columns. These systems are used as stand-alone instruments or can be integrated with downstream applications. For example, the MagNA Pure LC instrument (Roche Diagnostics) has been integrated with the LightCycler (Roche Diagnostics) for the performance of real-time PCR.[9] The COBAS AmpliPrep system can be integrated with either the COBAS AMPLICOR or COBAS TaqMan systems (Roche Diagnostics)[11] for conventional or real-time PCR analysis, respectively. Alternatively, the nucleic acid isolation system may become one process of a fully automated molecular diagnostic system with essential elements comparable with any standard automated clinical chemistry analyzer, such as barcode data entry, sample clot detection, level sensing, and internal control detection.

Besides the dedicated instruments described above, open systems are also available and are amenable to the setup of liquid handling steps according to the end-user's specifications for automated nucleic acid isolation. Examples of such systems

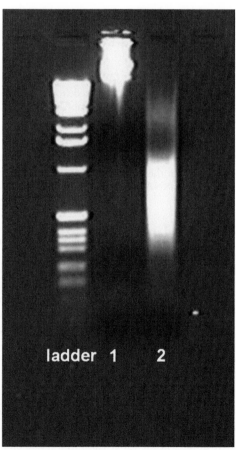

Figure 4-1

Assessment of DNA quality by gel electrophoresis. DNA extracted from whole blood specimens was resolved on 1% agarose gel. Extracted DNA consists of a pool of DNA fragments with varying sizes and appears as smears on gel electrophoresis. High quality DNA extractions are associated with high molecular weight fragments as shown in lane 1. Lane 2 illustrates the pool of DNA extracted from a degraded whole blood sample whereby the molecular weights of the DNA fragments are much reduced.

ladder   1   2

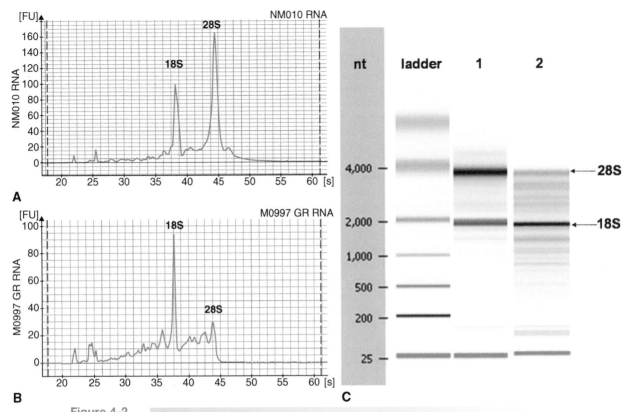

Figure 4-2

Assessment of total RNA quality by gel electrophoresis and densitometry. Total RNA extracted from whole blood specimens was analyzed by the Agilent 2100 bioanalyzer using the RNA 6000 Nano LabChip (Agilent Technologies). The gel electrophoretogram (**C**) is a simulated image based on the densitometry results. Extracted total RNA appears as a smear with two prominent bands corresponding to the 18S and 28S rRNA, respectively. High quality total RNA extractions, as shown in (**A**) and lane 1 in (**C**), are associated with high 28S/18S rRNA ratios with broad size distribution of the other RNA species. With RNase degradation as shown in (**B**) and lane 2 of (**C**), there is a reduction in the 28S/18S rRNA ratio and the overall RNA signal. There is also a shift toward shorter fragments of RNA. nt, nucleotides (see Color Plate 2).

include those from Tecan (Durham, NC)[12] and the Biomek series from Beckman Coulter (Fullerton, Calif.).[10] Although there are many operational advantages to the adoption of automated protocols of nucleic acid isolation, the implementation of an automated protocol should not be conducted without a detailed evaluation of the analytical performance of the protocol. A number of studies have now revealed that certain automated protocols do not perform as well as manual methods for nucleic acid isolation.[2,5,18] Another issue to consider is the possibility of cross-contamination of specimens. Most systems evaluated to date have been shown to be free from the problem of cross-contamination.[2,9] The clinical implications of the analytical performance of the nucleic acid isolation protocols on the molecular diagnostic testing need to be carefully considered before such protocols are adopted.

ISOLATION OF CIRCULATING NUCLEIC ACIDS

Blood is the most common specimen type in a diagnostic laboratory because it is more readily available than a biopsy specimen. Consequently, nucleic acid extraction from blood is commonly performed. Nucleic acids may be extracted from whole blood, buffy coat, plasma, or serum. Blood leukocytes contribute the bulk of the nucleic acids that could be isolated from whole blood and buffy coat. Therefore the isolation of

DNA or RNA from such specimens follows the general principles discussed in the sections above. On the contrary, as described in Chapter 1, circulating nucleic acids are the DNA and RNA molecules that are present in plasma and serum, external to intact cells. Because these nucleic acid molecules demonstrate certain physical properties that are different from the properties of nuclear DNA and RNA molecules found within cells, a number of additional issues need to be considered with regard to their isolation. Consequently, we are devoting this section to the discussion of specific issues related to the isolation of circulating nucleic acids.

Although circulating nucleic acids are present in amounts that are readily detectable by modern molecular techniques, such as real-time quantitative PCR, their concentrations are several orders of magnitude lower than in a tissue biopsy specimen or in a whole blood sample. For example, the typical DNA concentration in the plasma of a healthy volunteer is 100 to 1000 copies per milliliter of plasma.[14] As a result, an important factor affecting the successful adoption of plasma-based molecular diagnostics lies in maximizing the yield of circulating nucleic acids during the isolation procedure. Consequently, to maximize the amount of circulating DNA or RNA that could be extracted with the use of commercial nucleic acid extraction kits, it is preferable to scale up the volume of sample to be used in each extraction. Examples of such modified protocols are detailed in the indicated references.[4,20]

Other issues that are relevant to maximizing the yield or minimizing the loss of circulating nucleic acids during the isolation procedure include considerations involving the (1) size of the DNA or RNA fragments, (2) stability of the molecules, (3) effects of delayed sample processing, (4) specimen choice, and (5) type of anticoagulant. Both DNA and RNA exist in circulation as short fragments. Approximately 80% of DNA molecules in plasma, whether they are derived from a tumor, a fetus, or the background blood cells, are 180 bp or less in length.[1] Similarly, plasma RNA molecules that are associated with a tumor, a fetus, or background blood cells are found to be fragments of the corresponding full-length transcript.[24] Moreover, there is a preponderance of the 5′ ends of the transcripts. As such, the protocols selected for the isolation of circulating DNA and RNA should favor the isolation of low molecular weight fragments. Another related issue is the potential lability of plasma nucleic acids. Plasma DNA has been shown to be stable in unprocessed whole blood up to 24 hours at room temperature.[21] Surprisingly, plasma RNA has also been shown to be stable in unprocessed whole blood collected in tubes with ethylenediaminetetraacetic acid (EDTA) for up to 24 hours when stored at 4 °C.[21] This is in contrast to the rapid degradation seen with purified RNA.[21] The unexpected stability of circulating RNA molecules is possibly a result of its association with particulate matter as has been demonstrated by previous studies.[21] However, in contrast to short-term storage, the concentration of fetal DNA in harvested serum specimens decreased by 0.66 copy per milliliter for each month of storage.[15] More marked degradation upon long-term storage was seen in plasma RNA such that preservation by agents such as Trizol LS (Invitrogen, Carlsbad, Calif.) has been recommended by some investigators.[25]

Another potential pitfall in the isolation of circulating nucleic acids relates to the need to minimize the interference from nucleic acid molecules derived from the background blood cells.[16] For most applications of circulating nucleic acid analysis, the molecules of interest are those released from a tumor, fetus, or transplanted organ. However, these molecules are present in the circulation among a high background of other DNA and RNA species contributed by the blood cells.[16] As a result, the molecules of interest form the minority population. Because a low frac-

tional concentration of the DNA and/or RNA of interest would affect the reliability of their detection, measures are taken to minimize the amount of background nucleic acid concentrations. In this regard, the choice of plasma over serum specimens, the prevention of delays in the separation of whole blood, and the choice of anticoagulants are relevant issues. The concentration of total DNA is markedly higher in serum than in plasma.[16] The excess DNA was most likely released from blood cells during the clotting process. Consequently, plasma may be the preferred specimen type in the analysis of disease-associated DNA molecules that are present in the circulation as a minor fraction. Plasma should be separated from whole blood promptly to minimize the release of DNA from blood cells.[14] EDTA has been found to be the anticoagulant of choice because cellular integrity is better maintained, and hence, the release of DNA from blood cells is less than with citrate or heparin as the anticoagulant.[14] As discussed above, DNA and RNA in EDTA plasma remained stable in the unprocessed whole blood for up to 24 hours at room temperature and 4 °C, respectively.[21] The ability to eliminate background plasma DNA also requires efficient removal of cells from the plasma by the blood processing protocol.[6]

The above is a brief account of a number of issues to consider in the isolation of circulating nucleic acids. For further details, the reader may refer to the indicated review.[3] The authors' laboratory has developed plasma nucleic acid isolation protocols that take into account the factors discussed above, and the interested reader could refer to the indicated references.[4,20] Several of the discussed factors affect the concentration of plasma DNA and/or RNA appreciably and to a variable extent during each analysis, with ultimate implications for the analytical precision of the test. When different laboratories adopt different protocols, the plasma DNA and RNA concentrations cannot be comparable among these laboratories. Hence, standardization of these preanalytical and analytical issues may need to be considered in a similar light as that for any traditional clinical laboratory analysis.

ETHICAL ISSUES SURROUNDING EXTRACTION OF NUCLEIC ACIDS

As in other areas of molecular diagnostics, sensitive ethical issues arise in extraction and storage of nucleic acids. Some issues for discussion are highlighted in Ethics Box 4-1.

ETHICS Box 4-1   Ethical Issues Surrounding Extraction of Nucleic Acids

Our DNA is a unique fingerprint of ourselves. Information related to health or disease and biological relationships can be derived from the study of DNA. Hence, stored DNA is a valuable resource for the study of diseases and relationships in families or for research. Varying scales of DNA "banking" have been practiced. This ranges from the archiving of routine specimens in molecular diagnostic laboratories to research collections involving specific disease or ethnic groups to sizable commercial collections. Because the study of one's DNA may reveal certain attributes about the individual and his or her related community, the conduct of such DNA banking activities has been subjected to much discussion and debate.[22]

Concerns include how such DNA collections should be established[23] and operational guidelines governing the access and use of the banked DNA.[22] The central theme revolves around how best the DNA resource could be used for the good of the public while protecting the interests of an individual or community. Specific issues include in what manner consent should be obtained, mechanisms whereby information could be

fed back to the donor, access rights of blood relatives, duration of storage, and to what extent personal information should be traceable from the specimen.

Widely divergent views have been expressed. For example, blanket consent is favored by some so that the DNA resource could be made available for the conduct of research in a timely and efficient manner.[22] Others have argued that donors should be given a choice with each subsequent intended sample use because it would be impossible to provide "informed" consent when the nature of the future use was not known.[23] Yet others have raised additional issues, for example, how consent could be obtained from a group of individuals, such as ethnic or patient groups, when a study may reveal characteristics about the group in general. This is a sample of many viewpoints expressed on the issue of consent alone. Debates on the pertinent issues of DNA banking are ongoing, and laboratory practice guidelines can be established only when consensus with those issues is reached.

REFERENCES

1. Chan KCA, Zhang J, Hui AB, Wong N, Lau TK, Leung TN, et al. Size distributions of maternal and fetal DNA in maternal plasma. Clin Chem 2004;50:88-92.

2. Chiu RWK, Jin Y, Chung GTY, Lui WB, Chan ATC, Lim W, et al. Automated extraction protocol for quantification of SARS-Coronavirus RNA in serum: an evaluation study. BMC Infect Dis 2006;6:20.

3. Chiu RWK, Lo YMD. The biology and diagnostic applications of fetal DNA and RNA in maternal plasma. Curr Top Dev Biol 2004;61:81-111.

4. Chiu RWK, Lo YMD. Noninvasive prenatal diagnosis by analysis of fetal DNA in maternal plasma. In: Lo YMD, Chiu RWK, Chan KCA, eds. Clinical applications of PCR, 2nd ed. Totowa, NJ: Humana Press, 2006.

5. Chiu RWK, Lui WB, El-Sheikhah A, Chan ATC, Lau TK, Nicolaides KH, et al. Comparison of protocols for extracting circulation DNA and RNA from maternal plasma. Clin Chem 2005;51:2209-10.

6. Chiu RWK, Poon LLM, Lau TK, Leung TN, Wong EMC, Lo YMD. Effects of blood-processing protocols on fetal and total DNA quantification in maternal plasma. Clin Chem 2001;47:1607-13.

7. Chomczynski P, Sacchi N. Single-step method of RNA isolation by acid guanidinium thiocyanate-phenol-chloroform extraction. Anal Biochem 1987;162:156-9.

8. Connolly MA, Clausen PA, Lazar JG. RNA purification. In: Dieffenbach CW, Dveksler GS, eds. PCR primer. A laboratory manual, 2nd ed. New York: Cold Spring Harbor Laboratory Press, 2003:117-133.

9. Costa JM, Ernault P. Automated assay for fetal DNA analysis in maternal serum. Clin Chem 2002;48:679-80.

10. Greenspoon SA, Ban JD, Sykes K, Ballard EJ, Edler SS, Baisden M, et al. Application of the BioMek 2000 Laboratory Automation Workstation and the DNA IQ System to the extraction of forensic casework samples. J Forensic Sci 2004;49:29-39.

11. Hochberger S, Althof D, de Schrott RG, Nachbaur N, Rock H, Leying H. Fully automated quantitation of hepatitis B virus (HBV) DNA in human plasma by the COBAS ((R)) AmpliPrep/COBAS((R)) TaqMan ((R)) System. J Clin Virol 35:373-80, 2006.

12. Hourfar MK, Michelsen U, Schmidt M, Berger A, Seifried E, Roth WK. High-throughput purification of viral RNA based on novel aqueous chemistry for nucleic acid isolation. Clin Chem 2005;51:1217-22.

13. Kessler HH, Muhlbauer G, Stelzl E, Daghofer E, Santner BI, Marth E. Fully automated nucleic acid extraction. MagNA Pure LC. Clin Chem 2001;47:1124-6.

14. Lam NYL, Rainer TH, Chiu RWK, Lo YMD. EDTA is a better anticoagulant than heparin or citrate for delayed blood processing for plasma DNA analysis. Clin Chem 2004;50:256-7.

15. Lee T, LeShane ES, Messerlian GM, Canick JA, Farina A, Heber WW, et al. Down syndrome and cell-free fetal DNA in archived maternal serum. Am J Obstet Gynecol 2002;187:1217-22.

16. Lui YYN, Chik KW, Chiu RWK, Ho CY, Lam CW, Lo YMD. Predominant hematopoietic origin of cell-free DNA in plasma and serum after sex-mismatched bone marrow transplantation. Clin Chem 2002;48:421-7.

17. Panaro NJ, Yuen PK, Sakazu me T, Fortina P, Kricka LJ, Wilding P. Evaluation of DNA fragment sizing and quantification by the Agilent 2100 bioanalyzer. Clin Chem 2000;46:1851-3.

18. Schuurman T, van Breda A, de Boer R, Kooistra-Smid M, Beld M, Savelkoul P, et al. Reduced PCR sensitivity due to impaired DNA recovery with the MagNA Pure LC total nucleic acid isolation kit. J Clin Microbiol 2005;43:4616-22.

19. Smith C, Otto P, Bitner R, Shiels G. DNA purification. In: Dieffenbach CW, Dveksler GS, eds. PCR primer. A laboratory manual. 2nd ed. New York: Cold Spring Harbor Laboratory Press, 2003:87-115.

20. Tsui NBY, Ng EKO, Lo YMD. Molecular analysis of circulating RNA in plasma. In Lo YMD, Chiu RWK, Chan KCA, eds. Clinical applications of PCR, 2nd ed. Totowa, NJ: Humana Press, 2006.

21. Tsui NBY, Ng EKO, Lo YMD. Stability of endogenous and added RNA in blood specimens, serum, and plasma. Clin Chem 2002;48:1647-53.

22. World Health Organization. Review of ethical issues in medical genetics. Document WHO/HGN/ETH/00.4 2003.

23. Winickoff DE, Winickoff RN. The charitable trust as a model for genomic biobanks. N Engl J Med 2003;349:1180-4.

24. Wong BCK, Chiu RWK, Tsui NBY, Chan KCA, Chan LW, Lau TK, et al. Circulating placental RNA in maternal plasma is associated with a preponderance of 5′ mRNA fragments: implications for noninvasive prenatal diagnosis and monitoring. Clin Chem 2005;51:1786-95.

25. Wong SC, Lo ES, Cheung MT. An optimized protocol for the extraction of non-viral mRNA from human plasma frozen for three years. J Clin Pathol 2004;57:766-8.

REVIEW QUESTIONS

1. DNA isolation
   A. can be achieved by solid-phase extraction based on adsorption onto alumina.
   B. is a process that can be automated.
   C. must be followed immediately by DNA analysis, such as PCR, as purified DNA is not stable during storage.
   D. commonly involves the step of DNase digestion.
   E. is a challenging procedure because DNase is ubiquitous and can degrade DNA.

2. RNA isolation
   A. is a process that is comparatively easier than DNA isolation because RNA is more stable than DNA.
   B. procedures can only effectively extract rRNA and not mRNA from clinical specimens.
   C. can be achieved by liquid-phase extraction, which is readily adaptable to automated platforms.
   D. is best performed with fresh or adequately preserved clinical specimens because RNA is inherently unstable.
   E. may suffer from DNA contamination, but this is generally not an analytical concern.

3. Regarding the assessment of extracted nucleic acids,
   A. RNA yield can be assessed by determining the 28S/18S rRNA ratio.
   B. DNA yield is reflected by its absorbance at 280 nm.
   C. high quality DNA and/or RNA preparations are associated with high molecular weight fragments.
   D. densitometric methods allow the assessment of only nucleic acid yield.
   E. spectrophotometric methods are based on UV light absorbance by the phosphate backbone of nucleic acid molecules.

4. Regarding the isolation of circulating nucleic acids,
   A. plasma anticoagulated by heparin is preferred.
   B. protocols that favor the isolation of high molecular weight nucleic acid molecules are preferred to minimize the amount of fragmented DNA and RNA isolated.
   C. specimens are best stored as whole blood to preserve the integrity of the circulating nucleic acid molecules.
   D. this is technically challenging as a result of the relatively low DNA and RNA concentrations.
   E. serum is preferred over plasma in the study of tumor-derived nucleic acids.

5. DNA banking
   A. refers only to commercially operated collections of DNA samples.

B. is unlikely to be a concern for molecular diagnostic laboratories.

C. is governed by clearly defined guidelines.

D. involves asking individuals to waive all their rights to the donated sample.

E. involves many issues of ethical concern, such as consent, access rights, and duration of storage.

6. In contrast to liquid-phase DNA extraction methods, protocols based on solid phase are generally:

A. less amenable to automation.

B. more labor intensive.

C. more time consuming.

D. more imprecise.

E. less adaptable to extraction of large DNA quantities or large sample volumes.

7. Automated techniques for nucleic acid isolation

A. are available for DNA isolation only.

B. are usually based on the liquid-phase extraction protocols.

C. can hardly be integrated with downstream processes for nucleic acid analysis.

D. may lead to sample cross-contamination, which should be evaluated and considered.

E. always have better analytical performance than do manual methods.

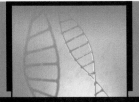

Chapter 5

Nucleic Acid Techniques

Carl T. Wittwer, M.D., Ph.D.
Noriko Kusukawa, Ph.D.

OUTLINE

Amplification Techniques
   Polymerase Chain Reaction—Target Amplification
   Other Forms of Target Amplification
   Other Approaches to Amplification
   Target Quantification After Amplification
Detection Techniques
   Generic Measurement and Visualization of Nucleic Acids
   Reporter Molecules and Labeled Probes
Discrimination Techniques
   Electrophoresis
   Alternatives to Electrophoresis
   Hybridization Assays—Principles
   Hybridization Assays—Examples
   Real-Time PCR
   Melting Analysis
   Comparison of Closed-Tube SNP Genotyping Methods
Ethical Issues
Conclusion

OBJECTIVES

1. Describe the measurement of isolated nucleic acids using ultraviolet absorbance.
2. Describe the action of restriction endonucleases on double-stranded DNA (dsDNA); give examples of several of these enzymes and their specific actions.
3. Devise a PCR method to detect a specific DNA sequence; include appropriate primers, thermocycling protocol, how contamination will be prevented, and appropriate controls.
4. Compare target amplification techniques with signal amplification techniques.
5. Contrast different target amplification methods.
6. Compare and contrast Northern and Southern blots.
7. Design a basic hybridization assay using a probe to assess a given clinical mutation; include the mutation to be assessed, the tissue used, the type of probe used, the detection method, and the necessary controls.
8. Relate the importance of stringency to a hybridization assay.

9. State the principle of basic nucleic acid electrophoresis; give examples of different electrophoretic techniques and their specific use in a molecular diagnostics laboratory.
10. State the principle of real-time PCR.
11. Discuss the need for and use of appropriate controls in the analytical phase of nucleic acid testing.

KEY WORDS AND DEFINITIONS

Amplification Methods: Techniques to amplify the amount of target, signal, or probe so that specific sequences can be readily observed.
Amplicon: The product of an amplification reaction, such as PCR.
Array: One or more measurement parameters used to distinguish different sequences. In spatial arrays, the parameters are physical distances, as in linear, two-dimensional, or three-dimensional arrays.
Detection Methods: Techniques to detect nucleic acid sequences, usually after purification and amplification.
dNTPs: Deoxyribonucleotide triphosphates (usually dATP, dCTP, dGTP, and dTTP), the building blocks of DNA.
Electrophoresis: Movement caused by an electrical field, often through a gel matrix. Polyacrylamide and agarose are common matrices used to separate DNA and RNA under an electric field.
Fluorescence: A physical property of some molecules toy emit light at a longer wavelength when excited at a shorter wavelength.
Heteroduplex: A DNA duplex with internal mismatches or loops.
Homoduplex: A perfectly matched DNA duplex.
Hybridization: The annealing or pairing of two DNA strands.
Insertion: An extra DNA sequence that is present in one sample compared with a reference sequence.
Intron: DNA sequence within a gene that is spliced out during mRNA processing.
Label: A modification that renders a molecule observable.
Northern Blot: A method for detecting specific RNA sequences with labeled probes after they have been separated by size using electrophoresis.

Oligonucleotide: A short single-stranded polymer of nucleic acid.

Polymerase: An enzyme that sequentially adds nucleotides onto a growing polynucleotide, usually requiring a primer and a template.

Polymerase Chain Reaction (PCR): An in vitro method for exponentially amplifying DNA.

Primer: An oligonucleotide that serves to initiate polymerase-catalyzed addition of nucleotides by annealing to a template strand.

Probe: A nucleic acid used to identify a target by hybridization.

Pseudogene: A genetic element that does not result in a functional gene product, usually because of accumulated mutations.

Real-Time PCR: Observation of PCR during amplification at least once each cycle.

Restriction Fragment Length Polymorphism (RFLP): A genetic polymorphism that results in changes in sizes of DNA fragments after restriction enzyme digestion and electrophoresis.

Sequencing: Any method that determines the exact order of bases in a DNA fragment.

Signal Amplification: Any method that increases the signal resulting from a molecular interaction that does not involve target amplification or probe amplification.

Southern Blot: A method for detecting DNA sequence variants after restriction enzyme digestion and size separation by electrophoresis. Hybridization with a labeled probe reveals sequence variants that result in a change in distance between restriction sites, including large insertions, deletions, and rearrangements.

Target Amplification: Any method for increasing the amount of target nucleic acid.

Molecular diagnostics requires techniques to detect extremely low concentrations of nucleic acids and to determine sequence variations that are minute changes in complex genomes, such as the human.[3,13] This chapter begins with a discussion of amplification techniques that are often necessary to observe or quantify nucleic acid sequences of interest. Then the tools used to detect or visualize nucleic acids are discussed. Finally, specific methodologies are described that allow identification, quantification, and/or segregation of individual nucleic acid species.

Developers of molecular diagnostic techniques are extremely competitive. Converts to one technique, instrument, or probe design often adopt a religious fervor and commitment. In this chapter, cute trade names and commercial references are omitted. Original research references for many of the techniques described here are available elsewhere.[14]

AMPLIFICATION TECHNIQUES

Achieving adequate detection limits is a central concern for clinical applications of nucleic acid analysis. Techniques that increase the (1) amount of the nucleic acid target, (2) detection signal, or (3) probe are referred to as **amplification methods.** Examples of amplification methods are listed in Table 5-1. In **target amplification,** the nucleic acid region around the area of interest is copied many times by in vitro methods. Areas outside the target are not amplified. In **signal amplification,** the amount of target stays the same, but the signal is increased by one of several methods, including sequential hybridization of branching nucleic acid structures and continuous enzyme action on substrate that may be recycled. Finally, in **probe amplification,** the probe (or a product of the probe) is amplified only in the presence of the target. Amplification techniques

TABLE 5-1	Amplification Techniques		
Techniques	**Amplification Type**	**Enzymes Needed**	**Thermal Cycling**
Polymerase chain reaction (PCR)[8]	Target	DNA polymerase (thermostable)	Yes
Ligase chain reaction (LCR)	Target	DNA ligase (thermostable)	Yes
Transcription-based amplification system (TAS)	Target	Reverse transcriptase RNA polymerase	Yes
Transcription-mediated amplification (TMA); self-sustained sequence replication (3SR); nucleic acid sequence-based amplification (NASBA)	Target	Reverse transcriptase RNA polymerase RNase H	No
Strand displacement amplification (SDA)	Target	*Hinc*II DNA polymerase I (exonuclease deficient)	No
Loop-mediated amplification (LAMP)	Target	DNA polymerase	No
Whole genome amplification (WGA) or multiple displacement amplification (MDA)	Target	φ29 DNA polymerase	No
Antisense RNA amplification (aRNA)	Target	T4 DNA polymerase Klenow S1 nuclease T7 polymerase	No
Branched DNA (bDNA)	Signal	Alkaline phosphatase	No
Serial invasive signal amplification	Signal	Cleavase	No
Rolling circle amplification (RCA)	Probe	T4 gene 32 protein	No

often achieve more than a million-fold amplification in less than an hour.

Polymerase Chain Reaction—Target Amplification

When the amount of target nucleic acid is increased by synthetic in vitro methods, target amplification is said to occur. The **polymerase chain reaction (PCR)**[8] is the best known and most widely applied of the target amplification methods. Because of the commercial availability of thermostable DNA **polymerases,** kits, and instrumentation, this method has been widely adopted in research and is also routinely used in the clinical laboratory.

Details of the PCR Process

PCR requires (1) a thermostable DNA polymerase, (2) deoxynucleotides of each base (collectively referred to as **dNTPs**), (3) the target sequence, and (4) a pair of **oligonucleotides** (referred to as **primers**) complementary to opposite strands flanking the sequence to be detected. In the first step, target duplexes are denatured into single strands by heat (Figure 5-1). When the mixture is cooled, primers provided in great excess (usually more than a million times the concentration of the initial target) specifically anneal to complementary sequences on the target. Once the primers are annealed, the action of the polymerase synthesizes two additional DNA strands containing the primers as the 5′ ends. The primers are placed close enough together so that the polymerase extends each strand far enough to include the priming site of the other primer. Usually the optimum temperature for polymerization is at an intermediate temperature between the denaturation and annealing temperatures. The second cycle also begins with denaturation, but now there are twice as many strands (the original genomic DNA and the extension products from the first cycle) available for primer annealing and subsequent extension. The temperature cycling is continued among (typically) three temperatures: (1) a high temperature sufficient to denature the target sequence, (2) a low temperature that allows annealing of the primers to the target, and (3) a third temperature that is optimum for polymerase extension. The instrument that takes samples through the multiple steps of changing temperature is known as a thermocycler.

Repetitive thermocycling results in the exponential accumulation of the short product (consisting of primers and all intervening sequences). If the efficiency of each cycle is optimal, the number of target sequences doubles each cycle (efficiency = 2.0). PCR efficiency depends on the primers and the temperature-cycling conditions, along with the presence or absence of polymerase inhibitors. Amplified products accumulate exponentially in the beginning cycles of PCR. At some point, however, the efficiency of amplification falls, and eventually the amount of product plateaus (Figure 5-2) either from exhaustion of components or from competition between primer and product annealing (i.e., the single strands of product are at such high concentrations that they anneal to each other rather than to the primers). The **S**-curve shape is similar to the logistic model for population growth. In a typical PCR reaction using 0.5 μmol/L of each primer, the maximum DNA concentration achievable is about 10^{11} copies/μL.

With the addition of an initial reverse-transcriptase (RT) step to form cDNA from the RNA that is present in the

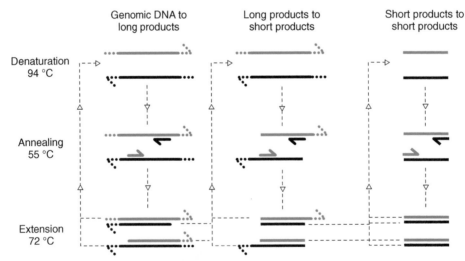

Figure 5-1

Schematic diagram of the PCR. Repetitive cycles of denaturation, annealing, and extension are paced by temperature cycling of the reaction. Two primers (indicated as short segments with half arrow heads) anneal to opposite template strands (long heavy lines) to define the region to be amplified. Extension occurs from the 3′ ends (indicated with half arrow heads). In each cycle, genomic DNA is denatured and annealed to primers that extend in opposite directions across the same region, producing long products of undefined length. Long products generated by extension of one of the primers anneal to the other primer during the next cycle, producing short products of defined length. Any short products present also produce more short products. After n cycles, up to 2^n new copies of the amplified region are present (n long products + $[2^n − n]$ short products + 1 original genomic copy). A similar approach can be used to amplify RNA targets by initial reverse transcription of the RNA template to produce the DNA template.

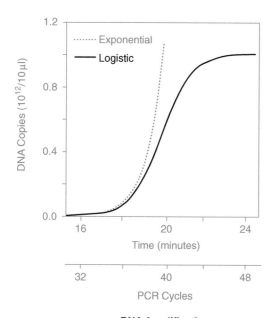

DNA Amplification

Figure 5-2

Exponential and logistic curves for DNA amplified by PCR. A doubling time of 30 seconds is assumed for PCR. That is, given the equation $N_t = N_0 e^{rt}$, in which N_t is the amount of DNA at time t and N_0 is the initial amount of the DNA, r is 1.386 min^{-1} for PCR. A carrying capacity of 10^{11} copies of PCR product per microliter was used, assuming that the reaction is primer limited at one third the primer concentration (initially at 0.5 μM, or 10^{11} primer molecule pairs per microliter). Starting with only one target copy, it takes only 23 minutes (46 cycles) to amplify the target to saturation.

(Modified with permission of the publisher from Wittwer CT, Kusukawa N. Real-time PCR. In Persing DH, Tenover FC, Versalovic J, Tang YW, Unger ER, Relman DA, White TJ [eds.], Molecular microbiology: Diagnostic principles and practice, Washington, DC: ASM Press, 2004:71-84. © 2004 ASM Press.)

sample, RNA targets are amplified into DNA copies. The reverse transcription and DNA amplification steps are usually catalyzed by two different polymerases, but some thermostable enzymes (such as the *Tth* polymerase) have both DNA polymerase and reverse transcription activities so that both steps are performed in the same tube with the same enzyme.

After amplification, the products are detected by various methods. Simple gel **electrophoresis** with ethidium bromide staining may suffice. When greater accuracy is required, one of the primers can be fluorescently **labeled** so that after PCR the fragments can be sized on a *DNA sequencing* device. Alternatively, some form of hybridization assay is used to verify or analyze the amplified product. Automated methods are always attractive, and closed-tube methods are particularly advantageous in the clinical laboratory. Adding a fluorescent dye or probe before amplification allows thermocyclers equipped with optical detection to analyze the reaction as it progresses (**real-time PCR**) or after the reaction is complete (end point measurement) without need to process the sample for a separate analysis step.

PCR Kinetics and Rapid Cycling

It is natural to think about PCR in terms of three events—(1) denaturation of double-stranded target, (2) annealing of target

and primers, and (3) extension of the DNA strand from the primer—occurring at three temperatures, each requiring a certain amount of time. Indeed, it is common to perform PCR by holding the reaction mixture at three different temperatures (for instance, denaturation at 94 °C, annealing at 55 °C, and extension at 72 °C). Standard thermocycling instruments that use conical tubes focus on accurate temperature control of the heating block at equilibrium, not on the dynamic control of the sample temperature. As a result, sample temperatures are not well defined during transitions, and long cycle times have become standard to ensure that the sample reaches target temperatures. Reproducibility between instruments and manufacturers is poor, and PCR may require 2 to 4 hours to complete a typical 30-cycle amplification.

The kinetics of PCR suggest that *controlled transitions* between temperatures with minimal or no pauses (temperature plateaus) provide a better paradigm of PCR amplification (Figure 5-3). Denaturation, annealing, and extension are very rapid reactions as shown by experiments in capillaries. The use of temperature "spikes" at denaturation and annealing, instead of extended temperature plateaus, allows for rapid cycling with the appropriate instrumentation. The actual time required for PCR depends on the size of the product, but when it is less than 500 base pairs (bp), a 30-cycle amplification is easily completed in 15 to 30 minutes. Furthermore, rapid amplification improves specificity. Figure 5-4 shows PCR amplification of a 536-bp fragment of β-globin amplified at different cycling speeds. With conventional slow cycling, many nonspecific products are generated (cycling profile A). These products disappear as the cycling time is decreased (profiles B, C, and D). In fact, amplification yield and product specificity are optimal when denaturation and annealing times are minimal.

Initial denaturation of genomic DNA may be required before PCR cycling, depending on how the DNA sample was prepared. Either boiling the sample or an initial denaturation step of 5 to 10 seconds before PCR cycling may be necessary. During PCR, however, denaturation is very rapid. Even for long PCR products, denaturation is complete in less than 1 second after the denaturation temperature is reached. Anything greater than a denaturation time of "0" only serves to degrade the polymerase. If longer denaturation times are required, either the sample is not reaching temperature or heat-activated polymerases are being used.

Product specificity is optimal when annealing times are less than 1 second. Longer annealing times may be required, however, when the primer concentrations are low. The required extension time for each cycle depends on the length of the PCR product. Extension is not instantaneous, although it is much faster than common practice would suggest. Extension rates of *Taq* polymerase under optimal conditions are 50 to 100 bases per second. Despite its common use, a 5- to 10-minute final extension is not rational. Products can be as small as 40 bp to about 40 kb. To amplify products longer than 5 kb, mixtures of polymerases that include some 3'-exonuclease activity to edit mismatched nucleotides are usually used.

Instead of separate annealing and extension temperatures, both processes can be carried out at the same temperature, resulting in two-temperature, instead of three-temperature, cycling. Although this simplifies the demand on instrumentation and programming, it limits the choice of primers and requires a longer extension time at suboptimum temperatures.

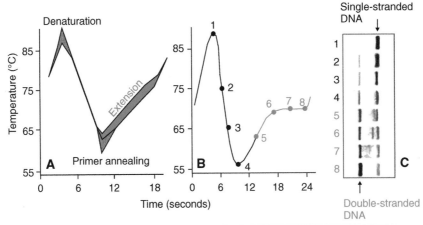

Figure 5-3

A visual demonstration of PCR kinetics. The three phases of PCR (denaturation, annealing, and extension) occur as the temperature is continuously changing (panel A). Toward the end of PCR temperature cycling, the reaction contains single- and double-stranded PCR products. When different points of the cycle are sampled (by snap cooling the mixture in ice water, panel B) and analyzed, the transition from denatured ssDNA to dsDNA is revealed as a continuum (panel C). Progression of the extension reaction can be followed by additional bands appearing between the ssDNA and dsDNA (time points 5 to 7). (Modified with permission from Wittwer CT, Herrmann MG: Rapid thermal cycling and PCR kinetics. In Innis M, Gelfand D, Sninsky J [eds.], PCR applications, San Diego: Academic Press, 1999:211-229. © 1999 Academic Press.)

PCR Optimization and Primer Design

In addition to the temperature-cycling conditions, the specificity of PCR depends on the choice of primers and the Mg^{++} concentration. The choice of primers often dictates the quality and success of the amplification reaction. To select primers, the sequence of the target must be known. Some guidelines for primer selection are intuitive and helpful:

1. Avoid primers that anneal to themselves or to other primers. Particularly avoid complementation at the 3′ end of primers, and especially do not use a primer that has reciprocal 3′ end complementation.
2. Choose primers that are specific to your target. Avoid simple sequence repeats and common repeated sequences, such as *Alu* repeats. If your target has close relatives, design your primers so that they will anneal only to your intended target. Targets that you want to avoid include **pseudogenes** (for genomic DNA) and related bacterial or viral strains (for microorganisms).
3. Avoid primers that have sequences complementary to internal sequences of the intended product, especially at the 3′ ends of the primers.
4. Use primers between 18 and 25 bases that are matched in melting temperature (Tm) to each other. A primer greater than 17 bases long has a good chance of being unique in the human genome.
5. Unless you have a reason to amplify longer targets, choose a product length less than 500 bases. Shorter products amplify with higher efficiency.
6. As a final test, do a search for sequences similar to your primers that are present in the background DNA likely to be present in your assay (http://www.ncbi.nlm.nih.gov/BLAST/). Many primer selection programs are available, both commercially and freely obtained over the Internet. However, very few if any of the selection rules often used have been empirically tested.

With the human genome sequenced, it should be possible to vastly improve primer selection. Given two primers, an entire genome search for mispriming sites could rule out primer pairs with the potential to produce undesired PCR products. For exponential PCR, priming sites must be oriented appropriately within a close distance. Amplification of the desired target is favored by choosing a small product size and rapid cycling.

Detection Limits of PCR

When PCR is performed under optimal conditions, a single copy of the target can be detected. In practice, however, the statistical probability of distributing at least a single copy from a dilute template solution into the PCR must be considered. The Poisson distribution indicates that if, on average, one target copy will be present per tube, 37% of the tubes will have no target, 37% will have one target, and the remainder will have more than one. If there is an average of two copies per tube, approximately 14% of the tubes will have no template and will provide a false-negative result. About five copies on average are necessary for 99% of the tubes to include at least one copy. This limitation of low copy analysis holds true for any amplification technique.

Use of dilute solutions of template in the PCR is sometimes advantageous. For example, *digital PCR* is a technique that depends on an on-off signal resulting from either the presence or absence of template in each of many reaction compartments. Instead of conventional tubes, these compartments may be minute aqueous droplets in a water-in-oil emulsion, or *polonies* (PCR colonies) on a thin film of acrylamide gel.[5]

3′ End of PCR Products

Taq DNA polymerase and other polymerases have a terminal transferase activity that may add a single unpaired nucleotide

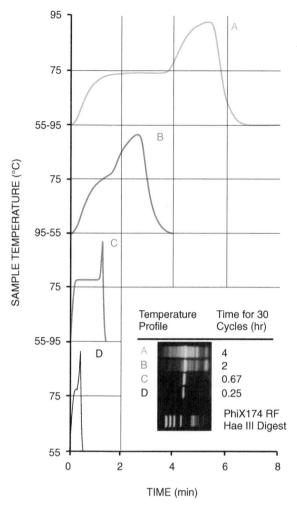

Figure 5-4
Rapid PCR improves product specificity. Samples were cycled 30 times through profiles A, B, C, and D. Increased specificity of amplification of a 534 bp β-globin fragment is seen with faster cycles (C and D). (Reprinted by permission of the publisher from Wittwer CT, Garling DJ: Rapid cycle DNA amplification: time and temperature optimization. BioTechniques 1991, 10:76-83. © 1991 Eaton Publishing.)

on the 3' end of PCR product strands. In the presence of all four dNTPs, dATP is preferentially added. This means that some percentage of the double-stranded products generated by PCR will not have blunt ends but a protruding A at one or both ends. Although this does not influence most detection protocols, it may complicate some systems that are able to distinguish products of similar size (that is, systems with high size resolution). Alternatively, this feature is useful for high-efficiency cloning and ligation of PCR products.

Contamination Control for PCR (False-Positive Results)

Because PCR can detect a single molecule of target sequence, a small amount of contamination in a sample easily produces a false-positive result. The greatest potential for contamination comes from the product of the amplification reaction, referred to as the **amplicon** (used interchangeably with *PCR product*). After amplification, each reaction mixture may contain as

many as 10^{12} copies of the amplicon. Thus minute aerosol droplets contain more than enough target for robust amplification. Amplicons can contaminate reagents, pipettes, and glassware. It is easy to turn a laboratory into a Dr. Seuss fiasco.[12] Experience has dictated the use of laboratory procedures that minimize contamination by amplicons. These include the use of (1) physically separated areas for preamplification and post-amplification steps, (2) positive-displacement pipettes to minimize aerosol contamination, and (3) prealiquoted reagents. The most effective way of all is to not let the product out of the tube. Methods that perform amplification, detection, and characterization in a closed tube eliminate the risk of product contamination. Even with these precautions, a negative control or blank (all reactants minus target DNA) is one of the most important controls for PCR.

In combination with the precautions listed above, it is possible to chemically modify the amplicon so it becomes an unsuitable template for further amplification. One of the commonly practiced chemical modifications is to substitute deoxyuridine 5' triphosphate (dUTP) for deoxythymidine 5' triphosphate (dTTP) in amplification reactions, which results in incorporation of U in place of T in the amplified product. A bacterial enzyme, uracil-N-glycosylase (UNG), degrades DNA that contains U. Because U is not normally found in DNA, only amplicons will be susceptible to degradation by UNG treatment. During a brief incubation step before amplification, uracil-containing DNA strands that are carried over from previous amplifications are enzymatically degraded and cannot serve as substrates for further amplification. UNG is then inactivated during the first denaturation cycle so newly formed amplicons can accumulate normally during the reaction. However, UNG may regain activity, even after multiple cycles of amplification, if the temperature of the reaction mixture drops below 55 °C. Residual UNG activity may also affect the detection limit if amplified products are held at room temperature before detection.

Inhibition Control for PCR (False-Negative Results)

PCR is a resilient process and does not require highly purified nucleic acid. In practice, however, clinical samples may contain unpredictable amounts of impurities that inhibit polymerase activity. To ensure reliable amplification in clinical analyses, some form of nucleic acid purification is often used. The idiosyncratic nature of PCR inhibitors within clinical specimens requires demonstration that the sample (or preparation of nucleic acid purified from it) will allow amplification. A control nucleic acid sequence, usually different from the target, can be added to the sample (or to nucleic acid extracted from the sample). Failure to amplify this control indicates that further purification of the sample is required to remove inhibitors of the reaction.

Hot Start Techniques

In practice, PCR sensitivity and specificity are compromised by the formation of unintended low molecular weight artifacts. This process is initiated before PCR when the primers, template, and polymerase are all together at temperatures below the annealing temperature of PCR. Even at low temperatures, if a primer momentarily anneals to another primer or to an undesired target region, *Taq* DNA polymerase may extend the complex. If the extension product, in turn, is primed and extended, then unintended, double-stranded products can be formed (e.g., primer dimers) that serve as amplification templates throughout the reaction. Primer-dimers can be distinguished from the intended target by their molecular weight or Tm, but they also influence the efficiency of the intended amplification and decrease the sensitivity of the assay.

The formation of primer-dimers can be minimized in several ways. All limit the activity of polymerase until the temperature is increased (thus the strategy is often collectively called *hot start*). One method of hot start involves the use of antibody (or an aptamer) to bind and inactivate the polymerase at room temperature. The binding agent is released upon heating, allowing polymerase activation. Another method uses wax or paraffin to create a physical barrier between the essential components in the reaction. This barrier may be created by putting some of the reaction components into the bottom of the tube and overlaying them with molten wax. Cooling solidifies the wax, and the missing components (usually the polymerase, or magnesium, which is essential for polymerase activity) can be placed on top. The wax melts when the temperature reaches 60°C to ~80°C, and all components are mixed together by convection while the molten wax floats on top and prevents evaporation of the sample. Various commercial wax beads encasing one or more critical components are available. Finally the polymerase itself can be modified so that it is activated by heat, usually requiring an extended initial denaturation period.

Asymmetric PCR and Allele-Specific PCR

Conventional PCR uses primers that are present in equal amounts, thereby ensuring that the majority of the products are double-stranded amplicons. *Asymmetric PCR* uses different concentrations of the two primers to generate more of one strand than of the other. For instance, the use of primer A at 0.5 µmol/L and primer B at 0.005 µmol/L produces mostly single-stranded DNA (ssDNA) extended off the more abundant primer. This is useful for sequencing purposes or making single-stranded probes. Yield of the product, however, may be low. With less extreme ratios (e.g., primer A at 0.5 µmol/L and primer B at 0.2 µmol/L), the yield is mostly preserved, with one strand produced in enough excess to make it more available for probe hybridization.

Another variant method called *allele-specific PCR* enables preferential amplification of one genetic allele over another. The 3′ end of one primer is placed at the polymorphic site and is extended readily only if it is completely complementary to the target. This strategy is used for distinguishing a gene from its pseudogenes and for genotyping of SNPs. Allele-specific PCR is also a common method for determining haplotypes.

Other Forms of Target Amplification

A large number of other methods for target amplification have been developed and are described briefly below. Citations to the original research literature are available elsewhere.[14]

Ligase Chain Reaction

The ligase chain reaction (LCR) uses four oligonucleotides and a DNA ligase. Two of the oligonucleotides anneal directly adjacent to each other on the target. When they are joined (ligated), they form a target for the remaining two oligonucleotides (and vice versa). As in PCR, temperature cycling is used, and the target is ideally doubled each cycle. The ligase chain reaction requires that the exact sequence of the region to be amplified is known.

Transcription-Based Amplification Methods

Transcription-based amplification methods are modeled after the replication of retroviruses. These methods are known by various names including (1) nucleic acid sequence-based amplification (NASBA), (2) transcription-mediated amplification (TMA), and (3) self-sustained sequence replication (3SR) assays. They amplify their target without temperature cycling (isothermally) and use the collective activities of reverse transcriptase (RT), RNase H, and RNA polymerase. As illustrated in Figure 5-5, the method may be applied to single-stranded RNA or dsDNA targets. An RT is used to synthesize a cDNA strand from the template RNA with a primer that has an RNA polymerase promoter sequence as a 5′ tail. The RNA strand of the RNA-DNA duplex is then digested with RNAse H, followed by synthesis of dsDNA with an opposing primer. The promoter sequence on the dsDNA then promotes transcription of multiple copies of single-stranded RNA by the RNA polymerase, completing the cycle. As in PCR, all reagents can be included in one mixture, and amplification is exponential, with completion in less than an hour. Unlike PCR these methods do not require temperature cycling (except for an initial heat denaturation if a DNA template is used). The method is particularly advantageous when the target is RNA (e.g., HIV and HCV in blood bank nucleic acid testing).

Strand Displacement Amplification

Another isothermal amplification technique is strand displacement amplification (SDA). After heat denaturation of DNA in the presence of four primers, dCTP, dGTP, dUTP, and a modified deoxynucleotide (dATPαS), two enzymes are added, an exonuclease-deficient polymerase and a restriction enzyme. The two flanking primers that enter into exponential amplification have a restriction site added to their 5′ end and get nicked by the restriction enzyme, allowing displacement of strands that are in turn primed, extended, and nicked. Deoxy-ATPαS is used so that the restriction sites include a hemiphosphorothioate linkage to allow single-strand nicking, instead of cutting through the double strands.

Loop-Mediated Amplification

The target amplification methods presented so far produce a defined length of RNA or DNA according to the placement of the primers. In loop-mediated isothermal amplification (LAMP), multiple populations of repeated DNA structures in the shape of a stem and loop (stem-loops) are produced, and concatenated structures of variable length and branching are generated. After DNA denaturation, the process is isothermal, requiring four primers and a polymerase. Two of the primers each recognize two distinct sequences on the target DNA, resulting in loops forming at the end of extension products. Repeated strand displacement DNA synthesis results in the final mixture of products.

Whole Genome and Whole Transcriptome Amplification

Instead of specific amplification of one target to improve sensitivity, methods that amplify all genomic DNA or mRNAs are

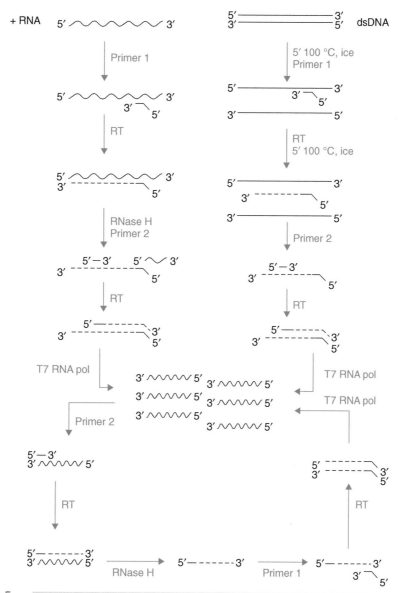

Figure 5-5

Schematic diagram of the NASBA method applied to single-stranded RNA and dsDNA. The method is based on the extension of primer 1 (containing a T7 promoter) by RT, degradation of the RNA strand by RNase H (or heat denaturation for dsDNA), synthesis of the second strand of DNA by RT, and RNA synthesis by T7 RNA polymerase (pol). With RNA synthesis, the system enters the cyclic phase. *Solid lines, DNA; dashed lines, newly synthesized DNA; wavy lines, RNA.*
(Reprinted by permission of the publisher from vanGemen B, Kievits T, Nara P, et al.: Qualitative and quantitative detection of HIV-1 RNA by nucleic acid sequence-based amplification. AIDS 7(Suppl 2): S107-S110, 1993. © 1993 Rapid Science Publishers.)

useful when the target is in short supply. For example, *multiple-displacement amplification* uses exonuclease-resistant random hexamers and a highly processive polymerase to amplify DNA nonspecifically. Initial DNA denaturation is not necessary, and the reaction proceeds isothermally. Similarly, it is possible to generically amplify mRNA by use of a poly(T) primer modified with an RNA polymerase promoter. After reverse transcription, second-strand DNA synthesis, and transcription, antisense RNA is produced. Both whole genome and antisense RNA amplification are also useful as nucleic acid purification methods before amplification or detection.

Other Approaches to Amplification

It is not always necessary to amplify the target DNA sequence or a cDNA sequence complementary to an RNA target. Instead of target amplification, both signal amplification and probe amplification are then used.

Signal Amplification: Branched-Chain DNA

Instead of increasing the concentration of target, signal amplification techniques use nucleic acids to magnify the detection signal. The branched-chain DNA (bDNA) method is one of these techniques in common use. The bDNA approach hybridizes the target nucleic acid to multiple capture probes affixed to a microtiter well. This is followed by hybridization to a series of (1) "extender," (2) "preamplifier," and (3) amplifier probes. The final, highly branched amplifier probe includes multiple copies of signal-generating enzymes that act on a chemiluminescent substrate to produce light. Nucleotide analogs isoC and isoG (isomers of C and G that are complementary to each other but not to other nucleotides) are often used to increase the specificity of the signaling cascade.

Serial Invasive Amplification

When two probes overlap on one target, certain structure-specific nucleases will cleave the DNA. The cleaved fragment, in turn, can lead to invasive cleavage of a secondary probe that has the appropriate sequence and is in the shape of a hairpin. The hairpin shape allows the probe to function as a fluorogenic indicator by virtue of having a reporter-quencher pair of dyes that are separated when cleavage occurs. This serial sequence of events (primary invasion and cleavage, followed by secondary invasion and cleavage of an indicator probe) is known as the serial invasive signal amplification reaction. After DNA denaturation, cooling, and the addition of enzymes, the reaction is run at a temperature at which both the primary and secondary reactions recycle.

Probe Amplification—Rolling Circle Amplification

If a primer is annealed to a closed circle of DNA in the presence of a processive, displacing polymerase, the complement of the circle will be synthesized over and over again with displacement of the tandem repeats. If two primers are used in opposite orientation, progressively more complex branches will be formed in an exponential reaction. The rolling circle is formed by ligation of the two ends of a linear probe on template DNA. Ligation may happen directly, after polymerization through a gap, or after annealing of an additional, allele-specific oligonucleotide.

Target Quantification After Amplification

Molecular diagnostic assays may be qualitative (presence and/or absence of a target or definition of a genotype) or quantitative (the original concentration of a target sequence in the sample). When amplification is part of the assay, many analytical variables need to be carefully controlled for accurate and precise quantification. Variations in (1) extraction efficiency, (2) presence of enzyme inhibitors, (3) lot-to-lot variation in enzyme and reagent performance, and (4) day-to-day variation in reaction and detection conditions need to be addressed in methods that attempt to yield a quantitative result.

Quantitative analysis at the end point of amplification is usually carried out by use of calibrators with known amounts of target or a target mimic. Quantification of sample nucleic acid may be accomplished by comparison with an *internal standard* of known amount that is added at the time of sample processing to control for efficiency of nucleic acid purification. Examples of internal standards are (1) DNA fragments, (2) plasmids, and (3) RNA packaged into synthetic phage or virus particles to mimic the assay of real viruses (so called *armored RNA*). One such strategy uses a *competitor* template that is amplified by the target primers but generates an amplicon with sequence or size different from that of the expected amplicon.

This competitor template is added in varying amounts to replicates of the sample before amplification. When the target and competitor are present at equal concentrations, the amounts of the two different products will also be the same. The competitor is present in the same tube as the sample, so any variation in enzyme activity affects both products identically. This method is not frequently used in clinical applications because of the requirement for multiple assays on each patient sample.

Real-time PCR is a simpler and more powerful approach to quantification than end-point assays. The reaction is monitored each cycle, and the profiles of the curves are used to calculate initial target concentrations. Real-time PCR is described in further detail in later sections of this chapter.

DETECTION TECHNIQUES

Molecular diagnostics requires both generic and specific detection techniques and quantitative measurements. That is, there is a need for both (1) generic measurement or visualization of nucleic acid and (2) discrimination and quantification of specific nucleic acid sequences. The latter task usually involves the use of reporter molecules and nucleic acid sequences.

Generic Measurement and Visualization of Nucleic Acids

To measure or visualize nucleic acids generically, two approaches are commonly used: ultraviolet (UV) absorbance and dye staining.

UV Absorbance

Nucleic acid molecules absorb UV light maximally at 260 nm owing almost entirely to the constituent bases. This absorbance is used to measure the nucleic acid content of a solution. DNA double helices have lower molar absorptivity than would be measured from the equivalent number of nucleotide monomers, and when DNA is denatured into single strands (ssDNA) (e.g., by extremes of heat or pH) absorptivity increases. If a dsDNA preparation is pure, a 50-mg/L solution has an absorbance of 1.0 at 260 nm. Single-stranded nucleic acids (DNA or RNA) have a greater absorbance so only about 30 mg/L gives an absorbance of 1.0. More exact estimates for oligonucleotides are based on dinucleotide contributions. It is common to assess the purity of a nucleic acid preparation by its ratio of absorbances at 260 nm and 280 nm (*260 : 280 ratio*). In contrast to nucleic acids, proteins absorb maximally at 280 nm. A pure preparation of nucleic acid should have a 260 : 280 ratio of 1.7 to 2.0, depending on base content. Lower values suggest significant protein contamination.

Fluorescent Staining of Nucleic Acids

Fluorescent stains that bind to nucleic acid are 1000 to 10,000 times more sensitive than absorbance measurements. The best known example of a nucleic acid dye is ethidium bromide, a positively charged, intercalating dye for dsDNA and to a lesser extent, ssDNA and RNA. Cyanine dyes, such as SYBR Green I, are also popular stains for nucleic acids because they do not fluoresce unless they are bound to nucleic acids, thus providing very low background. With the appropriate optics, single molecules of DNA can be visualized with cyanine-based nucleic acid stains.[6] Nucleic acid dyes can detect DNA and RNA in gels or in solution (such as in real-time PCR).

Reporter Molecules and Labeled Probes

UV absorbance and fluorescent dyes in themselves do not discriminate between different nucleic acid sequences (i.e., they are not sequence specific). Specificity in nucleic acid assays almost always comes from the hybridization of two complementary nucleic acid strands. Many types of reporter molecules have been covalently attached or incorporated into nucleic acid to form probes. These probes are used to reveal the physical presence or location of sequences complementary to the nucleic acid portion of the probe.

Radioactivity

The first probes used in nucleic acid detection were radioactively labeled. Radioactive labels are still favored in some research settings because of the sensitivity obtained with probes of high specific activity. The most frequently used isotopic labels are ^{32}P and ^{33}P, which are incorporated into the probe by enzymatic reactions. *Nick translation* is a classical method of labeling dsDNA fragments. Nicks are introduced randomly into each strand of DNA by DNase I, and the resulting 3′ OH groups form priming sites for DNA polymerase. Labeled nucleotides are incorporated as the polymerase extends the strand by digesting and removing the unlabeled strand. Another method of labeling dsDNA is *random priming,* in which the nucleic acid is denatured and allowed to anneal with short hexamer oligonucleotides of random sequence. The 3′ end of an annealed hexamer forms the initiation site for the DNA polymerase, which incorporates labeled nucleotides using single-stranded regions of the DNA as the template. Labeled nucleic acid can also be synthesized by PCR, or if a labeled RNA is desired, it can be prepared by use of a dsDNA fragment containing a promoter sequence for RNA polymerase and incorporating radiolabeled ribonucleotides by transcription.

Additional enzymatic reactions are useful for labeling oligonucleotides. T4 polynucleotide kinase may be used to label the 5′ end of an oligonucleotide with ^{32}P or ^{33}P. Alternatively, terminal deoxynucleotidyl transferase (TdT) is used to add labeled nucleotides onto the 3′ end in a *tailing* reaction. No template is required, and the number and type of nucleotides are controlled by the reaction conditions. This results in a somewhat longer probe than the original oligonucleotide, with additional labeled bases at the 3′ end. The sensitivity that is achieved with radioactive nucleic acid probes is largely determined by the extent of incorporation of the radiolabel. Radioactively labeled probes have a short half-life limited by isotopic decay and radiolysis of the nucleic acid. This inherent instability, along with concerns of radioisotope safety and disposal, restricts the use of radioactive probes in the clinical laboratory.

Indirect Probe Detection

The first practical example of nonradioactive probes used a biotin-labeled analog of dUTP. Despite the altered steric configuration, this nucleotide is incorporated by both DNA polymerase and terminal transferase. Other functional groups, such as digoxigenin, may also be used as affinity labels through chemical linkage to a dUTP and incorporation into polynucleotides. Alternatively, oligonucleotide probes have been labeled during synthesis with biotin or amino linkers for subsequent attachment to indicator molecules. Labels at either the 5′ or 3′ end of the molecule are usually preferred because central modifications may interfere with hybridization.

Biotin and other affinity labels do not generate detectable signals on their own but require high-affinity binding partners that are labeled, often with enzymes. The high-affinity binding partners are usually antibodies, or in the case of biotin, avidin or streptavidin. These binding molecules can be linked to enzymes—such as horseradish peroxidase or alkaline phosphatase—thus connecting a single target (nucleic acid) to a single enzyme. Enzyme activity is monitored according to the enzyme substrate used by use of chemiluminescent, photometric, or fluorescent detection.

Affinity labels also are used to capture and localize targets to an area of a solid support. For example, biotinylated probes are affixed to a streptavidin-coated surface. After incubation with the target nucleic acid, a second probe is added, which is either directly labeled with **fluorescence** or conjugated through an affinity label to an enzyme. Any background or nonspecific localization of reagents results in amplification of an undesired signal along with the desired signal, and these methods usually require multiple separation and washing steps to decrease the background.

Fluorescent Labels

Advances in oligonucleotide synthesis and fluorescence detection systems have made fluorescently labeled probes the preferred reporter for nucleic acid analysis. Many fluorescent labels are now available, allowing color multiplexing for applications such as (1) DNA sequencing, (2) fragment length analysis, (3) DNA **arrays,** and (4) real-time PCR (all reviewed later in this chapter). Techniques such as (1) fluorescence polarization, (2) fluorescence resonance energy transfer (FRET), and (3) fluorescence quenching can provide additional detection specificity. Fluorescence polarization has been used to distinguish free from bound label if the molecular rotation of the probe changes upon binding. Molecular rotation primarily depends upon the size of the molecule so binding of a small probe onto a large target results in a polarization increase that can be measured. FRET techniques depend on the distance between two spectrally distinct fluorescent labels. The two labels are either brought closer together through hybridization or end up farther apart, often through hydrolytic cleavage of a dual-labeled probe. Finally, fluorescence quenching or augmentation can occur with hybridization of a fluorescent oligonucleotide to its target. The effect depends on the specific fluorescent dye and the inherent quenching from G residues in the target and/or probe. Alternatively, quenching moieties can be purposely incorporated into the probe.

DISCRIMINATION TECHNIQUES

Three general categories of nucleic acid discrimination techniques will be reviewed:

- Electrophoretic separation: Provides physical separation of individual nucleic acid species based on molecular weight and shape
- Alternatives to electrophoresis: Determines the size or sequence of nucleic acids without use of electrophoresis. Examples are high-performance liquid chromatography (HPLC) and mass spectrometry
- Hybridization assays: Provides visualization of specific nucleic acids out of a background, usually by use of probes

Some techniques use both electrophoresis and hybridization.

Electrophoresis

Electrophoresis is the most commonly used method for DNA and RNA analysis. Both DNA and RNA are negatively charged and will migrate toward the anode (the positively charged electrode) when an electrical field is present within an appropriately buffered solution. Separation of different nucleic acids occurs when mixtures are allowed to travel through a neutral sieving polymer under the electrical field. Separation is primarily based on molecular weight, with smaller molecules traveling faster through the polymer than larger ones (Figure 5-6). When very large molecules (≥50 kb) have to be separated, pulsed electrical fields are employed to help move these molecules through the polymer matrix. Separation also occurs based on the physical conformation, or shape, of the molecule. For instance, single-stranded molecules may fold into secondary structures, and double-stranded molecules may form heteroduplexes, nicked strands, or superhelical circular structures. Separation based on shape can provide useful information, but it can also confuse size-based analysis. For instance, because RNA generally has a high degree of secondary structure, electrophoresis of RNA is usually performed under denaturing conditions to abolish these structures. Electrophoresis of DNA is performed under nondenaturing or denaturing conditions depending on the application. The result of an electrophoretic separation provides the basis of interpretation of many clinical assays.

Agarose and *polyacrylamide* are the two types of polymers commonly used in electrophoresis. Several chemical variants of the polymers are commercially available and are tailored for different separation ranges and applications. The choice of polymer and polymer concentration (usually expressed as % w/v) is dictated by (1) the size of nucleic acid to be separated, (2) the resolution that is required, and (3) how you will visualize and analyze the result. Using various concentrations, an agarose gel can separate nucleic acid fragments as small as 20 bp to more than 10 Mb (10,000 kb), including chromosomes of yeast, fungi, and parasites. However, the resolution of separations in agarose is limited, usually to a size difference of 2% to 5%. Agarose polymers are cast in trays (often commercially supplied as precast gels) and submerged in buffer. The gels are permeable to fluorescent nucleic acid–binding dyes, and results of electrophoresis are recorded by a photographic image of the stained gel under UV illumination.

Polyacrylamide polymers are suited for high-resolution separation (down to about a 0.1% size differences) of short molecules (up to about 2 kb) and are the primary polymer for single-stranded nucleic acid separation, such as DNA **sequencing.** Polyacrylamide is used either as a linear polymer solution, which is filled in capillaries (*capillary electrophoresis*), or as cross-linked gels, which are cast between two plastic or glass plates (*slab gel electrophoresis*). Polyacrylamide gels are permeable to fluorescent stains, and silver staining of nucleic acids can also be used. In addition, the optical clarity of polyacrylamide polymers makes them ideal for visualizing emission signals from fluorescently labeled fragments using laser-induced fluorescence detection.

Table 5-2 lists common electrophoresis-based techniques described further in this section.

Restriction Fragment Length Polymorphism

DNA extracted from a cell is extremely long and is usually cut into shorter fragments before electrophoresis to aid the analysis. Restriction endonucleases cut dsDNA into fragments of reproducible size; the same enzyme produces the same fragments in different specimens if the specimens contain the same DNA sequence. If an alteration in the DNA abolishes or creates a cleavage site recognized by the enzyme (or changes the spacing between two cleavage sites), then electrophoresis of

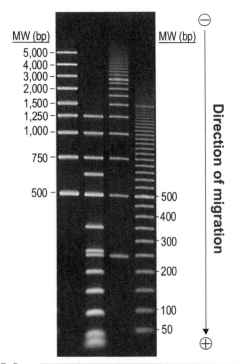

Figure 5-6

A photograph of multiple DNA fragments after agarose gel electrophoresis (1% w/v, SeaKem LE agarose gel) showing the separation of dsDNA molecules by size.
(Photograph courtesy of Lonza Bioscience, Rockland, Me.)

TABLE 5-2	Commonly Used Electrophoresis-Based Techniques	
Techniques Using Electrophoresis		**Primary Application**
PCR/Restriction fragment length polymorphism (RFLP)		Detection
PCR (RT-PCR) fragment analysis		Detection
Southern blotting		Detection
Northern blotting		Detection
Heteroduplex migration assay (CSGE)		Scanning
Single-strand conformation polymorphism analysis (SSCP, SSCA)		Scanning
Denaturing gradient gel electrophoresis (DGGE)		Scanning
Temperature-gradient electrophoresis (TGGE and TGCE)		Scanning
DNA sequencing		Detection
Single-nucleotide extension assay (SNE)		Detection
Oligo ligation assay (OLA)		Detection
Muliplex ligation-dependent probe amplification		Quantification

digested fragments will reveal those changes (or polymorphisms) in fragment length: hence, the name **restriction fragment length polymorphism (RFLP).**

PCR/RFLP

Many sequence alterations are on fragments that can be amplified by PCR, making RFLP analysis very simple. After PCR the products are digested with one or more restriction enzymes and analyzed by electrophoresis. For example, if a sample has a mutation that disrupts an enzyme recognition site, this can be distinguished from a sample that does not have the mutation. Such an assay will produce one uncut PCR fragment when the mutation is present and two shorter fragments when the mutation is absent (Figure 5-7). If the mutation is present as a heterozygote (one normal and one mutant copy of DNA), then one long and two shorter fragments will be observed. Usually, it is possible to design the assay so that the fragments can be easily resolved by agarose electrophoresis and visualized by staining the gel with a fluorescent DNA-binding dye, such as ethidium bromide. One variant of this method uses reverse-transcribed mRNA, which lacks the **introns** that would be present in the DNA. In this way, multiple exons can be analyzed in one PCR reaction.

PCR Product Length Analysis

Some DNA alterations involve (1) **insertions,** (2) deletions, (3) rearrangements, and (4) changes in the number of repeat

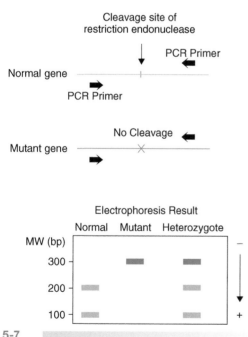

Cleavage site of
restriction endonuclease

Figure 5-7

An example of PCR-RFLP. A DNA fragment amplified by PCR carries a site (a unique sequence of generally four or more bases) that is recognized and cleaved by a restriction endonuclease. If a mutation is present, this site is altered and is no longer recognized by the enzyme. Electrophoresis reveals that the fragment from a normal specimen was indeed cut by the enzyme, generating two fragments shorter than the original length, whereas the fragment from a homozygous mutant was not cut and the original length of the amplicon was preserved. In a heterozygous mutant, both the original fragment and the shorter fragments are visible.

sequences. If these alterations reside within a fragment that is able to be amplified reliably by PCR, then variation in the length of the amplified fragment will indicate these structural alterations. Enzyme digestion is not necessary in many of these assays. The length differences may be large and easily picked up with agarose gel electrophoresis or small enough to require a denaturing polyacrylamide matrix. Fluorescent labels may be incorporated into the product during the PCR to simplify detection of the fragment lengths. These techniques are commonly used in the diagnosis of inherited diseases (Chapter 9) and in identity assessment (Chapter 10).

Direct analysis of PCR products by electrophoresis (without enzyme digestion) can also be directly diagnostic (e.g., for the presence of a bacterium, virus, or fungus in a specimen). The specificity of the amplification reaction is verified by the known size of the fragment. Internal negative and positive controls are employed in this part of the analytical phase to control for potential contamination and to establish detection sensitivity. Direct PCR product analysis by electrophoresis is also frequently used in the clinical laboratory to query the quality of intermediary steps before final detection. For example, electrophoresis can answer questions such as, Was the nucleic acid isolated successfully? How well was it purified? Did the amplification work? How specific was the PCR?

Southern Blotting

When a DNA alteration spans a large region that is not easily amplified by PCR, **Southern blotting** (or Southern blot analysis) can be used to detect the alteration (Figure 5-8). In this technique, (1) the original sample DNA (rather than an amplified fragment) is digested by a restriction endonuclease, (2) the DNA fragments are separated by agarose electrophoresis, and (3) the fragments are transferred to a solid support followed by (4) selective visualization of fragments by hybridization of labeled probes. A nylon or nitrocellulose membrane (or filter) is usually used as the support. Details of the transfer process differ, but most methods use acid treatment to fragment the DNA (thus making it smaller and easier to elute from the gel), followed by alkaline denaturation (single strands bind to membranes much more efficiently) and neutralization. Original methods of transfer relied on capillary action, with the filter placed in contact with the gel and absorbent paper stacked on top to blot the transfer buffer and DNA onto the filter. Typically, this process was allowed to proceed overnight. Vacuum or pressure systems are often used to speed the transfer. After transfer, DNA is permanently immobilized on the filter by baking or UV cross-linking. The filter is then incubated with a single-stranded probe that forms a stable complex with its complementary target affixed on the filter. If the original DNA was of good quality and if restriction enzyme treatment was complete, the fragments of interest will be visualized on film (autoradiographic or chemiluminescent) or directly on the filter (photometric) (see Figure 5-8). Ten to 50 μg of genomic DNA is usually sufficient for detection. The procedure was named after its inventor, E. M. Southern. Southern blot analysis reveals polymorphisms in the DNA sequence based on the RFLP profile made visible by probes. It can also detect large structural alterations, such as deletions, duplications, insertions, and rearrangements. Southern blotting is labor intensive and takes much longer than PCR.

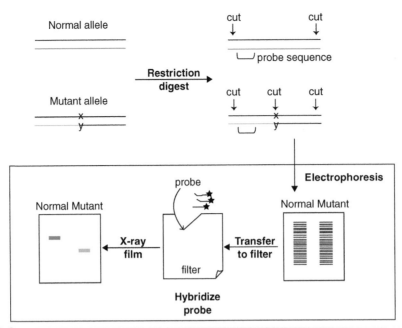

Figure 5-8

Schematic of Southern blotting. Genomic DNA is isolated from a normal specimen and from a mutant specimen carrying the polymorphic allele (x, y). The mutant allele generates a new site that is recognized by the enzyme. The normal specimen does not have this site. After restriction enzyme digestion of genomic DNA, both samples are separated by agarose electrophoresis. At this point, no discrete bands are visible over the background of many fragments that are generated by the enzyme. DNA is transferred to a filter and hybridized with a short DNA probe that is radioactively labeled. This probe hybridizes to the genomic sequence on one side of the polymorphic site. After exposing the filter to x-ray film, a smaller, digested band is seen in the specimen with the mutant allele compared with the larger fragment seen in the normal specimen.

Northern Blotting

Northern blotting was not named for its inventor, but as a companion technique that uses RNA rather than DNA as the test nucleic acid. RNA is transferred from the gel after electrophoresis onto a solid support followed by hybridization with a specific labeled probe. Because RNA molecules have defined lengths and are much shorter than genomic DNA, it is not necessary to cleave RNA before electrophoresis. However, because of the secondary structure of RNA, it is necessary to perform electrophoresis under denaturing conditions, usually with formaldehyde or formamide buffers in agarose gels. RNA extracted from cells consists primarily of ribosomal and transfer RNA. The mRNA comprises only 1% to 2% of total cellular RNA. After electrophoresis and staining, intact RNA reveals two clearly visible bands of ribosomal RNA. Electrophoresis of about 10 μg of RNA is usually sufficient to see the mRNA of interest after hybridization with a probe. Northern blotting provides information about the size of mRNA transcripts. Although only partly quantitative, the relative concentration of a particular transcript can be estimated by reference to a constitutively expressed control transcript, such as actin.

Heteroduplex Migration Analysis

Heteroduplex migration analysis (also called conformation-sensitive gel electrophoresis, CSGE) reveals the presence of mutations by the altered electrophoretic mobility of a dsDNA fragment that contains one or more mismatched bases (a **heteroduplex**) versus one that is perfectly matched (a **homoduplex**). Originally described as a PCR artifact, heteroduplex migration analysis has become a popular mutation-scanning technique, primarily because of its technical simplicity. With this technique, the dsDNA generated by PCR is denatured and then allowed to reanneal, followed by electrophoresis under slightly denaturing conditions (e.g., 15% urea, 40 °C) on polyacrylamide gels. Detection is performed by silver staining of the gel or by fluorescence detection if one of the PCR primers is labeled. Heteroduplexes usually tend to migrate more slowly than homoduplexes during electrophoresis (Figure 5-9). Whereas mutant alleles are often present as heterozygotes in a clinical specimen, homozygous mutations require mixing with wild-type DNA for the mutations to be detected.

This technique has the ability to detect the presence of a single nucleotide polymorphism in a fragment as large as 600 bp. The principal factor influencing the sensitivity of this technique is the combination of the mismatched bases. Greater mobility differences (relative to the homoduplex) occur with some combinations of mismatches than with others.

This technique and other mutation-scanning methods are useful when a wide variety of sequence alterations might be present. Particularly when most of the samples tested are wild type ("normal"), it is more economical to scan for the presence of mutations before performing specific genotyping or DNA sequence analysis.

Single-Strand Conformation Polymorphism Analysis

Single-strand conformation polymorphism analysis (SSCP or SSCA) is another electrophoresis technique used to scan for unknown variants in nucleic acid sequence. Similar to hetero-

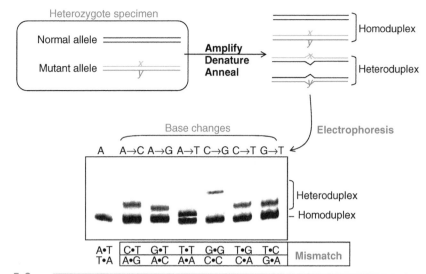

Figure 5-9

A schematic of heteroduplex migration analysis. When amplified DNA from a heterozygous specimen is denatured and cooled, the fragments anneal in four combinations. Electrophoresis on a specialized polyacrylamide gel reveals the presence of heteroduplexes by extra band(s) appearing above the homoduplex band.

duplex analysis, it first requires PCR amplification. The amplicon is then diluted, denatured with heat and formamide, and the resulting ssDNA is separated by nondenaturing polyacrylamide electrophoresis (usually run at 4 °C). During electrophoresis the single-stranded molecules fold into three-dimensional structures according to their primary sequence. Electrophoretic mobility then becomes a function of size and shape of the folded single-stranded molecules. If the sequence of a reference sample differs from that of the fragment being tested, even by only a single nucleotide, often at least one of the strands, if not both, will adopt different conformations and exhibit a unique banding pattern (Figure 5-10). Since its introduction in 1989, SSCP has become a popular mutation-detection strategy. Results are visualized by silver staining of the gel or by fluorescent detection using labeled primers during PCR. Unlike heteroduplex migration analysis, there is no need to mix reference materials to detect the presence of a homozygous mutant specimen. Reports on the sensitivity of the SSCP technique have been variable, and detection rates seem influenced by the GC content of the fragment and the assay conditions. Different conditions may be required to detect all mutations, making multiple runs sometimes necessary for one target sequence. Furthermore the results of SSCP are difficult to interpret when one sequence gives rise to multiple single-stranded conformations, some of which may be difficult to see, depending on the amplification and electrophoresis conditions. It is also difficult to establish reliable protocols for fragments greater than ~200 bp.

Denaturing Gradient Gel Electrophoresis

Denaturing gradient gel electrophoresis (DGGE) is yet another technique to scan for unknown variants in nucleic acid sequence. Separation of a PCR product is performed at a constant temperature with a gel that includes a concentration gradient of denaturants, such as urea, along the direction of electrophoresis. If the sequence of the PCR product is known,

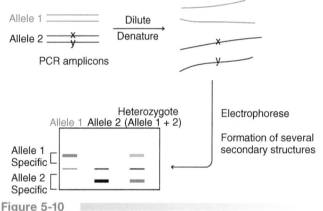

Figure 5-10

A schematic of SSCP. PCR amplicons carrying the polymorphic site (shown as x and y) are diluted and then denatured to form single-stranded fragments. During electrophoresis they assume secondary structures. When conditions are right, polymorphisms are detected by differential band patterns compared with a known sample.

the detection rate of mutations can reach 100%. However, creating identical gels is challenging, making routine implementation difficult. Depending on the melting characteristics of the product, it may be necessary to attach an artificial GC-rich sequence (GC *clamp*) to one end of the fragment to provide optimum separation.

Temperature-Gradient Electrophoresis

Temperature-gradient electrophoresis is similar to DGGE. Instead of using denaturants, a spatial or temporal temperature gradient is used to provide the denaturing effect. Initial designs placed an electrophoresis gel over an insulated metal plate with a linear temperature gradient established perpendicular or parallel to the direction of electrophoresis (temperature-gradient gel electrophoresis, or TGGE). Separation occurs according to size, shape, and thermal stability of the nucleic acids. If the temperature gradient is established perpendicular to the direction of electrophoresis, intramolecular conformational changes show up as continuous transition curves, and strand separation leads to discontinuous transitions. Heteroduplexes are detected by a shift of the transition curves to lower temperatures.

Temperature gradients have also been applied during capillary electrophoresis. A portion of the capillary array is placed inside a heating chamber whose temperature is computer controlled to generate a gradual heat ramp (typically a 10 °C ramp at 0.5 °C to ~0.7 °C/min). Similar to the heteroduplex migration assay, PCR products are first denatured, reannealed, and then injected into the capillary. The electrophoresis polymer solution contains an intercalating dye, and nucleic acids are detected by fluorescence. The presence of a heteroduplex is detected by a change in the peak profile, which under certain conditions may show all four possible duplexes as peaks (Figure 5-11). The technique detects the presence of heteroduplexes well and allows many samples be run at the same time. However, as with heteroduplex migration analysis, a homozygous mutant sample is difficult to discriminate from a homozygous normal sample without mixing the two together to form heteroduplexes.

DNA Sequencing

DNA sequencing, once strictly a research technique, is now routinely performed in the clinical laboratory. The actual nucleic acid sequence of a DNA fragment can be determined and compared with a reference sequence with an error rate of 0.1% (one misidentified base in 1000). Often the sequence is analyzed on both strands (sense and antisense), which will provide even greater accuracy. Any deviation from the reference sequence is identified using computer programs matching the sequences. Base changes resulting in an altered amino acid code, stop codons, deletions, or insertions can be identified. The most common sequencing strategy uses PCR in the first step to amplify the region of interest, followed by a variation of the chain-termination reaction developed by F. Sanger in the late 1970s.[9] This reaction (also referred to as the Sanger reaction) generates fragments that are terminated at various lengths by the incorporation of one of the four dideoxynucleotide base analogs (Figure 5-12) during extension from the sequencing primer (Figure 5-13). Dideoxynucleotides lack the 3′ hydroxyl group (OH) and the 2′OH on the pentose ring, and because DNA chain growth requires the addition of deoxynucleotides to the 3′ OH group, incorporation of this base analog terminates chain growth. The most common method for generating these terminated fragments is *cycle sequencing*, repeating the steps of annealing, chain extension and termination, and denaturation by temperature cycling, similar to PCR. The fragments generated are tagged with a fluorescent dye (by use of either labeled primers or labeled terminator dideoxynucleotides), then separated by denaturing polyacrylamide gel or capillary electrophoresis, and detected by fluorescence detection as the fragments travel past the detector (Figure 5-14). When fluorescently labeled primers are used, four tubes are needed for separate termination reactions. If only one color is used, then each termination reaction mixture is electrophoresed in a separate lane or capillary. If four colors are used, then the termination reactions are combined before electrophoresis, and only one capillary is necessary. Alternatively the use of four terminators of different colors makes it possible to streamline the process down to one tube for the termination reactions and one capillary. About 600 bases can be resolved in a 2½-hour run on a capillary electrophoresis instrument that can process

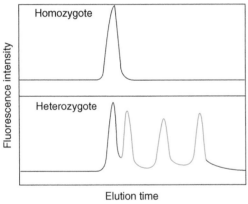

Figure 5-11
An example of TGCE. The PCR fragments are denatured and annealed before the electrophoresis (see diagram in Figure 5-10). Only one peak is visible for the PCR product of a normal homozygous specimen, whereas all four possible duplexes are visible and separated from each other in a heterozygous mutant specimen. The shape of the elution profile (rather than the elution time) is used to compare unknowns with control samples.

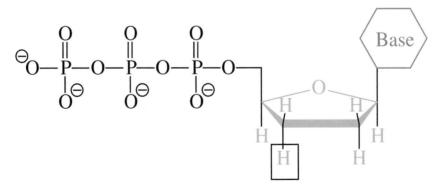

Figure 5-12
A dideoxynucleotide. Notice the absence of the 3′ OH that is usually present in standard deoxynucleotides.

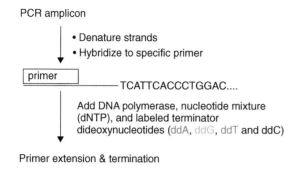

PCR amplicon
• Denature strands
• Hybridize to specific primer

primer ——— TCATTCACCCTGGAC....

Add DNA polymerase, nucleotide mixture (dNTP), and labeled terminator dideoxynucleotides (ddA, ddG, ddT and ddC)

Primer extension & termination

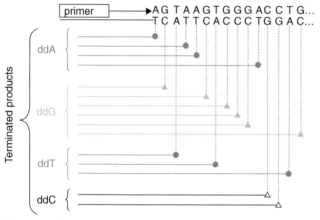

Figure 5-13
The chain-termination reaction (Sanger). A PCR amplicon is dena-tured and then hybridized to a specific oligonucleotide primer. As the DNA polymerase extends the primer by incorporating bases (dNTPs) complementary to the template, it occasionally incorporates a terminator base analog (ddA, ddG, ddT, or ddC) that stops further extension. The result is a mixture of extended products with varying lengths. Each terminator base may be labeled with one of four different fluorescent tags (shown as different symbols in the diagram). Alternatively, the primer can carry four different fluorescent tags in individual chain-termination reactions (containing only one ddNTP) performed in separate tubes. The original procedure incorporated a radioactive dNTP during extension, allowing monochromatic detec-tion of the truncated fragments that were electrophoresed in four sep-arate lanes, each for one of the terminator bases (see Figure 5-14).

96 or 384 samples in parallel. DNA sequencing in the clinical laboratory is most commonly used in infectious disease testing, such as genotyping of human immunodeficiency virus (HIV) for drug resistance and of hepatitis C virus (HCV) to establish prognosis and appropriate therapy.

Recent advances in throughput allow sequencing of an entire bacterial genome in one operation. Massively parallel amplification in microscopic polonies or emulsion droplets[4] is followed by extension reactions that are observed with fluores-cence or *pyrosequencing* (see next section on Alternatives to Electrophoresis). However, complete sequencing of only one gene (exons and splice sites) in the clinical laboratory for the detection of disease-causing mutations is still an expensive proposition. This is especially true for population screening (in which the majority of samples will not have a mutation), but also for patients with symptoms of the disease. Therefore in

genetic testing, DNA sequencing is often performed only after an initial *mutation scanning assay* has determined the exons that need to be sequenced or otherwise genotyped.

Single Nucleotide Extension Assay
Also known as *single-base primer extension* or *minisequencing*, single nucleotide extension (SNE) assays involve the annealing of an oligonucleotide primer to a single-stranded PCR ampli-con at a location that is immediately adjacent to, but does not include, the site of the SNP, followed by enzymatic extension of the primer in the presence of polymerase and dideoxynucleo-tide terminators without dNTPs. Each of the four terminators is labeled with a unique label so that it is possible to detect which base was incorporated. SNE assays can be multiplexed on automated DNA sequencing instruments by varying the lengths of the primers so that each SNP is resolved by size in one electrophoresis run. There are also many SNE **detection methods** other than electrophoresis, including (1) photometric detection on microtiter plates, (2) product-capture detection systems on DNA microarrays, (3) bead hybridization assays detected by flow cytometry, (4) solution-based fluorescence polarization detection systems, and (5) mass spectrometry. SNE assays are useful when the gene of interest contains a relatively large number of disease-causing SNPs. SNE assays do not work well if there are polymorphisms in the primer-binding site. Nor are they usually designed to detect polymor-phisms at a position other than immediately adjacent to the 3′ end of the primer.

Oligo Ligation Assay
Another assay format frequently used in the clinical laboratory for SNP detection is the oligonucleotide ligation assay (OLA). Two oligonucleotide probes are hybridized to adjacent sequences of amplified target DNA, with the known SNP site positioned at the end of one probe (Figure 5-15). DNA ligase covalently joins the two probes only if both probes are perfectly hybridized to the target including the polymorphic base. A probe match-ing the normal base and another probe matching the mutant base are usually prepared. These two can be discriminated by differential electrophoretic mobility by varying the number of modifying tail units attached. These tails were initially non-complementary poly A or poly C tails, but now consist of pen-taethylene oxide (PEO) units. The probe hybridizing to both alleles (the *common probe*) provides the reporter molecule, usually a fluorescent label. Multiplexing of SNP detection is achieved by attaching different fluorescent labels to the common probes and also varying the numbers of tail units on the allele-specific probes. Following ligation, probes for multiple SNP sites are separated by denaturing polyacrylamide electro-phoresis in the presence of labeled size standards.

Multiplex Ligation-Dependent Probe Amplification
Muliplex ligation-dependent probe amplification[11] or MLPA is a convenient method for relative quantification of up to 30 to 50 targets. The method is particularly useful to screen for dele-tions or duplications of multiple exons within a gene. For each target, two probes are designed that hybridize adjacent to each other so that they are in position to be ligated. The two probes have unique tails that do not hybridize to the target and that are the same between targets. After hybridization and ligation, the probes are amplified by PCR with a common primer pair

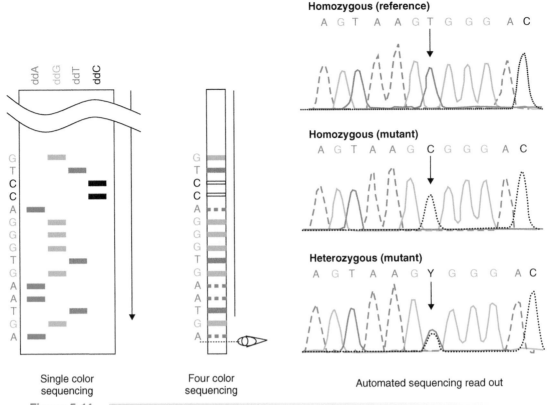

Figure 5-14

Schematic of DNA sequencing. Extension products generated by the chain-termination (Sanger) reaction are separated using four lanes (if only one label is used), or using one lane (if different color dyes are used for each of the terminator reactions). The four-color strategy is amenable to automated end-point fluorescence detection (shown by the eye icon) for both slab gels and capillary electrophoresis. The direction of fragment migration is from top to bottom. The sequence is read from bottom to top in the gels and from left to right for the automated sequence. Examples of a reference sample (homozygous *T* at the polymorphic site), a mutant sample (homozygous *C*), and a heterozygous mutant sample (*T* and *C*) are shown. *Y* indicates a pyrimidine (*T* or *C*).

(complementary to the tails). One of the primers is fluorescently labeled at its 5′ end. Because probes of different lengths are used, multiple PCR products of different sizes are produced and separated on a sequencing gel. The relative peak heights or areas of each target are compared for relative quantification.

Alternatives to Electrophoresis

Newer technologies that replace assays traditionally performed by electrophoresis are emerging. Some of these are attractive alternatives for the clinical laboratory because they are amenable to automation with less hands-on time. These include pyrosequencing, mass spectrometry, and HPLC.

Pyrosequencing

Pyrosequencing is a method to determine the nucleic acid sequence of short segments without the use of electrophoresis. A sequencing primer is hybridized to a single-stranded template that is usually generated by PCR. Four enzymes—a DNA polymerase, ATP sulfurylase, luciferase and apyrase—and two substrates—adenosine 5′ phosphosulfate and luciferin—are included in the reaction mixture (Figure 5-16). One of the four dNTPs is added to the reaction (dATPαS is substituted for

dATP because it is incorporated by the polymerase, but is not a luciferase substrate). If the base is complementary to the template strand, DNA polymerase catalyzes its incorporation. Each incorporation event is accompanied by release of a pyrophosphate (PPi) so that the quantity of PPi produced is equimolar to the amount of incorporated nucleotide. The release of PPi is monitored by conversion of PPi and adenosine 5′ phosphosulfate into ATP by the ATP sulfurylase, and ATP in turn drives conversion of luciferin into oxyluciferin, which generates visible light. The light produced is proportional to the number of nucleotides incorporated. Apyrase, which is a nucleotide-degrading enzyme, continuously degrades ATP and unincorporated dNTP. This switches off the light in preparation for the next dNTP addition. As the process is repeated by adding one dNTP at a time, the complementary DNA strand is built, and the nucleotide sequence is determined (see Figure 5-16). Because the technique can be automated, it is useful when the sequences of a large number of short segments need to be determined.

Mass Spectrometry

Matrix-assisted laser-desorption ionization time-of-flight (MALDI-TOF) mass spectrometry has been used to detect

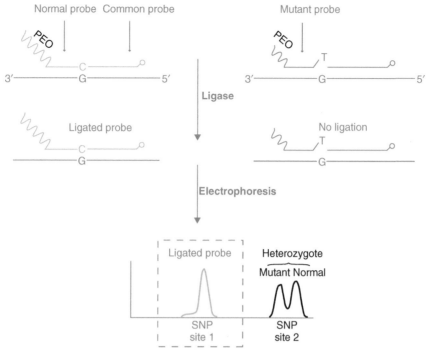

Figure 5-15

Oligo ligation assay. A probe specific to the normal allele (C) is shown hybridized onto a normal DNA sample (G). This probe also is attached to a mobility modifying tail (PEO). Hybridized next to the normal-allele probe is the common probe that is labeled with a fluorescent tag. In the presence of ligase, the two probes are covalently joined to generate a longer probe. The mutant-allele specific probe (T) with a shorter PEO tail also hybridizes to the normal DNA sample, but is not ligated to the common probe because of the mismatched base at its 3' end. Electrophoresis and end-point, laser-induced detection reveals the ligated normal-allele probe, which can be differentiated from the significantly shorter common probe alone (not shown on the graph) or from a ligated mutant-allele probe because of the different lengths of PEO tails. Multiple SNP sites can be analyzed in one electrophoresis assay by varying the tail lengths (e.g., SNP site 2 in the graph) or by use of multicolor fluorescence tags.

sequence polymorphisms. With mass spectroscopy, no label is necessary because the alleles differ in mass. After isolation of genomic DNA, a specific DNA fragment including the polymorphic site is amplified by PCR. Heat-labile alkaline phosphatase is added to the reaction to dephosphorylate any residual nucleotides, preventing future incorporation and interference with the primer extension assay. Samples are then heated to inactivate the alkaline phosphatase. An extension primer is hybridized directly or closely adjacent to the polymorphic site. Appropriate unlabeled deoxynucleotides and/or dideoxynucleotides are incorporated through the polymorphic site and terminated with the incorporation of a dideoxynucleotide generating allele-specific diagnostic product of different mass. Salt is removed from the sample, and ~10 nL of it is spotted onto an array coated with 3-hydroxypicolinic acid. This is placed into the MALDI-TOF, which measures the mass of the extension products. Once the mass is measured, the genotype is determined (Figure 5-17). Despite its complexity, automated systems are available that are capable of processing 384 to 1536 samples in a batch.

High-Performance Liquid Chromatography

HPLC is commonly used for separating and purifying oligonucleotides. Separation is usually based on ion-pair, reversed-phase chromatography and is particularly useful for purifying fluorescently labeled probes guided by absorbance and fluorescent elution profiles.

A variant of this technology is denaturing HPLC (dHPLC). dHPLC is run at a single elevated temperature to partially denature dsDNA. Similar to heteroduplex migration analysis, dHPLC analyzes a mixture of PCR amplicons that are denatured and reannealed, revealing the presence of heteroduplexes as additional peaks that are shifted in retention compared with the homoduplex sample. To separate dsDNA, alkylated nonporous poly (styrene-divinylbenzene) resins are used, with a hydroorganic eluent containing an amphiphilic ion (e.g., triethylammonium ion) and a small hydrophilic counter ion (e.g., acetate). Retention of dsDNA is governed by electrostatic interactions between the positive triethylammonium ions adsorbed to the resin and the negative phosphodiester groups of DNA. An increase in the concentration of organic solvent (e.g., acetonitrile) in the mobile phase results in desorption of the amphiphilic ions and the dsDNA. UV is often used for detection; thus PCR amplicons do not have to be labeled. Multicolor laser-induced fluorescence scanners and mass spectrometers are alternative detectors. Limitations of dHPLC include sequential (one at a time) analysis and the need to analyze some samples at multiple temperatures when more than one melting domain is present.

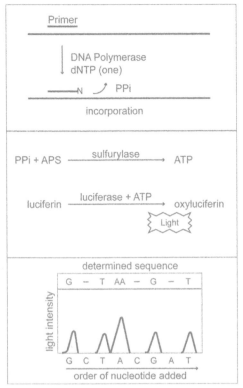

Figure 5-16

Schematic of pyrosequencing. Individual dTNPs are added one by one to the single-stranded template, a primer, and a polymerase. Pyrophosphate is generated if the dNTP is complementary to the next base on the template *(top)*. Any pyrophosphate produced reacts with adenosine-5′-phosphosulfate (APS) to produce ATP, which in turn generates light in the presence of luciferase *(middle)*. The sequence can be determined from the order of dTNP addition and the intensity of light produced.

Hybridization Assays—Principles

The second major category of nucleic acid discrimination techniques is **hybridization.** All hybridization assays are based on the ability of single-stranded nucleic acids to form specific double-stranded hybrids. The process requires (1) that probe and target nucleic acids are mixed under conditions that allow for specific complementary base pairing and (2) that there is a method to detect any resulting double-stranded nucleic acids. A **probe** indicates a nucleic acid whose identity is known, and the *target* or *sample* is a nucleic acid whose identity or abundance is revealed by hybridization. In some of the methods discussed here, hybridization occurs between a target in solution and a probe that is attached ("tethered") to a solid surface. In *homogeneous* or *real-time* techniques, both the probes and the targets are in solution, and hybridization and detection occur without washing steps. Some of the homogeneous methods also monitor the dissociation of hybridized duplexes under controlled heating, revealing the identities of the hybridized duplexes by *melting curve* signatures.

As with any assay, both positive and negative controls are necessary for validation of the analytical phase of hybridization assays. Positive controls contain sequences complementary to the probe, assess assay sensitivity, and ensure that the probe will hybridize to the target under the assay conditions. Negative controls without target sequence assess assay specificity and will detect positive contamination if present.

Hybridization Thermodynamics

The favored structure of DNA under physiological conditions is an ordered double-stranded helix held together by noncovalent interactions. The duplex structure is most stable when all opposing bases are complementary, allowing for maximal hydrogen bonding and base stacking. The noncovalent binding between two DNA strands is both specific (i.e., sequence

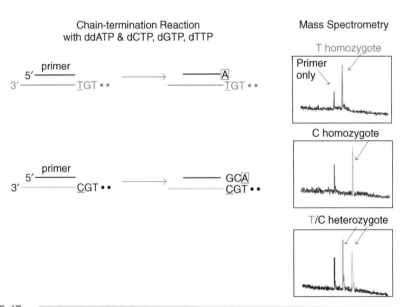

Figure 5-17

Sequence polymorphism analysis by mass spectrometry. The underlined base is the polymorphic site in the template (T or C). The single-stranded template is primed and extended in the presence of three dNTPs and one ddNTP, producing fragments of different mass depending on the sequence. The boxed "A" in this example indicates the incorporated terminator adenine base. The mass of terminated products is precisely measured by MALDI-TOF mass spectrometric data (relative intensity versus m/z).

dependent) and reversible. Denaturing conditions (such as high temperature [>90 °C], formamide, or extremes of pH) favor dissociation of the double-stranded molecule into two separate random coils (Figure 5-18). On removal of the denaturant, single strands attempt to rejoin to re-form duplexes, strongly favoring interactions that maximize complementary base pairing. Because temperature is the denaturant most easily manipulated, double- to single-strand transformation is referred to as *melting,* and the temperature at which one half of the DNA is melted is referred to as the *melting temperature,* or *Tm,* of the duplex. Duplexes with mismatched base pairs are less stable than those with a perfect sequence match and thus melt at a lower temperature. The reverse process, in which two complementary strands recombine to form a stable duplex molecule, is referred to as *annealing* or *hybridization.* Hybridization can occur between DNA strands, RNA strands, and strands of nucleic acid analogs (such as peptide nucleic acids, also known as PNA), in all combinations.

Stringency and Mismatches

The hybridization environment defines the degree of base pair mismatch that can be tolerated in a duplex structure. The tolerance (or lack thereof) for mistakes in base pairing is referred to as the *stringency* of a hybridization reaction. Conditions of high stringency (low salt concentration, high formamide, and high temperature) require exact base pairing. As the stringency is lowered (high salt concentrations, low formamide, and low temperature), more and more base pair mismatches can be tolerated in a duplex. The stringency of a hybridization reaction is determined by the hybridization conditions and the subsequent washing steps designed to remove nonspecifically interacting nucleic acid. In real-time PCR and melting analysis, the hybridization solution is the buffer in which PCR occurs, and there are no separate washing steps.

Hybridization Kinetics

The kinetics of solution-phase hybridizations are second order, being proportional to the concentrations of both hybridizing strands. The rate-limiting step is nucleation, where a small number of base pairs are formed in the correct orientation, followed by a rapid "zippering" of complementary sequences. In the case of a probe present in great excess to the target, hybridization proceeds as a pseudo–first order reaction, depending only on the concentration of the target. However, the time required to hybridize the probe to a given fraction of the target remains proportional to the probe concentration. For example, during PCR the concentration of primers is much greater than that of the target, and the reaction rate during each annealing step depends on the concentration of available single-stranded product, but the time required to anneal primers to a certain fraction of the target is proportional to the primer concentration.

The availability of nucleic acids for hybridization also is an issue. As the temperature cools during thermocycling, PCR primer annealing competes with the formation of double-stranded product. As the concentration of product increases during PCR, some double-stranded product is formed before primer annealing can occur (see Figure 5-3). Similarly, when double-stranded probes are used at high concentrations, probe self-annealing interferes with probe-target hybridization. Available hybridization sites also are limited by intramolecular secondary structure of the probe or target (e.g., as seen in SSCP).

In addition to probe concentration and availability, the length of the probe and the complexity of the nucleic acids affect hybridization rates. Rates are directly proportional to the square root of the probe length and inversely proportional to complexity, defined as the total number of base pairs present in nonrepeating sequences. Mismatches up to about 10% have little effect on hybridization rates.

The rate of the hybridization reaction is influenced by many factors in the reaction environment, most notably temperature and ionic strength. Above the Tm, no stable hybrids are present, although transient complexes may form. As the temperature is lowered below the Tm, hybridization rates increase until a broad maximum occurs about 20 °C to 25 °C below the Tm. Hybridization rates also increase with the ionic strength. Divalent cations, such as Mg^{++}, have a much stronger effect than monovalent cations, such as Na^+ or K^+.

When the nucleic acid target or probe is immobilized on a solid support, the kinetics of hybridization are even more complex. Many of the preceding observations still hold true, but the rate and extent of solid-phase hybridization are lower than with solution-phase hybridization. Depending on the concentrations of the reactants, solid-phase hybridization can be either nucleation limited or diffusion limited. Optimal efficiency of solid-phase hybridization is achieved under conditions that facilitate diffusion of the probe to the support and that favor hybridization over strand reassociation if double-stranded probes are used. This usually means a small volume of hybridization solution and relatively low probe concentrations. In practice, solid-phase hybridization assays are empirically

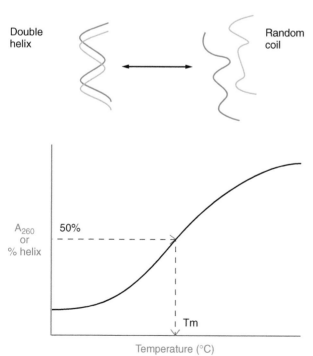

Figure 5-18
Melting curve of double-helical nucleic acid.
(Modified with permission from Piper MA, Unger ER: Nucleic acid probes: A primer for pathologists. Chicago, ASCP Press, 1989.)

designed. Time of hybridization and probe concentration are the two variables most frequently adjusted in the assay. Conditions that tend to maximize the extent of hybridization and minimize the background or nonspecific attachment of the probe are selected.

Probes

In a hybridization assay, the probe is analogous in its role and importance to the antibody in an immunoassay. As mentioned earlier, a probe is the nucleic acid whose identity is known and is used to reveal the identity or abundance of a target or sample. Like antibodies in immunoassays, probes are either unlabeled or labeled with one of a variety of reporter molecules, depending on the technique used to detect hybridization. Probes may be cloned (recombinant), generated by PCR, or synthesized (oligonucleotides). They may be DNA, RNA, or PNA, and single stranded or double stranded. Selection, purification, and labeling of probes are crucial to success of hybridization assays.

Cloned Probes

Cloned probes consist of a known segment of DNA inserted into a plasmid vector that is propagated by growth in a bacterium. Many different plasmid vectors are now available; pBR322 was one of the first in common use. The entire plasmid DNA (insert plus vector sequences) may be used as a probe, or the insert may be purified first from the vector sequences. The latter method is obviously more cumbersome, but may result in reduced background. The resulting probe is a dsDNA probe, and it must be denatured before use.

Some vectors contain RNA promoter regions adjacent to the inserted DNA sequence. These regions permit generation of RNA transcripts from the DNA insert. Because only one strand is copied during the RNA synthesis, single-stranded RNA probes are generated. Controlling the orientation of the insert in relation to the promoter region allows the production of transcripts in the "sense" direction (i.e., same as mRNA) or "antisense" direction (i.e., complementary to mRNA).

PCR-Generated Probes

PCR-generated probes are simple to prepare. During amplification, the PCR product typically is labeled with nucleotides that (1) are radioactive, (2) are fluorescent, or (3) have attached affinity labels. If desired, single-stranded probes are obtained by using a biotin-labeled primer, followed by solid-phase separation with streptavidin.

Oligonucleotide Probes

Oligonucleotide probes are even easier to obtain than PCR-generated probes. These probes are usually 15 to 45 bases of single-stranded nucleic acid that are chemically synthesized to a specified base sequence. Most commonly, they are DNA, but RNA and PNA oligonucleotides also have been used. Automated, efficient, and accurate methods of synthesis continue to lower the cost of production. Sequence information is now routinely available in public databases (e.g., the NIH genetic sequence database, GenBank[1]), and a similarity check for probe sequence can be performed using public algorithms (e.g., BLAST). Probe sequences must be carefully chosen to minimize cross-hybridization with pseudogenes (eukaryotes) or related species (bacteria and viruses). The Tm of the probe should allow both favorable hybrid stability and discrimination

between related sequences under the stringency of the assay. Oligonucleotide probes are often prepared with covalent attachment of a reporter molecule (such as fluorescent dyes) or affinity labels that allow them to be attached to solid supports. Probes used in homogeneous (real-time) PCR are usually oligonucleotides with a fluorescent label.

Estimating Tm of Oligonucleotide Probes

Significant progress in nearest neighbor stability calculations now allows probe Tm estimation to within 2 °C. A unified thermodynamic database has been compiled, and new parameters for all possible single mismatches and dangling ends have been estimated. Many software programs and Web sites are available for in silico Tm estimation.

Purity of Labeled Oligonucleotide Probes

The purity of labeled oligonucleotide probes is an important factor for success in hybridization assays and critical in homogeneous PCR assays. Commercial oligonucleotides with a fluorescent label are of variable purity. End users are well advised to assess the concentration and purity of all fluorescently labeled probes before use. A good method is to first calculate the predicted molar absorptivity (usually referred to in tables by the older term "extinction coefficient") of the oligonucleotide at 260 nm ($e_{260(oligo)}$) using nearest-neighbor absorbance values. These values have been tabulated and are used by many software programs to calculate the related value, nanomole per absorbance unit at 260 nm, or $nmol/A_{260(oligo)}$. Next the concentration of the fluorescent label (C_{fluor}) can be calculated from the molar absorptivities provided in the literature or by the supplier:

$$C_{fluor} = A_{\lambda max\ of\ fluor}/e_{\lambda max\ of\ fluor}$$

The concentration of the fluorescently labeled oligonucleotide is calculated as:

$$C_{oligo} = [A_{260} - (A_{\lambda max\ of\ fluor} \times e_{260(fluor)}/e_{\lambda max\ of\ fluor})]/e_{260(oligo)}$$

This equation takes into account the A_{260} contribution from the fluorophore. Similar equations for more than one label can be derived. The concentrations of fluorophore and oligonucleotide should be nearly equal (i.e., the ratio of fluorophore to oligonucleotide should be near 1). Acceptable ratios are between 0.8 and 1.2. Ratios less than 0.8 suggest incomplete labeling or destruction of the attached dye. Ratios greater than 1.2 suggest the presence of free dye. A ratio near 1 is a necessary but not a sufficient criterion of a pure probe. Co-elution of the A_{260} peak and the fluorescence peak on reversed-phase HPLC is additional evidence of purity.

Hybridization Assays—Examples

Hybridization reactions are divided into two broad categories: *solid-phase*, in which either probe or target is tethered to a solid support while the other is in solution, and *solution-phase*, in which both are in solution (Table 5-3). Somewhat surprisingly, nucleic acids bound on a solid matrix can still bind complementary nucleic acids. Solid-phase assays are useful because multiple samples are processed together, facilitating control, washing, and separation procedures. Hybridization on a solid support is, however, less efficient than solution-hybridization, and the kinetics are slower and more difficult to predict. Both solid-phase and liquid-phase assays are used routinely in the clinical laboratory. Solid-phase assays include dot blots, line probes, arrays, in situ hybridization, and Southern and Northern blotting.

Several classical hybridization methods used probe-target hybridization in solution, followed by either the removal of the unbound labeled probe (by exclusion chromatography or electrophoresis) or capture of the probe-target hybrid (by hydroxyapatite, magnetic particles, or other affinity capture methods). The signal from the labeled probe-target complex is then measured. For example, *hybrid capture* methods use a bound antibody that is specific for RNA-DNA hybrid molecules that are formed during solution-phase hybridization of a DNA sample and an unlabeled RNA probe. The assay has been adapted to a microtiter plate format for automation of washing and detection.

Recently solution hybridization has been combined with amplification, detection, and quantification all in the same

tube. Such closed-tube, real-time assays do not require any additions, washing, or separation steps.

Dot-Blot and Line-Probe Assays

Conventional hybridization assays on membranes are known as dot blots or line probes, depending on the geometry of the individual spots. The nucleic acids are applied with suction, using a commercially available manifold that results in a shape that is either round (dot) or elongated (line or slot). After immobilization the membrane is incubated with complementary nucleic acid at a constant temperature, followed by one or more washes to discriminate matched from mismatched nucleic acid. The method allows multiple probe-target hybridizations to be carried out simultaneously under identical conditions.

Two general formats are used for these assays: either multiple samples are affixed to the solid support and interrogated by a small number of probes ("sample-down"), or multiple probes are attached to the support and a small number of samples are used ("probe-down") (Figure 5-19). In the sample-down format, purified nucleic acid or amplified fragments from multiple samples are immobilized on the support.

In the probe-down format, unlabeled probes bound to the filter are allowed to interact directly with a specimen that carries the label (a technique also known as "reverse dot blot"). Alternatively, instead of having to label the sample, a set of secondary probes can be used for signal generation. Signal probes are attached to the filter only through sample-mediated

TABLE 5-3	Hybridization Assays
Solid-Phase Hybridization	• Dot-blot and line-probe assays • Arrays (microarrays and medium-density arrays) • In situ hybridization • Southern and Northern blotting
Solution-Phase Hybridization	• Real-time (or homogeneous) PCR • PCR melting analysis • Other classical techniques

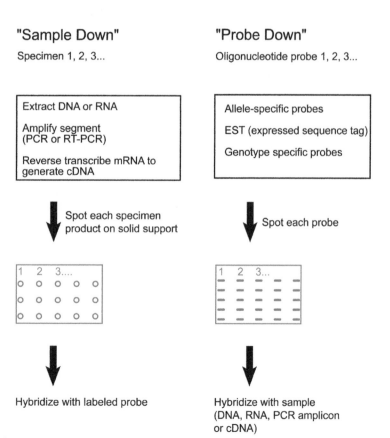

Figure 5-19

Two modes of dot-blot and line-probe assays. In the "sample-down" mode, DNA, cDNA, RNA, or amplified products are attached to the solid support and hybridized to labeled probes in solution. Alternatively, different probes are spotted onto the support ("probe-down"), and the sample is in solution.

hybridization; the sample nucleic acid forms a sandwich between the immobilized probe and the signal-generating probe. Similar assays have been developed substituting microtiter plate wells for filters. This requires chemical modification of the plastic wells to bind short DNA probes at one end, allowing the bound probes to hybridize to sample, but this approach is more amenable to automation of washing and detection.

Results of a dot-blot or line-probe assay are usually qualitative: if hybridization has occurred, a signal is generated at the specified spot and a simple yes or no interpretation is given. As the number of probes or samples increases, it becomes challenging to find a hybridization condition that provides high stringency for all probe-target combinations.

Arrays

Extending further the density of hybridization assays, microarrays (also called DNA arrays or DNA chips) were introduced in the mid 1990s.[10] Compared with dot-blot and line-probe assays, spot sizes in microarrays are decreased (typically to less than 200 microns in diameter) such that one array can contain thousands of spots. This dimensional change requires specialized detection equipment, software, and informatics to analyze the data. Microarrays are fabricated on solid surfaces (generally on glass, but sometimes on other supports, such as gel pads or coated gold surfaces) either by in situ synthesis of oligonucleotides or by physical spotting of probes with the aid of robotic arraying equipment or electronic addressing. (See also Chapter 6.) Because of their massively parallel capacity, microarrays have attracted tremendous interest among researchers who wish to monitor the whole genome (or at least a significant portion of the genome) for (1) identification of sequence polymorphisms and mutations and (2) quantification of gene expression. The development of expressed-sequence tag (EST) clone libraries has greatly contributed to the advancement of gene expression microarrays. ESTs are short sequences that are expressed in certain cells, tissues, or organs at different developmental stages (Figure 5-20). An example of a two-color comparative EST microarray used in gene expression studies is shown in Figure 5-21. Studying gene expression in tumors can lead to the discovery of new diagnostic or prognostic markers and novel therapeutic targets. For example, characteristic patterns of gene expression have been used to classify breast

tumors into clinically relevant subgroups. Expression microarrays have also identified specific signaling pathways in follicular lymphoma transformation, suggesting therapeutic targets. The promise of microarrays is accompanied by challenges, including the need for strict requirements for analytical controls and good experimental design.

Following the advent of high-density microarrays, arrays of lower density were introduced that still process more hybridization reactions than classical dot-blot or line-probe formats. Sometimes called *medium-density arrays*, these tools are emerging in the clinical laboratory for genetic disease, oncology, and pharmacogenetic testing of specimens for multiple mutations. Many companies are involved in the supply of microarray and medium-density array systems, and the industry is moving swiftly. The arrays do not need to be attached to a two-dimensional surface as long as their "address" can be decoded. For example, microspheres can be coded by fluorescence intensity in two different channels, while fluorescence in a third channel monitors hybridization. All channels can be read simultaneously using a flow cytometer. Some characteristics of arrays are listed in Table 5-4.

In Situ Hybridization

In situ hybridization is a specialized type of solid-support assay in which morphologically intact tissue, cells, or chromosomes affixed to a glass microscope slide provide the matrix for hybridization. The process is analogous to immunohistochemistry except that nucleic acids instead of antibodies are used as probes. The strength of the method lies in linking morphological evaluation with detection of specific nucleic acid sequences. When fluorescent probes are applied to metaphase chromosome spreads or interphase nuclei, the technique is referred to as fluorescent in situ hybridization or FISH. The technique allows rapid detection of numerical aberrations or translocations of chromosomes. FISH has also been combined with immunohistochemistry so that information on both the amount of protein expression and the gene dosage can be obtained on the same slide. In tissue, in situ hybridization is appropriate when localization of a target is important. Interpretation of the patterns requires experience in histology and histopathology. In situ hybridization can provide information on the amount of mRNA (or "gene expression") but not on the size or structure of the mRNA. As might be expected, hybridization within a tissue matrix is more variable than in solution or on well-characterized chemical surfaces.

Real-Time PCR

In real-time PCR, data are collected during nucleic acid amplification rather than at a single end point. The technique uses fluorescent reporter molecules and instrumentation that records fluorescence during thermal cycling. The data obtained provide information on the identity, quantity, and sequence of the nucleic acid sample. Fluorescent dyes or probes capable of signaling the relative quantity of DNA are added to the PCR mixture before amplification. The same reaction tube is used for amplification and fluorescence monitoring, and there are no sample transfers, reagent additions, or gel separation steps. This eliminates the risk of product contamination in subsequent reactions. Because the process is simple and fast, real-time PCR is replacing many conventional techniques in the clinical laboratory.

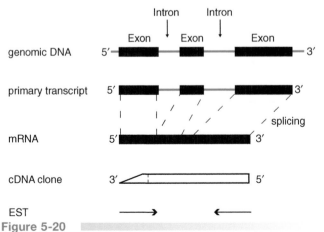

Figure 5-20
ESTs can be used as probes to identify expressed genes by hybridizing to mRNA or cDNA.

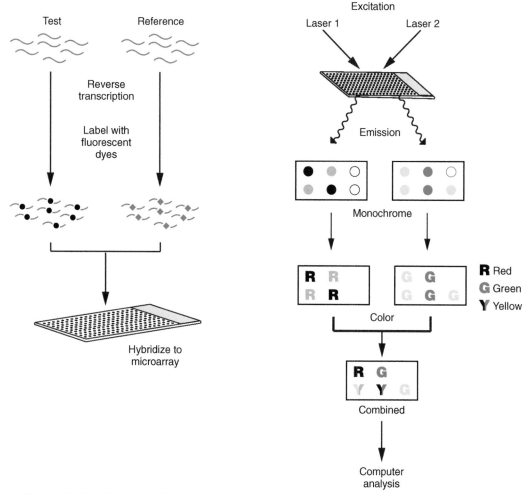

Figure 5-21

A two-color microarray experiment. An array of DNA clones representing ESTs is affixed to a glass slide. mRNAs in the test and reference specimen are converted into differentially labeled cDNA by reverse transcription and incorporation of two different fluorescent dyes. The two samples are hybridized together onto the array. The array is washed, and the image is captured twice, each time with a laser of a wavelength that excites one of the dyes but not the other. The monochromatic images are then converted to two colors (green for the test sample [G], and red for the reference [R]), and the images are combined. If the abundance of cDNA is the same in each of the two samples, then the composite spot will be shown as yellow [Y]. If one is in greater abundance, then that color will be preserved. Upregulation and downregulation of gene expression are then analyzed by software.

TABLE 5-4	Microarrays and Medium-Density Arrays		
Type of Array Surface	**What Is Tethered on the Array Surface**	**Hybridization**	**Detection**
Glass (microscope slides, silicon wafers) Chemically coated transducers (gold electrodes, gold-coated piezoelectric crystals) Microelectrodes coated with gel pads Microsphere beads (4 μm diameter, stained with fluorescent dye)	Oligonucleotide probes are synthesized either in situ (on-chip) or by conventional synthesis followed by on-chip immobilization Expressed-sequence tags (200-500 bases long) Sample DNA or cDNA (by electronic processing)	Typically the array is exposed to labeled sample DNA or labeled sample cDNA (and less frequently to labeled probes), hybridized, and the identity and/or abundance of complementary sequences is determined	Fluorescence detection: confocal or laser scanning devices, CCD cameras, near-infrared imaging, surface plasmon resonance imaging, flow cytometry (for microspheres) Other: electronic detection, mass spectrometry

Real-time PCR was first described using ethidium bromide to monitor the accumulation of a double-stranded PCR product with the fluorescence signal recorded once each cycle.[2] If target DNA is present, the fluorescence increases. How early during PCR one begins to see a signal depends on the initial amount of target DNA, and this provides a systematic method of quantification. Further, when fluorescence is continuously monitored as the temperature is increased, a melting curve is generated. Often the first derivative of this melting curve is plotted to visually aid a person in determining the position of the Tm. Melting analysis is used to verify the identity of the amplified product and to detect sequence variants down to a single base (Figure 5-22). Real-time PCR and melting analysis are considered "dynamic" hybridization assays in which the formation or dissociation of the probe-target duplex (or product duplex) is monitored in real time.

Dyes and Probe Formats for Real-Time PCR

Many different fluorescent reporter systems are used in real-time PCR, and some of the more common ones are shown in Figure 5-23. Many methods use probes with sequences complementary to the target. Others rely on the specificity afforded by PCR primers, and some have the additional option of melting analysis to verify the Tm of the probe or product.

Double-Stranded DNA Binding Dyes

Although ethidium bromide was the first dye used in real-time PCR, SYBR Green I is most widely used today. Introduced to real-time PCR in 1997, SYBR Green I has fluorescent properties similar to those of fluorescein, allowing the use of commonly available real-time optics. Both ethidium bromide and SYBR Green I exhibit an increase in fluorescence when bound to dsDNA (see Figure 5-23, row one), but the performance of SYBR Green I in real-time PCR surpasses that of ethidium bromide because of the very low background fluorescence of the free dye and because it better distinguishes double strands from single strands of nucleic acids. SYBR Green I is often used for real-time quantification when the specificity of a probe is not needed and the cost of probes is avoided.

One disadvantage of SYBR Green I is that it inhibits amplification at dye concentrations that are needed to saturate the amount of DNA usually produced by PCR. As a result, there is not enough SYBR Green I to go around and low Tm products are poorly detected in a multiplex amplification. Recently, alternative "saturating" DNA dyes that do not inhibit PCR have been developed. These dyes enable very simple solutions for genotyping and mutation scanning[7] that were previously not possible with SYBR Green I.

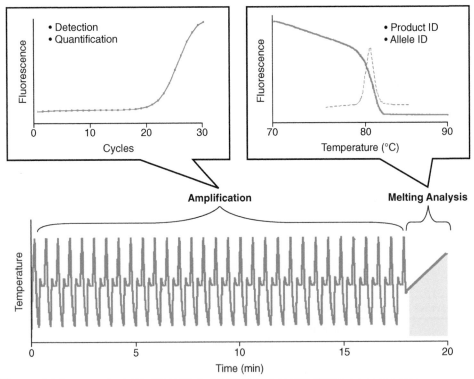

Figure 5-22

Real-time monitoring during amplification and melting analysis. The bottom panel shows a typical rapid-cycle temperature profile that is followed by a temperature ramp for melting analysis. When fluorescence is monitored during amplification once each cycle *(dotted lines),* it provides information on the presence or absence of specific target sequences and allows quantification of the target. When fluorescence is monitored continuously through the melting phase *(shaded area),* it can provide information that verifies target identification or establishes genotype.

(Modified with permission of the publisher from Wittwer CT, Kusukawa N. Real-time PCR. In Persing DH, Tenover FC, Versalovic J, Tang YW, Unger ER, Relman DA, White TJ [eds.], Molecular microbiology: Diagnostic principles and practice, Washington, DC: ASM Press, 2004:71-84. © 2004 ASM Press.)

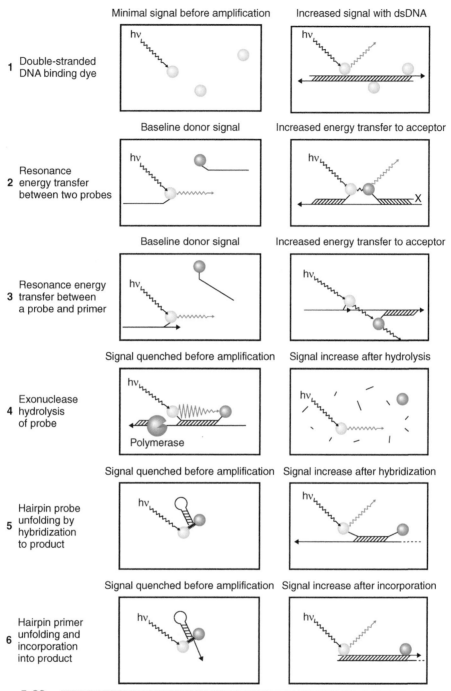

Minimal signal before amplification   Increased signal with dsDNA

1 Double-stranded
DNA binding dye

Baseline donor signal   Increased energy transfer to acceptor

2 Resonance
energy transfer
between two probes

Baseline donor signal   Increased energy transfer to acceptor

3 Resonance energy
transfer between
a probe and primer

Signal quenched before amplification   Signal increase after hydrolysis

4 Exonuclease
hydrolysis
of probe

Polymerase

Signal quenched before amplification   Signal increase after hybridization

5 Hairpin probe
unfolding by
hybridization
to product

Signal quenched before amplification   Signal increase after incorporation

6 Hairpin primer
unfolding and
incorporation
into product

Figure 5-23
Common probes and dyes for real-time PCR. *(1)* dsDNA dyes show a significant increase in fluorescence when bound to DNA (*hv* = excitation light). *(2)* Adjacent hybridization probes. FRET is illustrated between a donor and acceptor fluorophore. The "x" indicates termination of the 3′ end of the probe to prevent polymerase extension. *(3)* FRET between a labeled primer and a single hybridization probe. *(4)* Hydrolysis probes are cleaved between the reporter and quencher, resulting in increased fluorescence. *(5)* Hairpin probes are quenched in the native conformation, but increase in fluorescence when hybridized. *(6)* Hairpin primers retain their native, quenched conformation until they are incorporated into a double-stranded product.
(Modified with permission of the publisher from Pritham GH, Wittwer CT: Continuous fluorescent monitoring of PCR. J Clin Lig Assay 1998, 21:404-12. © 1998 Clinical Ligand Assay Society, Inc.)

Fluorescently Labeled Primers

Labeled primers also are used to monitor PCR. In one system, a primer with a 5′ hairpin is labeled with a fluorophore and a quencher so that fluorescence is quenched in the hairpin conformation. When the primer straightens out during PCR, fluorescence increases (see Figure 5-23, row six). If the sequence of the primer is carefully considered, the quencher moiety is not necessary. Nonhairpin primers with a single label also are used for detection and genotyping because of changes in fluorescence that occur with hybridization.

One advantage of fluorescently labeled primers over dsDNA dyes is that multiplexing is possible. However, with both dsDNA dyes and labeled primers, reaction specificity depends on the primers. Any double-stranded product that is formed will be detected, including primer-dimers. Therefore hot start techniques, temperature discrimination by collecting real-time data at a high temperature, and melting curve analysis to confirm the desired product are useful.

Probe-Specific Detection

The use of fluorescent probes in PCR provides an additional level of specificity to the process. Fluorescent probes that hybridize to PCR products during amplification change fluorescence by two possible mechanisms: (1) a covalent bond between two dyes is broken by hydrolysis or made through ligation, or (2) the fluorescence change follows reversible hybridization of the probe to the target. Following this distinction, when an irreversible covalent bond is involved, the probes are called *hydrolysis probes*. When probes reversibly change fluorescence on duplex formation, they are called *hybridization probes*. One major difference between the two probe types is that melting analysis is possible with hybridization probes, but not with probes that have been hydrolyzed.

Hybridization Probes. These probes change fluorescence upon hybridization, usually by fluorescence resonance energy transfer. Two interacting fluorophores may be placed on adjacent probes (see Figure 5-23, row two), or one may be placed on a primer and the other on a probe (see Figure 5-23, row three). Only one probe with one fluorophore may be necessary if the fluorescence is quenched by deoxyguanosine residues. Another single-labeled probe design uses thiazole orange attached to a peptide nucleic acid. In each of these designs, the fluorescence change with hybridization is reversible with melting.

Hydrolysis Probes. Fluorophore-labeled probes can be synthesized with a quencher molecule located in a position on the DNA that allows it to quench the fluorescence from the fluorophore molecule. If the probe is hydrolyzed between the fluorophore and the quencher during PCR, fluorescence will increase. The most common implementation uses the 5′-exonuclease activity of the DNA polymerase to hydrolyze the probe and dissociate the labels (see Figure 5-23, row four). This method has been simplified by putting the fluorophores on opposite ends of the probe. Hybrid-stabilizing agents, such as a minor-groove binder, can be added to the probe to make the system more robust. Dual-labeled probes can also be cleaved using a DNAzyme (a DNA molecule that acts as a catalyst) generated during PCR. Finally, irreversible ligation also has been used for homogeneous genotyping with a fluorescent readout. Hydrolysis probes generate fluorescence through changes in covalent bonds. The change in fluorescence signal is irreversible, and melting analysis of the hydrolyzed probe is not useful.

Mixed Mechanism Probes. Several probe systems appear to function by both hydrolysis and hybridization mechanisms. These include (1) hairpin probes, (2) self-probing amplicon primers, and (3) displacement probes. A hairpin probe functions similarly to a hairpin primer in that it is designed to increase in fluorescence when the distance between the quencher and the reporter increases upon target hybridization (see Figure 5-23, row five). Similarly, primers that result in self-probing amplicons have a hairpin that separates quencher from reporter when hybridized. Competitive displacement probes separate quencher and reporter by competitive hybridization. However, in all three cases, polymerases with exonuclease activity are usually used, and the labeled probes are potential substrates for exonuclease cleavage. Indeed, the fluorescence versus cycle number plots often resemble irreversible hydrolysis rather than reversible hybridization (Figure 5-24). Conversely, many exonuclease probes, especially probes labeled on each end, show significant hybridization signals.

Detection and Quantification in Real-Time PCR

When fluorescence is monitored once each cycle in the presence of SYBR Green I, the data closely follow the expected logistic shape discussed earlier (see Figures 5-2 and 5-24, top left). However, with hydrolysis probes, fluorescence is cumulative and continues to increase even after the amount of product reaches a plateau (see Figure 5-24, top middle). In contrast, reactions monitored with hybridization probes may show a decrease in fluorescence at high cycle number (see Figure 5-24, top right). Despite differences in curve shape, all real-time systems follow the amount of product being produced during PCR, and this information is used for detection and quantification.

Detection

A fluorescent signal that increases during PCR and follows one of the expected curve shapes suggests that the specific target is present and was amplified. In contrast, a signal that stays at background even after 40 to ~50 PCR cycles suggests that the target is absent and that no amplification occurred. Algorithms that analyze the entire curve are more robust than simple threshold methods. Adequate positive controls (to rule out inhibitory factors) and adequate negative controls (to rule out product contamination and nonspecific signal generation) are necessary. If the fluorescent signal is reversible with hybridization, melting analysis can be used to verify the expected Tm of the probe or product.

When specificity of the assay depends only on the primers ("primer-specific detection," as is the case when DNA dyes or labeled primers are used), the possibility of unexpectedly amplifying other targets or primer-dimers is a concern. One technique to eliminate or decrease the detection of unexpected targets is to acquire fluorescence during each cycle at a temperature just below the melting transition of the expected target. To illustrate the concept, Figure 5-25 shows a first-derivative melting curve of products at the end of a PCR that generated unexpected products along with the desired product. The signal was generated with SYBR Green I, a dye that detects all dsDNA. The plot reveals both lower Tm species that are unexpected products and a single Gaussian-shaped peak that is centered on the target's predicted Tm. If fluorescence is

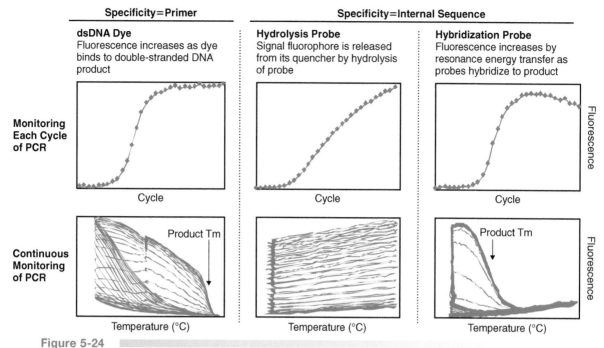

Figure 5-24

Monitoring in real time. The top row shows data collected once each PCR cycle, and the bottom row shows data collected continuously (five times per second) during all PCR cycles. Three different reporter systems are shown.

(Modified with permission of the publisher from Wittwer CT, Kusukawa N. Real-time PCR. In Persing DH, Tenover FC, Versalovic J, Tang YW, Unger ER, Relman DA, White TJ [eds.], Molecular microbiology: Diagnostic principles and practice, Washington, DC: ASM Press, 2004:71-84. © 2004 ASM Press.)

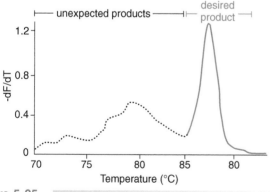

Figure 5-25

First-derivative melting curve showing the target (at high Tm, *solid line*) and nonspecific PCR products (at lower Tm, *dotted line*).

(Modified by permission of the publisher from Morrison TB, Weiss JJ, and Wittwer CT: Quantification of low-copy transcripts by continuous SYBR Green I monitoring during amplification. BioTechniques 1998, 24:954-63. © 1998 Eaton Publishing.)

acquired during each cycle at (in this case) 85 °C, the unexpected products will be denatured and will not contribute to the signal.

Multiplexing of detection is possible with probes that are labeled with different-color dyes or with probes that have different Tm. Examples in the clinical laboratory include probe multiplexing to detect the presence of more than one infectious organism or to discriminate an internal control template from the target.

Quantification

Real-time PCR offers a convenient and systematic approach to quantification by monitoring the amount of product each cycle. Perhaps the most popular clinical use of real-time PCR is in the assessment of viral load, particularly for HIV and HCV. The clinical need for quantification is well established, and real-time methods give rapid and precise answers. However, other amplification systems, particularly transcription-based and branched DNA methods, are also popular in this highly competitive field. Additional quantitative applications of real-time PCR include quantification of mRNAs (after reverse transcription) in gene-expression studies and assessment of gene dosage in genetics and oncology.

One of the advantages of real-time PCR is its large dynamic range. Figure 5-26, A shows an extended range of external calibrators in a typical real-time PCR. As the initial template concentration increases, the curves shift to earlier cycles. The extent of the shift depends on the PCR efficiency (Table 5-5). The cycle at which fluorescence rises above background correlates inversely with the log of the initial template concentration (Figure 5-26). This "cycle" is actually a *virtual* cycle that includes a fractional component determined by interpolation, which can be calculated by several methods. One method uses the maximum *second derivative* of the curve to determine the cycle number (Figure 5-27). The second derivative is derived

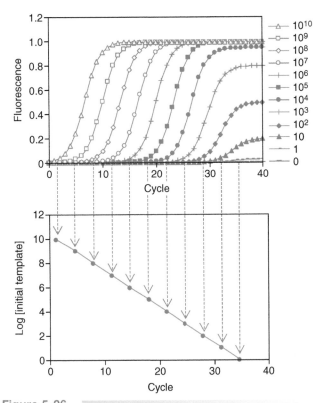

Figure 5-26
Quantification by real-time PCR. Shown are typical real-time curves for amplification reactions of varying initial target concentrations (panel A) and the log of the initial concentration plotted against the cycle number at which the signal rises above background (panel B) as calculated by the second derivative maximum (see Figure 5-27). (Modified with permission of the publisher from Wittwer CT, Kusukawa N. Real-time PCR. In Persing DH, Tenover FC, Versalovic J, Tang YW, Unger ER, Relman DA, White TJ [eds.], Molecular microbiology: Diagnostic principles and practice, Washington, DC: ASM Press, 2004:71-84. © 2004 ASM Press.)

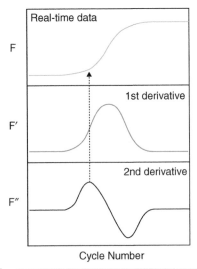

Figure 5-27
Finding the cycle number at which fluorescence rises above background. Real-time fluorescence data (F) from the amplification reaction are shown with the first (F') and second (F'') derivatives. The maximum of the second derivative corresponds to a defined point on the real-time data where the curve starts to rise.
(Modified with permission of the publisher from Wittwer CT, Kusukawa N. Real-time PCR. In Persing DH, Tenover FC, Versalovic J, Tang YW, Unger ER, Relman DA, White TJ [eds.], Molecular microbiology: Diagnostic principles and practice, Washington, DC: ASM Press, 2004:71-84. © 2004 ASM Press.)

TABLE 5-5	Relationship of PCR Efficiency and Amplification Curve Spacing
PCR Efficiency	**Cycles/Log [DNA]***
2.0	3.32
1.9	3.59
1.8	3.92
1.7	4.34
1.6	4.90
1.5	5.68

From Wittwer CT, Kusukawa N. Real-time PCR. In Persing DH, Tenover FC, Versalovic J, Tang YW, Unger ER, Relman DA, White TJ (eds.), Molecular microbiology: Diagnostic principles and practice, Washington, DC: ASM Press, 2004:71-84. © 2004 ASM Press.
*The number of cycles that separate each decade difference in initial template concentration (cycles/log [DNA]) is 1/log (efficiency). The calibration curve slope is the negative of this value (−1/log [efficiency]), assuming the log (initial template) is plotted on the x-axis as the independent variable and cycle number is plotted on the y-axis as the dependent variable.

from the shape of the curves, and there is no need to adjust baselines or worry about normalizing the fluorescence values. Alternatively, in *threshold analysis*, a fluorescence level is selected that intersects with the amplification curves, and the fractional cycle numbers are found by interpolation. In this case it is necessary to adjust the fluorescence baseline before comparing different samples. Usually an early cycle interval is chosen (e.g., cycles 5 to 10) to represent the baseline. In *arithmetic adjustment*, all baselines are adjusted to zero by subtracting a curve-specific constant. In *proportional adjustment*, each baseline is first adjusted to 1.0 by dividing by a curve-specific constant, followed by subtraction of 1.0 from all points to bring the baseline to zero. Amplification curves can also be *normalized* to between 0.0 and 1.0 with the equation $\Phi_{normalized} = (\Phi_{measured} - \Phi_{min})/(\Phi_{max} - \Phi_{min})$. However, even with appropriate baseline adjustment, threshold quantification will fail if the sample fluorescence does not reach the threshold (as may happen with low copy samples).

Calibration and Precision
The accuracy of real-time PCR quantification depends not only on the method chosen to analyze the curves, but also on the

quality of calibrators used. Purified PCR products quantified by spectrophotometry are easily obtained. When serially diluted, these can be used as calibrators. Alternatively, purified plasmids or genomic DNA are used as calibrators. Limiting dilution analysis to determine the amount of "amplifiable" DNA is seldom necessary. The precision of quantitative real-time PCR depends on the copy number. When the initial target concentration is low, imprecision is high. Part of the variance comes from stochastic limitations as defined by the Poisson distribution as described earlier. In addition, the PCR efficiency may be more variable at low copy numbers.

Melting Analysis

Not only can amplification, detection, and quantification be performed by homogeneous hybridization, but detailed genotyping information can also be obtained. Genotyping is best performed in the same tube by monitoring the melting of hybridized duplexes during controlled heating, producing a melting curve signature for the duplex. Such a signature monitors duplex binding over a range of temperatures in contrast to the single-temperature analysis of conventional hybridization techniques, such as dot blots or microarrays. The advantages of complete melting curves also apply when considering only homogeneous techniques. For example, methods that rely on hydrolysis for signal generation and/or those that acquire data only at one temperature generally result in more genotyping errors. Real-time amplification and melting analysis make up a powerful combination of techniques that only requires temperature control and sampling of fluorescence. Many other genotyping techniques require complex separation and/or detection equipment after PCR. Real-time PCR with melting curve analysis allows detection, quantification, and genotyping in less than 30 minutes (see Figure 5-22) without ancillary processing or additional equipment.

When fluorescence is monitored continuously within each cycle of PCR, the hybridization characteristics of PCR products and probes can be observed (see Figure 5-24, bottom panels). With SYBR Green I, the melting characteristics of the amplified DNA can identify the product. No hybridization information is revealed with hydrolysis probes, whereas the melting of hybridization probes is readily apparent. Probe melting occurs at a characteristic temperature that can be exploited to confirm target identity and to analyze sequence alterations under the probe. For routine testing in the clinical laboratory, a single melting curve is usually performed at the end of PCR instead of monitoring hybridization throughout the entire PCR process (see Figure 5-22).

Melting Protocols

Immediately after the last PCR cycle, the samples are momentarily denatured (90 °C to 94 °C), cooled to about 10 °C below the Tm range of interest, and finally heated at a ramp rate of 0.1 °C to 0.3 °C while continuously monitoring fluorescence. When hybridization probes are used, the cooling protocol should maximize formation of probe-target duplexes while minimizing formation of the duplex PCR product. Minor primer asymmetry (1:2 to 1:4) and use of 5′-exonuclease–deficient polymerases may be helpful. Rapid cooling (at rates of ~20 °C/s) to 10 °C above the Tm interest range, followed by slow cooling at 0.1 °C to 1.0 °C/s to 10 °C below the interest range, favors probe-target duplex formation of all alleles.

SNP Detection by Melting Curve Analysis

A hybridization probe-pair placed over a heterozygous polymorphism is shown in Figure 5-28. The reporter probe is complementary to the normal allele. As the temperature is increased, the mismatched mutant hybrid melts first, giving the first transition, followed by the matched normal hybrid. The Tms of both hybrids are easily seen in derivative plots. A well-optimized probe design will provide a Tm difference of 8 °C to ~10 °C for a single base mismatch under the probe.

SNP genotyping by melting curve analysis has been achieved with a variety of probe and dye methods.[14] The top row of

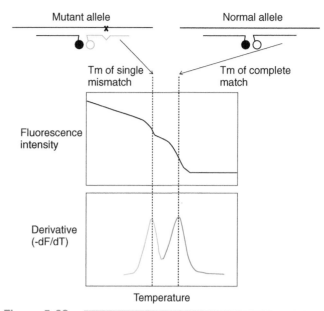

Figure 5-28

Melting curve SNP genotyping. A heterozygous specimen with an SNP under the probe is amplified and melted. Two temperature transitions are visible, one from the mutant allele that is mismatched with the probe and melts at a lower temperature and one from the normal allele that is completely matched with the probe and melts at a higher temperature. The derivative plot shows the Tms of both the mutant-probe and the normal-probe duplexes as peaks.

(Modified with permission of the publisher from Bernard PS, Pritham GH, Wittwer CT: Color multiplexing hybridization probes using the apolipoprotein E locus as a model system for genotyping. Anal Biochem 1999; 273:221-8. © 1999 Academic Press.)

Figure 5-29 shows the design of traditional hybridization probe pairs and the results of homozygous wild-type, mutant, and heterozygous samples that are well discriminated from each other. Virtually the same result is achieved by use of a single hybridization probe in which the fluorescent signal is quenched on the free probe but dequenched as it forms a hybrid with the target (second row). The third row shows a design in which no probe is used, and the signal is provided by either a labeled primer that is incorporated into the amplicon or a saturating DNA binding dye; the melting profile of the PCR product is used for genotyping. Finally the last row shows a design with an unlabeled probe and a saturating DNA binding dye. The last two methods are advantageous in that fluorescently labeled oligonucleotides are not required.

Mutation Scanning by Melting Curve Analysis

In earlier sections of this chapter, detection of heteroduplexes (either by electrophoresis or HPLC) was discussed as a means to scan stretches of DNA in which the presence of a polymorphism is suspected. Melting analysis with saturating dyes also has been used to detect heteroduplexes with equal or better sensitivity than these methods without the necessity of taking the amplified reaction mixture out of its tube.[7] Scanning sensitivity and specificity depend on melting resolution, and high-resolution melting instruments have recently become available. The melting data are normalized between 0% and 100% fluorescence, and the curves shifted in temperature to overlap at low fluorescence levels. An example of heteroduplex detection

| # Required | | Design | Derivative of Melting Curve |
Probes	Labels		
Two	Two	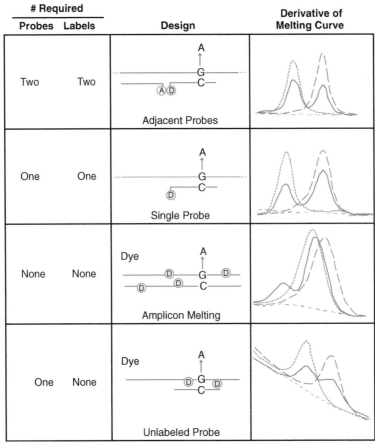 Adjacent Probes	
One	One	Single Probe	
None	None	Dye — Amplicon Melting	
One	None	Dye — Unlabeled Probe	

Figure 5-29

Four modes of SNP genotyping by melting analysis. The traditional hybridization-probe design *(top row)* uses a pair of probes, one labeled with an acceptor fluorophore (circle A) and the other with a donor fluorophore (circle D). The single hybridization probe design *(second row)* lacks the second probe. The amplicon melting design *(third row)* uses a saturating dsDNA binding dye. The two homozygotes, although close in Tm, can be differentiated on high-resolution instruments, and the heterozygote has an additional low-temperature transition caused by heteroduplexes. The unlabeled-probe design *(bottom row)*, similar to amplicon melting, does not require a covalently attached fluorescent label and requires a saturating DNA binding dye. However, because a probe is used, the derivative melting curves are better separated than with amplicon melting. Homozygous G allele *(dashed line in far right column)*, homozygous A allele *(dotted line)*, and the GA heterozygote *(solid line)*.

and SNP genotyping by melting curve analysis is shown in Figure 5-30. The PCR product was more than 500 bases in length, and the melting curves showed two clear melting domains. The SNP was present in the lower melting domain, and all genotypes were distinguishable. High-resolution melting analysis can scan genes for mutations and establish HLA genotypic identity.

Comparison of Closed-Tube SNP Genotyping Methods

There are many methods for SNP genotyping, and the method of choice depends on several factors, including turnaround time and throughput requirements. The necessities of high-volume genomic research are different from those of a clinical reference laboratory, a medical clinic, or the STAT laboratories of the future.

Methods for homogeneous SNP analysis in a closed-tube system differ greatly in their level of complexity (Figure 5-31).

The number of oligonucleotides required varies from 2 to 8. The simpler techniques do not require probes at all, although some of the more complex techniques require up to three labels or modifications on each probe. All of these methods use fluorescence and solution hybridization. Some of the methods that use melting analysis will detect more than two alleles if present; those based on allele-specific amplification or end-point analysis are limited to two.

The four simplest methods do not use fluorescently labeled probes. Amplicon melting requires only two primers and a saturating DNA dye (see Figure 5-29, row three). Unlabeled probe genotyping requires three oligonucleotides and a saturating DNA dye (Figure 5-29, bottom row). Allele-specific PCR requires three primers and is based on a preference by the polymerase to extend only a perfectly matched primer. By monitoring the reaction each cycle, genotyping and even allele frequencies in pools of DNA can be determined. Instead of real-time analysis, allele-specific PCR can incorporate a GC-

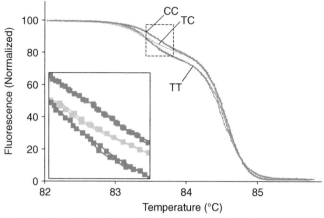

Figure 5-30
A single-nucleotide polymorphism demonstrated in a 544-bp fragment by melting analysis. Shown are high-resolution melting curves of PCR amplicons from the *HTR2A* gene locus carrying an SNP. Results are shown for six individuals, two different individuals for each of the three genotypes: wild-type homozygote (TT), mutant homozygote (CC), and heterozygote (TC). In the inset is a magnified portion of the data showing that all three genotypes can be discriminated.
(Modified by permission of the publisher from Wittwer CT, Reed GH, Gundry CN, et al. High-resolution genotyping by amplicon melting analysis using LCGreen. Clin Chem 2003;49:853-60. © AACC.)

clamp into the product of one allele so that alleles can be differentiated at the end of PCR by their Tm. Hybridization probe melting assays are intermediate in complexity. Designs with a single hybridization probe or a pair of probes are shown in Figure 5-29 (first and second rows).

The more complex closed-tube methods for SNP genotyping are end-point assays. In hybridization-probe–pair ligation, irreversible ligation of adjacent probes results in fluorescence resonance energy transfer. Allele-specific 5′-exonuclease and hairpin probes are commonly used methods. Self-probing amplicons and minor-groove binder 5′-exonuclease probes both require three modifications on two probes for SNP typing. Serial invasive signal amplification is a method of homogeneous genotyping that does not require PCR. Allele-specific PCR can be linked to hydrolysis of a dual-labeled probe by formation of a double flap gap. Finally, ligation can be used to join two ends of a long, single "padlock" probe if and only if both ends perfectly anneal to adjacent sites on the target. The resulting circle can be amplified by rolling circle amplification.

ETHICAL ISSUES

Molecular analysis can involve unique ethical issues. Some techniques such as gene sequencing and microarrays may provide information that was not requested by the physician. An example of the kind of issues that arise is given in Ethics Box 5-1.

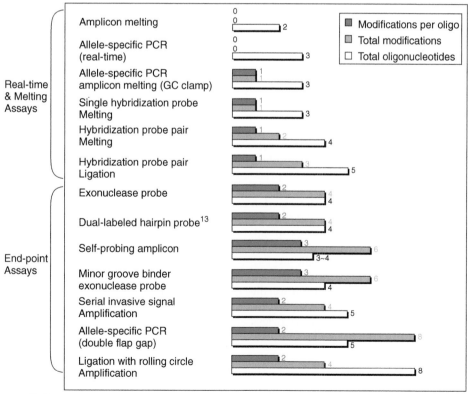

Figure 5-31
Closed-tube methods for SNP typing.[14] Methods are listed from top to bottom in ascending order of complexity. Modifications to oligonucleotides usually involve additions of a fluorophore or quencher, but occasionally 5′-tail additions of nucleotides. End-point and melting assays do not require signal acquisition during PCR. Melting analysis often detects more than two alleles, whereas the other techniques will detect only two.

ETHICS Box 5-1   Ethical Situation

You are responsible for performing an FDA-approved test for Factor V Leiden, a single base mutation that predisposes individuals to blood clots. The test uses a fluorescent probe over the mutation region and detects variants by a shift in the melting curve of the probe. In one patient, you notice that the melting curve shifts from wild type, but not by the amount expected for Factor V Leiden. You suspect a different sequence variant. You repeat the analysis and find the same results. A literature search reveals that such variants (other than the Leiden variant) have been reported by others and that it is not clear which if any of them might increase the risk of clots. Your laboratory is very busy, and there is pressure to turn out test results rapidly. You just listened to a talk by the laboratory manager about the need to control costs. What do you do?

You might rationalize that the result is not normal and that you should report the result as abnormal. This approach is problematic, however, because most sequence variants in the Factor V gene have no clinical consequences. Thus if you follow this course, the physician may erroneously put the patient on long-term anticoagulation (with rat poison!), a treatment that the patient may not need.

You might reason that the physician ordered a test for Factor V Leiden, and you have evidence that this patient does not have it. Thus you would believe it is acceptable to report the result as normal. But you believe that the patient's Factor V gene does not have the normal sequence, and this worries you.

Can you justify the expense of obtaining additional information about the DNA sequence of this patient's Factor V gene? Who has responsibility to do this? Should the patient be charged for additional sequencing of the gene? (The patient did not ask for sequencing; his physician ordered a test for Factor V Leiden.) Should the laboratory bear the expense of additional testing? Is it ethical at all to do testing beyond the test for Factor V Leiden that was ordered? Would an order from the patient's physician be adequate, or is the patient's informed consent necessary, given that the clinical significance of other variants in the gene may be unknown?

CONCLUSION

Molecular diagnostics remains a trendy, developing field in laboratory medicine. Current progress in nucleic acid techniques is extraordinary, driven by the promise of great return. Can drug therapy be tailored to each individual by appropriate molecular tests? Can diagnostic biochips parallel the microelectronics revolution, continuing to provide more information at less expense? Will complete genome sequencing for individual predisposition testing become a reality? Although we are still years away from the Star Trek tricorder, the time for immediate personalized diagnostics will come. To boldly explore these new frontiers, current and future analysis techniques will provide the starship. Indeed, the rate-limiting factor is usually in establishing the biological correlations, not the sophistication of the techniques to analyze nucleic acid. Nevertheless, simple, powerful, and cost-effective techniques will get us there sooner.

Techniques for molecular analysis often require multiple steps, including sample preparation, amplification, and analysis. As a result, successful automation is critical for their routine adoption in the clinical laboratory. However, to corruptly paraphrase Henry David Thoreau in *Civil Disobedience*—"I heartily adhere to the motto: The best automation is not needing to automate." The simplest techniques are often the best. As with immunoassays, methods that require separation and washing steps are being replaced with nonseparation methods that are rapid and homogeneous. These and other simple methods hold great promise for the clinical laboratory.

REFERENCES

1. Benson DA, Karsch-Mizrachi I, Lipman DJ, Ostell J, Rapp BA, Wheeler DL. GenBank. Nucleic Acids Res 2002;30:17-20.
2. Higuchi R, Fockler C, Dollinger G, Watson R. Kinetic PCR analysis: real-time monitoring of DNA amplification reactions. Biotechnology (N Y) 1993;11:1026-30.
3. Lander ES, Linton LM, Birren B, Nusbaum C, Zody MC, Baldwin J, et al. Initial sequencing and analysis of the human genome. Nature 2001;409:860-921.
4. Margulies M, Egholm M, Altman WE, Attiya S, Bader JS, Bemben LA, et al. Genome sequencing in microfabricated high-density picolitre reactors. Nature 2005;437:376-80.
5. Mitra RD, Butty VL, Shendure J, Williams BR, Housman DE, Church GM. Digital genotyping and haplotyping with polymerase colonies. Proc Natl Acad Sci U S A 2003;100:5926-31.
6. Perkins TT, Quake SR, Smith DE, Chu S. Relaxation of a single DNA molecule observed by optical microscopy. Science 1994;264:822-6.
7. Reed GH, Wittwer CT. Sensitivity and specificity of single-nucleotide polymorphism scanning by high-resolution melting analysis. Clin Chem 2004;50:1748-54.
8. Saiki RK, Gelfand DH, Stoffel S, Scharf SJ, Higuchi R, Horn GT, et al. Primer-directed enzymatic amplification of DNA with a thermostable DNA polymerase. Science 1988;239:487-91.
9. Sanger F, Nicklen S, Coulson AR. DNA sequencing with chain-terminating inhibitors. Proc Natl Acad Sci U S A 1977;74:5463-7.
10. Schena M, Shalon D, Davis RW, Brown PO. Quantitative monitoring of gene expression patterns with a complementary DNA microarray. Science 1995;270:467-70.
11. Schouten JP, McElgunn CJ, Waaijer R, Zwijnenburg D, Diepvens F, Pals G. Relative quantification of 40 nucleic acid sequences by multiplex ligation-dependent probe amplification. Nucleic Acids Res 2002;30:e57.
12. Seuss D. The cat in the hat comes back! Beginner Books, New York, 1958.
13. Stenson PD, Ball EV, Mort M, Phillips AD, Shiel JA, Thomas NS, et al. Human Gene Mutation Database (HGMD): 2003 update. Hum Mutat 2003;21:577-81.
14. Wittwer CT, Kusukawa N. Nucleic acid techniques. In Burtis CA, Ashwood ER, Bruns DE, eds. Tietz textbook of clinical chemistry and molecular diagnostics, 4th ed. St Louis: Saunders, 2006:1407-49.

REVIEW QUESTIONS

1. Target amplification techniques include:
   A. the PCR.
   B. the ligase chain reaction.
   C. transcription mediated amplification.
   D. strand displacement amplification.
   E. all of the above.
2. The PCR
   A. requires two primers in opposite orientations.
   B. cannot be adapted to RNA by including RT activity.
   C. cannot be performed in 15 minutes or less.
   D. requires three primers.
   E. requires a probe and two primers.
3. Fluorescent melting analysis of PCR products
   A. identifies products by their Tm rather than their size.
   B. can genotype single base changes in human DNA without probes.

C. can be performed with dyes that stain dsDNA.

D. can be used to verify the identity of the PCR product.

E. All of the above

4. Real-time PCR

A. uses gel electrophoresis or mass spectroscopy in final analysis.

B. is a technique for DNA sequencing.

C. collects data during temperature cycling.

D. cannot be used to quantify DNA.

E. cannot be used to detect more than one PCR product.

5. Which of the following is an example of a signal amplification technique?

A. PCR

B. Branched-chain amplification

C. Southern blotting

D. Northern blotting

E. Melting analysis

Chapter 6

Miniaturization: DNA Chips and Devices

Peter Wilding, Ph.D., F.R.C.Path., F.R.S.C., H.C.L.D. (A.B.B.)

OBJECTIVES

1. List the advantages of using microtechnology and nanotechnology in a molecular diagnostics laboratory.
2. Discuss the problems of hybridization microarrays, including those arising from the density of probes, interfering substances, and partial hybridization.
3. State the limitations of microdevices in regard to the amount of clinical material required.
4. Given a set of mutations within a disease genotype, design a hybridization microarray that could be incorporated into a hand-held device.

KEY WORDS AND DEFINITIONS

Array: A set of items that are randomly accessible by numeric index.
Microarray: A small piece of silicon, plastic, or glass onto whose surface has been fabricated a structured, two-dimensional array of compartments that are accessed by their position in the array.

Microfabrication: The collective term for the technologies used to fabricate components on a micrometer-sized scale.
Microfluidics: A multidisciplinary field comprising physics, chemistry, engineering, and biotechnology that studies the behavior of fluids at the microscale and mesoscale. It also concerns the design of systems in which such small volumes of fluids will be used.
Microtechnology: Technology with features near one *micrometer* (one millionth of a *meter*, or 10^{-6} meter, or 1 μm).
Minimum Feature Size: The dimension of the smallest feature actually constructed in the manufacturing process of a chip.
Nanotechnology: Technology that "involves research and technology development at the atomic, molecular, or macromolecular levels in the dimension range of approximately 1 to 100 nm. Nanotechnology research and development includes control at the nanoscale and integration of nanoscale structures into larger material components, systems, and architectures. Within these larger scale assemblies, the control and construction of their structures and components remains at the nanometer scale." (http://www.becon2.nih.gov/nstc_def_nano.htm).
Photolithography: A process used to transfer a pattern from a photomask to the surface of a substrate, such as silicon, glass, plastic, sapphire, or metal.

From the perspective of the clinical laboratory, miniaturization has been a long-term trend in clinical diagnostic instrumentation.[15] For example, capillary electrophoresis instruments, mass spectrometers, and point-of-care (POC) analyzers have been implemented on microchips of silicon, glass, or plastic.[18] This trend is continuing, as evidenced by the appearance of the very small devices resulting from developments made in the field of nanotechnology (see below). These devices are (1) approximately 100 μm in size, (2) employed in analytical measurement, and (3) fabricated using special forms that are designed for microdevices.

This chapter focuses primarily on microdevices rather than nanodevices because the latter have yet to make a significant entry into clinical laboratories. The readers should note, however, that several applications discussed later require only nanoliter (nL) quantities of a sample or deal with individual cells that may have cell volumes ranging from picoliter (pL) to nL. The chapter begins with critical definitions and a review of the key background of the field, followed by descriptions of applications of **microtechnology** that are relevant for clinical uses. The chapter concludes with a discussion, for those readers who have an interest in how such devices are fabricated, with description of some leading manufacturing techniques.

DEFINITIONS

A **microarray** is a small piece of silicon, plastic, or glass on the surface of which is a structured, two-dimensional **array** of compartments that are accessed by their position in the array.[8,28] Arrays are made by use of techniques similar to those used to fabricate computer chips; these techniques include printing, photolithography, and inkjet printing. Arrays of clinical relevance are fabricated by spotting or affixing biomolecules (such as oligonucleotides, cDNA, RNA, proteins, tissues, etc.) to the individual compartments of these microarrays. When segments of DNA molecules are affixed, the resultant arrays are known as (1) *gene chips,* (2) *DNA chips,* or (3) *biochips.* The individual segments are termed *probes,* and thousands of probes are contained on a single DNA chip. DNA chip technology is comparable with reverse dot blots (Chapter 5) in which unlabeled probes bound to filter paper are allowed to interact directly with a specimen that carries the label. Each of these is the "reverse" of Southern blotting technology in which fragmented DNA is attached to a substrate and then probed with a known gene or fragment.

Microchips have been designed for a range of chemical and biological analyses based on chromatography, electrophoresis, immunoassay, nucleic acid gene expression, and target and probe amplification.[9,14,15,18]

Nanotechnology, a term coined by Norio Taniguchi at the University of Tokyo in 1974, is used to describe rapidly emerging and converging technologies that are all based upon the scaling down of existing technologies to the next level of miniaturization. In 1981 Eric Drexler defined molecular nanotechnology as a technology based on the ability to build structures to complex, atomic specifications by means of mechanosynthesis; he published the first scientific article on the subject, "Molecular Engineering: An Approach to the Development of General Capabilities for Molecular Manipulation." Later in 1992, he authored the book *Nanosystems: Molecular Machinery, Manufacturing, and Computation.*

In 2000 the National Science and Technology Council (NSTC) expanded the definition of nanotechnology to:

> "*Nanotechnology* involves research and technology development at the atomic, molecular, or macromolecular levels in the dimension range of approximately 1 to 100 nanometers to provide fundamental understanding of phenomena and materials at the nanoscale and to create and use structures, devices, and systems that have novel properties and functions because of their small and/or intermediate size. The novel and differentiating properties and functions are developed at a critical length scale of matter typically under 100 nm. Nanotechnology research and development includes control at the nanoscale and integration of nanoscale structures into larger material components, systems, and architectures. Within these

TABLE 6-1	General and Medical Applications of Nanotechnology and Microtechnology	
General Applications	**Medical Applications**
Analytical chemistry	Basic research
Biotechnology	Disease discovery
Combinatorial chemistry	Drug development
Electronics	Drug manufacturing
Engineering	Gene expression
Environmental monitoring	Genomics
Fabrication	Genotyping
Fluidics	Medical diagnostics
Materials science	Medical screening
Pharmaceuticals	Nucleic acid analysis
Reactor technology	Proteomics
Robotics	
Waste minimization	

larger scale assemblies, the control and construction of their structures and components remains at the nanometer scale." (http://www.becon2.nih.gov/nstc_def_nano.htm).

Several leading scientists have discussed miniaturization and nanotechnology and the promises these technologies offer including (1) economy of scale, (2) ease of operation, (3) reliability of instrumentation, and (4) potential for microscale, massively parallel analyses (i.e., many analyses being performed simultaneously) (Table 6-1). Tremendous efforts are being invested in developing miniaturized devices.

BACKGROUND

Early efforts to reduce the volume requirements of clinical analyzers resulted in the modification of existing technology to use microvolume quantities of a sample. For example, in the 1970s the Chem-1 Analyzer (Technicon, Tarrytown, N.Y.) was modified to perform a single analysis on a sample volume of only 1.0 μL. Before this date, virtually all clinical analyzers used sample or reaction volumes in excess of 50 μL. By the 1980s, concerted efforts to develop hand-held devices led to the introduction of POC analyzers, such as the i-STAT system (iSTAT Corporation, East Windsor, NJ) in 1990 (Figure 6-1). This analyzer was one of the first such devices to include microfabricated electrodes and chemical sensors on silicon microchips. In addition, it featured a functional microsystem employing new fabrication technology that was associated with effective computer-based controls and monitoring capabilities. The use of photolithographic etching technology borrowed from the microelectronics industry illustrated to clinical scientists that microanalytical devices and components could be made in large numbers and be adapted effectively to include chemical components, electrodes, capacitors, and microfluidic features.

Engineering laboratories also have been successful in developing miniaturized components, such as miniature injection valves, actuators, and pumping systems that have been integrated into POC analyzers.[4] Notable efforts with distinct implications for the clinical laboratory community were microdevices for pH measurement fabricated from wafers of silicon. One of these devices facilitated the measurement of acidic metabolites, such as lactic acid from living cells confined

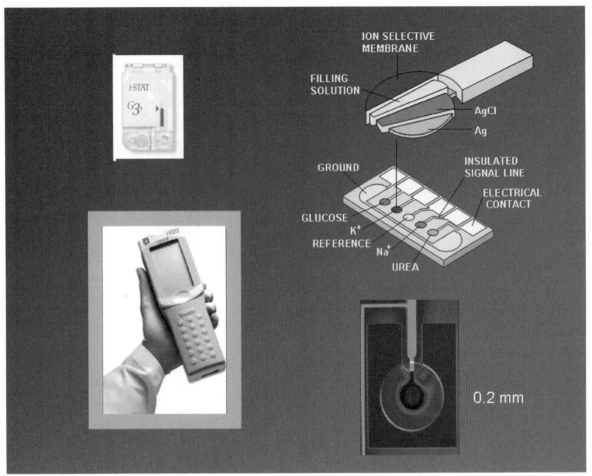

Figure 6-1
The i-STAT system showing a cartridge and the microchip-based electrode assembly.
(Reproduced by permission of i-STAT Corporation, East Windsor, N.J.)

to a flow chamber in silicon. The pH was measured using a light-addressable potentiometric sensor that detects attachment of protons to the chamber surface coated with protonatable silanol and amine groups. Using this device, the changes of metabolism in various forms of cells were monitored. In all of these developments, the exploitation of **microfabrication** techniques has been essential.

Since these early efforts, the scope of microtechnology has expanded markedly. In the early 2000s, development was driven by realization of the many potential benefits from microtechnology and by huge investments, particularly to support pharmaceutical research.[17] Hundreds of small companies worldwide have been created to exploit new fabricating techniques and to explore the potential benefit of being able to handle and process microsamples.[16,17] Notable developments that exemplify the direction of this rapidly developing field are (1) miniaturized total analytical systems (µTAS), (2) microarray-type devices for hybridization of deoxyribonucleic acid (DNA) and ribonucleic acid (RNA), and (3) microfluidic-based devices for capillary electrophoresis.

Clinical laboratorians require systems, not components, for analytical measurement. A challenge in developing microsystems is the necessity to provide associated components, such as valves and sensors, that are combined to maintain a micro-

environment. An additional requirement is the necessity for appropriate surface chemistry in microdevices to prevent adverse charges or chemical groupings on the surface that profoundly modify the behavior and function of the system. Moreover, some conventional methods and procedures (such as centrifugation of blood) are difficult to adapt to microscale, thus making it necessary to develop new ways to accomplish the related tasks (such as isolating cells or plasma from a blood sample).

Numerous excellent articles, books, editorials, and reviews cover the topic of microtechnology. A short list of some of the most relevant for a clinically oriented reader is presented in Table 6-2. Attention is drawn to three reviews published in 2002.[1,15,21,25] Authors of these reviews have pioneered the development of microtechnology, and their reports highlight the scope and magnitude of development that took place in the prior decade.

MICROFLUIDICS

The successful implementation of miniaturized systems into the clinical laboratory has required the development of systems for accurate and precise volume metering of fluids and reagents. Such movement of liquids on every microchip, regardless of the chip's function, is governed by the principles of the new science

TABLE 6-2	Significant Papers in Miniaturization of Relevance to Clinical Analyses		
Author(s)	**Year**	**Topic**	**Ref #**
Kricka	1998	Miniaturization of analytical systems	17
Ekins & Chu	1999	Microarrays: origins and applications	8
Wilding & Kricka	1999	Micro-microchips: how small?	26
Sanders & Manz	2000	Chip-based micro-systems	22
Reyes et al	2002	μ-TAS* theory and technology	21
Auroux et al	2002	μ-TAS* operations and applications	1
Verpoorte	2002	Microfluidic chips	25

*μTAS, *Miniaturized total analytical system.*

of **microfluidics.** Using the principles of microfluidics, workers have developed (1) miniature injection valves, (2) actuators, (3) pumping systems, and (4) mixing techniques.

Fluid Flow and Mixing

Controlled and precise flow of microliter or nanoliter volumes of fluids is needed for presenting a sample to a DNA microchip or a microarray and for carrying out procedures such as the polymerase chain reaction (PCR) or the labeling of a DNA fragment on a microchip. Thus an understanding of the principles of microfluidics is fundamental to the effective operation of DNA chips and microarrays. Microfluidics is a new science and a key functionality in the success of microdevices. It is defined as a branch of physics and biotechnology that studies the behavior of fluids at the microscale and mesoscale; the channels for fluid flow are in the range of nanometers (10^{-9} m) to micrometers (10^{-6} m), with volumes thousands of times smaller than a common droplet. At these small sizes, fluids behave differently than they do at larger sizes, and counterintuitive events happen. At large scales, for example, when two fluid streams (such as rivers) come together, the turbulence of the streams causes mixing. Thus when a yellow stream meets a blue one, we expect the resulting stream to very quickly become a green stream. At the microscale, turbulence is minimal, and special techniques are needed to accomplish mixing of two streams. The field of microfluidics is also concerned with the design of systems in which such small volumes of fluids will be used. For example, the gene chips and labs-on-a-chip are based on the transport of nanoliter or picoliter volumes of fluids through microchannels within a glass or plastic chip.

The success of microfluidics research is seen in the innovative designs of microdevices that have been constructed so that either stable fluid flow or chaotic mixing is achieved depending on the requirement. Adequate mixing of reagents or of sample with reagents is often critical for tests in molecular diagnostics. Some simple systems are based on the positioning of baffles in the flow stream; others achieve the mixing with complex three-dimensional serpentine structures or use of closed-loop devices. Furthermore, the design of microfluidic devices that facilitate rapid analysis of sequential samples without carryover or the separation of particulate materials (e.g., blood cells or bead preparations) has required meticulous study of flow character-

istics. Early studies in 1992 demonstrated techniques ("electro-osmotic" pumping or "electrokinesis") to control the movement of solutions in microcapillaries. Later in 1994, it was demonstrated that, by use of pressure, blood could be pumped through microchannels on a silicon microchip without causing obstruction of the channels. Subsequently the science of microfluidics has expanded greatly. In many devices, especially those involved with capillary electrophoresis, there is a requirement to accurately meter and mix nanoliter volumes of liquids with great precision followed by transfer of a small portion to a detection area. These activities are now characterized in terms of fluid dynamics, and future designs will be based on the understanding of these phenomena.[20]

As the designs of microdevices have developed, there has also been an increasing demand to exploit this technology for high-throughput screening, especially within the pharmaceutical industry. In an effort to accommodate this demand, creative designing has been necessary. Figure 6-2 shows a microchip that accommodates 96 capillary electrophoresis channels in one device.[23] Other developments have resulted in a device that allows for up to 384 parallel channels on one glass microchip (wafer). However, the problem with such designs is achieving convenient peripheral equipment that allows (1) filling of the multichannel devices; (2) the parallel, or sequential, monitoring of the fluid flow; and (3) the detection and quantitation of the various reactions. As a result, it is important to ensure that sample injection into microdevices occurs with as much precision and accuracy as the process requires. Ensuring that a sample is injected as a distinct bolus has initiated the design of numerous injection systems that are dictated by the pumping system being used. Electrokinetic pumping tends to employ T-shaped junctions where the fluid flow is controlled by application of differential voltages and pressure-based systems using rapid injection from syringes operated by pumps.

AC   To guide and control the flow of liquids on microchips, a number of microvalve systems have been developed. To date most have been microfabricated from silicon, although valves using plastic membranes have also been developed. Chip-based microvalve systems have been classified as either active microvalves (with an actuator) or passive (check) microvalves (without an actuator). The miniaturization of the active microvalve systems is restricted by the size of the actuator.

Actuators used for the active microvalve systems include solenoid plungers, bimetallic actuators, and piezoelectric actuators. However, numerous other principles have been employed, such as springs, pneumatic pressure, or electrostatic or electromagnetic forces. Other microvalve systems have been developed that employ a variety of principles, including hydrogel bistrips that are activated and deactivated by pH change, or a bistable gate valve actuated by electrolytically generated gas bubbles. However, none of these systems have been widely adopted even though one of them may well provide the basis for future analytical platforms.

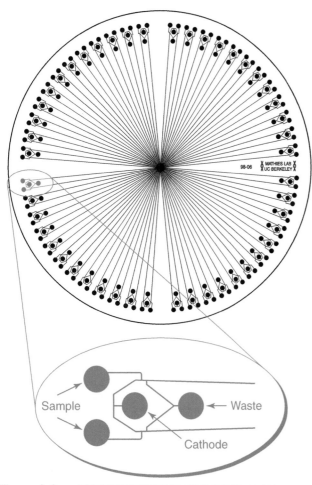

Figure 6-2

Design of a complex microfluidic device for parallel capillary electrophoresis. Figure shows the mask pattern for a 96-channel radial capillary electrophoresis microplate in glass. The separation channels with 200 μm twin-T injectors were masked to 10 μm width and then etched to form 110 μm wide by approximately 50 μm deep channels. The diameter of the reservoir holes is 1.2 mm. The distance from the injector to the detection point is 33 mm. The glass substrate is 10 cm in diameter.

(From Shi Y, Simpson PC, Scherer JR, et al. Radial capillary array electrophoresis microplate and scanner for high-performance nucleic acid analysis. Anal Chem 1999;71:5354-61.)

APPLICATIONS OF MINIATURIZATION

Microdevices and microtechnological developments have had their greatest impact in the field of genomics, and thousands of papers have been published describing their use in this arena. Recently DNA and RNA microarrays have been used to identify changes in malignant tissues that provide prognostic information and help to direct treatment of the malignancy. Among many emerging uses are bacterial identification and characterization of pathogens (e.g., of their sensitivity to drugs).

Miniaturization has been used in (1) devices for DNA amplification and characterization, (2) DNA (hybridization) arrays, and (3) devices for DNA sequencing.

DNA Amplification and Characterization

Early reports by Wilding, Kricka, and colleagues[6,26] established that DNA amplification using PCR was possible in a microchip. Several groups used elementary microchambers etched in silicon and demonstrated that effective amplification could be achieved. Subsequent reports indicated that this technology, which addressed the requirements of microfluidics, provided an effective and reliable amplification of nucleic acid on a microchip with an imprecision (coefficient of variation) of less than 10%. Using simple microchips, this degree of performance of PCR on a chip was attained with volumes of 10 to 50 μL of PCR reaction mixtures containing target DNA, DNA polymerase, DNA primers and the requisite nucleotides, and with heating by external thermocyclers. Using the latter, cycle times needed to (1) include adequate periods of heat to facilitate melting or denaturation of double-stranded DNA (at 95 °C), (2) anneal or bind the primers to the selected strand of DNA (at 55 °C), and (3) extend the selected strand from the nucleotides under the influence of the polymerase enzyme (e.g., Taq polymerase at 72 °C). Early efforts lacked evidence of the reliability, precision, and sensitivity of amplification, and it soon became apparent that other issues, such as surface chemistry and good heating control, had to be resolved before effective systems could be developed. Based on earlier work using glass capillary-based devices and forced air heating, it was assumed that very short cycling times for PCR would be achieved. However, forced air for thermocycling seems an unlikely basis for more complex devices.

Since the early demonstrations of microchip-based PCR, the large number of potential applications in the clinical laboratory made this an attractive field for commercial reasons. Microchip-based PCR and reverse-transcriptase PCR (RT-PCR) can be used in DNA sequencing and genetic analysis. Like other PCR systems, microchip-based PCR is sensitive to inhibitors of PCR (such as hemoglobin), but the microchips can incorporate steps to isolate DNA-containing elements (e.g., leukocytes) from the inhibitors.[27]

DNA chips designed specifically for sizing and quantification of small amounts of DNA have also been developed. As shown earlier, Figure 6-2 is an example of the level of complexity that these types of chips have achieved. Very successful DNA chips that facilitate sequential analysis of 12 samples now have widespread use. The design of some chips includes internal standards (a DNA ladder) and the ability to present the results in a pseudogel format to ease rapid assessment of results (see http://www.chem.agilent.com/Scripts/PCol.asp?lPage=50).

It was projected in the mid-1990s that chip-based devices would become more complex and combine nucleic acid amplification with detection of the amplified DNA and even preparation of the sample. As a result, the next generation of chip-based devices not only brought complexity but a clear awareness of the limitations and hurdles that microchip-based technologies present.

As of 2007, the majority of the benefits of using microchip-based devices for PCR are still perceived, rather than realized. It has been assumed since the first illustration of microchip-based PCR in the early 1990s that features such as (1) low-reagent consumption, (2) low-volume sample requirements, and (3) rapid cycle times would be a consequence of this technology. However, the ability to couple the PCR process with other features, such as sample preparation and detection of amplified

DNA, quickly initiated a drive to design and construct integrated devices that ultimately should provide convenient and inexpensive methods in the many fields in which molecular biology is practiced. The expected economy of scale of manufacturing has yet to be realized, but it is assumed that the pattern will follow that of the electronics industry, in which millions of microdevices are produced at low cost.

Many commercial and academic centers that are exploring this technology have already demonstrated the amplification by PCR of DNA targets from several biological systems, including the human genome, viruses, and microbes on miniaturized devices.[2] Newer developments have been directed toward total systems (Figure 6-3) that incorporate sample preparation, amplification, and detection. These developments achieve greater convenience and shorter cycle times for the PCR. Another approach used to achieve faster cycle time has been to use a microfluidic chip that pumps nanoliter (one one thousandth of a microliter) quantities of PCR-reaction mixture through a circular channel arranged over three heaters that facilitate denaturation, annealing, and extension during the PCR.

The fields in which the growth of microchip-based genomics have first emerged relate to drug development in the pharmaceutical industry, in which determination of inhibition or enhancement of nucleotide replication is important. Other early products include devices designed for the defense industry, in which the detection and identification of toxic agents is desirable. Another key area is the provision of products that facilitate the parallel operation of PCR on microsamples for the life sciences, in which production of sufficient amplicate is a required for sequencing studies.

DNA Hybridization Arrays
Hybridization arrays are now widely used in genomic research. Primarily, these arrays have been developed to meet the growing demands of pharmaceutical research. However, there are few academic centers today that do not have core facilities to prepare low- and high-density arrays to meet the requirements of academic research studying gene expression.

Design of DNA Microarrays
The basic principle underlying hybridization arrays is the immobilization of a DNA probe onto a planar (flat) surface of glass, silicon, or polymer material. The length of the DNA probe may vary greatly depending on the nature or role of the array. Attachment of probes to the surface has become a complex science involving coupling reagents, spacer molecules, and customized surface chemistry. Hybridization generally requires single-stranded DNA as a probe and DNA or RNA as a sample. To allow detection of successful hybridization, DNA or RNA from the sample is labeled with a fluorescent tag or with a tag, such as biotin, that will allow addition of a fluorescent marker at a later time. The time required for the hybridization process has varied from 24 hours in certain static systems to a few minutes in some of the newer devices with microfluidic flow and mixing features. When a single strand of DNA (such as ATCATG) matches a strand of RNA (in this case, UAGUAC), the two strands are "complementary" and will bind with each other. However, if the bases do not match, they will not bind. If large strands of DNA are used as the sample, some partial hybridization may occur, but use of multiple probes addressing different sections of the DNA will allow interpretation of the pattern of hybridization to the many probes on the surface.

The number of individual spots on a single array has varied from less than 10 on a glass slide to more than 10,000 per square centimeter in certain commercial products. Methods for creating or manufacturing arrays vary from simple spotting of a DNA probe solution with a micropipette to complex photolithographic techniques that allow for the light-mediated synthesis of a probe directly in each spot to create oligonucleotides up to 20 base pairs or more (Figure 6-4).[3,10,11] The density of spots achieved by this latter procedure can exceed 30,000 separate spots per square centimeter. With such high density, high-resolution readers are imperative.

The nature and length of the DNA probe attached to the chip surface vary greatly depending on the system. DNA strands of varying length, from complete DNA to very short oligomers, have been employed as well as a variety of labeling

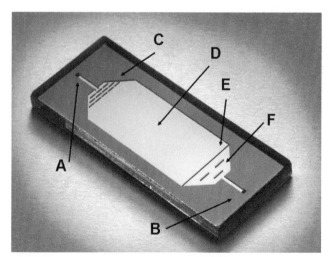

Figure 6-3
Silicon-glass microchip (14 × 35 mm) for cell isolation and PCR. By flowing 1.0 μL of whole blood into the chamber, WBCs are isolated on the filter bed. PCR is performed after releasing the cells back into the main microchip chamber. Thermocycling is achieved by external heating. The volume of the chamber is approximately 10 μL.
A, Entrance port to chip. **B,** Exit port from chip. **C,** Deflectors for forward flow. **D,** Chip chamber that is 80 μm deep and passivated with 2000 angstroms of thermal oxide. **E,** Filter bed having 667 pillars (10 × 20 μm, 3.3 μm gaps). **F,** Exit baffles.

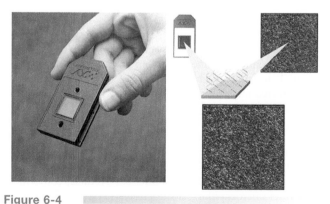

Figure 6-4
Microarray device showing principle and detail of high-density array.
(Courtesy Affymetrix Corp., Palo Alto, Calif.)

entities that allow successful hybridization to be detected. However, it is important that capture probes have similar melting temperatures if comparable hybridizations are to occur at all of the spots on the array.

Detection of Hybridization
Detection of the hybridization of fluorescently tagged DNA or RNA is effected with an array reader that identifies the location of the spot and quantifies fluorescence at that spot. When the array is a high-density one, the reader frequently uses confocal microscopy and considerable computing capacity. Because partial hybridization can occur, usually caused by use of an inappropriate length of probe or sample DNA, the fluorescent signal is modified. Therefore the interpretation of information from a high-density array is complex. More recent developments allow for scanning high-density arrays with lower cost devices. Several manufacturers now offer array readers with resolution of 1 μm or less.

AC

Other Modifications of Nucleic Acid Hybridization Arrays
In efforts to improve the specificity of hybridization, many techniques have been developed, including the use of microarrays created on electrodes that facilitate the selection of appropriate targets and the elimination of interfering molecules or other materials. A technique of so-called electronic stringency has been developed to achieve this.[5] Other expanding technologies based on hybridization arrays are those used for gene expression and gene mapping.[7] For this procedure, the assessment of sample quality is required to prevent the inappropriate use of expensive arrays. As a result, convenient microchip-based capillary electrophoresis devices have been developed that facilitate the assessment of DNA and RNA preparations and that are capable of providing a fast and accurate determination of the size and quantity of DNA or RNA fragments. One device analyzes up to 12 specimens in less than 30 minutes using only 1 mL of a sample and incorporates up to 13 internal standards. This device has also been adapted to facilitate testing of protein solutions.

Nucleic Acid Sequencing
The human genome project has been successful in the sequencing of the human genome (see Chapters 1 and 5) using conventional technology. However, it is now apparent that advancements made in microtechnology will provide another opportunity for the biologist eager to sequence DNA. Using long capillary channels fabricated in microfluidic devices of glass or silicon, several workers have demonstrated successful sequencing of up to 800 base pairs with a reported accuracy of 99%. The microdevices involved used 16-channel electrophoresis arrays, 40-cm-long microchannels, or a radially conformed 96-channel microcapillary electrophoresis system. Using such systems, a dramatic improvement in the speed of sequencing has been achieved, resulting in parallel sequencing separations of 450 bases in less than 15 minutes.

AC

Other Applications
Using the microenvironment of a microdevice to facilitate cell culture and the study of cellular behavior has resulted in several applications. For example, the incubation process of *Escherichia coli* in a gas-permeable PDMS microfluidic device has been monitored by fluorescence; also screening for agonists and antagonists in cultured cells has been achieved by monitoring calcium flux. In addition, using specifically designed filter systems or electrodes, it was shown that cells could be isolated by size or charge from other populations or surrounding media followed by a variety of treatments, such as immunoattachment, lysis, or DNA and RNA release. For example, the ability to create filter systems with selected pore sizes for isolation of white blood cells (WBCs) has been demonstrated starting with volumes of whole blood less than 5 mL.[27] Figure 6-5 illus-

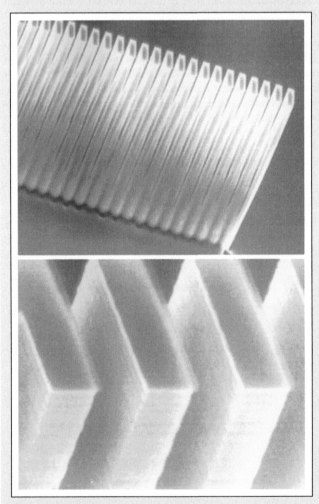

Figure 6-5
Microfiltration device made in silicon by reactive-ion etching. Upper picture shows low magnification of electron micrograph. Each pillar is 90 mm high. Lower picture shows detail of the gaps between filter elements (3.5 mm). Each pillar is 20 mm long and 10 mm wide, which allows easy passage of RBCs, but precludes large granulocytes.
(Courtesy Wilding P, Kricka LJ, University of Pennsylvania.)

trates the nature of a microfilter used for this purpose. Additional applications include the study of red blood cell (RBC) mobility and chemotaxis and locomotion of WBCs in a confined environment.

Other avenues of miniaturization are being pursued that have medical applications. These include the opportunity to manipulate analytes and cells to (1) provide improved methods of reagent and sample transfer; (2) mix aliquots using techniques such as electrokinesis; (3) isolate or separate macromolecules or cells by filtration and electrical charge; (4) ensure electronic stringency; and (5) use nanoparticles to measure biomolecules.

LIMITS OF MINIATURIZATION

Limits of miniaturization for clinical analyses include the concentration of the analyte to be measured and various surface effects.

Analyte Concentration

The limitations of miniaturization are invariably related to the concentration of the analyte or type of cell under study. If the device is capable of receiving only microliter quantities, then the final signal strength being measured will depend on the inclusion of an amplification process (e.g., PCR) or the ability to detect extremely low concentrations of analyte. For example, only 0.5 μL of whole blood is necessary to allow isolation of 500 WBCs, more than sufficient to provide genomic DNA for mutation detection by PCR. Similarly, submicroliter quantities of protein or DNA solutions provide adequate material for analysis by capillary electrophoresis. However, if the goal is to identify and isolate, from whole blood, infected WBCs that are present at an incidence of only 1 in 10 million uninfected WBCs, then quantities in excess of 10 mL of whole blood may be required just to encounter five cells. This does not provide the ideal situation for a microdevice.

An application in microchip technology that highlights the advantage of combining conventional technology with microtechnology is the use of a microfabricated filter to enhance the enrichment of fetal cells in a preparation to be used for genomic studies. In this study, the goal was to provide a sample that contained 5 to 50 nucleated RBCs (nRBCs) of fetal origin so that chromosomal or genomic studies could be performed. The starting specimen for this isolation and/or enrichment procedure was 20 mL of maternal blood, and so the 5 to 50 fetal nRBCs were being isolated from a matrix containing approximately 100 billion adult RBCs, 100 million adult WBCs, and 1.4 g of protein. The encouraging data resulting from this work are achieved only because microtechnology was used in combination with preparative steps using conventional technology (cell agglutination and immunoprecipitation with magnetic beads). Successful application of microtechnology in the clinical field will probably result in hybrid systems that exploit both conventional technology and microtechnology.

Surface Chemistry

Surface chemistry creates challenges for design of devices. Some details of surface chemistry are provided for interested readers.

AC An early discovery during the development of microchip PCR was the importance of surface chemistry in microchip operation and design.[24] This discovery demonstrated that PCR in silicon microchips was severely inhibited if the surface chemistry was unsuitable. These workers noted that the increase in surface area in microchips, relative to volume, could be twentyfold greater than with conventional tubes used for PCR. Moreover, if the surface was only partially coated, or if it existed as silicon, silicon nitride, or certain other substances, then it was very difficult to achieve reproducible or adequate amplification. However, successful and reproducible amplification could be achieved if the surface was subjected to coating with a suitable passivating layer (e.g., 2000 angstroms of silicon oxide). Passivation of the silicon surface has also been achieved with polymeric coatings of the microchip channels and chambers or by silanization of glass microchips followed by a coating of polyacrylamide.

Other studies have sought to employ other substrates with fewer problems, but the inherent one of increased surface-to-volume ratio always applies. One of the approaches has been to incorporate substances such as polyethylene glycol (PEG), polyvinylpyrrolidone (PVP), or epoxy compounds that significantly reduce or eliminate binding of analytes or key reagents to surfaces. Others have used silanization followed by coating of the channels or chambers with polymeric compounds. Additionally, microchip-based capillary electrophoresis devices constructed from polydimethylsiloxane (PDMS) and glass have been modified with a three-layer biotin-neutravidin sandwich coating, made of biotinylated IgG, neutravidin, and biotinylated dextran. By replacing biotinylated dextran with any biotinylated reagent, the modified surface can be readily patterned with biochemical probes, such as antibodies.

FABRICATION AND MATERIALS

For most devices employed in the clinical laboratory, conventional techniques of manufacture are used. However, microdevices and nanodevices require new techniques for their fabrication. This section discusses these technologies.

Computer chips are categorized by their **minimum feature size**—the dimension of the smallest feature actually constructed in the manufacturing process. The minimum feature size is continually getting smaller to pack more circuitry into the same space. For example, advanced chips in production in 2000 had minimum feature sizes of 180 nm, with chips with a size of 90 nm under development. This concept of a minimum feature size is also important in fabrication of microdevices because actual dimensions are determined by the choice of fabrication process. As discussed below, conventional photolithography (405 or 436 nm) is generally limited to features of approximately 1 μm. Deep ultraviolet (UV) (230 to 260 nm) lithography has a minimum feature size of 0.3 μm, and x-ray and e-beam are used to generate features as small as 0.1 μm.

For readers interested in how these devices are made, the following paragraphs describe the techniques used to manufacture, drill, and seal microdevices.

AC

Manufacturing Techniques

Photolithography on silicon, glass, and plastic surfaces and molding of polymers are commonly used to fabricate microdevices. Other processes in use or under investigation include (1) embossing, (2) laser ablation, (3) molding, and (4) atomic force microscopic etching.

Photolithography

Photolithography is the process of transferring geometric shapes on a mask to the surface of a silicon wafer. It involves a series of steps. First, a photomask defining the shapes of the structures to be etched on the silicon wafer is generated from larger drawings that have been accurately duplicated and reduced in size using computer-based programs (Figure 6-6). The silicon wafer is then oxidized to produce a thin surface layer of chemically resistant silicon dioxide that will allow coating with a photo resist material. The wafer is then evenly coated with a polymeric photo resist using a spin-coating procedure and patterned using a photomask and a UV light source. The photo resist is either a positive resist (photo resist in areas of the wafer exposed to light is rendered soluble) or a negative resist (photo resist in areas of the wafer unexposed to light is rendered soluble). The insoluble polymerized resist remaining on the wafer forms an image of the photomask on the silicon dioxide surface of the wafer. The wafer is now ready to have the oxide etched away either by a wet or dry etching process.

Wet Etching

Wet etching covers any form of etching in which etching is performed by immersing the silicon wafer or the glass or plastic surface in a bath of the chemical etchant. The chemical etchants are either isotropic or anisotropic. Isotropic etchants, such as hydrofluoric acid (HF), will etch a given material at the same rate whatever direction they are etching in and are less used because they are difficult to control and etch underneath the protective resist. By contrast, anisotro-pic etchants will etch at different rates in a given material depending on a number of factors, the most useful one being the crystal structure and orientation. Etching of glass is usually achieved using HF. Microstructures in glass can also be formed by laser ablation techniques.

Figure 6-7 illustrates how the angles of etching are controlled using an anisotropic etchant. The most widely used anisotropic etchant is potassium hydroxide (KOH). Most etchants will not etch impure silicon at the same rate

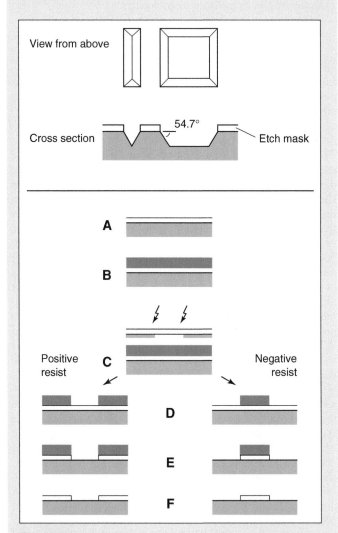

Figure 6-7
Schematic of the etching process used in photolithographic-based fabrication.
Upper box: Anisotropic etch of silicone by KOH using silicon nitride mask.
Lower box: **A,** Silicon wafer (*light blue*) with etch mask (white). **B,** Application of photo resist (*dark blue*) onto etch mask. **C,** Exposure of photo resist through photomask. **D,** Positive and negative photo resist after development of resist. **E,** Removal of etch mask. **F,** Removal of photo resist, leaving either the pattern present in the photomask or its opposite patterned into the etch mask.

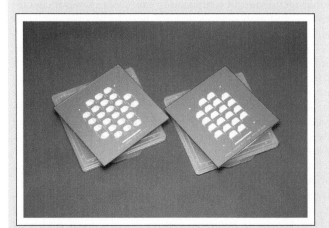

Figure 6-6
Two glass photomasks (approx 125 × 125 mm) showing patterns for multiple PCR devices to be fabricated in silicon.

as pure silicon; this fact can be used to the advantage of the engineer. An example of this would be that if a small part of the silicon substrate is doped with boron, the doped section will not be etched as fast as the normal silicon; if an isotropic etchant is used, the silicon beneath the boron-doped area will be etched away. The main disadvantage with using this doping method is that it alters the electrical properties of the silicon so that fabricating and micro-electronic devices on the same substrate will be much more difficult.

Dry Etching

This type of etching does not use any chemicals directly on the wafer; instead the most popular method involves accelerating ions toward the wafer to be etched. These ions will etch more in the direction in which they are traveling. This method is called reactive ion etching (RIE). RIE is an anisotropic etching method because the direction of the etching controls the rate of etching (see Figure 6-7). In the final steps, the photo resist and the silicon oxide layers are removed to give the final etched silicon wafer. By using multiple masks and sacrificial layers that permit undercutting to produce movable components, it is possible to fabricate complex, multicomponent structures on the surface of a silicon wafer. All of these fabrication steps are performed in a clean room environment, thus permitting the production of sterile devices suitable for in vivo or clinical application.

Molding of Polymeric Materials

LIGA is a German acronym (Lithographie, Galvanoformung, Abformung) standing for the main steps of the process; it involves (1) deep x-ray lithography, (2) electroforming, and (3) plastic molding. These steps make it possible to mass produce microcomponents at a low cost.

In practice, the LIGA process provides a way to manufacture a mold for a microstructure. It consists of the following steps. First, a resist-coated substrate is patterned using a mask and a source of synchrotron radiation (oriented x-rays). Secondly, after development, the resist structure is electroplated. This electroforming produces a metal microstructure (a negative replica of the structure), and this is then used as the mold for the final structure. Advantages of the LIGA process are that high aspect ratios are attained (e.g., lateral dimensions of a few micrometers and vertical dimensions of up to 1000 µm), and the molds are able to be used to prepare multiple replicas of the structure in a variety of materials (e.g., polyimide, polymethylmethacrylate [PMMA]).

Direct molding using a silicon master and a thermoplastic fluoropolymer (e.g., Hostaflon) at 150 °C and at a pressure of 50 kg/cm² has been employed to fabricate channels for performing electrophoresis. The plastic molded part is then clamped between two plates to complete the sealing of the channel.

Other Fabrication Techniques

Other methods have also been employed to create microfluidic devices in various polymeric materials. Laser abla-

tion of PDMS has been used to create elastomeric molds that pattern structures[13] or nickel molds produced from a silicon master pattern device from acrylic polymers or polystyrene.[29] Other devices for capillary electrophoresis of DNA samples have been made by compression molding of polycarbonate against a silicon master. In some of these devices using polymeric materials, such as polyimides, the molding has been coupled with metallization layers to allow the production of electrodes inside or outside the fluidic channels.[19] With all of these structures, there is a need for bonding or sealing processes that allow the formation of channels or chambers.

Incorporation of Electronic Components

Another requirement in certain microchips is the incorporation of electronic components, such as electrodes. So-called bioelectronic chips have been constructed that use arrays of platinum electrodes (80 µm in diameter) coated with streptavidin. By modifying the charge applied to the electrodes, molecules such as DNA or RNA are differentially attracted to, or displaced from, the electrode surfaces.[5,12]

Drilling

Mechanical, ultrasonic, and laser drilling are processes also used to fabricate chambers in microdevices. Laser drilling is particularly suited for drilling very small size holes (e.g., less than 2 µm using a deep UV excimer laser). This type of drilling is of increasing importance for the manufacture of devices used for high-throughput systems that are used for ion-channel studies on isolated cells in the pharmaceutical industry in which exact holes of approximately 1 µm are required. In these situations, the contours of the small holes being created and the surrounding surface area are critical to success, and the demanding criteria are rarely met by silicon with its crystalline structure.

Chambers have also been drilled through glass by means of an electrodischarge process in which the glass is submerged in an alkaline solution (e.g., NaOH) and a needle (30-µm diameter tip) contacting the glass and a negative potential applied (40 volts).

Bonding and Sealing

Sealing structures to produce liquid-tight enclosures (chambers and channels) is a key step in the fabrication of a microdevice. Several different processes are available depending on the materials employed. However, in nearly all cases, some method of surface cleaning is necessary before the bonding process. Bonding techniques include anodic (glass to silicon) at high temperature, eutectic (silicon to silicon) with gold as a sealant, and direct bonding or clamping. When nanoliter volumes are involved, the choice of chemistry and bonding technique is critical.

THE FUTURE

The future of nanotechnology and microfabrication in the clinical field, particularly where it will impact the clinical laboratory, is difficult to forecast. However, because the necessity to reduce analytical costs is a constant theme, there is little doubt that products of this technology will be implemented and used. Moreover, as the demand grows for increased effort at the point of care, coupled with the growing demand to achieve low-cost, high-throughput screening for malignancies and other diseases, it is inevitable that microtechnology will be a developing science for many years. Forecasting which subdisciplines in laboratory medicine will be the first to benefit is more difficult. The advances made in microcapillary electrophoresis, nucleic acid amplification, and the many detection techniques suggest that molecular pathology will benefit first, but that many other subdisciplines will soon follow. The application of nanostructures and the manipulation of molecular architecture to facilitate clinical assays have already commenced with the use of nano-sized beads as labels for ligands or antibodies and for the modification of surface chemistry. However, it will be necessary for these technologies to surpass current achievements using present-day techniques and to compete on an economic basis in the ever-demanding world of healthcare.

REFERENCES

1. Auroux PA, Lossifidis D, Reyes DR, Manz A. Micro total analysis systems. 2. Analytical standard operations and applications. Anal Chem 2002;74:2637-52.
2. Belgrader P, Benett W, Hadley D, Long G, Mariella RJ, Milanovich F, et al. Rapid pathogen detection using a microchip PCR array instrument. Clin Chem 1998;44:2191-4.
3. Bowtell DDL. Options available-from start to finish-for obtaining expression data by microarray. Nature Genet 1999;21 (Suppl.):33-7.
4. Burns MA, Mastrangelo CH, Sammarco TS, Man FP, Webster JR, Johnsons BN, et al. Microfabricated structures for integrated DNA analysis. Proc Natl Acad Sci U S A 1996;93:5556-61.
5. Cheng J, Sheldon EL, Wu L, Uribe A, Gerrue LO, Carrino J, et al. Preparation and hybridization analysis of DNA/RNA from E. coli on microfabricated bioelectronic chips. Nat Biotechnol 1998;16:541-6.
6. Cheng J, Shoffner MA, Hvichia GE, Kricka LJ, Wilding P. Chip PCR. II. Investigation of different PCR amplification systems in microfabricated silicon glass chips. Nucleic Acids Res 1996;24:380-5.
7. Eggers M, Erlich D. A review of microfabricated devices for gene-based diagnostics. Hematol Pathol 1995;9:1-15.
8. Ekins R, Chu FW. Microarrays: their origins and applications. Trends Biotechnol 1999;17:217-8.
9. Elvidge G. Microarray expression technology: from start to finish. Pharmacogenomics 2006;7:123-34.
10. Fodor SP, Rava RP, Huang XC, Pease AC, Holmes CP, Adams CL. Multiplexed biochemical assays with biological chips. Nature Biotechnol 1993;364:555-6.
11. Fodor SP, Read JL, Pirrung MC, Stryer L, Lu AT, Solas D. Light-directed, spatially addressable parallel chemical synthesis. Science 1991;251:767-73.
12. Gilles PN, Wu DJ, Foster CB, Dillon PJ, Channock SJ. Single nucleotide polymorphic discrimination by an electronic dot blot assay on semiconductor microchips. Nature Biotechnol 1999;17:365-70.
13. Grzybowski BA, Haag R, Bowden N, Whitesides GM. Generation of micrometer sized patterns for microanalytical applications using a laser direct-write method and microcontact printing. Anal Chem 1998;70:4645-52.
14. Hoheisel JD. Microarray technology: beyond transcript profiling and genotype analysis. Nat Rev Genet 2006;7:200-10.
15. Kricka LJ. Miniaturization of analytical systems. Clin Chem 1998;44:2008-14.
16. Kricka LJ, Fortina P. Microchips: An all-language literature survey including books and patents. Clin Chem 2002;48:1620-2.
17. Kricka LJ, Nozaki O, Wilding P. Micromechanics and nanotechnology: implications and applications in the clinical laboratory. J Intnl Fed Clin Chem 1994;6:52-6.
18. Li SFY, Kricka LJ. Clinical analysis by microchip capillary electrophoresis. Clin Chem 2006;52:37-45.
19. Metz S, Holzer R, Renaud P. Polyimide-based microfluidic devices. Lab Chip 2001;1:29-34.
20. Ramsey JD, Jacobson SC, Culbertson CT, Ramsey JM. High-efficiency, two dimensional separations of protein digests on microfluidic devices. Anal Chem 2003;75:3758-64.
21. Reyes DR, Lossifidis D, Auroux PA, Manz A. Micro total analysis systems. 1. Introduction, theory, and technology. Anal Chem 2002;74:2623-36.
22. Sanders GHW, Manz A. Chip-based microsystems for genomic and proteomic analysis. Trends in Anal Chem 2000;19:364-78.
23. Shi Y, Simpson PC, Scherer JR, Wexler D, Skibola C, Smith MT, et al. Radial capillary array electrophoresis microplate and scanner for high-performance nucleic acid analysis. Anal Chem 1999;71:5354-61.
24. Shoffner MA, Cheng J, Hvichia GE, Kricka LJ, Wilding P. Chip PCR. I. Surface passivation of microfabricated silicon-glass chips for PCR. Nucleic Acids Res 1996;24:375-9.
25. Verpoorte E. Microfluidic chips for clinical and forensic analysis. Electrophoresis 2002;23:677-712.
26. Wilding P, Joos T, Kricka LJ, Shi L. Guidelines for terminology for microtechnology in clinical laboratories. Pure Appl Chem 2006;78:677-684.
27. Wilding P, Kricka LJ. Micro-microchips: just how small can we go? Trends Biotechnol 1999;17:465-8.
28. Wilding P, Kricka LJ, Cheng J, Hvichia G, Shoffner MA, Fortina P. Integrated cell isolation and polymerase chain reaction analysis using silicon microfilter chambers. Anal Biochem 1998;257:95-100.
29. Zhao XM, Xia YN, Whitesides GM. Soft lithographic methods for nanofabrication. J Mater Chem 1997;7:1069-74.

REVIEW QUESTIONS

1. DNA microchips can be made from
   A. glass.
   B. polymers.
   C. silicon oxide–coated silicon.
   D. glass coated with a passivation material.
   E. all of the above.

2. Hybridization on a DNA array should always employ
   A. complete DNA strands.
   B. uniform exposure of the sample with the probes.
   C. DNA strands with different melting temperatures.
   D. control of stringency with an electrical field.
   E. DNA strands less than 10 oligomers.

3. Attachment of a DNA strand to a complementary DNA probe on a microarray is influenced by
   A. pH.
   B. ion concentration.
   C. probe attachment to the chip.
   D. length of the probe.
   E. all of the above.

4. The nature of the surface chemistry in a PCR chip
   A. reflects the low surface-to-volume ratio.
   B. may lead to inconsistent results.
   C. is unimportant.
   D. cannot be modified.
   E. all of the above.

5. Amplification of genomic DNA using microtechnology is limited by
   A. sample size.
   B. low levels of analyte concentration.
   C. protein.
   D. hemoglobin.
   E. all of the above.

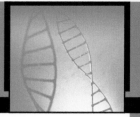

Chapter 7

Design and Operation of a Molecular Diagnostics Laboratory

Anthony A. Killeen, M.D., Ph.D.
Elaine Lyon, Ph.D.

OUTLINE

OBJECTIVES

1. Design a molecular diagnostics laboratory as in new construction; use appropriate labels to mark specific rooms and their purpose, and diagram airflow.
2. Discuss the factors involved in choosing a test menu for a molecular diagnostics laboratory, including financial considerations, clinical utility, and turnaround times.
3. Describe the requirements and reasons for comprehensive individual informed consent for genetic testing, and compare these with the requirements for informed consent for other types of laboratory testing.
4. Define the recommended qualifications of a molecular diagnostics laboratory director.
5. Describe methods that will alleviate the issue of amplicon contamination in a molecular diagnostics laboratory.
6. Write a procedure for a molecular diagnostics test that covers required information about specimen collection, reagents, instrumentation, safety precautions, and ethical issues.
7. List and define the components of a quality assurance program in a molecular diagnostics laboratory.
8. List the steps involved in placing a reagent into service in a molecular diagnostics laboratory.
9. State the rationale for using control specimens that test preanalytical, analytical, and postanalytical processes with all patient samples; provide examples of each type of control.
10. List the information that must be included on a genetics test result report.
11. Describe the ethical issues surrounding reporting results of genetics tests and list procedures that are used to deal with these issues.
12. Understand the rules of federal regulatory agencies concerning procedure writing, results reporting, recordkeeping, retention of samples, and proficiency testing in a molecular diagnostics laboratory.

KEY WORDS AND DEFINITIONS

Amplicon: Amplified pieces of nucleic acid; may contaminate reagents or samples in the laboratory.

Analyte-Specific Reagent (ASR): Reagents that are used in the assessment of biochemical substances in biological specimens; in regard to genetics testing, an ASR is the key ingredient of a specially designed in-house genetics assay.

Assay Controls: Samples or specimens that test preanalytical, analytical, and postanalytical processes and components of assays.

Centralization: In regard to molecular diagnostics laboratory design, the sharing of equipment, reagents, personnel, and space for various clinical disciplines represented in a clinical laboratory, such as infectious disease (clinical microbiology) and inherited disease (genetics) testing.

College of American Pathologists (CAP): An organization of board-certified pathologists that provides programs for proficiency testing and laboratory accreditation.

Decentralization: The use of separate and distinct laboratory space, equipment, reagents, and personnel for each clinical application of molecular laboratory testing, such as infectious disease, inherited disease, and molecular oncology testing.

In-House Assay: A laboratory assay that is developed within a laboratory using "homemade" reagents and ASRs and designed to respond to a need for a specific laboratory diagnosis.

Proficiency Testing: The process by which the same samples are analyzed by many laboratories, with the results from each laboratory evaluated to determine the quality of laboratory performance; all testing processes should be assessed.

Quality Assurance (QA): The practice that encompasses all endeavors, procedures, formats, and activities directed towards ensuring that a specified quality is achieved and maintained.

Quality Control: The assessment of laboratory performance by testing assay controls and the statistical analysis of assay control values.

Quality Improvement: A process that uses a structured procedure to identify the causes of problems and to recommend appropriate remedies.

In design and operation, molecular diagnostics laboratories have much in common with other areas of clinical laboratories. This chapter will not dwell on those common areas, but will highlight issues unique to a molecular diagnostics laboratory.

CENTRALIZATION OR DECENTRALIZATION?

Molecular techniques are of importance in clinical diagnostics in most disciplines of laboratory medicine and pathology, and their applications will continue to grow in essentially all areas of testing. These considerations raise a fundamental question in the design of a laboratory system: should each discipline that uses molecular techniques have its own molecular laboratory space or is a centralized molecular laboratory a more suitable model to deliver molecular testing services? The answer will depend to a large degree on local factors, but has significant implications for the overall costs and efficiencies of providing molecular testing services. The major argument in favor of **centralization** is the efficiencies achieved through sharing of equipment, reagents, personnel, and space. In favor of **decentralization,** the adoption of molecular techniques in areas as diverse as microbiology and inherited diseases requires a broad range of specialist skills and knowledge that may be difficult to develop in a centralized laboratory. In addition, certain molecular tests may be integral to the activities of another laboratory, thereby precluding their performance in a central molecular testing facility. As a compromise, many hospital laboratories use a dual system in which a central laboratory performs tests in areas such as molecular genetics and molecular oncology, whereas molecular techniques for advanced microbial identification and characterization are performed in the existing microbiology laboratory.

CHOOSING A TEST MENU

In choosing the molecular tests to offer, the laboratory needs to consider (1) the test's diagnostic accuracy, (2) its clinical utility, (3) the local demand for the test, (4) the resources available for its performance, (5) the skills and interests of the personnel (particularly the laboratory director), (6) the likelihood of the test being financially viable, (7) whether the test is, in whole or part, patented or has other intellectual property restrictions, and (8) the ability of the laboratory to deliver acceptable turnaround times.

Diagnostic accuracy (or clinical validity) confirms that the analyte is associated with the disorder or disease. It is most often established by large clinical research studies. If such studies are not available, the individual clinical laboratory should establish the association before offering the test. Clinical utility relates to the usefulness of the test, such as aiding or ruling out a diagnosis, determining a therapy, or providing information that is useful in family planning.

Local demand for testing will most likely come from clinicians who are looking for tests to aid in patient diagnosis and management. Such demands should be carefully evaluated to ensure that it is reasonably clear that the clinician's expectations will be met and that the volume of testing will make it

cost effective. Higher volume tests tend to improve the overall financial stability of a laboratory because the fixed costs become a smaller proportion of the individual test cost. Conversely, it seldom makes financial sense to offer low-volume tests unless reimbursements are sufficiently high to cover the costs. However, volumes may increase if the laboratory becomes a regional or national referral center for a test. If a clinician has expertise in a clinical area that stimulates test ordering, it is possible that offering a laboratory test may enhance the ability of the clinical service to attract increased recognition, more patients, research support, and other external funding. Thus what seems at first to be a low-volume test may with time become an important item in the laboratory's and institution's repertoire.

Expectations for turnaround time, and therefore the frequency with which tests must be performed, vary with the analyte. For example, tests for infectious agents usually require a shorter turnaround time than do tests for chronic, inherited diseases. Expectations of a short turnaround time tend to increase the analytical cost per sample, while at the same time indicating the need to offer a test in-house rather than send samples to an external laboratory.

SPACE AND DESIGN CONSIDERATIONS

The major consideration in the physical layout of a molecular diagnostics laboratory, other than adequate space, is a design that prevents or controls contamination. The use of polymerase chain reaction (PCR) and other target amplification methodologies (which make multiple copies of a piece of DNA) introduces an important potential source of laboratory error, namely, contamination of the laboratory with **amplicons** from previous reactions. These amplified pieces of nucleic acid will be introduced in the laboratory environment when a tube containing amplification product is opened and a small amount of the solution becomes an aerosol. Without careful laboratory technique, amplicons are spread to new samples and reagents by airborne droplets, gloves, skin, door handles, pens, paper, and pieces of equipment, such as pipettes. Because each amplicon is a target to be replicated in a subsequent amplification reaction, an amplicon that contaminates a new patient sample or a reagent solution has the potential to lead to an erroneous result, typically a false-positive value. Contamination of the laboratory by amplicons is a serious problem that often requires extensive cleaning to remove, and every precaution should be taken to prevent this problem.

Historically the design of the laboratory has been an important factor in controlling contamination, and the most common design feature that is unique to the molecular diagnostics laboratory has been use of (two) separate rooms for (1) sample processing, reagent preparation, and nucleic acid isolation, and (2) performance and analysis of target amplification reactions. Some laboratory designs incorporate a positive pressure air control system to prevent airflow from the amplification analysis room into the sample processing and reagent preparation rooms. The air from the analysis room may be vented directly to the exterior of the laboratory building. Implementation of such design features is easier when planning new construction than when attempting to adapt space in an older building for use as a molecular diagnostics laboratory. If multiple rooms are unavailable, consideration should be given to the use of laminar flow hoods that contain an ultraviolet (UV) light. UV-induced cross-linking of DNA minimizes the effects of amplicon contamination during sample setup.

Other methods of preventing contamination involve meticulous laboratory practice by personnel. The flow of operations from sample receipt to amplified product analysis involves a sequential series of steps that tend from "clean" to "contaminated." It therefore follows that there should be no movement of reagents or equipment in the reverse direction to this flow. For example, pipettes that are used in the postamplification area should never be introduced into a preamplification area. Laboratory coats that are worn in the postamplification area should be removed before entering a pre-PCR area. Gloves should be discarded after use in the post-PCR area. Laboratory benches should be regularly cleaned using amplicon decontaminating agents, such as solutions of bleach or commercial preparations.

An alternative approach to reducing contamination is to modify the procedures that are used. Such modifications include (1) reagent strategies, (2) closed analytical systems, and (3) use of methods that do not involve making copies of DNA or RNA. A reagent strategy is the use of uracil in PCR combined with preincubation of samples with uracil N-glycosylase (UNG) to degrade copied DNA that might have entered the samples from previous PCR (Chapter 5).[20] Commercially available systems have been developed that use a closed analytical system (i.e., reaction tubes that are analyzed without being opened). An example is the use of real-time PCR with melting analyses (Chapter 5). Finally, alternatives to PCR that do not involve making many millions of copies of the DNA (target amplification) avoid that risk of contamination by copied DNA.[15] These methods were described in Chapter 5. Depending on the laboratory space (particularly if only limited space is available) and the desired test menu, use of such techniques may be preferable to target-amplification methods.

OPERATIONAL CONSIDERATIONS

As mentioned previously, only operational details that are specific for a molecular diagnostics laboratory are discussed here. Many of these involve regulatory issues that are relevant to practice within the United States and vary among jurisdictions within the United States and among countries. They are provided here for general guidance along with reminders of requirements that apply to all testing.

Documents, Records, Sample Retention

Compared with other laboratory testing, molecular testing has some unique information needs and sample storage requirements. Requisitions, consent, records, and sample retention are reviewed in this section. As for other testing in the clinical laboratory, specific requirements for molecular testing vary among regulatory and accrediting agencies.

Requisitions

As with all requests for testing, the requisition form should indicate the (1) patient identifying information, (2) ordering physician's name and contact information, (3) sample type, (4) time of collection, and (5) test to be performed. For genetic testing, it is common that the requisition form will solicit information on relevant family history that is often provided as a hand-drawn pedigree diagram. When familial gene variants (mutations) are known, the variant and the relationship

of the patient to the proband (the first family member to be diagnosed or tested) should be included. Additionally, clinical history may be needed, such as history of bleeding in thrombophilia testing. Such information often is essential for test interpretation and should be available to the testing laboratory.

Consent for Genetic Testing and Privacy of Medical Records

Much more attention is given in the medical literature to the need for informed consent for genetic testing than to most areas of laboratory testing. The principal reason for this is that by testing for inherited disorders, information may be obtained that has diagnostic or risk implications for other family members. In addition, genetic testing may indicate a high probability of development of symptomatic disease later in life in patients who appear well at the time of testing. Patients and families may be stigmatized by a diagnosis of genetic disease and may suffer discrimination in employment and in insurability. Although the number of documented cases of such discrimination is small, the fear of adverse consequences of genetic testing is quite common. For these reasons, obtaining informed consent for genetic testing is a common practice and is required by law in many states.[13] Although the physician or other healthcare provider ordering the testing usually obtains the consent, the laboratory is responsible for providing information about the test, such as its appropriate use and limitations. It is also recognized that different genetic tests have different burdens associated with them. For example, confirmation of inherited thrombophilia (and risk of blood clots) by detecting the factor V Leiden gene variant has less stigmatization than predicting presymptomatically that a person will develop a more serious disorder, such as Huntington disease, later in life. For this reason, laboratories may choose to not request a formal consent for factor V Leiden testing,[11] but may decide to require it for Huntington disease testing, particularly in the absence of clinical symptoms.[4]

Record Keeping

Under current U.S. federal guidelines, the following records must be retained for at least 2 years for all laboratory testing: (1) specimen requisitions, (2) patient test results and reports, (3) instrument printouts, (4) accession records, (5) **quality control** records, (6) instrument maintenance records, (7) **proficiency testing** records, and (8) **quality improvement** records. Laws concerning records and chain of custody for paternity and forensic testing vary by state; it is the responsibility of the director to ensure that all applicable regulations are met.

Retention of Extracted Nucleic Acids

Under current federal law, there is no minimum length of time for which an extracted sample of DNA or RNA must be stored after analysis is complete, although regulations do exist for retention of the primary sample. Because extracted samples tend to be of small volume (measured in microliters), many laboratories retain samples indefinitely. Depending on local policies, deidentified residual specimens may be used for validation of new assays or assay improvements. However, some states, acting out of concerns for genetic privacy, have proposed or enacted legislation that requires destruction of samples for genetic testing after analysis is complete. These laws vary widely and often specify exceptions (e.g., for samples used in forensic work). Laboratory directors are responsible for following the requirements of their own jurisdictions.

Personnel

The qualifications of personnel are determined by regulatory agencies and by the availability of suitable staff. In the United States, the qualifications for director, technical supervisor, and medical technologists are provided in the Clinical Laboratory Improvement Amendments.[3]

Directorship

The laboratory director should be qualified to direct a high-complexity laboratory. Under current U.S. regulations, federal law requires no formal experience in molecular diagnostics. However, because of the need to issue an interpretation of many molecular diagnostic test results, the director should ideally have training that includes experience in at least one major area of molecular laboratory activity, such as molecular genetics, oncology, infectious diseases, or identity testing. The expertise of the director may need to be complemented by additional personnel with appropriate training, including associate directors with expertise in areas of relevance to the test menu (e.g., hematopathology, genetics, and microbiology). Specialized molecular pathology certification for director level MDs and PhDs are available through Molecular Genetics Pathology fellowships of the American Board of Pathology, the American Board of Medical Genetics, and the American Board of Clinical Chemistry, among others.

Technical Personnel

The most suitable educational background for a medical technologist in a molecular diagnostics laboratory is completion of a medical technology training program, including training or experience in molecular diagnostics. In the past, few medical technology programs produced graduates with specific skills in molecular diagnostics, and thus there is often a need for extensive on-the-job training of newly hired personnel. Medical technology programs have, however, incorporated molecular training in their curricula.

Individuals with skills in molecular biology, but without formal training in medical technology, may be an alternative source of personnel in some geographical areas, but their employment may be contingent on local legal standards for employment within a clinical laboratory (e.g., state licensure requirements). Such individuals often have a strong theoretical background and possibly extensive laboratory experience (often in a research setting), but it is important to recognize that there are specific skills acquired in a formal medical technology program. The clinical laboratory is a different environment from a research laboratory, and this is particularly true in the areas of quality control and exacting use of standard procedures. Various certification and specialty programs have come into being to meet the need for qualified personnel.

Reporting of Results

Specific guidelines for reporting molecular pathology test results in the United States are available in the "Molecular Pathology Checklist" from the **College of American Pathologists (CAP)**.[8] In general, information that should be included in reports of genetic testing include (1) the details of the

methods used including all probes and restriction enzymes, (2) locus and gene variants tested, (3) the findings, and (4) an interpretive report. The report should include the diagnostic sensitivity and diagnostic specificity (Chapter 8) of the test. Infectious disease tests may need to distinguish between latent, persistent, and active disease states.[5] Limits of detection should be reported for infectious disease and oncological applications. In quantitative tests, testing indications may include prognosis, therapeutic decisions, or therapeutic monitoring.[7] Reports may include an absolute value (often expressed as copy numbers or international units [IU]), a relative number (expressed per copy of a reference gene), or a change from a previous result.

For genetic tests, clinical sensitivity may refer to the ability to detect gene variants associated with disease. When testing is incomplete because not all possible disease-causing variants are examined, the report should indicate the false-negative rate. For example, the recommended panel for cystic fibrosis carrier screening in the U.S. population includes a basic set of only 25 of the greater than 1000 known disease-causing variants. Testing for this abbreviated panel detects 85% to 90% of disease-causing variants in Caucasians, making the false-negative rate 10% to 15%. In the case of an individual with a negative test result, the report should include the risk that the patient carries a disease-causing variant despite the negative test result.[12] A combination of family history and test results may be used to achieve this estimate. In many cases the clinical sensitivity and specificity can only be estimated, indicating the need for further clinical research.

The reports should also include analytical sensitivity and specificity. A cause for a reduced analytical sensitivity or specificity in genetic testing is the presence of rare sequence variants that interfere with the assay. In designing an assay, databases should be searched for common sequence variants to prevent this inherent limitation of nucleic acid testing and to increase the analytical specificity.

When genetic testing is based on linked genetic markers, the report should indicate the false-negative and false-positive rates arising from recombination between the test locus and the disease locus. This is inferred from the known genetic distance between the loci.

In the case of some genetic diseases, the genotype-phenotype relationship varies with the variant and the pattern of inheritance (e.g., dominant versus recessive inheritance, Chapter 9), and the report should include an appropriate discussion of the findings relevant to the observed gene variants. For example, some variants in *CYP21* (the steroid 21-hydroxylase gene)—such as gene deletion—are associated with severe, classic congenital adrenal hyperplasia, whereas other variants, such as V281L, in the same gene are associated with the late-onset form of the disease, which is characterized by milder symptoms of androgen excess in females.[14] In the case of Huntington disease, some variants are associated with a lower likelihood of disease, or an onset later in life, than are others (Chapter 9).[16,18] The report should include information that relates the specific variant to phenotypes, penetrance, and pattern of inheritance. It is also common practice to include in reports of genetic testing a statement that genetic counseling may be appropriate for the patient and family.

Laboratories that perform genetic studies occasionally encounter families in which the laboratory findings are inconsistent with the reported paternity. These situations should be discussed with the clinician or genetic counselor to determine whether specimens were correctly labeled and the family relationships accurately reported on the requisition form. If there is a possibility of a sample mix-up, new samples should be obtained. In cases of demonstrated nonpaternity, it may not be possible to determine the risk of a genetic disease to an offspring, and the report should indicate this, giving an inconclusive result. The issue of nonpaternity or undisclosed adoption is clearly one that has to be approached with great discretion by the genetic counselor or other professional who is responsible for communication of the test result to the patient or family.

Patients, fearing discrimination, sometimes request that genetic testing be performed without informing their health insurance companies and without having the results entered into the medical record. In such situations, the genetics results are often stored in a shadow chart maintained by the patient's physician in a private office or similar location. This practice is problematic for various reasons. (1) A complete medical record may be needed in an emergency, and the absence of essential medical information may delay appropriate medical therapy. Storing portions of the record in separate locations undermines the integrity and usefulness of the medical record. (2) As a practical matter, the reason for a clinic visit and some mention of the test result usually appears elsewhere in the medical record (e.g., in correspondence between physicians), and therefore the test results are rarely eliminated from the formal medical record. (3) From a legal perspective, the medical record includes all information relevant to a patient's care, even if that information is stored in an alternative location. The entire medical record should be available to authorized personnel.

The immediate resolution to these issues is to ensure that the complete medical record is secured and that hospital employees and others access only information that is needed for patient care. All employees should be made aware of policies related to confidentiality of patient records and the importance of adhering to principles of patient privacy. In the United States, this is not just an ethical requirement, but also a legal one under the Health Insurance Portability and Accountability Act of 1996 (HIPAA).[9] Respect of patient privacy should make the use of shadow records unnecessary. More global solutions to fears of genetic discrimination require introduction of legislation that forbids such discrimination, particularly in employment and insurability.[19]

Reporting Results Obtained by Use of Analyte-Specific Reagents

In the United States, laboratory methods that involve the use of **analyte-specific reagents (ASRs)** (which include many molecular test methods) necessitate a disclaimer on test reports since these reagents are not cleared by the FDA. The language should include the statement that "this test was developed and its performance characteristics determined by (laboratory name). It has not been cleared or approved by the U.S. Food and Drug Administration."[10] This statement is not required for tests that have been cleared by the FDA for use in clinical diagnostics. The language of the statement may be misinterpreted by some insurance payers as meaning that the test was performed for research purposes. To prevent this misperception, many laboratories include an additional statement to the effect that the test was not performed as a research test or that approval is not required by the FDA. Specific wording addressing this is recommended by the CAP molecular pathology inspection checklist.[8]

Quality Assurance and Quality Improvement

Quality assurance (QA) is involved with the monitoring of all laboratory processes. It is defined as the practice that encompasses all endeavors, procedures, formats, and activities directed toward ensuring that a specified quality is achieved and maintained. Some of the components of a QA program in a molecular diagnostics laboratory include testing of new reagents, use of **assay controls,** development of written laboratory procedures, and participation in proficiency testing. Quality improvement is a process that uses a structured procedure to analyze performance and recommend ways to improve its quality.

Testing of New Reagents

Because of the relatively high reliance on **in-house assays** in molecular diagnostics laboratories, it is still quite common for laboratories to produce their own reagents. Careful preparation of all reagents is essential; however, certain reagents, such as PCR primers and Southern blot probes, are particularly critical. Commonly, these are produced by the laboratory or by commercial suppliers that may vary in the degree of process control of the reagent manufacturing. Before any reagent is placed into service, it is necessary to verify that it performs to specification. The concentration and the purity of primers and probes are routinely determined by spectrophotometry with a ratio of absorbances at 260 nm and 280 nm (A260/A280) between 1.8 and 2.0. Results using the new reagents should be compared with results from a previous lot. This comparison should contain known positive and negative controls or as many of the possible genotypes as are available. Additional validation steps are often used: in the case of Southern blot probes that are cloned in plasmids, it may be possible to verify the identity of the probe by examining the restriction digestion pattern of the plasmid or by sequencing the cloned insert. In the case of PCR primers, the sequence of the PCR product is determined to confirm that the expected gene sequence is being amplified. The laboratory should retain documentation on the locus, sequence, origin, restriction map, presence of polymorphisms, presence of cross-hybridizing bands, and other relevant information for each probe or primer set that it uses. Such information is often invaluable in resolving unusual or unexpected results.

Assay Controls

As a matter of routine quality assessment, control specimens that test preanalytical, analytical, and postanalytical processes should be used with all patient samples. For typical target-amplification tests in microbiology and oncology, positive and negative control samples should be taken through the (1) extraction, (2) amplification, and (3) detection portions of the analysis to ensure that established limits of detection and/or quantification are being met. Any amplification reaction should include a blank control that contains all reagents but not an amplifiable template as a means to identify amplicon contamination.

Laboratories that perform genetic testing for inherited diseases use controls for amplification and detection, but not necessarily for extraction. Genomic control DNA samples containing specific variants are often rare. Additionally, a failed extraction is obvious by the lack of amplification of any allele. However, samples that show poor amplification should be reextracted since one allele may be amplified preferentially at very low DNA concentrations. Ideally, control materials containing all tested variants and the corresponding wild-type alleles should be analyzed with every patient run to confirm that the analytical method is producing accurate results. For certain genetic tests, in which a limited number of known disease-causing variants are tested, both disease-causing variants and wild-type controls are included with each analytical run. However, many genes of interest include a large number of disease-causing variants so that it is not always practical to run a control for each with every analytical run. In such a situation, a reasonable compromise must be achieved that ensures that the analytical method detects all disease-causing variants. This might be accomplished, for example, by testing all control samples when new lots of critical reagents are first placed in service, and thereafter by rotating a different set of controls with each run. Control materials containing known disease-causing variants are available from several sources. These include cell and DNA repositories, such as the one maintained by Coriell Laboratories, and synthesized control materials, such as oligonucleotides or plasmids. Synthetic controls are often designed to contain all disease-causing variants of a particular gene in a single reaction. These "supercontrols," if they are compatible with the PCR primers (Chapter 5), are taken through the entire extraction, amplification, and detection process. Alternatively, they serve as a detection control for all mutant alleles.

Appropriate controls must be considered for each assay type. If the assay detects the presence or absence of a PCR product, amplifying a reference sequence will control for potential PCR inhibitors. This type of control could be either co-amplified with the product of interest or amplified separately. A co-amplified control often uses primers homologous to the target, with the internal sequence being different enough (e.g., in size) to distinguish the control from the amplicon. These "competitive" controls compete with the target for the primers. If being used quantitatively, the competitor may limit the sensitivity or dynamic range of the assay. Heterologous co-amplified reference sequences (often a segment of β-globin) also may be amplified preferentially and therefore need to be used at a minimum concentration. Reverse-transcriptase PCR (RT-PCR) for mRNA is often used in molecular hematopathology tests to detect gene breakpoints associated with malignancy. An RT control is necessary to ensure adequate preparation of cDNA. Analytical methods that produce quantitative results (e.g., for HIV-1 viral load measurement or *bcr/abl* gene rearrangement) should include appropriate calibrators and controls. These calibrators need to have similar PCR efficiencies as the target. Calibrators are either co-amplified in the same reaction tube or used to generate an (external) calibration curve.[7] Sources of calibrators and controls include commercial manufacturers and in-house developed materials, which must also be thoroughly analyzed before use.

Control results are analyzed for statistical significance (mean, standard deviation [SD], and CV) in a manner similar to quantitative controls for hematology or chemistry testing. For example, in a qualitative assay for an infectious agent using real-time PCR, laboratories monitor the crossing point (Chapter 5) of the pool

used as a positive control. This allows detection of change in the amplification efficiency of the reaction. Similarly, monitoring of the melting points of wild-type and variant controls helps to identify unusual variants that have melting points outside the accepted control ranges for the control sequences.[17]

Procedures

Standard operating procedures are required for every process in the clinical laboratory. Procedures for specimen processing include specimen type and collection and transport requirements (see also Chapter 3). As a result of lability of RNA, specimens for RNA-based assays should be received in the laboratory within 72 hours. Specialized collection tubes that stabilize RNA upon collection have recently been developed and hold promise to reduce mRNA degradation. Technical procedures include not only the order of steps to perform a molecular test, but also probe and primer sequences and the reference sequence used for assay design. Instrument maintenance procedures should include calibration for detection instruments and temperature monitoring and temperature transition rates for thermal cyclers. Variations that occur between reaction well positions and between instruments are one source of seemingly sporadic amplification failures. Safety procedures should alert laboratory personnel to proper handling of toxic chemicals used in molecular procedures, such as acrylamide, phenol, or ethidium bromide. Safety precautions detail handling of radioactive material (typically ^{32}P) used for labeling probes or primers. However, radioactivity is increasingly being replaced by chemiluminescent or fluorescent chemistry.

Procedures should be developed to handle ethical issues involved in molecular testing. For example, genetics laboratories often employ or contract with genetic counselors who help with proper test ordering and interpretation. A procedure should outline their roles and how to document communication with healthcare professionals and laboratory personnel. Laboratories should consider their position on performing testing for children being placed for adoption. Although children will have the state's required newborn screening, adoptive parents may want to test a child with no symptoms for conditions not routinely tested by newborn screening (such as cystic fibrosis) since the family history is unknown.[1] Similarly a policy should be developed for testing asymptomatic children for adult-onset diseases. This issue is illustrated by Huntington disease testing, in which parents may want to know if their children carry the altered gene (Chapter 9). Since symptoms usually are not present until into the third or fourth decade or beyond, the general belief is that the children should make the decision as they become an adult.[2] An ethical dilemma in testing for inherited diseases is the implication of the test result for family members (see Ethics Box 7-1). Laboratories should consider these issues and have written policies that address them.

Correlation with Other Laboratory Results

For testing in areas such as molecular oncology, inherited disorders, and posttransplantation bone marrow engraftment, it is common that other testing is performed on the sample. This may include morphologic studies, flow cytometry, or cytogenetic evaluation. Where possible, the results of molecular diagnostic tests should be compared with those from other tests to ensure that results are consistent or that inconsistent results are fully investigated before a final report is issued. Such prac-

<table>
<tr><td>

ETHICS Box 7-1   Ethical Considerations

Ethical considerations in the operation of a molecular diagnostics laboratory often deal with the privacy of medical records. For infectious diseases, privacy issues are of concern for diseases that carry a social stigma. In genetic testing, privacy issues are at times in conflict with the ability to properly interpret results that need to be considered in a family context. Patients should be encouraged to discuss laboratory results with others who may be affected as well.

Imagine a scenario in which a grandparent suffers from an autosomal-dominant, adult-onset disease, such as Huntington disease. The parent has a 50% risk, but is asymptomatic and chooses to not be tested. An adult child of that parent is at 25% risk, and he wants to be tested by the DNA test. Detecting the expansion in the child would also indicate that the (asymptomatic) parent is at risk. In this case the child's right to know must be weighed against the parent's right not to know.

Ensuring appropriate testing also has ethical consequences. Although recommendations exist that discourage testing minors for adult-onset conditions, parents and/or clinicians may insist on testing. In these cases laboratories may need to respect the decisions of the clinicians or have policies defining the conditions in which testing would be refused.

The main ethical concern for the laboratory, however, is to ensure the integrity of results. Every effort should be made to resolve discrepancies and to correct procedures that are at high risk for human error. The laboratory personnel must always remember that therapeutic and disease-management decisions are based on the results from the laboratory. Since genetic results should not change over time, the patient may be tested once in his or her lifetime. Therefore the laboratory has only one chance to get the right result.

</td></tr>
</table>

time will identify problem areas, such as increasing failure rates or increasing turnaround times (TAT), thus allowing corrections to be made. TAT priorities should be given to some infectious disease tests and any fetal testing. Collecting and linking laboratory results and data from other areas of the healthcare system has the potential to lead to better service to patients and the community.

SUMMARY

The design and operation of a molecular diagnostics laboratory have several unique aspects that differ from those in other clinical laboratories. The choice of a central facility versus discipline-specific molecular diagnostics laboratories will have a large impact on overall cost and efficiencies. In choosing a test menu, careful attention should be paid to costs, reimbursement, expected volumes, turnaround times, and the expertise required of personnel. The use of target-amplification methods requires careful attention to laboratory design and workflow.

Operational details that are specific to a molecular diagnostics laboratory include regulatory issues related to genetic information that may vary between jurisdictions, personnel qualifications and availability, and the ability to report genetic results based on appropriate statistical calculations. Use of appropriate quality control materials and participation in a PT program that challenges all phases of the analytical process are essential for successful operation of a molecular diagnostics laboratory.

tice should be an integral component of the laboratory's quality assurance program.

Proficiency Testing[6]

The major proficiency testing (PT) program in the United States is provided by the CAP. U.S. laboratories that hold a certificate under the Clinical Laboratory Improvement Act must be enrolled in an acceptable PT program if one is available. Because of the limited number of tests that are covered in organized PT programs, it is often necessary for laboratories to perform some other kind of PT. These must be performed at least semiannually. If no formal PT program exists, acceptable alternatives include participation in ungraded PT challenges, sample exchange with other laboratories performing the test, split sample analysis with another in-house method or by another technologist using the same method, testing of assayed materials, regional pools, and clinical validation by chart review or other means. Wherever possible, the PT program should cover the entire testing process. In the case of molecular diagnostics, this should include nucleic acid extraction, sample analysis, and interpretation of the results, including (if appropriate) calculation of risk of disease. As in all laboratory areas, the results of all PT challenges must be documented and reviewed by the laboratory director or designee.

Quality Improvement

Laboratories should continually identify ways to improve their testing. PT as described above is not only a quality control, but a quality improvement measure as well. It allows the laboratory to compare results, technologies, and interpretations from multiple laboratories. Monitoring other indicators for trends over

REFERENCES

1. [Anon] Genetics Testing in Adoption. Joint Statement of the American Society of Human Genetics and the American College of Medical Genetics. Am J Hum Genet 2000;66:761-7.
2. [Anon] Points to consider: Ethical, legal and psychosocial implications of genetic testing in children and adolescents. American Society of Human Genetics Board of Directors and American College of Medical Genetics Board of Directors. Am J Hum Genet 1995;57:1233-41.
3. Clinical Laboratory Improvement Amendments. http://www.cms.hhs.gov/clia/ (accessed February 26, 2007).
4. Clinical and Laboratory Standards Institute/NCCLS. Molecular Diagnostic Methods for Genetic Diseases; Approved Guideline. CLSI/NCCLS document Mm01-A (ISBN 1-56238-395-7). Wayne, Pa: National Clinical and Laboratory Standards Institute, 2000.
5. Clinical and Laboratory Standards Institute/NCCLS. Molecular Diagnostic Methods for Infectious Diseases; Approved Guideline. CLSI/NCCLS document MM03-A2 (ISBN 1-56238-596-8). Wayne, Pa: National Clinical and Laboratory Standards Institute, 2006.
6. Clinical and Laboratory Standards Institute/NCCLS. Proficiency Testing (External Quality Assessment) for Molecular Methods. CLSI/NCCLS document MM14-A (ISBN 1-56238-581-X). Wayne, Pa: National Clinical and Laboratory Standards Institute, 2005.
7. Clinical and Laboratory Standards Institute/NCCLS. Quantitative Molecular Methods for Infectious Diseases; Approved Guideline. CLSI/NCCLS document MM06-A (ISBN 1-56238-508-9). Wayne, Pa: National Clinical and Laboratory Standards Institute, 2003.
8. College of American Pathologists. Commission on Laboratory Accreditation. Laboratory Accreditation Program. Molecular Pathology Checklist. http://www.cap.org/apps/docs/laboratory_accreditation/checklists/molecular_pathology_october2005.doc (accessed February 26, 2007).
9. Department of Health and Human Services, Centers for Medicare & Medicaid Services, The Health Insurance Portability and Accountability Act of 1996 (HIPAA) http://www.cms.hhs.gov/HIPAAGenInfo/ (accessed February 26, 2007).
10. Department of Health and Human Services, Food and Drug Administration. Medical devices; classification/reclassification; restricted devices; analyte specific reagents. Final rule. Fed Register.

1997(Nov 21);62243-45 [21CFR809, 21CFR864] http://www.fda.gov/cdrh/oivd/index.html (accessed February 26, 2007).

11. Grody WW, Cutting GR, Klinger KW, Richards CS, Watson MS, Desnick RJ. Laboratory standards and guidelines for population-based cystic fibrosis carrier screening. Genet Med 2001;3:149-54.

12. Grody WW, Griffin JH, Taylor AK, Korf BR, Heit JA (ACMG Factor V Leiden Working Group). American College of Medical Genetics Consensus Statement on Factor V Leiden Mutation Testing. Med Genet 2001;3:139-48.

13. Johnson A. Genetic Privacy. Genetics Brief, National Conference of State Legislatures, Denver, Colo, 2002 http://www.ncsl.org/programs/health/genetics/geneticprivacy.pdf (accessed February 26, 2007).

14. Keegan CE, Killeen AA. An overview of molecular diagnosis of steroid 21-hydroxylase deficiency. J Mol Diagn 2001;32:49-54.

15. Killeen AA. Principles of molecular pathology. Totowa, NJ: Humana Press, 2004.

16. Kremer B, Goldberg P, Andrew SE, Theilmann J, Telenius H, Zeisler J, et al. A worldwide study of the Huntington's disease mutation. The sensitivity and specificity of measuring CAG repeats. N Engl J Med 1994;330:1401-6.

17. Mahadevan, MS, Benson PV. Factor V null mutation affecting the Roche LightCycler Factor V Leiden assay. Clin Chem 2005;51:1533-5.

18. Potter NT, Spector EB, Prior TW. Technical standards and guidelines for Huntington disease testing. Genet Med 2004;6:61-5.

19. Silvers A, Stein MA. Human rights and genetic discrimination: protecting genomics' promise for public health. J Law Med Ethics 2003;31:377-89.

20. Udaykumar, Epstein JS, Hewlett IK. A novel method employing UNG to avoid carry-over contamination in RNA-PCR. Nucleic Acids Res 1993;21:3917-8.

REVIEW QUESTIONS

1. Unidirectional workflow is necessary in a molecular laboratory to
   A. prevent contamination.
   B. improve workflow efficiency.
   C. meet reagent storage requirements.
   D. reduce cleaning measures.
   E. prevent sample mix-up.

2. Factors that would discourage offering a new test include
   A. local expertise.
   B. proven clinical utility.
   C. low complexity and low cost.
   D. restricted licensing.
   E. short turnaround times.

3. Reports should include all of the following elements except
   A. gene locus.
   B. disease-causing variants (mutations) tested.
   C. genotype-phenotype correlation.
   D. analytical sensitivity and specificity.
   E. sample retention policy of the laboratory.

4. Calibrators for quantitative assays must
   A. be developed by a certified governmental agency.
   B. have similar PCR efficiencies as the target.
   C. be radioactively labeled.
   D. contain multiple disease-causing variants (mutations).
   E. be competitive against the target.

5. Correlating molecular results with a cytogenetic evaluation is useful for
   A. a triplet repeat disease, such as Huntington disease.
   B. a "mutation panel" for cystic fibrosis.
   C. translocations, such as Bcr/abl in malignancies.
   D. monitoring a bone marrow engraftment from an identical twin.
   E. confirming parentage.

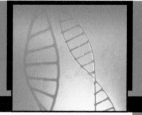

Chapter 8

Introduction to Evidence-Based Molecular Diagnostics

David E. Bruns, M.D.
Christopher P. Price, Ph.D.
Patrick M.M. Bossuyt, Ph.D.

OBJECTIVES

1. List five reasons for performing a laboratory test.
2. State the purposes for practicing evidence-based medicine (EBM) and evidence-based laboratory medicine.
3. List and describe the four key diagnostic questions addressed by the decision-making process in laboratory medicine.
4. Describe the five major goals involved in evidence-based laboratory medicine studies.
5. Design a diagnostic accuracy study; specify the inclusion and exclusion criteria and other items in the methods section of the standards for reporting of diagnostic accuracy (STARD) checklist.
6. Compare and contrast internal and external validity in relation to a diagnostic accuracy study.
7. Discuss the STARD initiative including it uses, its components, and its application in the clinical laboratory.
8. Explain the need for outcomes studies in medical practice.
9. Design a randomized controlled trial (RCT); specify the subjects and interventions; determine which outcomes are to be assessed.
10. List the five components of a systematic review of a diagnostic test.
11. Define "cost" in relation to healthcare and list five methods for evaluating the economic impact of a diagnostic test.
12. State how economic evaluations are perceived by different groups including patients, laboratory practitioners, clinicians, insurance companies, and society.
13. Discuss the usefulness of clinical practice guidelines and clinical audits.
14. List four components of a clinical audit.
15. Discuss how the principles of evidence-based laboratory medicine can be applied to routine laboratory practice.

KEY WORDS AND DEFINITIONS

Bias: Systematic error that occurs when there is constant overestimation or underestimation of a measured value as opposed to random error, which is unpredictable.

Clinical Audit: The review of case histories of patients against the benchmark of current best practice; used as a tool to improve clinical practice.

Clinical Practice Guidelines: Systematically developed statements to assist practitioner and patient decisions about appropriate healthcare for specific clinical circumstances; in the laboratory, guidelines may include goals for accuracy, precision, and turnaround time of tests.

Diagnostic Accuracy: The closeness of agreement between values obtained from a diagnostic test (index test) and those of a reference standard (gold standard) for a specific disease or condition; these results are expressed in a number of ways, including sensitivity and specificity, predictive values, likelihood ratios, diagnostic odds ratios, and areas under receiver operating characteristic (ROC) curves.

Evidence-Based Laboratory Medicine: The application of principles and techniques of EBM to laboratory medicine; the conscientious, judicious, and explicit use of best evidence in the use of laboratory medicine investigations for assisting in decision making about the care of individual patients.

Evidence-Based Medicine (EBM): The conscientious, judicious, and explicit use of the best evidence in making decisions about the care of individual patients.

External Validity: The degree to which the results of a study can be generalized to other patients.

Index Test: In diagnostic accuracy studies, the "new" test or the test of interest.

Internal Validity: The degree to which the results of a study can be trusted for the population of patients in the study; depends on the experimental design, research design, instruments used, calibration, etc.

Molecular Diagnostics: A field of laboratory medicine in which principles and techniques of molecular biology are applied to the study of disease.

Outcomes: Results related to the quality or quantity of life of patients; examples include mortality, morbidity, functional status, length of stay in a hospital, and costs.

Outcomes Studies: Studies performed to determine if a medical intervention (such as a specific laboratory test) will improve health outcome (clinical or economic or both).

Randomized Controlled Trial (RCT): An experimental study in which study participants are randomly allocated to an intervention (treatment) group or an alternative treatment (control) group.

Reference Standard: The best available method for establishing the presence or absence of the target disease or condition; this could be a single test or a combination of methods and techniques.

STARD: Standards for reporting of diagnostic accuracy; a project designed to improve the quality of reporting the results of diagnostic accuracy studies.

Systematic Review: A methodical and comprehensive review of all published and unpublished information about a specific topic to answer a precisely defined clinical question.

Validity: (In research) The degree to which a measure is measuring what it is supposed to measure or the degree to which the study is able to answer the study question; validity requires reliability and accuracy.

The recent strides in molecular biology have provided powerful new ways of looking at health and disease. The most apparent impact of this work is in molecular diagnostics. A parallel impact has come to medicine from the field of clinical epidemiology. This revolution has been called by several names, most commonly "**evidence-based medicine**" **(EBM)**. EBM uses principles of clinical epidemiology to find the best available evidence for use in the care of patients. Molecular biology and EBM come together in the field of molecular diagnostics. It is critical that standards of EBM be used to characterize the new tools from molecular biology.

In this chapter, we consider the relationships among molecular diagnostics, laboratory medicine, and **evidence-based laboratory medicine.** We explore principles that underlie:

- How to assess the **diagnostic accuracy** of tests
- How to use clinical **outcomes studies**
- Ways to evaluate the *economic value* of medical tests
- How to conduct **systematic reviews** of diagnostic tests
- How to use **clinical practice guidelines**
- When and how to conduct **clinical audits**

These principles provide a foundation for the rational and appropriate use of tests performed in the molecular diagnostics laboratory.

CONCEPTS, DEFINITIONS, AND RELATIONSHIPS

Molecular diagnostics is a field of laboratory medicine in which the principles and techniques of molecular biology are applied to the study of disease. Molecular diagnostic tests are used in the diagnosis, prognosis, screening, and monitoring of disease and in identifying optimal treatment strategies for conditions ranging from acute infections to cancer and inherited diseases. In this section, we discuss the role of laboratory medicine and evidence-based laboratory medicine in molecular diagnostics.

What Is Laboratory Medicine?

The term "laboratory medicine" refers to the discipline involved in the selection, provision, and interpretation of diagnostic testing that uses, primarily, samples from patients. The field includes clinical service, research, and teaching activities and clinical administration. Testing in laboratory medicine may be directed at (a) *confirming* a clinical suspicion (which could include *making* a diagnosis), (b) *excluding* a diagnosis, (c) assisting in the *selection, optimization,* and *monitoring* of treatment, (d) providing a *prognosis,* or (e) *screening* for disease in the absence of clinical signs or symptoms. Testing is also used to establish and monitor the severity of a physiological disturbance.

The field of laboratory medicine includes such areas as clinical chemistry and its traditional subdisciplines (including toxicology and drug monitoring, endocrine and organ-function testing, and "biochemical" genetics), microbiology, hematology, hemostasis and thrombosis, blood banking (transfusion medicine), immunology, clinical genetics, and identity testing. In some parts of the world, laboratory medicine also encompasses cytology and anatomical pathology (histopathology). Molecular pathology is now becoming integrated into all of these specialties. The analytical components of these specialties are delivered from central laboratories or through a more distributed type of service (point-of-care testing [POCT]) or both. Information management and interpretation (including laboratory informatics) are key aspects of the laboratory medicine service, as are activities concerned with maintaining quality (e.g., quality control and proficiency testing, audit, benchmarking, and clinical governance).

From the physician's and the patient's perspective, there is no distinction among the many specialties of laboratory medicine. Moreover, the repertoire of more than one specialty invariably will be called upon when making a clinical decision. Boundaries between and among the parts of the clinical laboratory have blurred with the increasing emphasis on use of chemical and "molecular" testing. Molecular diagnostics testing has evolved beyond human genetic testing to include infectious disease testing, cancer diagnostics, and identity testing, activities that were formerly associated almost solely with, respectively, clinical microbiology, hematology, and blood bank laboratories. Successful contribution to these areas requires an understanding of the principles of laboratory medicine and close collaboration with clinical microbiologists, hematologists, and others who have specialized expertise in those areas of laboratory medicine.

Molecular Diagnostics, Laboratory Medicine, and Evidence-Based Laboratory Medicine

In this chapter, we review the new influences on molecular diagnostics and laboratory medicine from the fields of clinical epidemiology and EBM. Clinical epidemiologists have developed study designs to quantify the diagnostic accuracy of the tests developed in laboratory medicine and study methods to evaluate the effect and value of laboratory testing in healthcare. Practitioners of EBM focus on use of the best available evidence from well-designed studies in the care of individual patients. EBM rephrases problems in the clinical care of patients as structured clinical questions, looks for the available evidence, evaluates the quality of clinical studies, evaluates the clinical implications of the results, and provides tools to help clinicians optimally use those results in the care of individual patients. Application of these principles to laboratory medicine constitutes evidence-based laboratory medicine.

EVIDENCE-BASED MEDICINE—WHAT IS IT?

This brief section contains a definition of EBM and describes its goals and key practices. Following this, evidence-based laboratory medicine will be addressed.

Definition and Goals of Evidence-Based Medicine

Among the definitions proposed for EBM, the foremost probably is "*the conscientious, judicious, and explicit use of the best evidence in making decisions about the care of individual patients.*"[21] The word *judicious* implies use of the skills of experienced clinicians to put the evidence in context and to recognize patient individuality and preferences. A goal of EBM is "*to incorporate the best evidence from clinical research into clinical decisions.*" The word *best* implies the necessity for critical appraisal. The words *making decisions* indicate why the principles of EBM can, and must, be applied in laboratory medicine because laboratory medicine is one of the fundamental tools used in making decisions in the practice of medicine.

Since the introduction[10] of the term "evidence-based medicine" in 1991 by Gordon Guyatt (initially in an editorial in *ACP Journal Club* and in a supplement to *Annals of Internal Medicine*), volumes have been written on the topic. A December 2006 PubMed search for the term returned nearly 24,000 articles. The papers address every area of medicine and activities, such as disease management. Compared with practitioners in many of these areas, workers in clinical laboratories were late in embracing the activities of EBM, but numerous evidence-based studies are now influencing the practice of laboratory medicine.

The Practice of Evidence-Based Medicine

Guyatt and colleagues[12] summarized the practice of EBM as follows:

> An evidence-based practitioner must understand the patient's circumstances or predicament; identify knowledge gaps and frame questions to fill those gaps; conduct an efficient literature search; critically appraise the research evidence; and apply that evidence to patient care.

The efficient practice of EBM requires:
- A knowledge of the *clinical process* and conversion of a clinical goal into an answerable question
- Facility to generate and critically appraise information to generate knowledge
- A critically appraised knowledge resource
- Ability to use the knowledge resource
- A means of accessing and delivering the knowledge resource
- A framework of clinical and economic accountability
- A framework of quality management

AC   The identification of a clinical goal provides the foundation of the service provided by the healthcare professional. In the area of laboratory medicine, as described later in this chapter, the goal can be expressed in terms of answering a clinical question. Knowledge of the characteristics of these investigations is needed to decide which test to use, when to use it, and how to interpret the results.

Finding and appraising knowledge that is relevant to the question requires awareness of the information resources available, ready access to them, and an ability to critically appraise the relevance of the available data.

A knowledge resource in the form of systematic reviews (see later in this chapter) should provide the critically reviewed evidence of the efficacy, benefits, limitations, and risks from using a test, intervention, or device. Access has classically been through scientific journals and textbooks, and electronic communication of various sorts (including textbooks and journals) is making access faster and more up-to-date.

Knowledge on the use of a test or intervention ultimately has to be placed in the context of a clinical and economic accountability framework and ensuring the highest quality and lowest risk to patients. Clinical audit is a key element of meeting this objective.

EVIDENCE-BASED MEDICINE AND LABORATORY MEDICINE

When a patient has symptoms or signs of a health problem, the clinician establishes hypotheses about their cause. Competing hypotheses must be resolved. After decisions are made about the nature of the condition, the process of care may then involve further decisions depending on the nature of the problem or disease. The services of laboratory medicine are one of the tools at the disposal of the clinician to answer the questions posed by the hypothesis and to help make decisions.

The tools provided by laboratory medicine are called *diagnostic* tests, but tests are used far more broadly than in making a diagnosis. As mentioned above and discussed below, they are also used in making a prognosis, excluding a diagnosis, monitoring a treatment or disease process, and screening for disease. Thus the word "diagnostic" is used (often unknowingly) in a much broader sense.

What Is Evidence-Based Laboratory Medicine?

Evidence-based laboratory medicine is simply the application of principles and techniques of EBM to laboratory medicine. A clinician requesting an investigation has a question and must make a decision. The clinician hopes that the test result will help to answer the question and assist in making the decision. Thus a definition of evidence-based laboratory medicine could be *"the conscientious, judicious, and explicit use of best evidence in the use of laboratory medicine investigations for assisting in decision making about the care of individual patients."* It might also be expressed more directly in terms of health outcomes as *"ensuring that the best evidence on testing is made available and the clinician is assisted in using the best evidence to ensure that the best decisions are made about the care of individual patients and lead to increased probability of improved health outcomes."* As discussed later, outcomes can be clinical, operational, economic, or any combination of these effects.

Types of Diagnostic Questions Addressed in Laboratory Medicine

The decision-making process involves one of four scenarios typified by these questions (Figure 8-1):

• What is the diagnosis?
• Can another diagnosis be ruled out?
• What is this patient's prognosis?
• How is the patient doing?

In the first scenario, a diagnosis is being sought. Diagnostic conclusions lead to a decision and some form of action, which often involves an intervention. The intention is that the cascade from diagnostic question through result, decision, and action should lead to an improved outcome. An example of this scenario occurs when a rapid nucleic acid test reveals the presence of herpes simplex virus (HSV) DNA in the spinal fluid of a patient with suspected HSV encephalitis. In such cases, antiviral treatment can be initiated rapidly without need for a brain biopsy to make the diagnosis. The test in this scenario is referred to as a "rule-in test."

In the second scenario, the test result excludes a diagnosis; this is referred to as a "rule-out test." The actions resulting from

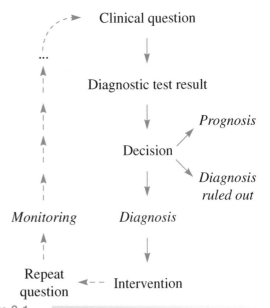

Figure 8-1

Schematic representation of four common decision-making steps in which the result of an investigation is involved.

excluding a diagnosis will invariably involve the evaluation or creation of another hypothesis. In the example of HSV above, when a test for HSV DNA in spinal fluid is negative, empirical therapy can be stopped, and the possibility of alternative diagnoses must be pursued more vigorously.

The third use of an investigation is for prognosis, which may be considered as the assessment of risk, and complements the diagnostic application. For example, the measurement of the concentration of human immunodeficiency virus (HIV) RNA in plasma following initial diagnosis of HIV infection can be used to predict the time interval before immune collapse if the condition is not treated.

The fourth broad use of a test result is concerned with patient management. For example, a test result may be used to select therapy. Other tests may be used to assess the outcome of the therapy and whether the therapy should be continued. In a woman with metastatic breast cancer, tests of the HER-2/*neu* gene or gene product will indicate whether Herceptin therapy is likely to be worthwhile for the patient (see Chapter 13). Gene variants that govern the rate of drug metabolism are used to determine the appropriate dose of a drug (see Chapter 12). Similarly, analysis of the primary HIV RNA sequence in a patient with HIV infection can reveal resistance to specific drugs. Combination antiviral therapy will be selected based on this information (see Chapter 11).

In each of these examples, three components are present: a *question*, a *decision*, and an *action*. Identifying these three components proves to be critical in designing studies of utility or outcomes of testing (see later in this chapter). They are also important in audit (see below) of the use of investigations. The recognition of these three components has led to the definition of an *appropriate test request* as one in which there is a clear clinical *question* for which the result will provide an answer, enabling the clinician to make a *decision* and initiate some form of *action* leading to a health benefit.

Using the Test Result

The key criterion for a useful test is that the result can lead to a change in the probability of the presence of the target condition. This is true even for genetic tests, because the presence of a mutation may or may not lead to clinical disease and may or may not predict its severity (see Chapter 9).

Test Results Alone Do Not Produce Clinical Outcomes

In most cases testing must be followed by an appropriate intervention to produce a desired outcome. A test result alone may provide reassurance or an understanding of the origin of one's complaint, but even this may require explanation and reassurance from a physician. Because of the difficulty of documenting that testing improves patient outcomes, most research in laboratory medicine addresses only the analytical characteristics and diagnostic performance of tests and not the effects of tests on patients' lives. This restricted research leads to poor understanding and lack of appreciation of the contribution of tests to improved outcomes. Nonetheless, studies of outcomes are being done, and more are needed (see Outcomes Studies later in this chapter).

INFORMATION NEEDS IN EVIDENCE-BASED LABORATORY MEDICINE

Studies in the field of evidence-based laboratory medicine have five major goals:

1. Characterization of the *diagnostic accuracy* of tests by studying groups of patients
2. Determination of the value of testing (*outcomes*) for people who are tested
3. *Systematic reviewing* of studies of diagnostic accuracy or outcomes of tests to answer a specific medical question, and to provide the core information for clinical guidelines
4. *Economic evaluation* of tests to determine which tests to use
5. *Audit* of performance of tests during use (of guidelines) to answer questions about their use

The following sections of this chapter provide brief introductions to the principles of how to gain these critical types of information that are needed for patient care.

CHARACTERIZATION OF DIAGNOSTIC ACCURACY OF TESTS

Users of tests need information about the extent of agreement of the test's results with the correct diagnoses of patients. Researchers thus compare results from the new test with the results obtained from the gold standard test for the condition. The gold standard test is called the **reference standard.** The results of the comparison can be expressed in a number of ways, including diagnostic sensitivity and specificity. We will refer to such studies as diagnostic accuracy studies.

Study Design

In studies of diagnostic accuracy, the results of one test (often referred to as the **index test,** the test of interest) are compared with those from the reference standard (the best current practice) to arrive at a diagnosis. A reference standard can be any method for obtaining additional information on a patient's health status. This includes not only laboratory tests, imaging

tests, and function tests but also data from the history, physical examination, and genetics.

The *reference standard* is the best available method for establishing the presence or absence of the target condition (the suspected condition or disease for which the test is to be applied). The reference standard can be a single test or a combination of methods and techniques. Thus in evaluating a genetic test for porphyria, the reference standard might be a test for porphobilinogen. Alternatively, it could be more rigorous and include a set of findings on a group of tests of various porphyrins and related metabolites. Obviously the apparent diagnostic accuracy of the test will be affected by the quality of the reference standard.

The reference standard can include clinical follow-up of tested patients. Thus in evaluating a molecular test for the presence of enterovirus species in spinal fluid of patients with signs of meningitis, the reference standard might be a one-time viral culture; instead, it could also be a combination of culture and clinical course of the illness over several days.

There are several potential threats to the *internal* and *external* **validity** of a study of diagnostic accuracy. Poor **internal validity** (problems in the design of the study) will produce **bias,** or systematic error, because the estimates of diagnostic accuracy differ from those one would have obtained using an optimal design for the study. Poor **external validity** limits the generalizability of the findings because the results of the study, even if unbiased, do not correspond to settings encountered by the person using the results of the study. For example, studies done exclusively in older men may not be applicable to women of a childbearing age seen by an obstetrician who would like to use the results of the study.

The ideal study examines a consecutive series of patients, enrolling all consenting patients suspected of the target condition within a specific period. All of these patients then undergo the index test and then are evaluated by the reference standard. The term "consecutive" refers to total absence of any form of selection, beyond the definition (determined at the start of the study) of the criteria for inclusion (and exclusion) in the study, and requires explicit efforts to identify and enroll patients qualifying for inclusion.

AC Alternative designs are possible. Some studies first select patients known to have the target condition and then contrast the test results of these patients with those of individuals in a control group. This approach has been used to characterize the performance of tests in settings in which the condition of interest is uncommon as in many single-gene inherited disorders. It is also used in preliminary studies to assess the potential of a test before embarking on prospective studies of a series of patients. With this design, the selection of the control group is critical. If the control group consists of healthy individuals only, diagnostic accuracy of the test is likely to be overestimated. The control group should include patients in whom the disease is suspected but is excluded.

In the ideal study, the results of all patients tested with the test under evaluation are contrasted with the results

Continued

of a single reference standard. If the reference standard is not applied to all patients, then *partial verification* exists. In a typical case, some patients with negative test results (test-negatives) are not verified by an expensive or invasive reference standard, and these patients are excluded from the analysis. This may result in an underestimation of the number of false-negative results.

A different form of verification bias can happen if more than one reference standard is used, and the two reference standards correspond to different manifestations of disease. This study design can produce *differential verification bias*. Suppose test-positive patients are verified with further testing and test-negative patients are verified by clinical follow-up. An example is the verification of suspected appendicitis, with histopathology of the appendix versus natural history as the two forms of the reference standard. A patient is classified as having a false-positive test result if the additional test does not confirm the presence of disease after a positive index test result. Alternatively a patient is classified as a false-negative if an event compatible with appendicitis is observed during follow-up after a negative test result. Yet these are different definitions of disease because not all patients who have positive test results by the reference standard would have experienced an event during follow-up if they had been left untreated. The use of two reference standards, one pathological and the other based on clinical prognosis, can affect the assessment of diagnostic accuracy. It can also lead to variability among studies that depend on the proportions of patients verified with each of the two standards.

There is a long-standing debate on whether or not clinical data should be provided to those performing or reading the index test. This is especially so when that test has a subjective component. If a pathologist interpreting a liver biopsy knows that the patient carries the mutation associated with hemochromatosis, the interpretation of the biopsy may be affected. Withholding such diagnostically relevant information is known as blinding or masking. Some clinical information is often routinely known by the reader of the test, such as when radiologists see the patients on whom they are performing a test or a pathologist is told the site from which a biopsy is obtained. A similar concern occurs in the molecular diagnostics laboratory. For example, trained individuals must interpret studies of gene rearrangement for assessment of clonality in patients suspected to have leukemia or lymphoma. Most interpreters will know not only the site of the biopsy but also the histological findings. To try to withhold such information in the context of a study of diagnostic accuracy may create an artificial scenario that has no counterpart in patient care. Thoughtful attention to this question is important in the early phases of designing a study of diagnostic accuracy. For most study questions, masking is preferable because knowledge of the results will tend to increase agreement of the result of the studied (index) test with the reference standard (test).

The severity of disease in the studied patients with the target condition and the range of other conditions in the other patients (controls) can affect the apparent diagnostic accuracy of a test. For example, if a test that is designed to detect early cancer is evaluated in patients with clinically apparent cancer, the test is likely to perform better than when used for persons who do not yet show signs of the condition. This problem has been called "*spectrum bias*." Similarly, if a test is developed to distinguish patients with the target condition from patients with a similar condition, it may be misleading to use healthy subjects as controls, rather than patients with similar symptoms, when evaluating the diagnostic accuracy of the test.

The Reporting of Studies of Diagnostic Accuracy and the Role of the STARD Initiative

Complete and accurate reporting of studies of diagnostic accuracy should allow the reader to detect the potential for bias in the study and to assess the ability to generalize the results and their applicability to an individual patient or group. Reid et al[19] documented that most studies of diagnostic accuracy published in leading general medical journals either had poor adherence to standards of clinical epidemiological research or failed to provide information about adherence to those standards. A later study showed similar problems in studies of genetic tests. These reports led to efforts at the journal *Clinical Chemistry* in 1997 to produce a checklist for reporting of studies of diagnostic accuracy. The quality of reporting in that journal increased after introduction of this checklist, though not to an ideal level.

The work of Lijmer et al[15] showed that poor study design and poor reporting are associated with overestimation of the diagnostic accuracy of evaluated tests. It indicated the necessity to improve the reporting of studies of diagnostic accuracy for all types of diagnostic tests. This led to an initiative on standards for reporting of diagnostic accuracy (**STARD**)[4] aimed at improving the quality of reporting of diagnostic accuracy studies. The key components of the STARD document are a checklist of items to be included in reports of studies of diagnostic accuracy (Figure 8-2) and a flow diagram to document the flow of participants in the study (Figure 8-3).

AC   The STARD initiative has been endorsed by numerous journals (such as *Journal of the American Medical Association [JAMA]* and *Annals of Internal Medicine*) and published in many of them, including all the major journals of clinical chemistry and other leading journals including *Radiology* and the *British Medical Journal (BMJ)*. A separate document explaining the meaning and rationale of each item and briefly summarizing the available evidence was published in *Annals of Internal Medicine* and *Clinical Chemistry*.[5] The STARD group plans to prepare updates of the STARD document when new evidence on sources of bias or variability becomes available. In the experience of the editor of *Clinical Chemistry*, one of the authors of this chapter (DB), use of the checklist has increased the information content of all manuscripts to which it has been applied, and use of the flow diagram has led to correction of errors in many manuscripts.

Section and Topic	Item #		On page #
TITLE/ABSTRACT/ KEYWORDS	1	Identify the article as a study of diagnostic accuracy (recommend MeSH heading sensitivity and specificity).	
INTRODUCTION	2	State the research questions or study aims, such as estimating diagnostic accuracy or comparing accuracy between tests or across participant groups.	
METHODS		Describe	
Participants	3	The study population: The inclusion and exclusion criteria, setting and locations where the data were collected.	
	4	Participant recruitment: Was recruitment based on presenting symptoms, results from previous tests, or the fact that the participants had received the index tests or the reference standard?	
	5	Participant sampling: Was the study population a consecutive series of participants defined by the selection criteria in items 3 and 4? If not, specify how participants were further selected.	
	6	Data collection: Was data collection planned before the index test and reference standard were performed (prospective study) or after (retrospective study)?	
Test methods	7	The reference standard and its rationale.	
	8	Technical specifications of material and methods involved including how and when measurements were taken, and/or cite references for index tests and reference standard.	
	9	Definition of and rationale for the units, cutoffs and/or categories of the results of the index tests and the reference standard.	
	10	The number, training, and expertise of the persons executing and reading the index tests and the reference standard.	
	11	Whether or not the readers of the index tests and reference standard were blind (masked) to the results of the other test and describe any other clinical information available to the readers.	
Statistical methods	12	Methods for calculating or comparing measures of diagnostic accuracy, and the statistical methods used to quantify uncertainty (e.g. 95% confidence intervals).	
	13	Methods for calculating test reproducibility, if done.	
RESULTS		Report	
Participants	14	When study was done, including beginning and ending dates of recruitment.	
	15	Clinical and demographic characteristics of the study population (e.g. age, sex, spectrum of presenting symptoms, comorbidity, current treatments, recruitment centers).	
	16	The number of participants satisfying the criteria for inclusion that did or did not undergo the index tests and/or the reference standard; describe why participants failed to receive either test (a flow diagram is strongly recommended).	
Test results	17	Time interval from the index tests to the reference standard, and any treatment administered between.	
	18	Distribution of severity of disease (define criteria) in those with the target condition; other diagnoses in participants without the target condition.	
	19	A cross tabulation of the results of the index tests (including indeterminate and missing results) by the results of the reference standard; for continuous results, the distribution of the test results by the results of the reference standard.	
	20	Any adverse events from performing the index tests or the reference standard.	
Estimates	21	Estimates of diagnostic accuracy and measures of statistical uncertainty (e.g. 95% confidence intervals).	
	22	How indeterminate results, missing responses, and outliers of the index tests were handled.	
	23	Estimates of variability of diagnostic accuracy between subgroups of participants, readers, or centers, if done.	
	24	Estimates of test reproducibility, if done.	
DISCUSSION	25	Discuss the clinical applicability of the study findings.	

Figure 8-2
STARD checklist.

General example

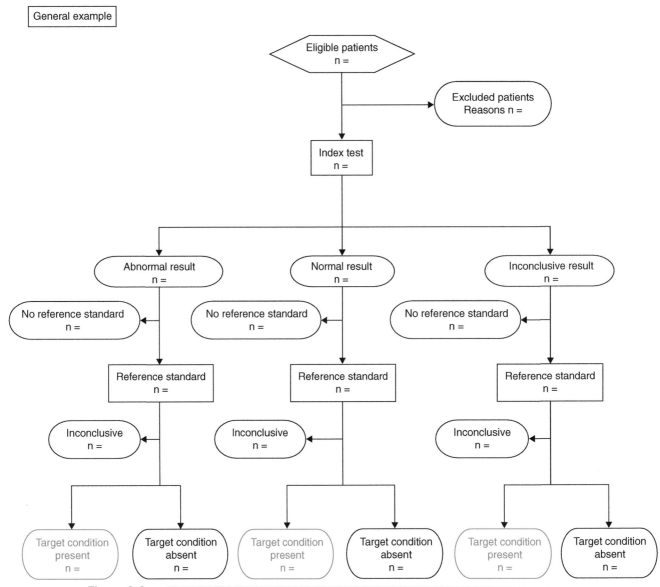

Figure 8-3
An example of a STARD flow diagram. The appearance of a flow diagram will vary among studies because it depends on the design of the study.

Use of the STARD initiative is recommended for all reports of studies of diagnostic accuracy. Most if not all of the content of STARD also applies to studies of tests used for prognosis, monitoring, or screening. A related checklist, called REMARK,[16] has been developed for the reporting of tumor marker prognostic studies.

OUTCOMES STUDIES

Medical and public health interventions are intended to improve the well-being of patients, the population at large, or population segments. For therapeutic interventions, patients are interested, for example, not only if a drug decreases blood pressure (a risk factor), but more importantly whether it decreases the risk of heart attack, stroke, and cardiovascular death.

On the diagnostic side of medicine, most patients have little interest in knowing their serum cholesterol concentration unless that knowledge will lead to actions that improve their quality or quantity of life. People want improved **outcomes.** We may think about how molecular testing fits into this paradigm. For example, a test result (such as the finding of HSV DNA in spinal fluid) may suggest the need for a life-saving therapeutic intervention for an existing disease. Other tests, such as a test that identifies a mutation in the gene for factor V, may lead to a change in treatment or life-style that will decrease risk of developing deep vein thrombosis or pulmonary embolism. Other test results can provide valuable reassurance, as when a genetic test indicates that a family member does not carry a mutation (such as the *BRCA* mutation associated with familial breast cancer). In still other cases, a laboratory test may provide prognostic information that allows the patient to better plan for the future despite an unfavorable prognosis. Similarly, it may reassure the patient that symptoms are not signs of serious disease and thus allow him or her to better manage the symptoms without fear. The test-related *outcomes* in these examples range from preventing imminent death to being better able to plan for death.

What Are Outcomes Studies?

Outcomes may be defined as results of medical interventions in terms of health or cost. "Patient outcomes" are results that are perceptible to the patient.[2] Outcomes that have been studied commonly include mortality, complication rates (such as the hospital-acquired infection rate), length of stay in the hospital, waiting times in a clinic, cost of care, and patients' satisfaction with care. Test results themselves are not generally considered to be outcomes. Nonetheless, an improved test will improve outcomes when the outcomes depend on making the correct diagnosis. (This may be difficult to establish if no successful treatment exists for the diagnosed condition or if the condition and conditions with which it is confused are treated in the same way.) Some tests are increasingly being used as surrogate markers of outcomes in intervention studies when a strong relationship has been documented between the test result and morbidity or mortality; a common example is the use of viral loads in studies of antiviral drugs for AIDS.

Outcomes studies must be distinguished from studies of prognosis. Studies of the prognostic value of a test ask the question, "Can the test be used to predict an outcome?" By contrast, outcomes studies ask questions such as, "Does use of the test improve outcomes?" For example, a study of the prognostic ability of a test might ask the question, "Does amplification of the *ERBB2* gene (HER2/neu) in breast cancer cells correlate with mortality rate?" (It does.) An outcomes study might ask, "Is the mortality rate of patients with breast cancer decreased when physicians alter therapy based on results of tests for *ERBB2* amplification (which decreases response to hormonal therapy)?"

Many test attributes are amenable to studies of outcomes. Studies can address not only the test availability, relative to nonavailability, but also such attributes as the methodology used for a measurement, the analytical quality of test performance (e.g., precision), the turnaround time (as for rapid molecular microbiology tests), and the method of reporting of test results (e.g., with or without extensive interpretation of the results of genetic tests for hereditary disease).

Why Outcomes Studies?

Outcomes studies have taken on considerable importance in medicine. On the therapeutic side of medicine, few drugs can be approved by modern government agencies (or paid for by healthcare organizations or health insurers) without **randomized contralled trials (RCTs)** of their safety and effectiveness. Increasingly, diagnostic testing is entering a similar environment in which physicians, governments, commercial health insurers, and patients demand evidence of effectiveness of diagnostic procedures. To appreciate this, one need only recall the enormous interest in controversies about the value of mammography and the effectiveness of measuring prostate-specific antigen in serum. These issues (and many others) hinge on demonstration of improved outcomes.

In the United States, the important Joint Commission on Accreditation of Healthcare Organizations (JCAHO, see www.jointcommission.org) defines *quality* as increased probability of *desired outcomes* and decreased probability of *undesired out-*

comes. If a healthcare organization, or a unit of it, such as the molecular diagnostics laboratory, wishes to propose that its quality is high or that it contributes to the quality of the institution, the message is clear: demonstrate improved outcomes.

Design of Studies of Clinical Outcomes

The RCT is the de facto standard for studies of the health effects of medical interventions. In these studies, patients are randomized to receive either the intervention to be tested or an alternative (typically either a placebo or a conventional treatment), and an outcome is measured. RCTs have been used to evaluate therapeutic interventions, including drugs, radiation therapy, and surgical interventions, among others. The measured outcomes vary from hard evidence, such as mortality and morbidity, to softer evidence, such as patient-reported satisfaction and surrogate end points typified by markers of disease activity (e.g., viral load as mentioned earlier).

The high impact of RCTs of therapeutic interventions led to scrutiny of their conduct and reporting. An interdisciplinary group (largely clinical epidemiologists and editors of medical journals) developed a guideline known as CONSORT[17] for the reporting of these studies. Although initially designed for trials of therapies, CONSORT provides useful reminders when designing or appraising outcomes studies of tests in clinical chemistry and molecular diagnostics. The key features of the guideline are a checklist (Figure 8-4) of items to include in the report and a flow diagram (see Figure 8-5 for an example) of patients in the study.

AC   The optimal design of an RCT of a diagnostic test is not always obvious. A classical design is to randomize patients to receive or not receive a test and then to modify therapy from conventional therapy to a different therapy based on the test result in the tested patients. This approach leads to interpretive problems.[3] For example, if the new therapy is always effective, the tested group will always fare better even if the test is a coin toss because only the tested group had access to the new therapy. The conclusion that the testing was valuable would thus be wrong. A similar problem occurs if the tested group had merely an increased access to the therapy. (A possible example is the apparent benefit of fecal occult blood testing in decreasing the incidence of colon cancer where the tested group is more likely to undergo colonoscopy and removal of premalignant lesions in the colon. A random selection of patients for colonoscopy might achieve results similar to the results for the group tested for fecal occult blood.) This problem will lead to the erroneous conclusion that the test itself is useful. By contrast, if the new therapy is always worse than the conventional treatment, patients in the tested group will do worse, and the test will be judged worse than useless, no matter how accurate it is. Similarly, if the two treatments are equally effective, the outcomes will be the same with or without testing; this scenario will lead to the conclusion that the test is not good, no matter how diagnostically accurate it is. When a truly better therapy becomes available, the test may prove to be valuable, so it is important to not discount the test's

Continued

Checklist of items to include when reporting a randomized trial

PAPER SECTION And topic	Item	Description	Reported on page #
TITLE & ABSTRACT	1	How participants were allocated to interventions (*e.g.*, "random allocation," "randomized," or "randomly assigned").	
INTRODUCTION Background	2	Scientific background and explanation of rationale.	
METHODS Participants	3	Eligibility criteria for participants and the settings and locations where the data were collected.	
Interventions	4	Precise details of the interventions intended for each group and how and when they were actually administered.	
Objectives	5	Specific objectives and hypotheses.	
Outcomes	6	Clearly defined primary and secondary outcome measures and, when applicable, any methods used to enhance the quality of measurements (*e.g.*, multiple observations, training of assessors).	
Sample size	7	How sample size was determined and, when applicable, explanation of any interim analyses and stopping rules.	
Randomization -- Sequence generation	8	Method used to generate the random allocation sequence, including details of any restriction (*e.g.*, blocking, stratification).	
Randomization -- Allocation concealment	9	Method used to implement the random allocation sequence (*e.g.*, numbered containers or central telephone), clarifying whether the sequence was concealed until interventions were assigned.	
Randomization -- Implementation	10	Who generated the allocation sequence, who enrolled participants, and who assigned participants to their groups.	
Blinding (masking)	11	Whether or not participants, those administering the interventions, and those assessing the outcomes were blinded to group assignment. When relevant, how the success of blinding was evaluated.	

Figure 8-4
CONSORT checklist.

potential based on a study with a new therapy that offers no advantage over the old therapy.

Bossuyt and colleagues[3] describe a study design to determine whether ultrasound testing of the fetus can be used to identify those women with growth-restricted fetuses who can be safely managed at home rather than in the hospital. In a common study design, women with fetuses showing intrauterine growth restriction (IUGR) are randomized to receive Doppler ultrasound. Women with positive test results would be kept in the hospital and those with negative test results would go home. Women in the control arm would stay in the hospital, the usual approach. One can see here that if some women benefit from home care, whereas all other women do equally well with either of the two treatments, home-care patients will

do better regardless of the intrinsic value of the ultrasound test. Thus patients in the tested arm will fare better, and the testing itself will erroneously be declared a success. By contrast, a proper interpretation would be that the strategy worked well, and a testable hypothesis might be generated from the study that all patients can be sent home without testing.

Alternative designs have been described to address the question of use of ultrasound in women with IUGR.[3] In one design, all patients undergo the new test, but the results are hidden during the trial. Patients are randomized to receive or not receive the new therapy. In this design, the new test should be adopted only if there is an improvement in patient outcome caused by switching to the new therapy and if that improvement in outcome is associated

Statistical methods	12	Statistical methods used to compare groups for primary outcome(s); methods for additional analyses, such as subgroup analyses and adjusted analyses.	
RESULTS Participant flow	13	Flow of participants through each stage (a diagram is strongly recommended). Specifically, for each group report the numbers of participants randomly assigned, receiving intended treatment, completing the study protocol, and analyzed for the primary outcome. Describe protocol deviations from study as planned, together with reasons.	
Recruitment	14	Dates defining the periods of recruitment and follow-up.	
Baseline data	15	Baseline demographics and clinical characteristics of each group.	
Numbers analyzed	15	Number of participants (denominator) in each group included in each analysis and whether the analysis was by "intention-to-treat." State the results in absolute numbers when feasible (e.g., 10/20, not 50%).	
Outcomes and estimation	17	For each primary and secondary outcome, a summary of results for each group, and the estimated effect size and its precision (e.g., 95% confidence interval).	
Ancillary analyses	18	Address multiplicity by reporting any other analyses performed, including subgroup analyses and adjusted analyses, indicating those pre-specified and those exploratory.	
Adverse events	19	All important adverse events or side effects in each intervention group.	
DISCUSSION Interpretation	20	Interpretation of the results, taking into account study hypotheses, sources of potential bias or imprecision, and the dangers associated with multiplicity of analyses and outcomes.	
Generalizability	21	Generalizability (external validity) of the trial findings.	
Overall evidence	22	General interpretation of the results in the context of current evidence.	

Figure 8-4, cont'd
CONSORT checklist.

with the test outcome. For example, the improvement may be larger in the subgroup that had positive test results on ultrasound compared with the subgroup that had negative test results.

An RCT is not always feasible. Alternatives to the RCT include studies that use historical or contemporaneous control patients in whom the intervention was not undertaken. Other studies include patients with and patients without the outcome of interest. These studies are called case-control studies. Uncertainty about the comparability of the controls and the patients in such designs is a threat to the validity of these studies.

Researchers have turned to other methods for exploring the outcomes of testing strategies. To address the multitude of available options when several tests are available, decision analysis has been proposed. These studies rely on a model that links data on diagnostic accuracy with data on health outcomes. Patients with true-positive test results receive the benefits of treatment for the target condition, in contrast with patients who have true-negative test results. On the other hand, those with false-positive test results undergo the risk of the side effects associated with treatment, without the benefits.

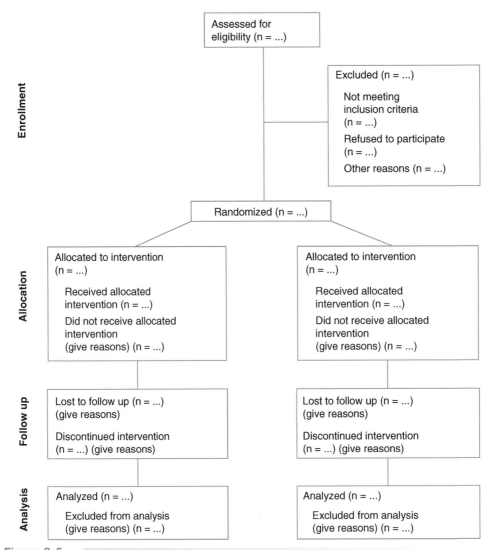

Figure 8-5
An example of a CONSORT flow diagram for patients in an RCT.

SYSTEMATIC REVIEWS OF DIAGNOSTIC TESTS

Systematic reviews are recent additions to the medical literature. In contrast to traditional "narrative" reviews, these reviews aim to answer a precisely defined clinical question and to do so in a way that is transparent and designed to minimize bias. Some of the defining features of systematic reviews are (1) a clear definition of the clinical question to be addressed, (2) an extensive and explicit strategy to find all studies (published or unpublished) that may be eligible for inclusion in the review, (3) criteria by which studies are included and excluded, (4) a mechanism to assess the quality of each study and, in some cases (5) synthesis of results by use of statistical techniques of meta-analysis. By contrast, traditional reviews are subjective, are rarely well focused on a clinical question, lack explicit criteria for selection of studies to be reviewed, do not indicate criteria to assess the quality of included studies, and rarely can use meta-analysis.

The explicit methodology of systematic reviews suggests that persons skilled in the art of systematic reviewing should be able to reproduce the data of a systematic review, just as researchers in molecular biology or biochemistry expect to be able to reproduce published primary studies in their fields. This concept strengthens the credibility of systematic reviews, and workers in the field of EBM generally consider well-conducted systematic reviews of high-quality primary studies to constitute the highest level of evidence on a medical question.

AC
Why Systematic Reviews?

The explosion of research and the vastness of the medical literature are such that no one can read, much less digest, all relevant work. The massive amount of new technology, the poor quality of narrative reviews, and the necessity to provide an accurate digest for practicing clinicians constitute the background to the call for a more systematic review of literature.

Systematic reviews can achieve multiple objectives. They can identify the number, scope, and quality of primary studies by using an extensive search strategy; provide a summary of the diagnostic accuracy of a test; compare the diagnostic accuracies of tests; determine the dependence of reported diagnostic accuracies on quality of study design; identify dependence of diagnostic accuracy on characteristics of the patients or of the method for the test; identify areas that require further research; and recognize questions that are well answered and for which further studies may not be necessary.

Conducting a Systematic Review

Systematic reviewing is time consuming and requires multiple skills. Usually a team is required, and the team should include at least one person experienced in the science and art of systematic reviewing. The team must agree on the clinical problem to be tackled and on the scope of the review.

An early step in preparation for performing a systematic review is to identify whether a similar review has been undertaken recently. Among other things, such a search will help to focus the review. The Cochrane Collaboration provides an excellent resource of reviews, but unfortunately few are reviews of diagnostic tests. The Database of Abstracts of Reviews of Effectiveness (DARE), which is run by the Centre for Reviews and Dissemination at the University of York in the United Kingdom, contains reviews of some diagnostic tests. A third resource is the Bayes Library of Diagnostic Studies and Reviews, which is associated with the Cochrane Collaboration (http://www.bice.ch/engl/content_e/bayes_library.htm, accessed December 3, 2006). Other resources include electronic databases such as PubMed and Embase, and recent clinical practice guidelines, which are likely to cite systematic reviews that were available at the time of the guidelines' development (see section on guidelines later in this chapter).

The review team must develop a protocol for the project. A protocol should include, in addition to a title, background information, composition of the review group, and a timetable:

- The clinical question(s) to be addressed in the review
- Search strategy
- Inclusion and exclusion criteria for selection of studies
- Methodology of and checklists for critical appraisal of studies
- Methodology of data extraction and data extraction forms
- Methodology of study synthesis and summary measures to be used

Description of all of the details is beyond the scope of this chapter, and only some highlights will be discussed. Review of the literature on systematic reviews is recommended before embarking on such an exercise.

The Clinical Question and Criteria for Selection of Studies

Among the steps in conducting a systematic review of a diagnostic test, the most important is the identification of the clinical question for which the test result is required

to give an answer and thus formulation of the question that forms the basis of the review. Two types of questions can be addressed in a systematic review in diagnostic medicine: one type is related to the diagnostic accuracy of a test and the other to the clinical value (to patients or to others) of using the test. The questions that arise are similar in structure, but require different approaches. Examples:

Type 1 question regarding diagnostic accuracy of a test:

In patients attending a clinic for treatment with warfarin, how well does the identification of a variant form of the drug metabolizing enzyme CYP2C9 predict bleeding complications as assessed by clinical observation?

Type 2 question regarding the value of a test in improving patient outcomes (called a phase 4 evaluation of a test by Sackett and Haynes[20]):

In clinic patients treated with warfarin, how well does use of testing for variant forms of CYP2C9 perform as a guide to dose of warfarin in decreasing the frequency of bleeding complications that comes to medical attention?

Note that each question identifies (1) the patient's problem (need for warfarin) and the setting (clinic), (2) the test being used (test for CYP2C9 alleles), (3) the reference standard for the diagnosis or outcome (clinical observation, current practice [i.e., not having the test available], or both), and (4) an outcome (bleeding complications).

More complex questions often arise. For example, a type 1 question may involve comparing the diagnostic accuracies of two or more tests, or it may address the improvement in diagnostic accuracy from adding results of a new test to results of an existing test or tests. A complex type 2 question may involve the utility of testing for variant drug metabolizing enzymes to reduce clinic visits by helping to establish optimum drug dosages. In all cases, however, it is usually best that the clinical question be specific and focused on defined clinical scenarios and clinical settings.

The clinical question leads to inclusion and exclusion criteria for studies to be included in the review. These criteria include the patient cohort and setting in which the test is to be used and the outcome measures to be considered. These are all important because both the "patient setting" and the nature of the question affect the diagnostic performance of a test.

Until recently, methodologists interested in systematic reviews have focused on studies of the effects of interventions, especially drugs, on patient outcomes. That work is generally applicable to systematic reviews of diagnostic tests that start with a question of the second type above. Unfortunately for systematic reviews of diagnostic tests, it is unusual at present to find more than one study on any combination of a test and an outcome. We therefore focus on systematic reviews of the diagnostic accuracy of tests.

When the questions to be addressed are defined, the review group must agree on the scope of the review. Irwig et al (http://www.cochrane.org/docs/sadtdoc1.htm)

Continued

(accessed December 3, 2006) summarized the two main approaches to defining the scope of a systematic review of studies of diagnostic accuracy:

- Restrict the review to studies of high quality directly applicable to the problem of immediate interest to the reviewer.
- Explore the effect of variability in study quality and other characteristics (setting, type of population, disease spectrum, etc.) on estimates of accuracy, using subgroup analysis or modeling.

The second approach is more complex, but allows estimates of such things as the applicability of estimates of diagnostic accuracy to different settings and the effect of study design and inherent patient characteristics (e.g., age, sex, and symptoms) on estimates of a test's diagnostic accuracy.

Search Strategy

Searching of the primary literature is usually carried out in three ways: (1) an electronic search of literature databases, (2) hand searching of key journals, and (3) review of the references of key review articles. It is usual to search both Medline and Embase because the overlap between the two can be as low as 35%. Searching of databases is a detailed exercise, and the help of a librarian or information scientist is recommended. An incorrectly structured search can generate a large number of irrelevant references and miss crucial references. Guidance that is tailored to searching for studies of diagnostic accuracy in the published literature is available in Irwig et al. http://www.cochrane.org/docs/sadtdoc1.htm (accessed December 3, 2006).

Additional studies may be found in the "gray" literature that is not indexed by the major databases. These sources include theses, conference proceedings, technical reports, and monographs. Consultation with individuals active in the field may uncover studies in these sources and studies that are being prepared for publication.

Data Extraction and Critical Appraisal of Studies

Identified papers should be read independently by two persons and data extracted according to a template. A checklist of items to extract from primary studies in preparing a systematic review on test accuracy is available online at http://www.cochrane.org/docs/sadtdoc1.htm (accessed December 3, 2006). The STARD checklist[4] (see Figure 8-2) can also be used as an additional guide in designing the template.

The quality of studies must be assessed as part of the systematic review. Rating schemes for the quality of primary studies have been concerned mostly with studies of therapeutic interventions. These schemes have focused on the type of study design, with large RCTs routinely considered to have the highest level of quality, and other designs given lower ratings. Different types of clinical questions (such as questions related to diagnostic approaches) often require different types of study design, however. Thus a randomized trial, though ideal for studies of the effects of interventions, is not the most appropriate design to study whether

(for example) computerized or human reading of cervical smears is better (or to study the natural history of a disease or the cause of a disease, etc.). Moreover, a study may use a good design but suffer from serious drawbacks in other dimensions, such as the number of patients lost to follow-up. Thus adequate grading of the quality of studies must go beyond the categorization of study design. An instrument to evaluate the quality of diagnostic test accuracy studies in systematic reviews has recently been developed.[23]

Summarizing the Data

The characteristics and data from critically appraised studies should be presented in tables. The data should include sensitivities, specificities, and likelihood ratios wherever possible. These can then be summarized in plots that provide an indication of the variation among studies. The summary should also include an assessment of the quality of each study, using an explicit scoring system. A review should also present critical analysis of the data highlighted in the review.

Meta-Analysis

It may be possible to undertake a meta-analysis if data are available from a number of similar studies (i.e., asking the same question in the same type of patients and in the same or similar clinical settings). Meta-analyses can explore sources of variability in the results of clinical studies, increase confidence in the data and conclusions, and signal when no further studies are necessary. For guidelines on conduct of meta-analyses of RCTs, see the quality of reporting of meta-analyses (QUORUM) statement at http://www.consort-statement.org/QUOROM.pdf (accessed December 3, 2006).

Although meta-analyses are hampered in diagnostic research by the paucity of high-quality primary studies, the quality of these studies is improving. For descriptions of meta-analytical techniques in diagnostic research, including the summary ROC curve, see papers by Irwig et al[13,14] and Deeks[8] and the book chapter by Boyd and Deeks.[6]

ECONOMIC EVALUATIONS OF DIAGNOSTIC TESTING

Healthcare costs worldwide have surged in recent decades. For example, the United States spent $1,678,900 million dollars on healthcare in 2003 or 15.3% of its gross domestic product (see http://www.cms.hhs.gov/NationalHealthExpendData/, accessed December 3, 2006). Although the direct laboratory costs are small in comparison, the tests have a profound influence on medical decisions and therefore total costs.

A Hierarchy of Evidence

A hierarchy of evidence regarding clinical tests[11] begins with assessment of the test's technical performance and proceeds through the study of the test's diagnostic performance to an identification of potential benefits and thus to economic evaluation. This hierarchy of evidence can also be seen in the context of the data that are required to make decisions about the implementation of a test. It therefore lies at the heart of the process of policy making and service management. Economic evaluation provides a means of evaluating the comparative costs of alternative care strategies and providing a means of evaluating health outcomes at the highest level in terms of life years gained and social benefit.

Methodologies for Economic Evaluations

Health economics is concerned with the *cost* and *consequences* of decisions made about the care of patients. It therefore involves the identification, measurement, and valuation of both the costs and the consequences. The process is complex and is an "inexact science." The approaches to economic evaluation include (1) cost minimization, (2) cost benefit, (3) cost effectiveness, and (4) cost utility analysis (Table 8-1).

Cost minimization can be considered as the simplest approach and provides the least information; it is an evaluation of the costs of alternative approaches that produce the same outcome. In the area of diagnostic testing, it is applicable only to the cost of alternative suppliers of the same test, device, or instrument. It is therefore a technique that is limited to the procurement process in which the specifications of the service are already established and the outcomes clearly defined. It might be considered as providing the "cost per test," an often quoted parameter that is not, however, a true economic evaluation because it does not identify an outcome except the provision of a test result.

Cost-benefit analysis determines whether the cost of the benefit exceeds the cost of the intervention and therefore whether the intervention is worthwhile. The value of the consequence or benefit is assessed in monetary terms; this can be quite challenging because it may require the analyst to equate a year of life to a monetary amount. There are a number of methods, including the "human capital approach," which assesses the individual's productivity (in terms of earnings) and the "willingness to pay approach," which is more of a modeling approach having determined by questionnaire what individuals are prepared to pay. Cost-benefit evaluation is not widely used, but it might have some value in comparisons of different testing modalities.

Cost-effectiveness analysis looks at the most efficient way of spending a fixed budget, and the effects are measured in terms of a natural unit. The ultimate natural unit is the life year, but more practical measures include reduction in the frequency of

hypoglycemic episodes or number of strokes prevented. Surrogate measures with clear relationships to morbidity and mortality have also been used (e.g., change in blood pressure). When assessing an intervention, the number of cases of disease prevented may be used as a measure of benefit. Investigative and treatment strategies may be compared for outcome measures (e.g., cost per ulcer cured and cost per patient treated).

Cost-utility analysis includes the quality and the quantity of the health outcome, or in other words, looking at the quality of the life years gained. The cost of the intervention is assessed in monetary terms, but the outcomes are expressed in "quality-adjusted life years" (QALYs). Cost-utility analysis has seen little use in the study of diagnostic tests probably because of the complexity of the clinical process involving both diagnostic tests and treatment necessary to produce a measurable clinical outcome. It has, however, been used to assess the utility of some screening programs. The inclusion of a quality of life component can affect choices among alternatives and have a major impact on the cost effectiveness.

When tests increase both the cost and benefit, decisions about their use will depend on factors such as willingness to pay and other political and individual pressures. A figure of $50,000 per QALY has been used in the United States as a reference point. That figure reflects a decision by the U.S. Congress to approve dialysis treatment for end-stage renal failure, which has a cost of about that amount per QALY. Although providing useful comparative data, there are concerns about the use of tables of cost per QALY.

The underlying issue of economic evaluations is to compare the costs that will be incurred with an estimate of the gain, and for this there are four possible findings and three possible decisions:

- Test more costly but providing greater benefit—possibly introduce depending on overall gain
- Test more costly but providing less benefit—do not introduce test
- Test less costly but providing greater benefit—introduce test
- Test less costly but providing less benefit—possibly introduce test depending on the size of the loss in the benefit and the magnitude of savings (which may be able to produce a demonstrably greater benefit if spent on a different intervention or test)

These options have been expressed graphically in a two-dimensional plot called the "cost-effectiveness plane" with cost on the horizontal axis and benefit on the perpendicular axis.

TABLE 8-1	Approaches to Economic Evaluations	
Type of Evaluation	**Effect or Outcome**	**Decision Criteria**
Cost minimization	Identical outcomes	Least expensive alternative
Cost benefit	Improved effect or outcome	Effect evaluated purely in monetary terms
Cost effectiveness	Common unit of effect but differential effect	Cost per unit of effect (e.g., dollars per life years gained)
Cost utility	Improved effect or outcome	Outcome expressed in terms of survival and quality of life

AC

Quality of Economic Evaluations

In exactly the same way as for studies on diagnostic performance and for outcomes studies, there is a minimal set of criteria for evaluating an economic study of a diagnostic test. A suggested list of criteria includes[9]:

- Clear definition of economic question including perspective of the evaluation (e.g., perspective of a patient or society or an employer or a health insurance company or a hospital administrator; long-term versus short-term perspective)

Continued

- Description of competing alternatives
- Evidence of effectiveness of intervention
- Clear identification and quantification of costs and consequences including incremental analysis
- Appropriate consideration of effects of differential timing of costs and benefits
- Performance of sensitivity analysis (How sensitive are results to changes in assumptions or in input [e.g., cost of drugs or expected benefit in life years]?)
- Inclusion of summary measure of efficiency, ensuring that all issues are addressed

Reviews of economic evaluations of diagnostic tests have shown poor adherence to the criteria outlined above, with only about half of the evaluated papers meeting the criteria.

Perspectives of Economic Evaluations

The perspective from which an economic evaluation is performed affects the design, conduct, and results of the evaluation. The perspective may, for example, be that of a patient, a payer (government health agency or health insurance company), or society. The perspective may be long term or short term. The perspective is a practical consideration when attempting to assess the benefit of a particular test or device as part of a more complex clinical protocol. Perspective is also important in relation to many of the routine decisions made about a diagnostic test. The questions below illustrate the importance of perspective:

- What is the cost of the test result produced on analyzer A compared with analyzer B? This is the type of evaluation that is done when making a deal. It is a simple procurement exercise, but if the extra expense of an automated method is exactly offset by its lower personnel costs, a technologist and a financial administrator may have different views.
- What is the cost of the test result produced by laboratory A compared with laboratory B? This question must take into account additional factors, such as logistical issues associated with sample transport and the level of communication support provided by the laboratories. Users of the test results may have a different perspective than do the providers.
- What is the cost of the test result produced by POCT compared with testing in a laboratory? This question is more complicated because POCT may be seen by physicians as providing faster results and thus saving their time and being cost saving.
- Will provision of rapid enterovirus testing of spinal fluid reduce the length of patients' stays in the hospital and thus decrease hospital costs? From the laboratory's perspective, this new test will increase cost; from the hospital administrator's perspective, it is a cost-saving measure.

Think about the perspectives suggested in the following additional questions: Will replacing culture for a pathogen with a rapid molecular test offer greater compliance with therapy on the part of *patients* by providing results at the time of the clinic visit? Will it save money for the patients' *employers* by reducing employees' time away from work for physician appointments? Will it save time for the physician and thus money for the *clinic*?

Will it improve disease management (perhaps by facilitating counseling at the time of the clinic visit) for the *patient*? Will it save money for the *health system* by improving disease management and thus decreasing the burden of the complications associated with infection? Will it provide benefit for *society* by decreasing society's healthcare costs (for hospitalizations) and increasing patients' functioning and contributions to society?

AC Most economic evaluations of diagnostic tests will have a perspective beyond the bounds of the laboratory if the value of the test is to be appreciated and understood. Unfortunately, many economic studies look solely at the costs of producing the test result. The studies overlook the potential value of the key objective of producing the result more quickly so that a decision can be made immediately and a treatment instituted or changed. When a test is proposed to reduce the use of other resources within the hospital (e.g., use of drugs or blood products or other expensive diagnostic technology), the expectation is that the clinical outcome will be unchanged (e.g., the patient is not put at risk by using less blood or the less expensive technology). When provision of a test result may have a longer-term impact, as in management of chronic disease, use of intermediate measures of outcome may be especially important. Modeling can be used to assess the impact of a particular testing strategy on a health system or on society; this has been done for molecular testing for chlamydia in the at-risk population.

Choice of Outcome Measures

Tests are not always evaluated in terms of life years gained. When members of a family have multiple endocrine adenomas, the family members undergo (annual or more frequent) screening to allow early detection of treatable tumors. With the advent of genetic tests for the syndromes, many family members can be shown to not have inherited the mutation that predisposes to the tumors. In these family members, the high cost of annual screening is avoided. Thus an important outcome measure is the decreased cost and morbidity of frequent testing for tumors in those who are not at risk.

Surrogate clinical markers and surrogate economic markers may have a place. The use of surrogate markers of clinical outcome (such as lowering of the concentration of HIV RNA in plasma) requires the existence of a clear, demonstrated relationship between the marker and morbidity and mortality. Even if such a relationship is demonstrated, changes in the surrogate do not reliably lead to changes in the associated patient-important outcome. This limits the strength of inferences from such studies.

Although short-term studies of tests have been done, rigorous economic evaluations of the long-term use of most tests are rare. Long-term costs and benefits, as in management of a chronic condition such as diabetes, may be influenced by other (confounding) factors. Assessing these costs and benefits is challenging, and to identify the role of the tests is particularly difficult. Here again modeling may be of help.

Use of Economic Evaluations in Decision Making

The stream of new tests in laboratory medicine requires frequent decisions about whether or not to implement them. Economic evaluations can help in making these decisions. The finite resources for healthcare require use of an objective means of determining how resources are allocated and how the efficiency and effectiveness of service delivery can be improved.

AC   Use of economic evaluations faces several challenges. First, the laboratory medicine budget is usually "controlled" independently of the other costs of healthcare. This is often referred to as "silo budgeting." In practical terms, the budget for testing is established independently of the budgets for all of the other services, including budgets for which the contemplated diagnostic test might be able to provide savings. Second, achievement of a favorable outcome (e.g., from a reduction in length of stay or a decrease of admissions to the coronary care unit) is of use from a management standpoint only if the potential savings can be turned into "real money" (leveraged). Third, the introduction of a new test or testing modality will undoubtedly lead to a change in practice, and so the benefits can be achieved only if the change in practice can be implemented. Finally, even if the desired cost savings are achieved, silo budgeting ensures that the savings are seen in a budget different from the laboratory's, and the laboratory budget shows only an increased cost. Fortunately the drawbacks of silo budgeting are being recognized, and a broader view of health economics seems to be developing in some healthcare settings.

Economic evaluations can provide the objective measure of what can be achieved and the standard against which the change in practice can be audited after implementation.

CLINICAL PRACTICE GUIDELINES

The patient-centered goals of evidence-based laboratory medicine cannot be reached by primary studies and systematic reviews alone. The results of these investigations must be turned into action. Increasingly, health systems and professional groups in medicine have turned to the use of clinical practice guidelines. Guidelines are a tool to facilitate implementation of lessons from primary studies and systematic reviews. Important motivations for development of guidelines have been to decrease variability in practice (and improve the use of best practices) and to decrease the (often prolonged) time required for new information to be used for the benefit of patients and for prevention of disease.

Most guidelines have been developed primarily for use by clinicians. Publication of guidelines on the Internet and descriptions of them in articles in the popular press have led to their use by patients and their families.[7] The development of such guidelines is a challenging new area. Unfortunately, there is an absence of guidance on the development of laboratory-related guidelines. A start in this direction for laboratory medicine has appeared recently.[18]

What Is a Clinical Practice Guideline?

A widely quoted definition of clinical practice guidelines comes from a report of the U.S. Institute of Medicine. "Clinical practice guidelines are systematically developed statements to assist practitioner and patient decisions about appropriate healthcare for specific clinical circumstances." This definition appears broad enough to accommodate the laboratory-related guidelines that are appearing in the literature and on the Internet. Guidelines of various sorts have long addressed issues of concern to laboratorians, such as requirements or goals for accuracy, precision, and turnaround time of tests. The new focus of modern clinical practice guidelines, such as recent ones on laboratory testing in diabetes[22] and liver disease, is the patient in the "specific clinical circumstances" referred to in the definition of clinical practice guidelines. The new ingredient in development of these guidelines is a tool kit from EBM and clinical epidemiology, which allows the guidelines to grow in a more transparent way from well-conducted primary studies and systematic reviews.

A Transparent Process Must Be Used in the Development of Guidelines

In the absence of a transparent process for development of a guideline, the credibility of the guideline is compromised and can be legitimately questioned. When guidelines are developed by a professional group (such as specialist physicians or laboratory-based practitioners), the recommendations (e.g., to perform a diagnostic procedure in a given setting) may be suspected of promoting the welfare of the professional group. By contrast, when guidelines are prepared under the auspices of healthcare payers (governments and insurance companies), the recommendations may be suspected of being cost-control measures that may harm patients. Some ethical considerations are indicated in Ethics Box 8-1.

ETHICS Box 8-1   Ethical Considerations in Development of Guidelines

The process of guideline development requires the use of judgment. It is not surprising that the recommendations in different guidelines often do not agree. This raises concerns that personal financial interests may have influenced the guidelines.

Some questions that arise are listed below for discussion.

Should we allow companies that are affected by recommendations in guidelines to support the development of those guidelines? The most recent Canadian Diabetes Association guidelines were developed with support from 11 pharmaceutical companies. The sponsors were not involved in the development of the guidelines, and one may wonder how the guidelines could have been developed without some form of financing. But are you concerned about the effect of the corporate support on the guidelines?

How can guideline developers adjust for the known facts that positive results are reported in medical journals more commonly than negative results and that published reports pay more attention to benefits from an intervention than to harm from the intervention? Will this invariably bias the guidelines in favor of interventions (such as genetic tests) that are of uncertain value?

Should organizations that develop guidelines require guideline developers to provide information about their potential conflicts of interest, such as owning stock in companies in the field? Is it adequate for such information to be reviewed by the organization and then kept in a confidential file? Should the information be made public despite its perceived confidential nature?

Steps in the Development of Guidelines

The development of guidelines is best undertaken with a step-by-step plan. One such scheme is shown in Figure 8-6. For a detailed discussion of guideline development, see Bruns and Oosterhuis[13] or Oosterhuis et al.[18]

AC

Selection and Refinement of a Topic

The critical importance of this first step is analogous to the importance of the corresponding step in development of a systematic review. The scope must not exceed the capabilities (in time, funding, and expertise) of the group, the topic must not be without evidence (or the guideline will lack credibility), and the area must be one requiring attention (or the guideline will have little value and will attract no attention).

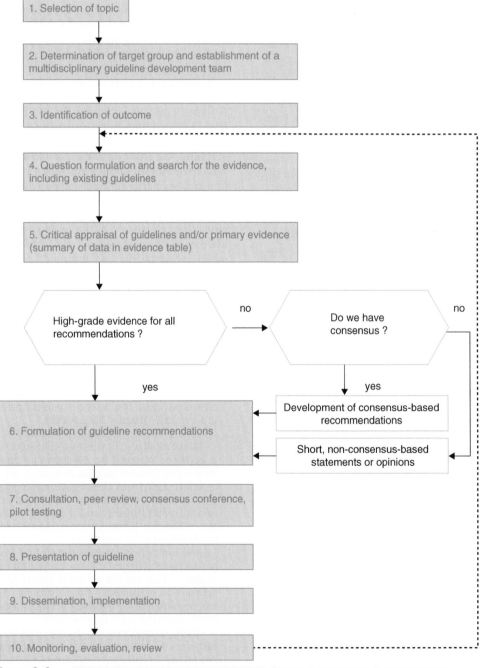

Figure 8-6

Steps in development of a clinical practice guideline.
(Modified from Oosterhuis WP, Bruns DE, Watine J, Sandberg S, Horvath AR. Evidence-based guidelines in laboratory medicine: principles and methods. Clin Chem 2004;50:806-18.)

Guidelines can address clinical conditions (such as diabetes and liver disease), symptoms (chest pain), signs (abnormal bleeding), or interventions, whether therapeutic (coronary angioplasty and aspirin) or diagnostic (such as a genetic test for susceptibility to breast cancer). The priorities for a guideline should be: Is there variation in practice that suggests uncertainty? Is the issue of public health importance, such as in the increasing problem of diabetes and obesity? Is there a perceived necessity for cost reduction?

The critical issues to be addressed must be identified and distinguished from those that may be considered peripheral or simply beyond the scope that can reasonably be included. Ideally, this process involves a multidisciplinary group, with clinicians, laboratory experts, patients, and likely users of the guidelines. The scope will be affected by the staff (if any) and the amount of financial support available to the guideline group. The time and cost are usually underestimated.

Determination of Target Group and Establishment of a Multidisciplinary Guideline Development Team

The intended audience must be identified: Is it nurses, general practice physicians, clinical specialty physicians, laboratory specialists, or patients?

The team should include representatives of all key groups involved in the management of the target condition. In development of guidelines in laboratory medicine, teams ideally include relevant medical specialists, laboratory experts, methodologists (for expertise in statistics, literature search, critical appraisal, and guideline development), and those who deliver services (such as nurse practitioners and patients for guidelines on home monitoring of glucose; laboratory technologists and managers for a guideline that addresses the performance of a test in the molecular diagnostics laboratory).

As the composition of guideline development groups affects recommendations, with those who perform procedures more likely to recommend their use, potential conflicts of interest of all members must be noted. The role, if any, of sponsors (commercial or nonprofit) in the guideline development process must be agreed upon and reported. Ideally, staff support is available for arranging meetings and conference calls and assisting with publication and other forms of dissemination (e.g., audioconferences).

A minimum group size of six has been recommended. Making the team larger than 12 to 15 persons can inhibit the airing of each person's views. A recommended tool is the use of subgroups to focus on specific questions, with a steering committee responsible for coordination and the production of the final guidelines. Other ways of using subgroups can be envisioned.

Identifying and Assessing the Evidence

When available, well-performed systematic reviews form the most important part of the evidence base for guidelines. Systematic reviews are necessary when there is expected to be variation among studies, sometimes attributable to effects too small to be measured. Where no systematic reviews exist, the group effectively must undertake to produce one. The level of evidence supporting each conclusion in the review will affect the recommendations made in the guidelines.

Translating Evidence into a Guideline and Grading the Strength of Recommendations

The processes for reaching recommendations within an expert group are poorly understood. For clinical practice guidelines, the process may involve balancing of costs and benefits after values are assigned and the strength of evidence is weighed. Conclusive evidence for recommendations is only rarely available. Authors of guidelines thus have an ethical responsibility to make very clear the level of evidence that supports each recommendation.

There are schemes available for grading the level of evidence, and one of them should be adopted and used explicitly. A rather simple one, with a rather typical four levels (A through D), is shown in Table 8-2. More complex schemes are shown in Table 8-3 and Box 8-2. For a recent and different approach, see the GRADE scheme.[1] The level of evidence does not always predict the strength of a recommendation because recommendations may either follow directly from clinical studies or be extrapolated from the results of the studies. For example, multiple studies supporting use of a drug may have been done well, and a competent systematic review may be available so that the evidence may be graded as high. However, if the study was done in adults and the guideline is for children, the strength of the recommendation may be low.

Level A evidence is rare in guidelines on the use of diagnostic tests. The recommendations made in the National Academy of Clinical Biochemistry (NACB) guidelines on laboratory testing in diabetes[22] were graded by the scheme of the American Diabetes Association, a scheme similar to that in Table 8-2 except that level D is referred to as level E. As shown in Figure 8-7, the vast

TABLE 8-2	A Scheme for Grading of Strength of Recommendations in Clinical Guidelines
Level	Characteristics
A	Directly based on meta-analysis of RCTs or on at least one RCT
B	Directly based on at least one controlled study without randomization or at least one other type of quasiexperimental study or extrapolated from RCTs
C	Directly based on nonexperimental studies or extrapolated from RCTs or nonrandomized studies
D	Directly based on expert reports or opinion or experience of authorities or extrapolated from RCTs, nonrandomized studies, or nonexperimental studies

From Shekelle PG, Woolf SH, Eccles M, Grimshaw J. Clinical guidelines: developing guidelines. BMJ 1999;318:593-6.

Continued

TABLE 8-3	Categories of Evidence Supporting Guidelines (A-E) and Quality of Evidence on Which Recommendation Is Based (I-IV) as Used by the American Association for the Study of Liver Disease

Category	Explanation
I	Evidence from multiple well-designed RCTs, each involving a number of patients to be of sufficient statistical power
II	Evidence from at least one large well-designed clinical trial with or without randomization, from cohort or case-controlled analytical studies or well-designed meta-analysis
III	Evidence based on clinical experience, descriptive studies, or reports of expert committees
IV	Not rated
A	Survival benefit
B	Improved diagnosis
C	Improvement in quality of life
D	Relevant pathophysiological parameters improved
E	Impacts cost of healthcare

From Dufour DR, Lott JA, Nolte FS, Gretch DR, Koff RS, Seeff LB. Diagnosis and monitoring of hepatic injury. II. Recommendations for use of laboratory tests in screening, diagnosis, and monitoring. Clin Chem 2000;46:2050-68.

System to Rate the Strength of a Body of Evidence

QUALITY OF PRIMARY STUDIES AND REVIEWS: RATING THE LEVEL OF EVIDENCE OF INDIVIDUAL ARTICLES

Ia Meta-analysis or systematic review based on at least several level Ib studies
Ib Diagnostic trial or outcome study of good quality
II Diagnostic trial or outcome study of medium quality, insufficient patients, or other trials (case-control, other designs)
III Descriptive studies, case reports, other studies
IV Statements of committees, opinion of experts, etc., review, not systematic

RATING OF THE STRENGTH OF THE EVIDENCE SUPPORTING GUIDELINE RECOMMENDATIONS

A Supported by at least two independent studies of level Ib or one review of level Ia ("it was shown/demonstrated")
B Supported by at least two independent studies of level II ("it is plausible")
C Not supported by sufficient studies of level I or II ("indications")
D Advice of experts, etc. (there is no "proof")

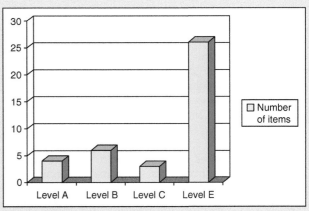

Figure 8-7
Level of evidence for recommendations in NACB guideline for testing in diabetes.[22]
(From Bruns DE, Oosterhuis WP. From evidence to guidelines. In Price CP, Christenson RH, eds. Evidence-based laboratory medicine: From principles to outcomes. Washington, DC: AACC Press, 2003.)

TABLE 8-4	Hierarchy of Criteria for Quality Specifications

Level	Basis
1A	Medical decision making: use of test in specific clinical situations
1B	Medical decision making: use of test in medicine generally
2	Guidelines—"experts"
3	Regulators or organizers of external quality assurance schemes
4	Published data on state of the art

From Fraser CG, Petersen PH. Analytical performance characteristics should be judged against objective quality specifications. Clin Chem 1999;45:321-3.

---

majority of the recommendations were graded only as level E (expert opinion) by the authors of the guidelines, and only three were graded as A. The high proportion of recommendations in the NACB document supported only by expert opinion is far from unique or peculiar to that document or to guidelines for diagnostic tests.

For analytical goal setting or "quality specifications" for analytical methods in guidelines, RCTs (outcomes studies) are rarely available. A different hierarchy of evidence (Table 8-4) may be useful for grading of such laboratory-related recommendations. The highest level of evidence is evidence related to medical needs.

Level 1B in Table 8-4 refers primarily to the concepts of within-person and among-person biological variation. Levels of optimal, desirable, and minimal performance for both imprecision and bias have been defined based on these concepts. When a test is to be used for monitoring, use of this type of quality specification for imprecision appears appropriate in guidelines. Failure to use this approach is difficult to justify because data on within-person and among-person biological variation are available for virtually all commonly used tests. The quality specifications relate directly to the ability to use assays for monitoring and the ability to use common reference intervals within a population. These may be considered patient-centered objectives in a broad sense if not in a narrow one.

Obtaining External Review and Updating the Guidelines

Three types of outside examiners can evaluate the guidelines:

- Experts in the clinical content area—to assess completeness of literature review and the reasonableness of recommendations
- Experts on systematic reviewing and guideline development—to review the process of guideline development
- Potential users of the guidelines

In addition, journals, sponsoring organizations, and other potential endorsers of the guidelines may undertake formal reviews. Each of these reviews can add value.

As part of the guideline development process, a plan for updating should be developed. The importance of this step is underscored by the finding that one of the most common reasons for nonadherence to guidelines is that the guidelines are outdated. Consistent with that finding, a study of clinical practice guidelines of the Agency for Healthcare Research and Quality showed that about half the guidelines were outdated in 5.8 years (95% confidence interval [CI] 5.0 to 6.6 years). No more than 90% of conclusions were still valid after 3.6 years (CI 2.6 to 4.6 years). These findings suggest that the time interval between completion and review of a guideline should be short.

CLINICAL AUDIT

The term "audit" is associated with a particular connotation in healthcare, namely *clinical audit*, and refers to the review of case histories of patients against the benchmark of current best practice. The clinical audit was proposed as a tool to improve clinical practice, and a recent study indicates that it can do so, though the effects are modest. A more general role for audit, however, is that it can be used as part of the wider management exercise of benchmarking of performance with the use of relevant performance indicators against the performance of peers.

Four distinct activities can be considered under the broad umbrella of an audit: (1) solving problems associated with the process or outcome, (2) monitoring workload in the context of controlling demand, (3) monitoring the introduction of a new test and/or changes in practice, and (4) monitoring the adherence with best practices (e.g., with guidelines).

The components of the audit cycle are depicted in Figure 8-8. All of the audit activities are found in the practice of evidence-based laboratory medicine, namely that there is a clinical question for which the test result should provide an answer and that the answer will lead to a decision being made and an action taken, leading to an improved health outcome. There should be evidence to support the use of the test in the setting for which it is being used.

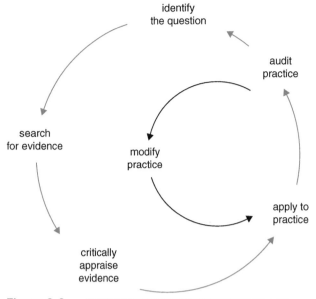

Figure 8-8
The audit cycle.
(From Price CP. Evidence-based laboratory medicine: supporting decision making. Clin Chem 2000;46:1041-50.)

AC
Audit to Help Solve Problems

All audits involve the collection of observational data and comparison against a standard or specification. In many cases a standard does not exist and maybe not even a specification; then it is important to establish a specification as the first stage of auditing a process. Such a specification may then generate observations, which can lead to the creation of a standard. At the outset, it provides the comparative measure against which to judge the performance data collected.

Solving a problem relating to a process may first involve collecting data on aspects of the process that are considered to have an influence on the outcome with the goal of identifying rate-limiting steps. For example, a study of turnaround times for STAT testing of spinal fluid for enterovirus might collect data on quality of patient identification, transport time, sample registration time, quality of sample identification, sample preparation time, analysis time, test result validation time, and result delivery time.

Monitoring Workload and Demand

The true demand for a test will depend on the number of patients and the spectrum of disease in each case in which the test is appropriate. The appropriateness of the test request is a valuable arbiter in situations in which workload or demand for tests is questioned. A portfolio of evidence helps to define the basis for the appropriate use of tests. When conducting an audit of workload for a test, it is possible to ask a number of questions, usually by questionnaire, that are directly related to the original generation of the evidence upon which the use of the test should be based (guidelines). These include:

- What clinical question is being asked?
- What decision will be aided by the results of the test?

Continued

- What action will be taken following the decision?
- What risks are associated with not receiving the result?
- What are the expected outcomes?
- Is there evidence to support the use of the test in this setting?
- And for tests ordered urgently, why was this test result required urgently?

This approach is likely to identify unnecessary use of tests, misunderstandings about the use of tests, and instances of use of the wrong test. With the advent of electronic requesting and the electronic patient record, it is possible to build this approach into a routine practice.

After receipt of the results from the questionnaire, a number of actions may follow depending on the findings from the survey. They are likely to include (1) feedback of results to the users, (2) re-education of users, (3) identification of unmet needs and research to satisfy, for example, a need for advice on alternative tests, (4) creation of an algorithm or guideline on use of the test, and (5) re-audit in 6 months time to review for change in practice. Any algorithm may be embedded in the electronic requesting package to provide an automatic bar to inappropriate requesting (e.g., to prevent liver function tests from being requested every day).

Monitoring the Introduction of a New Test

In this situation, the main objectives of the audit are to ensure (1) that the change in practice that is often appropriate upon the introduction of a new test has occurred and (2) that the outcomes originally predicted are being delivered. For example, a rapid molecular test may be introduced for enterovirus in spinal fluid to identify those children with meningitis whose condition is caused by the virus. Such patients can safely be sent home, whereas children with a negative test may have a more serious condition and should not be sent home. The early discharge of those children with positive test results (and compatible symptoms) allows savings in the hospital (and, of course, benefits for the patient and the family). Audit should determine if a positive test result is usually followed by early discharge from the hospital and that the clinical and medical outcomes are as predicted. Similarly the introduction of a rapid molecular test for methicillin-resistant *Staphylococcus aureus* (MRSA) can lead to earlier intervention and reduction in the infection rate in a hospital, with obvious benefits.

The development of any new test should lead to evidence that identifies the way in which the test is going to be used, including:

- Identification of the clinical question(s), patient cohort, clinical setting, etc.
- Identification of preanalytical and analytical requirements for the test
- Identification of any algorithm into which the test might have to be inserted (e.g., use in conjunction with other tests, signs, or symptoms)
- Identification of the decision(s) that is likely to be made on receipt of the result

- Identification of the action(s) likely to be taken on receipt of the result
- Identification of the likely outcome(s)
- Identification of any risks associated with introduction of a new test
- The evidence (and strength of that evidence) that supports the use of the test and the outcomes to be expected
- Identification of any changes in practice (e.g., deletion of another test from the repertoire, move to POCT, and reduction in laboratory workload)

This "summary of use" and portfolio of evidence forms the basis of the "standard operating procedure" for the clinical use of the test, the core of the educational material for users of the service, and the basis for conducting the audit.

Before auditing, the introduction of a new test must include a full program of education of users and necessary changes in the clinic and ward routines.

Monitoring Adherence to Best Practice

This is the scenario that probably best reflects the way in which the "clinical audit" was first envisaged and practiced. Typically, it is based on the review of randomly selected cases from a clinical team with the review undertaken by an independent clinician. This approach is the most likely to identify when a test has not been performed, and to identify unnecessary testing. The audit is best performed against some form of benchmark. The benchmark may be a local, regional, or national guideline. An appropriately written guideline will have taken into account the best evidence available. In that way, it removes differences of opinion that may exist between clinical teams.

In recent years, registers have been established to track the performance of health institutions and organizations. Typically, such registers are disease specific and will measure outputs at a high level (e.g., morbidity and mortality). In some cases (e.g., the UK Renal Registry), the data collected are extensive and include laboratory information. This depth of data is extremely helpful to the laboratory specialist because it begins to provide a basis for looking at issues such as the impact of the analytical performance of certain tests on clinical outcomes.

APPLYING THE PRINCIPLES OF EVIDENCE-BASED LABORATORY MEDICINE IN ROUTINE PRACTICE

The principles of EBM can underpin the way in which molecular diagnostics is practiced, from the discovery of a new diagnostic test through to its application in routine patient care. The principles provide the logic on which all of the elements of practice are founded. The tools of evidence-based laboratory medicine provide the means of delivering the highest quality of service in meeting the needs of patients and the healthcare professionals who serve them. The application of evidence-based practice is far more complex in the case of laboratory medicine than in the major area in which such principles have previously been applied, namely the pharmaceutical intervention.

The ways in which the test is used, once its efficacy has been demonstrated, will be embodied in the laboratory's handbook which, increasingly, will be electronic, fully searchable in real time, and built into clinical protocols and local care pathways. Such a handbook can then be supported by an information resource, again searchable, which will inform the clinician (and the patient) of the strength of evidence to support the use of the test in a specific situation.

The demonstration of improved outcomes, in addition to providing a validation of the test, also provides the data on which to undertake some form of economic analysis. This will show where the benefits are generated and what the costs and savings will be—costs to the molecular diagnostics budget and savings elsewhere in the health economy. This information will enable a business case to be produced, supporting a reimbursement strategy—the style of which will depend on the type of healthcare system. The real challenge, however, comes in identifying the changes in practice, which will undoubtedly have to be implemented should the test be introduced (e.g., to stop doing annual tests for endocrine tumors in family members shown not to carry the mutation associated with multiple endocrine neoplasia).

The evidence base then underpins the activities that ensure the maintenance of a high quality of service: (1) provision of a knowledge resource that summarizes the evidence and its application, (2) use of this resource in education and training of healthcare professionals, and (3) audit to ensure correct implementation and maintenance of good practice.

EBM expects clinicians to turn to primary studies of diagnostic performance and outcomes to guide decision making. However, as has been observed during the course of this chapter, there are few such studies available for diagnostic tests and devices. Furthermore, in the case of many tests, it will be difficult to undertake such studies because use of the markers has become embedded in routine practice and consensus guidelines. In these cases it will be necessary to depend on a more audit style of evaluation to attempt to validate the use of a test. Although this may appear as a limitation, it still embodies many of the principles of evidence-based practice in laboratory medicine, crucially, recognition of the question for which the test result is seeking to provide an answer. The focus on outcomes will certainly help to demonstrate the value of the laboratory medicine service.

REFERENCES

1. Atkins D, Best D, Briss PA, Eccles M, Falck-Ytter Y, Flottorp S, et al. (GRADE Working Group). Grading quality of evidence and strength of recommendations. BMJ 2004:1490.
2. Bissel MG. Laboratory related measures of patient outcomes: An introduction. Washington, DC: AACC Press, 2000:194pp.
3. Bossuyt PM, Lijmer JG, Mol BW. Randomised comparisons of medical tests: sometimes invalid, not always efficient. Lancet 2000;356:1844-7.
4. Bossuyt PM, Reitsma JB, Bruns DE, Gatsonis CA, Glasziou PP, Irwig LM, et al. Towards complete and accurate reporting of studies of diagnostic accuracy: the STARD initiative. Standards for Reporting of Diagnostic Accuracy. Clin Chem 2003;49:1-6.
5. Bossuyt PM, Reitsma JB, Bruns DE, Gatsonis CA, Glasziou PP, Irwig LM, et al. The STARD statement for reporting studies of diagnostic accuracy: explanation and elaboration. Clin Chem 2003;49:7-18.
6. Boyd JC, Deeks JJ. Analysis and presentation of data. In Price CP, Christenson RH, eds. Evidence-based laboratory medicine: From principles to outcomes. Washington, DC: AACC Press, 2003:115-36.
7. Bruns DE, Oosterhuis WP. From evidence to guidelines. In Price CP, Christenson RH, eds. Evidence-based laboratory medicine: From principles to outcomes. Washington, DC: AACC Press, 2003:187-208.
8. Deeks JJ. Systematic reviews in health care: Systematic reviews of evaluations of diagnostic and screening tests. BMJ 2001;323:157-62.
9. Drummond MF, O'Brien BJ, Stoddart GL, Torrance GW. Methods for the valuation of health care programs, 2nd edition. Toronto: Oxford University Press, 1997.
10. Evidence-Based Medicine Working Group. Evidence-based medicine. A new approach to teaching the practice of medicine. JAMA 1992;268:2420-5.
11. Fryback DG, Thornbury JR. The efficacy of diagnostic imaging. Med Decis Making 1991;11:88-94.
12. Guyatt GH, Haynes RB, Jaeschke RZ, Cook DJ, Green L, Naylor CD, et al. Users' Guides to the Medical Literature: XXV. Evidence-based medicine: principles for applying the Users' Guides to patient care. Evidence-Based Medicine Working Group. JAMA 2000;284:1290-6.
13. Irwig L, Macaskill P, Glasziou P, Fahey M. Meta-analytic methods for diagnostic test accuracy. J Clin Epidemiol 1995;48:119-30.
14. Irwig L, Tosteson ANA, Gatsonis C, Lau J, Colditz G, Chalmers TC, Mosteller F. Guidelines for meta-analyses evaluating diagnostic tests. Ann Intern Med 1994;120:667-76.
15. Lijmer JG, Mol BW, Heisterkamp S, Bonsel GJ, Prins MH, van der Meulen JH, Bossuyt PM. Empirical evidence of design-related bias in studies of diagnostic tests. JAMA 1999;282:1061-6.
16. McShane LM, Altman DG, Sauerbrei W, Taube SE, Gion M, Clark GM; Statistics Subcommittee of the NCI-EORTC Working Group on Cancer Diagnostics. Reporting recommendations for tumor marker prognostic studies (REMARK). J Natl Cancer Inst 2005;97:1180-4.
17. Moher D, Schulz KF, Altman DG for the CONSORT group. The CONSORT statement: revised recommendations for improving the quality of reports of parallel group randomized trials 2001. JAMA 2001;285:1987-91. Available at: http://www.consort-statement.org/Statement/revisedstatement.htm (accessed on December 3, 2006).
18. Oosterhuis WP, Bruns DE, Watine J, Sandberg S, Horvath AR. Evidence-based guidelines in laboratory medicine: principles and methods. Clin Chem 2004;50:806-18.
19. Reid MC, Lachs MS, Feinstein AR. Use of methodological standards in diagnostic test research. Getting better but still not good. JAMA 1995;274:645-51.
20. Sackett DL, Haynes RB. The architecture of diagnostic research. BMJ 2002;324:539-41.
21. Sackett DL, Rosenberg WMC, Muir Gray JA, Haynes RB, Richardson WS. Evidence-based medicine: What it is and what it isn't. BMJ 1996;312:71-2.
22. Sacks DB, Bruns DE, Goldstein DE, Maclaren NK, McDonald JM, Parrott M. Guidelines and recommendations for laboratory analysis in the diagnosis and management of diabetes mellitus. Clin Chem 2002;48:436-72.
23. Whiting P, Rutjes AW, Reitsma JB, Bossuyt PM, Kleijnen J. The development of QUADAS: a tool for the quality assessment of studies of diagnostic accuracy included in systematic reviews. BMC Med Res Methodol 2003;3:25.

REVIEW QUESTIONS

1. Among the following choices, the highest quality evidence on the effect of a test on patient outcomes is obtained from
   A. the opinions of a group of experts.
   B. an RCT.
   C. a case-control study.
   D. an observational study.
   E. polling of laboratories.

2. Testing in laboratory medicine is used for which of the following purposes?
   A. Confirming a clinical suspicion of disease or excluding a disease
   B. Screening for disease in people without symptoms
   C. Monitoring of treatment and selection of therapies
   D. Prognosis and risk assessment
   E. All of the above

3. The field of laboratory medicine includes which of the following activities?
   A. Provision of tests
   B. Selection of tests
   C. Interpretation of test results
   D. Research and teaching
   E. All of the above

4. EBM is the "conscientious, judicious, and explicit use of the best evidence in making decisions about
   A. how to save money in medicine."
   B. the care of individual patients."
   C. the diagnostic accuracy of tests."
   D. the impact of tests and drugs on outcomes."
   E. methods to characterize the efficacy of drugs."

5. Ideally, in studies of diagnostic accuracy,
   A. consecutive patients suspected of the target condition are studied.
   B. all patients undergo the index test and are evaluated using the reference standard.
   C. those performing the index test do not know the results of the reference standard.
   D. the affected patients have the stages of disease that the index test is intended to detect.
   E. All of the above

6. Which of the following is (are) items of the STARD checklist?
   A. Methods for calculating test reproducibility
   B. When the study was done
   C. Distribution of severity of disease
   D. Estimates of diagnostic accuracy and measures of statistical uncertainty
   E. All of the above

7. Which of the following may be measured as an outcome?
   A. Mortality
   B. Morbidity
   C. Patient satisfaction
   D. Length of stay
   E. All of the above

8. In the United States, the JCAHO defines "quality" as
   A. decreased cost per patient admission.
   B. increased probability of desired outcomes and decreased probability of undesired outcomes.
   C. patient satisfaction with care.
   D. decreased rate of medical errors.
   E. adherence to clinical practice guidelines.

9. Systematic reviews require all of the following, except
   A. an explicit clinical question to be addressed.
   B. an explicit and extensive strategy to find relevant studies.
   C. a meta-analysis of the results of the studies.
   D. criteria for inclusion and exclusion of studies.
   E. a mechanism to assess the quality of the studies.

10. A meta-analysis is
    A. a systematic review.
    B. synthesis of results by use of statistical techniques.
    C. a philosophical discussion of the results of a narrative review.
    D. required in all systematic reviews.
    E. not appropriate for use in systematic reviews.

11. Which of the following types of economic analyses can be used by clinical laboratories?
    A. Cost-minimization analysis
    B. Cost-benefit analysis
    C. Cost-effectiveness analysis
    D. Cost-utility analysis
    E. All of the above

12. Possible perspectives for economic analyses include
    A. the patient's perspective.
    B. the payer's perspective.
    C. society's perspective.
    D. long-term or short-term perspective.
    E. all of the above.

13. Clinical practice guidelines
    A. are systematically developed statements.
    B. are designed to assist practitioner and patient decisions.
    C. address appropriate healthcare.
    D. are concerned with specific clinical circumstances.
    E. all of the above

SECTION III

APPLICATIONS

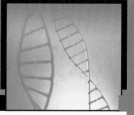

Chapter 9

Inherited Diseases

Cindy L. Vnencak-Jones, Ph.D.

OBJECTIVES

1. Describe the molecular diagnostic assays used to detect inherited diseases.
2. Compare and contrast dominant, recessive, and X-linked inheritance patterns including mode of transmission, expression in offspring, and parental carrier pattern.
3. Discuss cystic fibrosis (CF), including inheritance pattern, incidence in various ethnic populations, gene location, protein involved and its function, disease phenotypes, mutation classes, DNA assays, and ethical issues regarding DNA testing of CF.
4. Characterize the inheritance pattern, gene, and protein that are altered in hereditary hemochromatosis (HH); discuss the three common sequence variants and the phenotype associated with HH and list common clinical laboratory analyses that are used to identify hemochromatosis.
5. Address the challenges involved in DNA testing for carbamoyl phosphate synthetase 1 (CPS1) deficiency.
6. Describe the use of linkage studies in the assessment of CPS1 deficiency.
7. Characterize achondroplasia including inheritance pattern, specific gene alterations, protein involved, effects of altered protein, and the phenotype.
8. Discuss Charcot-Marie-Tooth (CMT) disease type 1, including inheritance pattern, gene and gene alteration, protein involved, and phenotypes.
9. Describe the inheritance pattern and phenotype of Huntington disease (HD) and discuss the genetic alteration and protein dysfunction that produce the symptoms.
10. Characterize the inheritance pattern, specific gene alteration, protein involved, effects of alteration in the protein, and phenotype of hemophilia A; list the routine coagulation laboratory analyses that are used to identify hemophilia A.
11. Describe Duchenne muscular dystrophy (DMD) in regard to inheritance pattern, genotype, and phenotype.
12. Explain the effect of premutation alleles on fragile X phenotype; describe the inheritance pattern, the genetic alterations, and the phenotype of fragile X syndrome.
13. List disorders in which mitochondrial DNA (mtDNA) is affected and state the specific defect in each.
14. Distinguish Prader-Willi syndrome (PWS) from Angelman syndrome (AS) based on imprinting.
15. Define complex disease and complex inheritance pattern.
16. State one complex disease and distinguish it from diseases caused by typical mendelian inheritance.
17. Characterize inherited breast cancer including inheritance pattern, genes involved, difficulty in assessing disease-associated mutations, and screening assays used.
18. Characterize inherited colon cancer including inheritance pattern, pathways and genes involved in the molecular basis of colon cancer,

common susceptibility syndromes, and phenotypes; describe a protein truncation test.

19. Describe a trinucleotide repeat expansion and the manner in which it leads to disease.
20. State the usefulness and ethical implications of genetic counseling in the presymptomatic diagnosis of genetic disease.
21. Resolve ethical conflicts involving predictive genetics testing.

KEY WORDS AND DEFINITIONS

Allele: An alternative form of a gene found at a specific location on a chromosome.

Anticipation: A progressive increase in severity and/or decrease in age of onset of a genetic disorder in subsequent generations of a family; associated with trinucleotide repeat disorders that are described in this chapter.

Autosomal Dominant: An autosomal dominant gene is one that is located on an autosome (that is, a chromosome that is not one of the sex chromosomes, X and Y) and that causes a specific phenotype to be expressed even if it is present only on one of the two autosomes (that is, it is heterozygous); an autosomal dominant disorder is one that is caused by an autosomal dominant disease-causing gene variant; it will be expressed in 50% of offspring if one parent is heterozygous for the gene; use of the word "dominant" typically refers to a phenotype.

Autosomal Recessive: An autosomal recessive gene is one that is located on an autosome and that causes a specific phenotype to be expressed only if it is present on both copies of the chromosome (homozygous); an autosomal recessive disorder is one that is caused by two copies of a recessive gene and will be expressed in 25% of offspring if both parents carry the recessive gene; use of the word "recessive" typically refers to a phenotype.

Crossing Over: See "Recombination."

Diploid: Having a full set of (paired) chromosomes (46 chromosomes in humans, half from each parent).

DNA Marker: A polymorphic locus that is easily assayed, yielding reproducible results.

DNA Methylation: The addition of a methyl residue to the 5 position of the pyrimidine ring of a cytosine base to form 5-methylcytosine and most often occurring at CpG DNA sequences; DNA methylation serves as a mode of gene regulation by preventing gene transcription.

Downstream: A DNA sequence located 3' to another DNA sequence.

Gene Deletion: A circumstance in which all or part of a gene is lost.

Gene Dosage: The number of copies of a particular gene; in most cases, there are two copies of each gene, thereby producing the expected amount of the protein product from that gene; in situations in which more or fewer copies of the gene are present, an increase or decrease in the protein product typically occurs.

Gene Duplication: A condition in which all or part of a gene is repeated.

Gene Inversion: A rearrangement of the gene or part of the gene causing the orientation of the DNA sequences in the gene to be reversed in relation to the flanking chromosomal DNA sequences; for example, the base sequence ACTG, if inverted, would be GTCA.

Haploid: Having a single set of chromosomes, as in gametes (eggs and sperm) (i.e., half the number of chromosomes present in a mature somatic cell); contrast with diploid.

Haploinsufficiency: In the presence of a loss-of-function DNA mutation, the remaining normal allele is unable to produce sufficient quantities of the specific gene's protein product, and disease or other change results.

Haplotype: The genetic makeup of a single chromosome; shortened from "haploid genotype."

Heterozygous: The presence of different versions of a gene (alleles) at the same locus on the two copies of a chromosome; for example, one copy of the gene may be the usual (wild-type) gene, and the other copy may contain a disease-causing change in the DNA.

Homologous Sequences: DNA sequences that share a similar order of DNA bases; if two sequences are 95% homologous, 95% of their bases are identical.

Homozygous: Having the same allele present on both chromosomes in the pair.

Imprinting: Process that leads to differential expression of a gene in an offspring, depending on whether the gene was inherited from the mother or the father.

Inheritance: The biological process through which an offspring acquires characteristics of its parents.

Linkage Studies: A method using DNA markers physically adjacent (i.e., "linked") to a disease gene; this "indirect" analysis allows the disease gene to be tracked through a family; in this way, the genetic status of at-risk individuals can be determined even when the identity of the disease-causing DNA sequence variant is unknown.

Meiosis: The two-step process of cell division that produces gametes (ova in females and sperm in males) with one half the number of chromosomes of the parent cell; contrast with mitosis.

Mendelian Inheritance: Patterns of heredity that abide by a set of laws relating to transmission of inherited characteristics and assortment of alleles.

Microsatellite Repeat Markers: Highly polymorphic DNA sequences of short repeats generally containing less than 6 bases; these repeats are widely prevalent in both coding and noncoding regions of the human genome.

Mitosis: Process of cell division that produces daughter cells with the same number of chromosomes as the parent cell; contrast with meiosis.

Mosaicism: The presence of two populations of cells in one individual, each with a different genotype.

Nondisjunction: Failure of chromosomes to separate during cell division.

Penetrance: The percentage of individuals with the disease genotype who develop symptoms of the disease; complete penetrance implies that all individuals who possess the abnormal genotype will develop the disease, whereas incomplete or reduced penetrance indicates that not all individuals who have the disease genotype will become symptomatic; incomplete penetrance of a disease suggests that other genetic loci and/or environmental factors influence or modify the development of the disease.

Preimplantation Genetic Testing: Determining the genotype of an embryo relative to a specific genetic disease before choosing to implant the embryo in the womb.

Premutation Allele: An allele with more copies of a trinucleotide (group of three nucleotides) than are present in a normal allele; for example, if the trinucleotide CAG is normally repeated 4 times (CAG CAG CAG CAG) in a certain gene, in a premutation allele of that gene it might be repeated 20 times; a premutation allele is at risk for expansion to a "full mutation" (that is, at risk to gain even more copies of the trinucleotide) and thus cause disease; some premutation alleles produce clinical symptoms that are different from the clinical symptoms associated with a full mutation allele in the same gene.

Recombination: Crossing over between DNA sequences resulting in the exchange of information between two alleles; this process occurs in meiosis between homologous chromosomes and during mitosis between sister chromatids; homologous recombination refers to this process when it occurs between similar sequences in corresponding regions; crossing over between misaligned yet similar sequences is called **unequal homologous recombination;** it is a mechanism to produce a duplication of the involved DNA segment on one chromosome and loss of the corresponding DNA (reciprocal deletion) on the other copy of that chromosome.

Skewed X-Inactivation: A process by which inactivation of the X chromosome (lyonization) is not random.

Uniparental Disomy: The inheritance of two copies of a mutant gene from one parent and no normal gene from the other parent.

Upstream: A DNA sequence located 5′ to another DNA sequence; contrast with downstream.

X-Linked: An X-linked gene is one that is present only on an X chromosome; an X-linked disorder is a phenotype for which expression is dependent on the sex of an individual; in an X-linked recessive disorder, females are carriers of an X-linked gene when one of their (two) X-chromosomes carries the gene variant, whereas males will exhibit the phenotype whenever they inherit the gene variant on their (single) X-chromosome.

The polymerase chain reaction (PCR) was first applied to the diagnosis of the inherited disease sickle cell anemia in 1985. Now more than 20 years later, numerous applications of PCR have been described. The invention of PCR coupled with advances in computer technology and the chemistry of fluorescent molecules have enabled the accelerated completion of the Human Genome Project and revolutionized the field of human genetics. The Internet has contributed to the growth of this discipline by enabling rapid exchange of information and unrestricted communication among investigators around the world. Society has become aware of the power of molecular genetic testing and of the ethical issues it raises (Ethics Box 9-1).

This chapter will review deoxyribonucleic acid (DNA) testing for some of the more common inherited autosomal recessive, autosomal dominant, and X-linked genetic diseases and discuss testing of several mitochondrial, **imprinting,** and complex diseases. Molecular testing for inherited diseases has impacted virtually every discipline of clinical medicine. In this rapidly evolving area of diagnostic testing, multiple methodologies are used to achieve similar diagnostic sensitivities and

ETHICS Box 9-1 Ethical Issues Associated with Genetic Testing

In conjunction with the scientific discoveries that have been made in the area of human genetics, equally explosive has been the public awareness of DNA and genetic diseases through the media and the Internet. During the next 20 years, we as scientists and as a society will debate various issues. Which genetic tests will be used for routine carrier or diagnostic screening? Who has a right to know the results of genetic testing? The insurance company? The employer? Will knowledge of this information cause discrimination or stigmatization? Once we begin to unravel the interaction between genetic and environmental factors, is it acceptable for insurance or healthcare coverage to be denied to the person who engages in a lifestyle that is likely to cause disease based on their genetic predisposition? How will the healthcare system absorb the cost of these expensive assays? Can the healthcare community be trained to understand complex principles of genetics and provide comprehensive counseling? Should a genetic makeup predisposing a person to aberrant behavior provide a defense in a court of law? To what extent will manipulation of genetic material be tolerated in our society? Will most couples undergo in vitro fertilization and preimplantation genetic screening to choose the embryo with the most desirable genes? Will cloning be allowed? Will embryonic stem cell research be routine? Although it is difficult to predict what the future will bring, one thing is clear: the future will be both scientifically and intellectually stimulating, yet no doubt controversial.

specificities. As in other areas of laboratory medicine, the methodology chosen by a molecular diagnostics laboratory is determined by the expected volume for the test, the availability of personnel to perform the assay, the current instrumentation within the laboratory, and the accessibility of funds for capital equipment.

DISEASES WITH MENDELIAN INHERITANCE

Autosomal Recessive Diseases

An individual with an **autosomal recessive** disease has inherited two abnormal **alleles** at a given locus by receiving one mutant allele from each carrier parent, and the disease-causing gene is on one of the autosomes (chromosomes 1 to 22) and not a sex chromosome (X or Y). Typically the carrier parent with one abnormal allele has no clinical features of the disease yet possesses a 50% risk of donating the mutant allele to his or her offspring. Matings in which both partners are carriers of an abnormal allele have a 25% chance of having a child with both normal alleles, a 50% chance of having a child that has received only one abnormal allele, and a 25% chance of having an affected child. The affected individual may be **homozygous,** with two copies of the same mutation, that is, the individual received one copy of the gene with the same sequence variant from each parent. Alternatively, an individual may be a *compound* **heterozygous** with two *different* mutations, having received a different mutation from each parent. In either of these two mechanisms, the end result is the same: the individual has no normal allele. The base sequences of the disease-causing variants (mutations) in the individual often determine the likely severity of the disease. In pedigrees illustrating autosomal recessive disorders, males and females typically are affected with equal frequency (Figure 9-1).

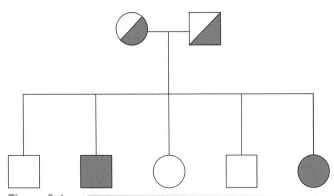

Figure 9-1
A pedigree illustrating autosomal recessive inheritance.

Cystic Fibrosis

Cystic fibrosis (CF) is one of the most common autosomal recessive diseases in people of Northern European ancestry, with an estimated incidence in the United States of about 1 in 3200 and a carrier frequency of about 1 in 29. The frequency of the disease within other ethnic populations is much lower, with an estimated incidence of 1 in 9200 in U.S. Hispanics; 1 in 10,900 in Native Americans; 1 in 15,000 in African Americans; and 1 in 31,000 in Asian Americans. CF is a multisystem disorder affecting the pulmonary, gastrointestinal, and reproductive organs.[19] However, the phenotypic expression of the disease is heterogeneous, variable between individuals, ranging from meconium ileus and severe respiratory disease in infants to mild pulmonary symptoms and no evidence of gastrointestinal problems even in adulthood. Morbidity and mortality of the disease are most related to (1) mucus accumulation, (2) recurrent infections with *Pseudomonas aeruginosa*, and (3) excessive inflammation in the lung. Although in the past CF resulted in death in early childhood, currently the median survival age is 32.2 years, with about 40% of individuals living past the age of 18. The increased survival age is largely caused by organ transplantation, improved nutrition, and new drug therapies and is likely to continue with the potential of successful gene therapy to the lung during the next decade.

The CF gene, located on 7q31.2 (long arm of chromosome 7 band 31.2), is extremely large, contains 27 exons, and produces a messenger ribonucleic acid (mRNA) transcript of approximately 6.5 kb. It codes for the CF transmembrane conductance regulator protein (CFTR) with 1480 amino acids.

AC   CFTR consists of two repeated motifs, each containing six hydrophobic transmembrane domains and one hydrophilic intracellular nucleotide-binding fold connected by a highly charged regulatory domain site. The molecule is located within the lipid bilayer, predominantly at the apical membrane of secretory epithelial cells where it serves as a cyclic adenosine monophosphate (cAMP)–activated chloride ion channel to regulate chloride ion conductance.

In addition to chloride conductance, the molecule is involved in transport of sodium, potassium, and ATP from the intracellular compartment to the extracellular surface. A routine sweat chloride concentration determination is considered necessary for the diagnosis of CF (>60 mmol/L in childhood; >40 mmol/L older than 15 years), although some individuals with *CFTR* mutations may have atypical presentations with borderline or normal results and associated physical findings of congenital bilateral absence of the vas deferens (CBAVD), pancreatitis, pulmonary disease, or nasal polyps. The wide clinical diversity among people with CF is due in part to varying effects that different mutations have on the CFTR protein. Although the type and location of the mutation within the *CFTR* gene vary, environmental factors and less characterized modifier genes also appear to be important in modulating the CF disease phenotype.

Because CF is an autosomal recessive disorder, the person with CF must have two mutant *CFTR* alleles to develop the disease. Some mutations are "private" and unique to a family, and others may be common among individuals with CF. *CFTR* mutations are divided into five classes. *Class 1* mutations produce defects in protein production. *Class 2* mutations are associated with defective processing of CFTR protein. In both cases, CFTR trafficking to the cell membrane does not occur, and both class 1 and class 2 mutations are typically associated with a severe phenotype. *Class 3* and *class 4* mutations have CFTR expression at the cell membrane, but channel activity is reduced. The reduced activity in class 3 variants is associated with defective regulation of the channel, whereas class 4 variants produce defective conduction. Class 3 mutations are associated with a more severe phenotype, and class 4 mutations with milder disease. *Class 5* mutations are associated with abnormal splicing of the *CFTR* (mRNA) and may be associated with a severe phenotype (for example, 621+1G>T) or a mild phenotype (2789+5G>A). The most common mutation, deltaF508 (deletion of the 3 nucleotides that code for the phenylalanine [F] at position 508 in the CFTR protein), seen in about 70% of CF chromosomes in Caucasians of Northern European descent, affects processing of CFTR and prevents its movement to and insertion in ("trafficking to") the apical membrane. Prevalent mutations G542X and W1282X cause premature termination of translation and thus truncation of the protein (at amino acids 542 and 1282, respectively). The frequently observed mutation G551D in which the glycine at position 551 is replaced by aspartic acid results in CFTR that reaches the apical membrane but that improperly regulates the chloride channel. For some sequence variants that have been found in *CFTR*, the relationship with CF is unknown.

DNA testing for the identification of *CFTR* mutations is performed for a variety of reasons (Box 9-1). DNA testing is performed to confirm the diagnosis of disease in individuals with equivocal sweat chloride results or in instances in which insufficient material is collected. Alternatively, if the diagnosis is already known, mutation analysis is often requested to help predict the prognosis since some genotype-phenotype correlations exist. At the same time, identifying the mutations segregating in a family enables prenatal testing or **preimplantation genetic testing,** determining the genotype of the embryo before implantation into the womb, and carrier or diagnostic testing for other at-risk family members. Similarly, state-sponsored

Referrals for *CFTR* Mutation Analysis

Confirm diagnosis
Determine prognosis
Family member testing
Newborn screening
Preconception couples
Expectant couples
Prenatal testing—at-risk fetus
Prenatal testing—echogenic bowel
Preimplantation diagnosis
Infertile male with CBAVD
Semen and oocyte donors

newborn screening programs have detected infants with CF and at the same time have identified at-risk family members and enabled genetic testing. In addition, newborn screening allows for early diagnosis and intervention, which has been associated with reduced severity of lung disease and increased survival. Some families referred for prenatal CF testing have no family history of CF. Rather, in these families, hyperechogenic bowel was identified in the fetus on routine ultrasonography. If echogenic bowel is detected, there is about a 3% to 5% risk that the fetus has CF.

The most challenging and controversial DNA testing was recommended in October 2001 by the American College of Obstetricians and Gynecologists (ACOG) in conjunction with the American College of Medical Genetics (ACMG) for CF carrier screening for expectant couples and couples considering having children. Testing for the more than 1300 mutations that have been identified in this gene would be a daunting task. For this reason, a core panel of 25 mutations was proposed as a minimum standard for CF carrier screening (for a list of the 25 mutations, see Table 14-1 in Chapter 14). One approach to testing for the common mutations is illustrated in Figure 9-2. The mutations included are those with an estimated prevalence of at least 0.1% of CF mutant alleles; this yields a CF carrier detection rate of about 88% for non-Hispanic Caucasians.[24] However, because of differences in the frequency of these mutations among ethnic groups, the detection rate is lower in Hispanic Caucasians (71.9%), African Americans (64.5%), and Asian Americans (48.9%) but higher in Ashkenazi Jews (94.1%). The social and technical issues surrounding this testing are complex. Some issues include: (1) the inability to detect CF carriers with *CFTR* mutations other than the 25 included in the screening panel, (2) the need for appropriate genetic counseling of patients before their consenting to the analysis, (3) the need for proper understanding of the possibility of a false-negative result, (4) stigmatization of being a "carrier" of a genetic disease, (5) threats to confidentiality of results, (6) effects on health insurability, and (7) possible increase in the number of abortions following the identification of previously unknown affected fetuses. In addition to these social and/or ethical issues, opposition to this screening panel has also arisen over the set of mutations included in the panel because those currently selected underrepresent the mutations found in minorities. It is likely that mutations in the *CFTR* screening panel will change as carrier screening evolves and the program is critically evaluated.

Hereditary Hemochromatosis

Hereditary hemochromatosis (HH) is an autosomal recessive disorder of iron regulation that is characterized by excess iron deposition in otherwise healthy tissue.[17] Affected individuals absorb approximately 3 to 4 mg of iron per day compared with the normal rate of 1 to 2 mg per day. Symptoms associated with this disease occur during mid to late adulthood, but the diagnosis of HH is often delayed because the early symptoms of weakness, lethargy, joint pain, and abdominal pain are nonspecific. Complications of the disease include hepatic cirrhosis, diabetes mellitus, hypopituitarism, hypogonadism, arthritis, and cardiomyopathy. The incidence of the disease is estimated to be about 1 in 200 to 400, making HH one of the most common genetic disorders known. However, the phenotypic expression of the disease is dependent on other genetic and environmental factors. The disease is more common in men than women, presumably because of the protective effect of iron loss during menstruation and pregnancy. In addition, regular blood donation is also protective against HH. However, increased alcohol consumption, dietary iron, and vitamin C (an enhancer of iron uptake) increase the likelihood of symptoms in an individual with the genetic predisposition for this disease.

Laboratory testing for hemochromatosis most often includes determination of transferrin saturation [(serum iron/total iron-binding capacity) × 100] and serum ferritin, with a saturation >55% to 60% considered abnormal for men, >45% to 50% abnormal for women, serum ferritin >400 μg/L (400 ng/mL) abnormal for men, and >200 μg/L (200 ng/mL) abnormal for women. These tests may be ordered singly or in combination. Subsequently a liver biopsy often follows to determine the amount of stainable iron and the degree of injury. Management of the disease includes therapeutic phlebotomy and dietary avoidance of medicinal iron, mineral supplements, excess vitamin C, and uncooked seafoods.

The HH gene, *HFE*, was cloned in 1996. Although *HFE* remains the primary gene associated with hemochromatosis, other genes have been mapped or cloned that are associated with dominantly inherited hemochromatosis (*SLC11A3, ferroportin1, and H-ferritin*) and with juvenile and rare autosomal recessive forms of hemochromatosis (*TFR2*). Additional genes associated with iron metabolism likely exist. The *HFE* gene protein, HFE, encodes a β_2-microglobulin–associated protein with structural resemblance to MHC class I proteins. The *HFE* gene contains seven exons spanning about 12 kb, yielding a mRNA product of 4.1 kb. Normal HFE binds to the transferrin receptor and reduces its affinity for iron-loaded transferrin. Interestingly, although HFE is widely expressed in the gastrointestinal tract, the most abundant immunohistochemical staining for the protein is in the intestinal crypt cells, where it has a distinct intracellular localization suggesting that its function is to sense the level of body iron stores and regulate, rather than directly participate in, iron absorption.

A common G-to-A base substitution results in a cysteine-to-tyrosine substitution at amino acid 282 (C282Y) in HFE, which disrupts disulfide bridges required for normal interaction with β_2-microglobulin on the cell surface and allows for high-affinity transferrin binding to the uncomplexed transferrin receptor. This mutation is found in about 80% to 85% of HH alleles, and the frequency of this allele is about 5% in Caucasians, 1% in Hispanics, and as low as 0.67% in African

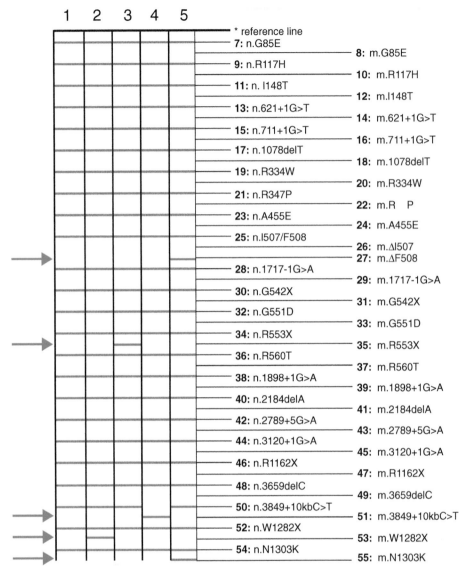

Figure 9-2

CF mutation-detection assay CF Gold 1.0 developed by Roche Diagnostics Corp. Thirty to 45 ng of patient DNA is amplified in a multiplex amplification reaction. Amplicons are denatured and hybridized to membrane-bound oligonucleotide probes specific for 25 normal (n) and corresponding mutant (m) alleles. *Lane 1* represents the pattern obtained from patient DNA in which none of the 25 common mutations is present; bands detected correspond only to normal alleles. *Lane 2* represents the pattern obtained from patient DNA in which mutation W1282X is present in one allele since bands corresponding to both nW1282X and mW1282X are present. In *lane 3*, mutation R553X is present in one allele since bands corresponding to mR553X and nR553X are present. *Lanes 2* and *3* could represent CF carriers or could represent DNA from patients with CF for whom only one of their two mutations is identified. In the latter case, the second disease-causing mutation must be a mutation other than one of the 25 represented in this panel. Conversely, *lane 4* represents patient DNA in which two copies of mutation 384910kbC>T are detected. Note that no band corresponding to n384910kbC>T is present. *Lane 5* represents DNA from a CF patient who is a compound heterozygote with mutation delta F508 present on one allele and mutation N1303K present on the second mutant allele. Detection of 5, 7, or 9 T polymorphism in intron 8 has not been determined in these patients, but can be performed by this assay. The strip contains oligonucleotide probes for the determination of this polymorphism in patient DNA above the reference line. However, before testing, this part of the strip is removed and is only performed as a reflex test if mutation R117H is detected (see Color Plate 3).

Americans. Although carriers of this mutation have been reported to have a twofold increased risk for acute myocardial infarction compared with noncarriers, they do not have higher transferrin saturation or ferritin than C282Y noncarriers.

A second base substitution of C-to-G in exon 2 resulting in a histidine (H) to aspartic acid (D) substitution at codon 63 (H63D) has been identified in a higher percentage of C282Y-negative HH patients than would be expected based on the frequency of this mutation in the population. This mutation is observed in 89% of HH chromosomes that do not have mutation C282Y compared with a frequency of 15% to 17% in Caucasian control *HFE* genes. With this alteration, *HFE* is expressed at the cell surface, but its interaction with the transferrin receptor is altered, resulting in more iron deposition within the cell. The frequency of mutation H63D is lower in African Americans (0.026) and Hispanics (0.10). Mutation H63D is associated with an increased risk of developing a mild form of hemochromatosis when inherited with a C282Y mutation, but appears to have little effect for causing disease when inherited by itself (wild type and/or H63D), which represents 2.5% of HH chromosomes, or when two copies of the mutation are inherited (H63D/H63D), which is seen in about 1.5% of HH patients. Although many compound heterozygotes (C282Y/H63D) in the general population are asymptomatic, H63D may contribute to disease when inherited with mutation C282Y since 4.5% of HH individuals have this genotype, although interestingly, these people display variability in liver histological findings and iron indices.

More recently a third common mutation in the *HFE* gene has been reported that is associated with a mild form of hemochromatosis. This A-to-T mutation results in a serine-to-cysteine substitution at codon 65 (S65C) in exon 2 and is in close proximity in the gene to the previously described H63D mutation. In one study, mutation S65C was detected in 2.49% of normal controls yet was identified in 10 of 128 (7.8%) of HH chromosomes that did not have mutations C282Y or H63D. Thus although C282Y is the primary mutation in *HFE* associated with HH, compound heterozygotes C282Y/H63D and C282Y/S65C have an increased risk of developing HH, thereby suggesting their role in the development of HH.

DNA analysis of the *HFE* gene is performed using a variety of methodologies and in most laboratories includes testing for mutations C282Y and H63D (Figure 9-3). Once *HFE* mutation analysis has confirmed the cause of HH in an individual, transferrin saturation, serum ferritin, and DNA testing of at-risk family members are used to identify those who may benefit from earlier treatment and dietary restrictions.

HH is illustrative of common problems in screening for genetic disorders. Since HH is a common disorder with serious consequences that are prevented with easy and inexpensive early intervention, population-based screening for HH has been considered. If DNA-based testing were to be used in an attempt to identify HH individuals, stigmatization and discrimination in the *HFE*-positive person could result. Moreover, many people with mutations will neither have nor develop disease, a phenomenon referred to as incomplete or reduced **penetrance**. Incomplete penetrance, or the lack of disease symptoms in an individual despite the presence of the gene mutation, suggests that other genetic and/or environmental factors influence or modify the pathogenesis of the disease. For this reason, phenotypic measurements of transferrin saturation

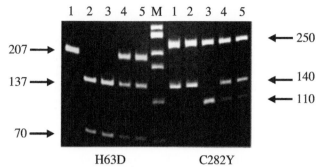

Figure 9-3

Detection of mutations H63D and C282Y in the *HFE* gene. Patient DNA is amplified by PCR using oligonucleotide primer pairs that flank either mutation H63D or C282Y, respectively. For detection of mutation H63D, 207-bp PCR products are digested with restriction endonuclease *Bcl*I and subjected to electrophoresis on a 5% polyacrylamide gel *(left)*. Mutation H63D results from a C-to-G base substitution and destroys a *Bcl*I site thereby preventing digestion of 207-bp fragments into 137-bp and 70-bp fragments. Detection of mutation C282Y uses digestion of 390-bp amplified products with restriction endonuclease *Rsa*I and electrophoresis on a 5% polyacrylamide gel *(right)*. Mutation C282Y results from a G-to-A base substitution and creates an *Rsa*I site within the amplicons cleaving 140-bp fragments to 110-bp and 30-bp fragments. In patient one *(lane 1)*, the H63D-specific 207-bp amplification products are not digested with *Bcl*I to yield wild-type bands of 137 bp and 70 bp, thereby indicating that the restriction site has been lost in both alleles. Conversely the C282Y-specific amplicons from patient one yield exclusively wild-type bands of 250-bp and 140-bp fragments. Genotype for patient one is interpreted as mutation H63D, wild-type C282Y on both alleles. Genotype for patient two *(lane 2)* is wild-type H63D, wild-type C282Y on both alleles. Genotype for patient three *(lane3)* is wild-type H63D, mC282Y on both alleles. Patient four *(lane 4)* is a compound heterozygote with mH63D, wild-type C282Y on one allele and wild-type H63D, mC282Y on the second allele. *Lane 5* represents control DNA heterozygous for mutations H63D and C282Y.

or serum ferritin could be more appropriate than genotypic studies for population-based screening for HH, but these results can also be misleading because iron overload occurs in a host of other conditions unrelated to hemochromatosis and mutations in *HFE*. For these and other reasons, national population-based screening programs have not been implemented. Research is being conducted to evaluate the prevalence, genetic, and environmental factors associated with HH and the personal and societal impact of screening and diagnosis. As this information is gathered, policies regarding the feasibility, logistics, and associated benefits of population screening may be developed.

Carbamoyl Phosphate Synthetase I Deficiency

Carbamoyl phosphate synthetase I (CPS1) deficiency is an autosomal recessive inborn error of metabolism with an estimated incidence of about 1 in 62,000 in the United States and 1 in 800,000 in Japan.[13] The frequency of the disease may actually be higher in regions of the world where marriages within families are common. Further, the estimated incidence of disease does not account for the undiagnosed neonates that die in the first few days of life, but may have had CPS1 deficiency (CPS1D). The affected newborn appears clinically normal, but within the first 24 to 72 hours develops vomiting and lethargy.

As blood ammonia concentrations continue to increase, coma and death are imminent unless treatment is initiated immediately. Although a delay in diagnosis and treatment is associated with a worse prognosis, the disease is rare, the symptoms are rather nonspecific, and diagnosis is often delayed. The condition is often first interpreted as sepsis. Once the correct diagnosis is made, administration of sodium benzoate and sodium phenylacetate is started. Hemodialysis may be required to further decrease ammonia concentrations and prevent irreversible brain damage and death arising from cerebral edema. Prospective treatment in at-risk newborns to prevent hyperammonemia improves neurological outcome. Laboratory findings include increased plasma ammonia, low plasma urea, decreased or absent plasma citrulline and arginine, normal urine orotic acid, and normal urine organic acids. The diagnosis is confirmed by a liver biopsy for measurement of CPS1 activity. In most affected individuals, CPS1 enzyme activity less than 20% of controls is consistent with CPS1D, and activity less than 5% results in neonatal presentation of disease. However, a few cases have been reported with partial CPS1 activity that was associated with late or adult presentation. The chronic phase of the disease is treated with a nitrogen-restricted diet, citrulline, and chronic sodium phenylbutyrate to reduce the blood ammonia. Management of this urea cycle disorder is complex and is most effective with immediate intervention and a multidisciplinary effort. Liver transplantation has been reported to correct the metabolic abnormalities.

The *CPS1* gene is mapped to 2q35, spans >120 kb, comprises 38 exons, and consists of a 123-nucleotide 5′-untranslated region, an open reading frame of 4500 nucleotides, and 1123 nucleotides in the 3′-untranslated region. Exons range in size from 56 to 260 bp in length, and introns range from 415 to 21,160 bp. The *CPS1* gene encodes a 165-kDa proenzyme that is transported into the mitochondria, where it is cleaved into the functional 160-kDa form. CPS1 is present in the mitochondrial matrix of hepatocytes and epithelial cells of the intestinal mucosa. CPS1 catalyzes the first step of the urea cycle by converting ammonia and bicarbonate to carbamyl phosphate. Through a series of enzymatic reactions, the toxic ammonia molecule is converted to the nontoxic water-soluble urea containing two amino groups, which is excreted in urine. In the absence of CPS1 or any of the other urea cycle enzymes, a hyperammonemic crisis ensues, and associated neurological tissue destruction and/or death occurs.

In contrast to DNA testing for HH, which is a widespread disorder with only three common mutations, or CF, a common disease with more than 1300 mutations, CPS1D represents a rare disorder with no common mutations. Rather, heterogeneous, or many different types of mutations throughout the gene, have been described including missense, deletion, insertion, and splicing mutations. Heterogeneous mutations for a rare disease make clinical testing for CPS1D challenging. Because of the low number of specimens received annually for testing, clinical laboratories cannot perform testing in batches to improve the efficiency of testing because turnaround times would not be acceptable. It is also not feasible for a clinical laboratory to sequence the very large *CPS1* gene in every family to identify the private mutations segregating in that family. For these reasons, DNA testing in a clinical laboratory for CPS1D involves indirect testing using **linkage studies**. Linkage studies use highly polymorphic microsatellite repeats, repeated DNA

sequences from 1 to 6 bases in length, that are physically linked to the disease gene to track a disease gene through a family (Figure 9-4). DNA testing is not used to make the diagnosis in the affected individual, but rather to determine the **haplotype,** or group of microsatellite markers linked to and flanking the abnormal *CPS1* genes segregating with the disease in the family. These studies, using highly polymorphic **DNA markers,** are performed without requiring knowledge of the actual disease-causing *CPS1* mutations in the family. Once haplotype analysis has been performed, this information is available for use on future at-risk fetuses to determine their status with regard to CPS1D.

To initiate these studies, once the diagnosis of CPS1D has been confirmed by enzymatic studies on the affected child, or is strongly suspected from abnormal laboratory results, DNA specimens are collected from the parents and the affected child. If the affected child died before collection of a peripheral blood sample, paraffin-embedded autopsy material is suitable for analysis. Within days, *CPS1*-linked DNA markers for the family are analyzed, markers for which the family is informative are identified, and the accuracy of future prenatal linkage studies is determined. When the family ultimately requests future prenatal testing, either chorionic villus tissue or cultured chorionic villus tissue or amniocytes from the fetus are submitted for analysis. Within a few days, the fetal DNA is tested with the DNA markers for which the family is informative, and a diagnosis regarding the CPS1D of the fetus is known. In most instances, the accuracy of the results approaches 99%.

Although considered highly accurate and rapidly applicable to all families regardless of the CPS1 mutation, linkage studies present challenges.

1. Linkage studies cannot determine the diagnosis of the affected child. These studies rely upon additional laboratory testing and clinical findings to identify this disease in the patient. An *accurate diagnosis* of CPS1D is essential before initiating DNA studies. For example, if the diagnosis in the affected child is incorrect and a disease-causing mutation is present in a gene other than *CPS1*, then linkage studies using DNA markers flanking the *CPS1* gene to predict the status of an at-risk fetus are totally irrelevant and will lead to erroneous conclusions. In such cases, a second child inheriting the same *CPS1* haplotypes from each parent may be misinterpreted as affected; the pregnancy may be terminated when tragically the fetus was normal. Alternatively, if the second child inherits different *CPS1* haplotypes from each parent, the fetus may be misinterpreted as being normal when in fact the fetus may have inherited the same unknown disease-causing mutation(s) as the previously affected child with an inaccurate diagnosis of CPS1D.

2. The family structure must be accurately reported. Since the **microsatellite repeat markers** used in the analysis are highly polymorphic, cases of *alternative paternity* are likely to be detected. Nonetheless, if the father of the affected child shared similar haplotypes with the father of the fetus, misinterpretation of the results would occur. This scenario could result in the termination of a normal pregnancy.

3. The phenomenon of *genetic recombination* creates the potential for incorrect diagnosis. This occurs with crossing over (*genetic recombination*) of DNA sequences on

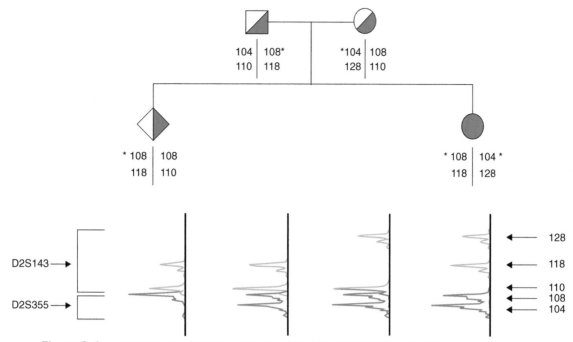

Figure 9-4

Electropherograms illustrating prenatal DNA-linkage studies on a family with CPSI deficiency D2S355 and D2S143 represent dinucleotide markers 4 cM 5' (D2S355) and 3 cM 3' (D2S143) to the *CPSI* gene, respectively. DNA samples from the affected child, parents, and fetus are amplified by PCR using oligonucleotide primer pairs specific for each marker, with one primer of each pair labeled with a fluorescent dye. Amplicons are subjected to electrophoresis on a 5% denaturing polyacrylamide gel on an ABI 377 DNA sequencer and analyzed using GeneScan software 3.1b3. The maternal haplotype donated to the affected child is 104,128, indicating that the mother's 108,110 allele is not linked to an abnormal *CPSI* gene. The paternal allele donated to the affected child is 108,118, indicating that the father's 104,110 allele is in repulsion with CPSI deficiency. The maternal allele donated to the fetus is 108,110. This allele is not linked to an abnormal *CPSI* gene. The paternal allele donated to the fetus is 108,118. This allele is linked to an abnormal *CPSI* gene. These results indicate that the fetus is a carrier of CPSI deficiency, but is not affected (see Color Plate 4).

homologous chromosomes during **meiosis,** between the *CPS1* gene and the linked, flanking polymorphic markers. When this leads to a haplotype in an affected fetus that is different from the haplotype in affected sibling(s), the affected fetus will be misdiagnosed as unaffected. Similarly, an unaffected fetus will be mischaracterized as affected if, through genetic recombination, it shares the haplotype of affected siblings.

4. One or both parents sometimes are *not informative* (i.e., are not heterozygous) for one or more of the DNA markers. This occurs despite the fact that the markers are highly polymorphic, and it prevents prenatal studies on future at-risk pregnancies or compromises the diagnostic accuracy of the results.

Autosomal Dominant Diseases

In **autosomal dominant** conditions, a single abnormal allele is sufficient to cause disease despite the presence of a normal allele. An individual with an autosomal dominant disease may have inherited an abnormal allele from an affected parent, or alternatively the mutant allele may have risen de novo as a new mutation during gametogenesis in an unaffected parent. The disease-causing gene is on one of the autosomes (1 to 22) and not on a sex chromosome (X or Y). An affected individual

possesses a 50% risk of donating the mutant allele to an offspring. Different mutations within the gene have varying effects on the protein so that affected individuals have variable clinical expression of the disease. In some instances, known mutant gene carriers have no clinical symptoms of the disease, as a result of reduced penetrance, yet still possess a 50% chance of having an affected child. Differences in phenotypic expression of the disease are most likely explained by the effect of other genes (modifier genes) and/or environmental influences. In pedigrees illustrating autosomal dominant **inheritance,** both males and females are affected, and male-to-male transmission is observed (Figure 9-5).

Achondroplasia

Achondroplasia is the most common form of human genetic dwarfism and is inherited as an autosomal dominant trait with complete penetrance, meaning that all individuals who have the mutation will express the disease.[11] Inheritance of two mutated alleles is lethal. The disease in heterozygotes is characterized by short-limbed dwarfism (rhizomelic form), macrocephaly (large head), frontal and biparietal bossing, and bowing of the lower extremities, but normal intelligence. Some infants with the disease have died within the first year of life from central apnea caused by compression at the craniocervical

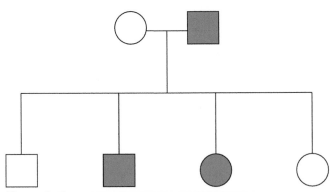

Figure 9-5
A pedigree illustrating autosomal dominant inheritance.

junction. Surgical decompression of the craniocervical junction decreases mortality and allows improvement in neurological function. The mean (and standard deviation) adult height is 131 (5.6) cm for men and 124 (5.9) cm for women. The life expectancy is about 10 years less than that for the general population. During the first 5 years of life, affected children are at risk of death from compression of the brainstem and/or the upper cervical spinal cord. Deaths in adults between 25 and 54 years of age are most often attributed to cardiovascular problems. Achondroplasia has an incidence of about 0.5 to 1.5 per 10,000 births and has been reported in individuals from different races and ethnic groups. More than 90% of affected individuals are born to parents of normal height. These represent sporadic cases arising de novo as new mutations during gametogenesis, and are often associated with advanced paternal age.

The gene for achondroplasia (*FGFR3*) is located on 4p16.3 (short arm of chromosome 4 band 16.3) and encodes the fibroblast growth factor receptor 3 (FGFR3). The primary mutation in achondroplasia results in a defect in internalization and degradation of the mutant receptor. Thus it is retained on the cell surface and has uncontrolled and prolonged activation in chondrocytes. Hence, chondrocyte maturation and terminal differentiation are inhibited.

AC   This protein contains three extracellular immunoglobulin-like domains, a single transmembrane domain, and an intracellular tyrosine kinase domain. FGFR3 is a tyrosine kinase receptor that when bound to 1 of 23 fibroblast growth factors (FGFs) coupled with heparin sulfate–bearing proteoglycans on the cell surface induces dimerization of receptor monomers, activates tyrosine kinase activity, and promotes phosphorylation of key tyrosine residues in the cytoplasmic domain, which in turn induces multiple signaling pathways. Precisely which FGFs serve as ligands for FGFR3 is not known, and FGFR3 may use different FGFs at different stages of development and at different locations of the growth plate. The target genes for FGFR3 are not well characterized, but FGFR3 is thought to negatively regulate chondrocyte proliferation and differentiation.

In the original report identifying the *FGFR3* gene as the cause of achondroplasia, 15 of 16 cases studied had a G-to-A transition mutation at nucleotide 1138 (G1138A); the only individual that did not have this mutation instead had a G-to-C transversion mutation at the same position (G1138C). Both mutations result in a glycine-to-arginine substitution in the transmembrane domain of FGFR3 at codon 380. The association of the G-to-A transition mutation at codon 380 with achondroplasia is well documented. This base pair may be prone to mutation, because a cytosine residue in a CpG dinucleotide is known to be a hot spot for transition mutations. If the cytosine residue is methylated (i.e., as 5-methylcytosine), it can spontaneously deaminate to thymine to introduce the change from a G:C base pair to an A:T base pair in subsequent replications of DNA. Since >98% of *FGFR3* mutations causing achondroplasia are G1138A, and about 1% are G1138C, DNA testing includes direct mutation analysis for both mutations. Postnatal testing is performed to confirm the diagnosis of achondroplasia. In addition, prenatal DNA testing may be requested in some situations. In unaffected couples who have had an affected child, the risk for germline mosaicism, or the presence of two populations of gametes (normal and with a mutation), is considered low, and their risk of a second affected child is minimal. By contrast, pregnancies involving mating between two affected individuals are not uncommon, and these couples have a 25% chance of having a child with two mutations.

Charcot-Marie-Tooth Disease

Charcot-Marie-Tooth (CMT) disease, sometimes referred to as hereditary motor and sensory neuropathies (HMSN), refers to a genetically heterogeneous group of hereditary neuropathies characterized by chronic motor and sensory polyneuropathy and demonstrating all patterns of **mendelian inheritance:** autosomal dominant, autosomal recessive, and X-linked.[5] The most common form of CMT, type 1A, is one of the most common autosomal dominant disorders in humans, with an estimated incidence of 1 in 2500. This disease is characterized by progressive distal muscle atrophy and weakness, depressed or absent deep tendon reflexes, high-arched feet, decreased nerve conduction velocity (generally <35 to 40 m/s), and nerve demyelination as visualized on biopsy specimens. The age of onset is within the first decade of life in 50% of individuals and before the age of 20 in 70% of all cases. However, despite a common genetic abnormality, phenotypic manifestations of the disease are variable even within a family, suggesting the influence of environmental factors or modifier genes at other loci. Lastly, as in achondroplasia, the phenotype of affected individuals who are homozygous for two abnormal CMT genes, having inherited an abnormal CMT gene from each of their parents, is more severe despite having nerve conduction velocities similar to heterozygotes (who have only one abnormal allele).

The CMT gene is on the short arm of chromosome 17 and specifically localized to 17p11.2-p12 (short arm of chromosome 17 between banding regions 11.2 and 12). The peripheral myelin protein gene, *PMP22*, was identified as a candidate gene for CMT type 1A in 1992. *PMP22* is contained within a 1.5-Mb monomer unit that is flanked by several low-copy repeat sequences. The presence of two copies of the gene on one chromosome, a **gene duplication,** is associated with disease and results from unequal meiotic crossing over caused by misalignment of similar, or homologous, DNA sequences. Breakpoints within the repeated sequences are variable between individuals, but 76% occur within a 1.7-kb "hot spot" for recombination where the DNA sequences are 98% homologous. The reciprocal deletion of this **crossing over** event, resulting in the loss of an allele and only one copy of the *PMP22* gene, is associated with a different condition, hereditary neuropathy with liability to pressure palsies (HNPP). Although the vast majority of individuals with CMT type 1A have *PMP22* gene duplications, point mutations have also been reported to cause disease.

A duplication of *PMP22* results in an extra copy of the gene. This altered gene copy number, or altered **gene dosage,** with three copies of the gene instead of two, results in more mRNA and ultimately more PMP22 protein. This overexpression of the PMP22 protein is considered the causative event for disease. Interestingly, individuals with trisomy 17p (three copies of the short arm of chromosome 17), who thereby also have an extra *PMP22* copy number, have clinical features consistent with CMT. PMP22 is a 160-amino acid transmembrane glycoprotein that contains four transmembrane hydrophobic regions and two extracellular domains with the amino and C termini exposed to the cytosol. It is predominantly localized in the compact portion of myelin.

> **AC**   PMP22 is predominantly expressed in myelinating Schwann cells of the peripheral nervous system where it is important in myelination and myelin stability and acts as a negative modulator of Schwann cell growth. From studies on transgenic mice, it has been proposed that when overexpressed, PMP22 accumulates in a late-Golgi and/or plasma-membrane compartment and uncouples myelin assembly from the underlying program of Schwann cell differentiation.

The *PMP22* gene duplication associated with CMT type 1A is detected by use of (1) Southern blot analysis, (2) fluorescence in situ hybridization (FISH) on interphase cells, or (3) PCR. Unique PCR products, not seen in samples from individuals who do not have the mutation, are seen with the CMT 1A duplication or the HNPP deletion; these products represent junction fragments formed from the recombination event between *PMP22* flanking repeated sequences. Alternatively, the detection of three alleles (CMT 1A) or conversely one allele (HNPP), rather than the expected two seen in normal control DNA following amplification of multiple microsatellite repeat markers in this region, offers another rapid and accurate use of PCR.

In families in which the duplication has been identified, testing of asymptomatic adult relatives is possible, and testing of minors is discouraged. Prenatal testing for this nonlethal, clinically variable, adult-onset disorder would be possible, but requires in-depth genetic counseling to review the ethical and psychological aspects of such studies. For the individual in which CMT is suspected but with no family history and in which no gene duplication has been identified, the risk of transmission of the disorder to their offspring is less clear. This individual could (1) have an undetected *PMP22* mutation, (2) be unaware of an affected biological father, (3) have CMT caused by an autosomal recessive or an X-linked gene, or

(4) have a similar disorder arising from an environmental effect.

Huntington Disease

Huntington disease (HD) is an autosomal dominant, late-onset neurodegenerative disorder with an incidence of about 1 in 10,000 in most populations of European origin.[2] The disease is progressive and characterized by frequent involuntary, rapid movements (chorea) and dementia with a median survival time of 15 to 18 years after the onset of symptoms. The mean age of onset is in the decade between 35 and 44 years, but approximately 25% of patients first display symptoms after the age of 50, and about 10% of cases have juvenile HD with the age of onset before 20 years. In the first few years of the disease, symptoms include mood disturbances, cognitive deficits, clumsiness, and impairment of voluntary movement. The next stage of the disease is associated with slurred speech (dysarthria), hyperreflexia, chorea, gait abnormalities, and behavioral disturbances including intermittent explosiveness, apathy, aggression, alcohol abuse, sexual dysfunction and deviations, and increased appetite. As the disease advances, bradykinesia (slowed movements), rigidity, dementia, dystonia, and dysphagia (difficulty swallowing) are present. In the late stages of HD, weight loss, sleep disturbances, and incontinence occur.

Through an international collaborative effort, the gene for HD, named huntingtin (symbol *HD*, alias IT15), was cloned and mapped to 4p16.3 (short arm of chromosome 4 band 16.3). The molecular basis of HD is an increase in the number of repeated glutamine-encoding CAG codons in exon 1 of the *HD* gene. The multiple copies of CAG are referred to as a "trinucleotide repeat," and the increase in number of the repeats is called an "expansion." Normal CAG repeats range from 10 to 27 copies of the sequence CAG; repeats of 28 to 35 are considered "mutable," and repeats of 36 to 39 are associated with reduced penetrance of the disease. Repeats of 40 or greater are always associated with disease (Figure 9-6). New mutations for HD (the presence of an affected individual in the absence of a family history) occur from expansion of CAG-mutable alleles and occur most commonly through expansion during paternal gametogenesis. The number of CAG repeats is inversely correlated with the age at onset of the disease. Individuals with onset as early as 2 years of life have a repeat number approaching 100 or greater and late-onset–disease individuals have repeat numbers of 36 to 39.

The onset of symptoms occurs at progressively younger ages in successive generations of affected families, a pattern called **anticipation.** Anticipation is explained by meiotic expansion of the unstable CAG repeat during transmission by the affected parent, resulting in an even higher CAG-repeat number in the offspring and an earlier age of onset. In addition, although 69% of affected father-child pairs show expansion, only 32% of affected mother-child pairs demonstrate expansion. Further, <2% of maternal expansions result in a change of >5 repeats, whereas up to 21% of paternal transmissions increase by >7 repeats. An increase in the CAG-repeat number is also associated with more rapid progression of disease and greater neuropathological severity in the striatum region of the brain. Interestingly, however, homozygotes with two expanded CAG-repeat alleles do not have more severe disease than heterozygotes or those individuals with only one abnormal HD allele.

The HD gene protein, also called huntingtin (htt), consists of 3144 amino acids, is expressed in all tissues, and

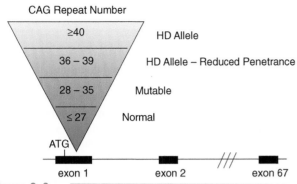

Figure 9-6

Schematic representation of the polyglutamine-encoding CAG repeat in exon 1 of the HD gene and associated alleles. A CAG-repeat number ≤27 is considered normal. CAG-repeat numbers of 28 to 35 are "mutable," and although they are not associated with an abnormal phenotype, these alleles are prone to meiotic expansion to an HD allele. CAG repeats of 36 to 39 are considered HD alleles but with reduced penetrance, indicating that both unaffected and affected patients have been reported with alleles of this size. CAG repeats ≥40 are associated with HD with complete penetrance.

predominantly resides in the cytoplasm with lesser amounts in the nucleus. In neurons, it is associated with synaptic vesicles and microtubules and is abundant in dendrites and nerve terminals. Huntingtin interacts with multiple proteins functioning in intracellular trafficking and cytoskeletal organization, thereby suggesting its role in these activities. Expansion of the CAG repeats results in elongation of the N-terminal glutamine tract and triggers the preferential loss of striatal neurons.

AC   The expansion of trinucleotide repeats is thought to occur by slippage in "hairpin-loop" structures during DNA replication. Hairpin loop structures are stretches of DNA that fold back on themselves and are shaped like a hairpin. These natural structures are like the "hairpin" probes illustrated in Chapter 5, Figure 5-23, panels 5 and 6. Trinucleotide repeats form stable hairpin structures, with mismatched base pairs in the stem of the hairpin structure during replication of DNA. Details of the mechanisms that produce expansions are under investigation.

The precise mechanism of disease has not been elucidated. However, expanded alleles are effectively transcribed and translated, but as a result of the increase in glutamine residues, the protein is misfolded. Thus abnormal folding may result in aberrant protein-protein interaction of mutant htt with any of its protein partners and could contribute to the pathogenesis of HD. In addition, truncated fragments of mutant htt, containing the amino terminus with expanded polyglutamine repeats, accumulate to form large aggregates in the nucleus (nuclear inclusions) and in other subcellular compartments. The aggregates are thought to be toxic to the cell and may also sequester proteins essential for cell viability (e.g., transcription factors) or may trigger degradation of specific factors through the ubiquitin-proteasome-dependent pathway.

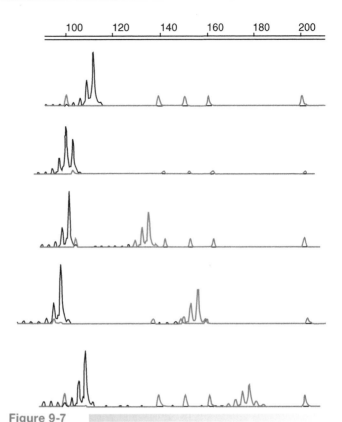

Figure 9-7

Electropherograms representing various patterns observed in patients referred for HD testing. The polyglutamine-encoding CAG repeat in exon 1 is amplified by PCR using flanking oligonucleotide primers, one of which is labeled with a fluorescent dye. Amplicons are subjected to electrophoresis on a 5% denaturing polyacrylamide gel on an ABI 377 DNA sequencer and analyzed using GeneScan software 3.1 b3. Amplicons 100 bp in length contain 18 CAG repeats and flanking DNA. Patient one (row 1, top) has amplicons 112 bp in length and has 22 CAG repeats on both HD alleles. Patient two (row 2) has 97-bp and 100-bp amplicons, corresponding to CAG repeats of 17 and 18. The diagnosis of HD is ruled out in these two patients. Patient three (row 3) has 97-bp and 133-bp amplicons corresponding to CAG repeats of 17 and 29. The results would not support a diagnosis of HD. However, a CAG repeat of 29 is mutable and can undergo meiotic expansion to an HD allele. Patient four (row 4) has CAG repeats of 19 and 38 as depicted by amplicons 103 bp and 160 bp in length. In the symptomatic patient, these results would support the diagnosis of HD. However, in the presymptomatic patient, the phenotype of this HD allele with reduced penetrance cannot be predicted with certainty. Patient five (row 5) has CAG repeats of 21 and 44 since amplicons 109 bp and 178 bp in length were detected. These results would confirm the diagnosis of HD. Genetic counseling regarding the implications of the DNA findings in patients three, four, and five is indicated (see Color Plate 5).

DNA testing for HD is performed by use of PCR, which allows the exact CAG-repeat number to be determined. The most common methodology for this assay involves the use of PCR with fluorescently labeled primers (Figure 9-7). Besides the technical and interpretive difficulties associated with HD testing, many ethical issues exist as well, primarily as they relate to presymptomatic testing (Ethics Box 9-2).

The approach used for HD has become the model for predictive testing for late-onset diseases, and similar formats have

---

ETHICS Box 9-2   **Ethical Issues Associated with Presymptomatic DNA Testing for HD**

- Patients must be 18 years of age.
- The decision to proceed with testing must be voluntary and informed.
- Genetic counseling regarding benefits and pitfalls of testing is required.
- A support partner is needed for the patient for counseling and the testing process.
- Diagnosis of HD in a family should be confirmed by DNA testing before presymptomatic testing.
- Psychiatric assessment of a patient is necessary before testing.
- Follow-up genetic counseling is recommended after delivery of results.
- Discrimination by insurance carriers or employers may occur following completion of testing.
- Prenatal testing of fetus is controversial; preimplantation diagnosis is available.

---

been applied to other late-onset inherited diseases, including autosomal dominant cerebellar ataxias, and less common, dominantly inherited, fatal familial insomnia. When an HD-causing expanded CAG-repeat allele is identified in an asymptomatic individual (≥40 years), determination of the number of CAG repeats allows counselors to tell the person the median age of onset of HD in individuals with that CAG-repeat number. Predictive testing should be performed only on adults and only with informed consent. Informed consent implies that the individual has been thoroughly counseled and clearly understands both the advantages and disadvantages of knowing the results. Advantages of having this test include but are not limited to the removal of uncertainty regarding whether they have or have not inherited the mutant allele and the feeling of relief for those who have not inherited a mutant HD allele. This information has the potential to help individuals appropriately plan their personal and career paths. Disadvantages of knowing this information include but are not limited to: (1) the feeling of "survivor's guilt" in those who learn that they have not inherited a mutant allele and other family members have; (2) fear from learning that they have inherited a mutant HD allele and will develop this incurable disease; (3) risk of discrimination in employment or health insurance coverage if the results are disclosed; (4) worry that they possess a 50% chance of passing this gene on to their offspring; and (5) uncertainty of developing disease if they have inherited a mutant HD allele containing 36 to 39 CAG repeats.

Importantly, the guidelines indicate that the individual should be accompanied by a trusted friend or loved one throughout the counseling and testing procedure. An important role for this person is to provide stability to the at-risk individual by being able to intimately discuss the situation and the information shared at the counseling sessions. Most importantly, when the results of the testing are revealed, the partner will be present and thus able to provide comfort and support as needed both then and in the following days, weeks, or months. Ultimately, however, it is the decision of the individual at risk to proceed with this testing and to accept both the benefits and pitfalls of knowing this information. The decision

to proceed must be his or hers, without coercion from family members, clinicians, friends, or employers.

Since catastrophic events, such as suicides or attempted suicides, have followed predictive testing, a psychiatric assessment is often part of the testing protocol. Before performing the mutation studies, it is important that the individual be considered mentally stable since the HD test results have precipitated depression. The results of the psychiatric evaluation influence the time of the DNA test, postponing it until the individual is considered mentally able to deal with the possibly devastating news. If possible before testing, the diagnosis of HD should be confirmed in an affected member of the family to be certain that the disease in the family is indeed HD. Excluding HD does not rule out a different dominantly inherited neurodegenerative disease in the family for which the individual likely retains a risk of development. Because HD is a delayed-onset disease, the risk of having a positive test result for an expanded CAG repeat decreases as an asymptomatic at-risk individual ages. Thus should the individual elect not to have predictive testing, the genetic counselor is available to provide information, based on the individual's age, regarding the probability that an HD mutation exists, which may provide some comfort.

Prenatal testing for HD is another complicated issue associated with this disease and may not be provided in all laboratories that perform routine HD testing. If a molecular genetics laboratory chooses not to provide prenatal testing (e.g., because of the possibility of termination of a pregnancy for a late-onset disorder or because it constitutes presymptomatic testing of the child should the parents choose not to terminate), it is the responsibility of the laboratory to identify an alternative source of testing to which the at-risk individual who wants testing will be referred. Preimplantation genetic testing for HD is an alternative that eliminates some of the controversy surrounding prenatal testing. Once PCR has been used to determine the HD CAG-repeat numbers in each embryo created through in vitro fertilization, only embryos with normal HD alleles are implanted. This methodology, combining direct mutation analysis and preimplantation genetic testing, eliminates the necessity for prenatal testing to determine the HD status of the fetus since the HD alleles of the fetus are known to be normal, and the need for decisions about termination of a pregnancy is eradicated. Further, this procedure does not require disclosing the HD status of the asymptomatic, at-risk parent.

X-Linked Diseases

In **X-linked** diseases, the mutant allele resides on the X chromosome. In X-linked recessive diseases, females are carriers of the disease, with one normal and one mutant allele, but typically are not affected. Males receiving the mutant allele from their mothers and having only one X chromosome have no normal allele and thus are affected. All daughters of affected males are carriers of a mutant allele. Carrier females have a 25% chance of transmitting their normal allele to a son, a 25% chance of having an affected son, a 25% chance of having a daughter who carries the mutant allele, and a 25% chance of having a daughter who receives their normal allele (Figure 9-8).

Roughly one third of all cases of X-linked disorders represent new mutations (that arise during formation of the egg). In these cases, the mother is not a carrier of a mutant allele and thus is not at risk for having subsequent affected children.

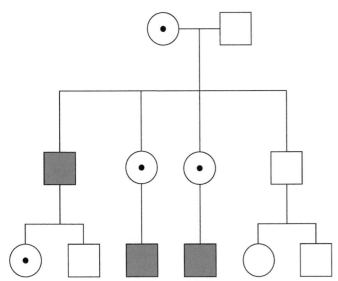

Figure 9-8
A pedigree illustrating X-linked inheritance.

In pedigrees associated with X-linked recessive conditions, typically only males are observed, and male-to-male transmission of the disease is not seen. In less common X-linked dominant diseases, one copy of the mutant allele is sufficient to cause disease despite the presence of a normal allele. Further, in males with only a mutant allele, these diseases are often lethal.

Hemophilia A

Hemophilia A is an X-linked recessive bleeding disorder caused by a deficiency of coagulation factor VIII (FVIII) and affects approximately 1 in 10,000 males worldwide.[8] The disease is characterized by prolonged bleeding after injuries or surgery, renewed bleeding after the initial bleeding has ceased, and, in severe cases, spontaneous bleeding into the joints. The severity of the disease is determined by the amount of FVIII coagulant activity present in the plasma; mild, moderate, and severe disease have corresponding FVIII activity levels of 5% to 30%, 1% to 5%, and <1% of control, respectively. In the individual with severe or moderate hemophilia A disease, the activated partial thromboplastin time (aPTT) will be prolonged, whereas all other routine coagulation test results are normal. In individuals with mild hemophilia A disease, however, aPTT is often normal. The age of diagnosis is typically earlier in patients with severe disease and a family history. Although most individuals with severe disease are diagnosed in the first year of life, those with mild disease may not be diagnosed until several years later. Although hemophilia A is an X-linked disease and typically appears in males, females with the disease have been reported. Some carrier females have severe disease caused by nonrandom, **skewed X-inactivation** in which the X chromosome with the mutant *FVIII* gene is not inactivated, but remains transcriptionally active while the normal allele is silenced. Alternatively, a female may have disease because she has a mutant *FVIII* gene on each of her X chromosomes.

The *FVIII* (symbol *F8*) gene is positioned on Xq28 (long arm of the X chromosome band 28). The gene spans more than 186,000 base pairs and includes 26 exons. A plethora of nucleo-

tide substitutions, **gene deletions,** insertions, and rearrangements throughout the *FVIII* gene have been reported. The variability in the type and location of the mutation in *FVIII* accounts for much of the clinical heterogeneity that is observed with this disease. Interestingly, although routine screening of the coding, splice junctions, promoter region, and polyadenylation site of the gene could detect the mutation in the majority of individuals with mild to moderate disease, the disease-causing mutation in about half of the patients with severe disease remained elusive for several years. Approximately 45% of individuals with severe disease have an inversion mutation arising from genetic recombination between a small intronless gene within intron 22, gene A, and one of two additional copies of the gene A located approximately 500 kb 5' or **upstream** from the *FVIII* gene. The mechanism for the inversion involves flipping of the tip of the X chromosome, allowing pairing between **homologous sequences** and genetic recombination between one of the upstream copies of gene A and the copy of gene A within intron 22. Consequently the *FVIII* gene is divided into two parts, with exons 1 to 22 widely separated and in an opposite orientation and thus inverted from exons 23 to 26. The majority (>75%) of inversion mutations involve the distal copy of gene A upstream from the *FVIII* gene as compared with the adjacent proximal copy of gene A. Genetic recombination between homologous intragenic and extragenic copies of gene A occurs as a new mutation and is 300 times more common during male meiosis than during female meiosis. This is explained by the fact that during male meiosis, Xq is unpaired with a homologue, and is able to flip on itself for an intrachromosomal recombination event. The role of this mutation as a primary cause of severe hemophilia A disease was subsequently confirmed by the analysis of DNA from individuals with hemophilia from around the world. Additionally, this mutation has been identified in the Chapel Hill dog colony with hemophilia A disease and presumably arose from the same mechanism of genetic recombination between homologous DNA sequences. Although the causative mutation in the majority of individuals is identifiable through a combination of various screening techniques, in 1% to 2% of individuals, no causative *FVIII* gene mutation is identified. These may represent individuals with mutations in upstream regulatory sequences or at other gene loci whose proteins interact with the FVIII molecule.

AC   FVIII is synthesized as a single polypeptide chain of 2351 amino acid residues and an approximate weight of 280 kDa. The encoded FVIII protein is predominantly produced in the liver, circulates in the plasma, and is stabilized through noncovalent binding to the complex multimeric glycoprotein von Willebrand's factor (vWF). In the intrinsic coagulation pathway, proteolytic activation of FVIII by small amounts of thrombin frees it from vWF, where it then participates as a cofactor with activated factor IX to catalyze the conversion of factor X to factor Xa. Factor Xa hydrolyzes and activates prothrombin to thrombin. As the concentration of thrombin increases, FVIIIa is ultimately cleaved by thrombin and inactivated. This dual action of thrombin on FVIII regulates the formation of the complex of factors FVIIIa, IXa, and X and thus regulates the clotting cascade. A deficiency of coagulation FVIII then leads to uncontrolled bleeding. The treatment for bleeding episodes is intravenous infusions of FVIII concentrate as quickly as possible to prevent pain, disability, and chronic joint disease. Children with severe hemophilia are given prophylactic infusions of FVIII concentrate to maintain their clotting activity above 1% and decrease the number of spontaneous bleeding episodes. As a result, clotting factor consumption has increased dramatically over the years and is quite costly, but has significantly decreased hemophilic arthropathy. However, management of 15% to 33% of severe and moderately affected individuals is complicated by antibody formation to exogenous FVIII caused by repeated infusions. The antibodies rapidly neutralize infused FVIII. Interestingly the antibodies produced by many individuals have hydrolytic activity toward FVIII. Management of the disease was further complicated in hemophilic individuals who had contracted human immunodeficiency virus (HIV) and/or hepatitis C virus (HCV) from contaminated plasma-derived FVIII concentrates in the early 1980s. Fortunately, with mandatory and improved screening for these and other viruses, these products are considerably safer, but fears are not completely alleviated. For these reasons, there is great interest in gene therapy for the treatment of hemophilia; several clinical trials have been completed, and others are underway.[12]

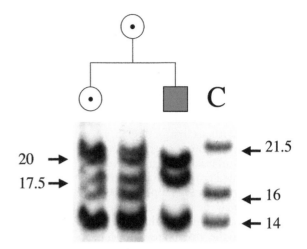

Figure 9-9
Southern blot analysis for the detection of a common inversion mutation present in the DNA of about 50% of patients with severe hemophilia A disease. Patient DNA is digested with restriction endonuclease BclI, blotted to a nylon membrane, and hybridized with a ³²P-labeled probe corresponding to sequences in intron 22 of the factor VIII gene. Autoradiography was at −70 °C for 24 hours. Normal control DNA (lane C) yields bands 21.5 kb, 16 kb, and 14 kb in length. The pattern observed for the affected male (shaded box) in this family yields an altered banding pattern with bands of 20 kb, 17.5 kb, and 14 kb. Bands of these sizes confirm the presence of an inversion mutation resulting from homologous recombination between a copy of gene A within intron 22 of the FVIII gene and the distal copy of gene A 5′ to the FVIII gene. DNA analysis of the patient's mother and sister indicates that they are carriers of the inversion mutation with bands at 21.5 kb, 16 kb, and 14 kb generated from their wild-type allele and bands at 20 kb, 17.5 kb, and 14 kb generated from their mutant allele. Identification of the inversion mutation in this family will facilitate accurate carrier screening in other at-risk females in this family.

A significant improvement in DNA testing for hemophilia A was the identification of the inversion mutation in families with severe disease. As a result, the carrier status of the mother of a sporadic case with a detectable inversion mutation could now be determined with certainty, and her risk for another affected son could be precisely predicted to be 25% (Figure 9-9). In addition, prenatal and carrier testing results would be completely informative and accurate. Subsequently a PCR assay for the detection of the inversion mutation was developed. It eliminated the necessity for labor-intensive and expensive Southern blot analysis and significantly improved turnaround times. For clinical samples, if the individual has a negative test result for a common inversion mutation, DNA sequence analysis of the FVIII gene is typically performed, and the turnaround time is about 4 to 8 weeks. Once the mutation segregating in the family has been identified, direct mutation testing for prenatal studies or the carrier status for other at-risk females in the family is available with a usual turnaround time of 2 weeks.

Duchenne Muscular Dystrophy
Duchenne muscular dystrophy (DMD) is an X-linked recessive disorder characterized by progressive skeletal muscle wasting.[18] The incidence of DMD is about 1 in 3500 male births, making it the most common severe neuromuscular disease in humans. The onset of DMD is typically before 3 years of age. It has symptoms of gait difficulty, progressive myopathic weakness

with pseudohypertrophy of calves, and grossly elevated serum creatine kinase (CK) as a result of degenerating fibers. Electromyography and muscle biopsy are used to confirm the diagnosis.

Most people with DMD are wheelchair bound by 10 to 15 years of age. Continual degeneration and regeneration of muscle eventually lead to the replacement of muscle tissue by adipose and connective tissue, causing progressive disease; death usually occurs before the age of 30 from respiratory or cardiac failure. Carrier females either are asymptomatic or have varying degrees of clinical symptoms depending on the degree of inactivation of the X chromosome harboring the mutant DMD gene in the various tissues where the DMD protein is expressed. Females with severe disease most often result from a carrier female with skewed lyonization or an X-autosome translocation involving the DMD gene.

The DMD gene is located on Xp21 (short arm of the X chromosome band 21) and is the largest gene in the human genome, spanning 2.2 megabases (Mb). It contains 79 exons and has multiple promoter regions. The protein product, dystrophin with 3685 amino acids, has a molecular weight of 427 kDa and represents approximately 0.002% of total striated muscle protein.

AC Dystrophin is a cytoskeletal protein associated with a protein complex, dystrophin-associated protein complex (DAPC), which in skeletal muscle plays a structural role connecting the actin cytoskeleton to the extracellular matrix, stabilizing the sarcolemma during repeated cycles of contraction and relaxation, and transmitting force generated in the muscle sarcomeres to the extracellular matrix. Without dystrophin, an integral component of DAPC, sarcolemmal integrity is compromised. As a result, there is an influx of extracellular calcium triggering calcium-activated proteases and fiber necrosis. Other roles for DAPC have also been proposed, indicating that several mechanisms may be involved in the DMD phenotype. Gene expression studies of diseased and normal muscle have revealed the overexpression of genes involved in muscle structure and regeneration processes. Further characterization of the genetic profiles of normal and diseased muscle may help elucidate the molecular mechanisms underlying the dystrophic changes and muscle hypertrophy seen in DMD individuals. Although not yet reality, technological advances in many areas of science and medicine suggest that gene therapy for DMD lies in the not so distant future.

Because of the tremendous size (2.2 Mb), complexity (8 promoters), and diversity of mutations within the *DMD* gene, DNA testing for DMD presents a challenge for clinical laboratories. Although DNA testing is often not required for diagnosis, because findings on immunohistochemical studies on a biopsy of muscle tissue are considered diagnostic, identification of the mutation causing the disease in a family is required for carrier detection of at-risk females and for prenatal testing. Intragenic deletions, often resulting in the loss of multiple exons within the gene, represent about 60% to 65% of all mutations. These deletions may affect the translational reading frame of the protein and lead to truncated and nonfunctional proteins. Duplications of gene sequences are observed in about 5% of affected individuals. Both deletions and duplications are rapidly detected by use of a combination of multiplex PCR reactions. Electrophoretic gels of the amplified DNA will show the loss of a band or bands or an increased intensity of one or more bands. Duplications in affected males and carrier females and deletions in carrier females can be more difficult to observe, but can be detected using an internal standard. Detection of the remaining 30% of mutations is tedious, labor intensive, and often beyond the scope of most clinical laboratories. Many of these mutations are within noncoding parts of the gene and are private (i.e., unique to a single patient). Such *DMD* gene mutations have been detected by use of one of a variety of reported techniques, including denaturing gradient gel electrophoresis, protein truncation test, heteroduplex analysis, single-strand confirmation polymorphism, and DNA sequencing.

Becker muscular dystrophy (BMD), a milder and less common form of muscular dystrophy with an estimated incidence of 1 in 18,500 births, is an allelic variation of DMD caused by different mutations within the *DMD* gene. About 55% of persons with BMD have deletions within the dystrophin locus, with those having deletions around the distal rod domain of dystrophin (exons 45 to 60) showing a more classic BMD phenotype and in some cases even remaining free of symptoms until their 50s. However, BMD individuals with deletions involving the amino-terminal domain of dystrophin (exons 1 to 9) have a more severe phenotype with an earlier age of onset and a more rapid progression of disease. Individuals with X-linked dilated cardiomyopathy (DCM) have also been shown to have mutations at the dystrophin locus. The pattern of mutations in dystrophin causing DCM is less well characterized, with alterations reported in various regions including the promoter region, exon:intron junction splice sites, and various exons throughout the gene.

When no deletion or duplication is detected, *DNA linkage studies* represent an alternative for carrier and prenatal testing. However, since the intragenic recombination frequency for this gene is estimated to be about 12%, these studies require the use of multiple intragenic and 5′ and 3′ flanking DNA markers for an accurate carrier or prenatal result. Particularly difficult are sporadic cases of DMD or BMD in which no other family member with DMD or BMD is known, and no mutation in the affected individual is detected. Generally, one third of sporadic cases are thought to represent a new mutation in the mother's gamete from which that individual was derived. Thus neither the mother nor female siblings would be carriers, and the risk to the mother for a second affected son would be considered minimal.

In mutation-negative families, carrier assessment involves measurement of serum CK activity and linkage studies. Carrier assignment, however, is not perfected. Linkage studies are complex, require participation of multiple family members, and are confounded by inaccuracy caused by meiotic **recombination** or germline **mosaicism.** Serum CK is, by definition, above the reference interval (defined as the 95th percentile of a healthy reference group of age-matched women) in ~1 of 20 noncarrier women. Moreover, serum CK decreases in DMD carrier women as they age. Thus for DMD and/or BMD families, identification of the mutation in the family best enables rapid and accurate direct mutation analysis for carrier and prenatal testing in that family.

Fragile X Syndrome

Fragile X syndrome is one of the most common inherited forms of mental retardation, with an estimated incidence of 1 in 3500 males and 1 in 9000 females.[23] The name of the condition reflects the cytogenetic abnormality of a breakpoint or fragile site in the X chromosome first noted in the leukocytes of some mentally retarded males following incubation of cells in cell culture media depleted of folate and thymidine. Further, this chromosomal marker segregated with mental retardation in families. The fragile site is localized to Xq27.3 (the long arm of the X chromosome band 27.3). Common clinical features associated with fragile X syndrome are mental retardation, delayed motor and speech development, macroorchidism, long face, prominent forehead and jaw, large ears, flat feet, and abnormal behavioral characteristics that include hyperactivity, hand flapping, temper tantrums, persevering speech patterns, poor eye contact, and occasionally autism. These features are often less frequent and milder in affected females than in affected males because of random X inactivation of their abnormal fragile X gene and expression of their normal gene in half of their tissue.

As a sex-linked disease, fragile X syndrome has a complicated inheritance pattern. Affected females are heterozygous for the mutation, and unaffected males transmit the mutation to their offspring. Fragile X syndrome is considered an X-linked dominant disorder with reduced *penetrance* (79% for males and 35% for females), but the penetrance of the disease appeared to increase in subsequent generations within a family. The *FMR1* (fragile X mental retardation) gene causes disease through an expansion of an unstable trinucleotide repeat sequence and was the first of numerous genes identified to cause disease via this mechanism.[7] The unstable CGG repeat is located in the 5'-untranslated region of *FMR1* in exon 1. The gene spans 38 kb, contains 17 exons, and encodes a 4.4-kb transcript. Alleles contain blocks of CGG repeats, usually 7 to 13 repeats in length, interrupted with single AGG trinucleotides. Allelic diversity results from the variable number and lengths of these CGG-repeat blocks. There are no distinct boundaries separating the repeat number categories, however. Normal alleles have 5 to 45 repeats; gray zone alleles have 46 to 54; **premutation alleles** have 55 to 200; and full mutation expansion alleles contain >200 repeats (Figure 9-10). Individuals with a normal number of CGG repeats do not have fragile X syndrome nor are they at risk of having an affected child. Alleles with 46 to 54 repeats are in the upper range of normal or are smaller-than-average premutation alleles. These individuals do not have fragile X syndrome, but may have a slightly increased risk of repeat instability and expansion to a full mutation in their offspring in some families. Premutation alleles are unstable and can expand to a larger allele in the premutation range when transmitted; alternatively, they can expand to a full mutation allele and thus lead to an offspring with fragile X syndrome. Premutation carrier females have a higher prevalence of premature ovarian failure (POF) as compared with females with normal CGG-repeat numbers in the general population. Interestingly, full mutation carrier females

and their noncarrier sisters appear to have no increased risk for POF. Moderate CGG expansion seen in premutation carrier females may affect neurocognitive functioning related particularly to attention-related tasks. Further, despite overexpression of *FMR1* in premutation carriers, the FMR1 protein, FMRP, appears to be significantly diminished, suggesting reduced translation efficiency. Thus FMRP levels in premutation carriers are negatively correlated with the repeat number, and overexpression of *FMR1* has a positive correlation with the repeat number. The risk of CGG expansion from a premutation to a full mutation allele is dependent on several factors including the number of pure uninterrupted CGG repeats, the number and position of interspersed AGG repeats, the haplotype background, and less-well characterized heritable factors. The CGG expansion most often occurs before zygote formation, but CGG expansion can occur very early in embryogenesis. Expansions of premutations to full mutations are largely confined to transmissions from females to offspring.

Like expansion of the CAG repeat associated with HD, the *FMR1* CGG expansion is thought to occur from slippage during DNA replication of the lagging strand as a result of hairpin formation within the expanded CGG-repeat sequence. In contrast, premutation repeat alleles in males remain stable in 16% of transmissions, decrease in size in 22% of transmissions, and expand to a larger premutation allele in 62% of transmissions. Premutation carrier fathers of premutation carrier females were previously thought to have a fairly normal phenotype with no clinical features of fragile X syndrome, although these males may have large ears and deficits in nonverbal tasks, which now is explained by reduced levels of FMRP. Further, older premutation carrier males may exhibit a neurodegenerative syndrome characterized by progressive intention tremor, parkinsonism, and generalized brain atrophy.[9] Although FMRP is decreased, increased concentrations of *FMR1* transcript may represent a gain-of-function effect and may play a

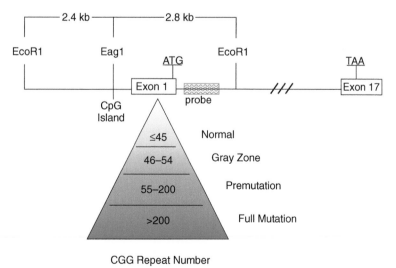

Figure 9-10
Schematic representation of the CGG repeat in exon 1 of *FMR1* and associated alleles. A CGG-repeat number less than or equal to 45 is normal. A CGG-repeat number of 46 to 54 is in the gray zone and has been reported to expand to a full mutation in some families. A CGG-repeat number of 55 to 200 is considered a premutation allele and is prone to expansion to a full mutation during female meiosis. A CGG-repeat number in excess of 200 is considered a full mutation and is diagnostic of fragile X syndrome.

role in this premutation tremor and/or ataxia syndrome. Mice with premutation CGG repeats in the *FMR1* gene have been shown to have intranuclear inclusions in distinct regions of the brain, suggesting the role of the *FMR1* gene in this process and providing a possible explanation of clinical features observed in symptomatic premutation carriers. Although expansion of a premutation to a full mutation is associated with maternal transmission, the sex of the fetus has no apparent effect on this process.

The fragile X phenotype occurs following expansion of the CGG repeat, hypermethylation of the DNA and histone deacetylation of the adjacent CpG island in the promoter region of the *FMR1* gene, transcriptional silencing of the gene, and ultimately no production of FMRP. Males with full expansion alleles but incomplete **DNA methylation**—"mosaic males"—may have severe mental retardation or a milder phenotype because some *FMR1* mRNA may be produced. *FMR1* mRNA is highly expressed in the testis and in the fetal and adult brain. FMRP is an RNA-binding protein with two RNA-binding motifs and is associated with translating polyribosomes as a part of a large ribonucleoprotein complex. Thus in cells from fragile X patients, hundreds of mRNAs exhibit abnormal translational profiles.

Although CGG expansion is the mechanism of disease in greater than 99% of all cases, a point mutation within the gene (I304N) and deletions have also been reported to cause disease in males having a clinical phenotype of fragile X syndrome. DNA testing for fragile X syndrome using Southern blot analysis (Figure 9-11) of peripheral blood enables detection of all possible genotypes (though not of all causes of fragile X as detected by cytogenetics). The use of methylation-sensitive restriction enzymes is explained in the legend of Figure 9-11. PCR analysis with capillary electrophoresis is used to complement the testing by providing the precise CGG-repeat number. (It may also be used as the first test, but when it fails to resolve two alleles in a female or to identify an allele in a male, the sample must be tested by Southern blot analysis because an expanded allele may be present that is too large to be amplified.) Chorionic villus samples or cultured amniocytes can be tested, but the methylation pattern expected in adult tissue may be absent.

As expected, as the CGG-repeat length increases, the risk of expansion from a premutation to a full mutation in premutation carrier females increases.[15] This information is most useful for determining the risk of an affected offspring during genetic counseling of a premutation carrier female. Although a woman with premutation CGG repeat of 55 to 59 is given about a 5% risk of expansion to a full mutation, a woman with a repeat length of 70 to 79 is given a 31% risk of expansion, and a woman with a CGG-repeat length >100 is given close to a 100% chance of expansion.

DISEASES WITH NONMENDELIAN INHERITANCE

Mitochondrial DNA Diseases

Mitochondria are organelles present in the cytoplasm of all eukaryotic cells of animals, higher plants, and some microorganisms. Mitochondria generate energy for the cellular processes by producing adenosine triphosphate (ATP) through oxidative phosphorylation (OXPHOS); they are important in

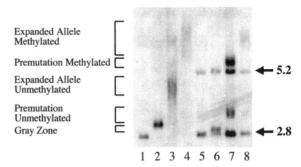

Figure 9-11

Southern blot analysis for the diagnosis of fragile X syndrome. Patient DNA is simultaneously digested with restriction endonucleases *EcoR*1 and *Eag*1, blotted to a nylon membrane, and hybridized with a ^{32}P-labeled probe adjacent to exon 1 of *FMR1* (see Figure 9-10). *Eag*1 is a methylation-sensitive restriction endonuclease that will not cleave the recognition sequence if the cytosine in the sequence is methylated. Normal male control DNA with a CGG-repeat number of 22 on his single X chromosome (*lane 1*) generates a band about 2.8 kb in length corresponding to *Eag*1-*EcoR*1 fragments (see Figure 9-10). Normal female control DNA with a CGG-repeat number of 20 on one X chromosome and a CGG-repeat number of 25 on her second X chromosome (*lane 5*) generates two bands, one at about 2.8 kb and a second at 5.2 kb. *EcoR*1-*EcoR*1 fragments approximately 5.2 kb in length represent methylated DNA sequences characteristic of the lyonized chromosome in each cell that is not digested with restriction endonuclease *Eag*1. DNA in *lane 2* contains a *FMR1* CGG-repeat number of 90 and is characteristic of a normal transmitting male. The banding pattern observed in *lane 3* is representative of a mosaic male with a single X chromosome with a full mutation (>200 repeats). However, the full mutation in some cells is unmethylated; in other cells, the full mutation is fully methylated, hence the term mosaic. In those cells in which the full mutation is unmethylated, digestion by both *Eag*1 and *EcoR*1 occurs, and in those cells in which the full mutation is fully methylated, digestion of the DNA by *Eag*1 is inhibited. The banding pattern observed in *lane 4* is diagnostic of a male with fragile X syndrome illustrating the typical expanded allele fully methylated in all cells. *Lane 6* is characteristic of a female with a normal allele and a CGG-repeat number of 29 and a larger gray zone allele with a CGG-repeat number of 54. *Lane 7* is the banding pattern observed from a premutation carrier female with one normal allele having a CGG-repeat number of 23 (band at about 2.8 kb) and a second premutation allele with CGG repeats of 120 to about 200 (band at about 3.1 kb). In premutation carrier females, in cells in which the X chromosome with the premutation allele is lyonized, the normal 5.2 kb *EcoR*1-*EcoR*1 band is larger because of the increased CGG-repeat number and is about 5.5 kb in length. *Lane 8* is diagnostic of a female with fragile X syndrome with one full expansion mutation allele that is completely methylated and transcriptionally silenced on one X chromosome but with a second normal allele with a CGG-repeat number of 33.

numerous cellular processes and play a role in apoptosis. The matrix of the mitochondrion is surrounded by a cardiolipin-rich inner membrane, and both are enclosed by a second outer membrane. Within the matrix are copies of the mitochondrial genome, mitochondrial deoxyribonucleic acid (mtDNA). Each mitochondrion contains between about 2 and 10 copies of mtDNA; so with hundreds of mitochondria per cell, an estimated 10^3 to 10^4 copies of mtDNA exist within each cell, with brain, skeletal, and cardiac muscle having particularly high concentrations.

The mtDNA is a double-stranded, circular molecule containing 16,569 base pairs that encodes 37 genes including two ribosomal RNAs (rRNA), 22 transfer RNAs (tRNA), and 13 subunits required for the OXPHOS system, with seven belonging to complex I, one to complex III, three to complex IV, and two to complex V.[20] The majority of the subunits involved in the OXPHOS system are encoded by nuclear DNA as are several nuclear gene products that regulate mitochondrial gene expression. Interestingly the mitochondrial genetic code is slightly different from the universal code. For example, in mtDNA, TGA codes for tryptophan rather than a termination codon, and all mitochondrial-encoded polypeptides contain codons requiring only the mitochondrial-encoded 22 tRNA molecules for translation rather than the 31 predicted by Crick's wobble hypothesis. The high copy number of mtDNA per cell coupled with a small genome and unique sequence variations between individuals makes mtDNA sequence analysis an ideal tool for forensic studies.

Inherited mitochondria-related diseases result from mutations in either nuclear DNA or the mitochondrial genome.[22] However, mitochondrial genetics are different from mendelian genetics in four important aspects.

(1) All mtDNA is maternally inherited. With mature oocytes having the highest mtDNA copy number per cell at 10^5 and sperm having the lowest mtDNA copy number per cell at 10^2 after fertilization, sperm mtDNA is selectively degraded so that only maternal mtDNA remains. Thus if a mother is carrying an mtDNA mutation, it will be transmitted to all of her children, but only her daughters can transmit the disease to their offspring. If an mtDNA mutation arises, it will exist among a population of normal mtDNA.

(2) Normal and mutant mtDNA copies coexist within the same cell. This coexistence is referred to as *heteroplasmy*.

(3) The proportion of normal and mutant mtDNA often varies among cells and tissues within the body. During cell division, the proportion of normal and mutant mtDNA can shift as mitochondria and their accompanying genomes are partitioned into daughter cells.

(4) The proportion of mutant mtDNA required within a cell, tissue, or organ system to result in a deleterious phenotype is variable, a phenomenon referred to as the *threshold effect*. The threshold for disease varies among people, tissues, and mtDNA mutations. As is evident, genetic counseling for families with mtDNA disorders is complicated by the inability to accurately predict phenotype caused by the phenomena of heteroplasmy and threshold effect.

Two types of mtDNA mutations exist, those that affect mitochondrial protein synthesis (tRNA and rRNA genes) and those within the protein-encoding genes themselves. Direct sequencing of mtDNA is considered the gold standard for mutation detection, but this methodology may be unable to detect a low percentage of mutant mtDNA in a heteroplasmic state. However, temporal temperature-gradient gel electrophoresis coupled with PCR and DNA sequencing detects heteroplasmic mutations as low as 4%. Although mtDNA mutations are now associated with a significant number of inherited diseases, acquired mtDNA deletions are associated with the aging process, and mitochondrial dysfunction is associated with neurodegenerative diseases. The most likely cause of somatic mtDNA mutations is via damage by oxygen free radicals produced as byproducts of aerobic metabolism.

Leber Hereditary Optic Neuropathy

Leber hereditary optic neuropathy (LHON) is the most common mitochondrial disease and the first linked to maternal inheritance through a mutation in the mtDNA. LHON is characterized by subacute loss of central vision of both eyes caused by focal degeneration of the retinal ganglion cell layer and of the optic nerve. After initial symptoms, both eyes are usually affected within 6 months. Approximately 50% to 60% of males and only 8% to 32% of females who possess the mtDNA mutation will actually develop this optic neuropathy. Nuclear-encoded factors that affect mtDNA expression, mtDNA products, or mitochondrial metabolism may modify the phenotypic expression of LHON. Genetic counseling in LHON is complicated in that the amount of mutant mtDNA transmitted by heteroplasmic females cannot be predicted, and testing cannot predict which individuals will develop visual symptoms.

LHON is a disorder caused by OXPHOS deficiency. Although more than 27 mutations have been associated with this disease, mtDNA mutations G3460A, G11778A, and T14484C represent 95% of those identified. Mutation G11778A was the first described, is the most common, and accounts for at least 50% of cases. In most affected individuals, LHON mutations appear to be homoplasmic, with only mutant mtDNA detected, but in 15% of cases, the mutations are heteroplasmic, with a mixture of both normal and mutant mtDNA detected. Each of the common mutations affects a subunit of the nicotinamide adenine dinucleotide:ubiquinone oxidoreductase in complex I of the OXPHOS pathway. However, the mechanism by which these mutations cause the LHON phenotype is not well understood.

Clinical DNA testing for these mutations is widely available and typically involves PCR amplification coupled with restriction endonuclease analysis and gel electrophoresis. If an individual's mtDNA is negative for the three common mutations, testing for other mtDNA mutations associated with LHON should be considered. DNA sequencing of all of the mtDNA-encoded complex I genes or of the entire mitochondrial genome may be required but should be employed only when clinical suspicion for LHON is high.

Leigh Syndrome

Leigh syndrome (LS), or subacute necrotizing encephalomyelopathy, is a progressive neurodegenerative disorder that eventually leads to death. In contrast to LHON, within the first few years of life individuals exhibit hypotonia, failure to thrive, psychomotor regression, ocular movement abnormalities, ataxia, and brainstem and basal ganglia dysfunction caused by severe dysfunction of mitochondrial energy metabolism. The clinical phenotype for LS is variable between people with the same pathogenic mtDNA mutation and largely results from differences in the percentage of mutant mtDNA among organs and tissues within each individual (Figure 9-12).

LS exhibits genetic heterogeneity, with disease-causing mutations identified in both nuclear and mtDNA, making both mendelian and maternal patterns of inheritance possible for this syndrome. Mutations in mtDNA genes (e.g., for ATPase6 [complex V], NADH dehydrogenase [complex I], and *tRNA*[Lys]), or nuclear-encoded genes affecting pyruvate dehydrogenase or respiratory chain enzyme complexes I, II, and IV have been reported. The most common biochemical abnormality

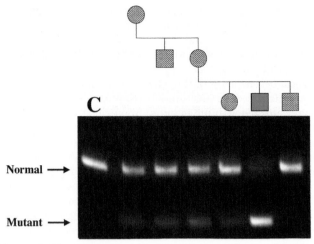

Figure 9-12

Detection of varying degrees of heteroplasmy for mtDNA mutation A8344G in a family with Leigh syndrome. mtDNA was extracted from a peripheral blood specimen from an affected male with Leigh syndrome and from family members. mtDNA was amplified using an oligonucleotide primer pair that flanks mitochondrial mutation A8344G. The A-to-G base substitution creates an *Nae*1 recognition site (GCCGGC), which is not present in normal control mtDNA (C). Amplicons from each member of the family and the control were digested with *Nae*1 and subjected to gel electrophoresis. The virtual absence of undigested amplicons in the affected male indicates the presence of almost 100% mutant mtDNA in the cells from this specimen and coincides with the severe phenotype of Leigh syndrome in this patient. In contrast, his sister, mother, and grandmother with 30%, 40%, and 20% mutant mtDNA suffer only from migraine headaches. His uncle, with 30% mutant mtDNA present, suffers with attention-deficit/hyperactivity disorder and learning disabilities. Heteroplasmy, or variation in the percentage of normal and mutant mitochondria, largely explains the observed phenotypic differences in this family.

(Courtesy Thomas W. Prior, Ph.D., Depts of Pathology and Neurology, Ohio State University, Columbus, Ohio.)

associated with LS is deficiency of cytochrome c oxidase caused by defects in the assembly of complex IV. The protein products from the *SURF-1* and *COX 10* genes play an important role in the assembly of complex IV, and mutations in these genes follow an autosomal recessive mode of inheritance.

Clinical testing for mitochondrially inherited LS uses direct sequencing of mtDNA-encoded genes. Because of the genetic heterogeneity of nonmitochondrially inherited LS and the need for mutation screening for a number of genes, clinical testing for LS is limited.

Imprinting Disorders

Imprinting refers to the differential marking or "imprinting" of specific paternally and maternally inherited alleles during gametogenesis, resulting in differential expression of those genes. Such imprints on the DNA during gametogenesis must be maintained through DNA replication in the somatic cells of the offspring, must be reversible from generation to generation, and must influence transcription. DNA methylation (Chapter 1) is the primary mechanism for genomic imprinting. The number of imprinted genes in the human genome is estimated to be less than 200, and most are clustered around imprinting control centers. Alterations in normal imprinting patterns can result in disease.

Prader-Willi and Angelman Syndromes

Prader-Willi syndrome (PWS) is characterized by hypotonia, obesity, short stature, small hands and feet, motor and mental retardation, and hypogonadism.[3] The syndrome is also associated with specific behavioral and psychopathological characteristics, which present challenging management issues. The disorder is relatively frequent, with an incidence of 1 in 10,000 to 15,000. Angelman syndrome (AS) is characterized by severe mental retardation, inappropriate bouts of laughter, absence of speech, gait ataxia, frequently microcephaly, and seizures.[25] The incidence of AS is estimated at about 1 in 12,000 to 20,000. As apparent from their characteristic physical findings, PWS and AS are clinically distinct syndromes; yet each results from one of several possible genetic changes involving chromosomal region 15q11-q13 (long arm of chromosome 15 within banding regions 11 and 13). Within this 4-Mb region, 2 Mb are imprinted, with gene expression dependent on parental origin. PWS results from the loss of paternally expressed genes in this region, and AS results primarily from the loss of a maternally expressed gene in this region.

The primary candidate gene for PWS is the paternally expressed *SNURF-SNRPN* locus. There is extensive DNA methylation at the CpG island upstream from this locus on the maternal allele, resulting in transcriptional silencing of this locus. The *SNURF-SNRPN* is a complex locus that contains multiple genes and a *cis*-acting regulatory region referred to as the imprinting center (IC). The IC controls resetting of parental imprints in the 15q11-13 region during gametogenesis.

AC   Also important are two polypeptides, SmN and SNURF, and a small nucleolar RNA (snRNA), *HBII-13*. SmN is involved in mRNA splicing in the brain, and SNURF (*SNRPN* upstream reading frame) is found in the nucleus, contains 71 amino acids, may bind RNA, and has a C-terminal motif similar to ubiquitin. HBII-13 is encoded from within intron 12 of SNURF and modifies RNA, perhaps mRNA and rRNA and snRNA. In addition, multiple imprinted and paternal-only expressed genes have also been identified in this region including *NDN*, which encodes necdin, a protein important for neuronal differentiation and a suppressor for cell proliferation; *IPW*, which encodes a 2.2-kb RNA, but is not translated into a polypeptide; *MKRN3*, which encodes makorin ring zinc-finger protein 3; and *MAGEL2*, which encodes melanoma antigen-like gene 2. These expressed genes may have additive roles in the phenotype of PWS.

The loss of normally expressed paternal genes in 15q11-q13 resulting in PWS occurs by one of several mechanisms (Table 9-1).

1. A de novo deletion. The deletion encompasses this area following *unequal homologous* recombination involving repeated homologous sequences in this

TABLE 9-1	Molecular Mechanisms and Tests for Prader-Willi and Angelman's Syndromes*			
Molecular Mechanism	Angelman's Syndrome (Frequency)	Prader-Willi Syndrome (Frequency)	Methylation-Specific PCR Result	Possible Detection Methods
Deletion cytogenetics (~4 Mb) of chromosome 15q11-13	70% (maternal)	65%-70% (paternal)	Abnormal	High-resolution or FISH
Uniparental disomy	7% (paternal)	25%-30% (maternal)	Abnormal	PCR for microsatellite analysis
Imprinting center defect	3%	~5%	Abnormal	IC sequencing
UBE3A mutation (specific to AS)	11%	N/A	Normal	UBE3A sequencing
Chromosomal rearrangement in chromosome 15q11-13 region	<1% (maternal)	<1% (paternal)	Normal	High-resolution cytogenetics or FISH
No detectable abnormality	~11%	Very few cases	Normal	N/A

*Modified from a table prepared by Allison Presley, MD, University of Virginia.

region. The subsequent zygote is monosomic for these genes by possessing only the maternal copy. De novo deletion accounts for 65% to 75% of cases of PWS.

2. **Uniparental disomy.** In these patients, although two copies of the genes located in 1q11-q13 exist, both are maternal in origin (arising in most cases from meiosis I **nondisjunction,** when homologous chromosomes fail to separate) and subsequent loss of the third, paternal-derived chromosome 15 (through mitotic loss postzygotically). This mechanism of chromosome loss rescues the zygote from trisomy 15, a condition that is incompatible with life. Although in this situation the fetus is genetically complete with two chromosome 15s (disomy), both chromosomes are from the same parent (uniparental) with a loss of paternal-expressed loci in the critical imprinted region 15q11-q13. Uniparental disomy accounts for 25% to 30% of cases of PWS.

3. Microdeletions encompassing the paternal IC. These microdeletions account for about 5% of cases of PWS.

4. Abnormal imprinting without detectable DNA mutation. A microdeletion containing the IC prevents this cis-acting control center from resetting the imprint in the germline. These mutations, if present on the maternal chromosome of phenotypically normal fathers, will be transmitted to offspring as the paternal chromosome and result in a child with PWS.

5. Chromosomal rearrangements disrupting the genes in the 15q11-q13 region. These chromosomal rearrangements account for less than 1% of PWS cases.

The primary maternally expressed gene in the PWS and/or AS critical region is UBE3A, although a second gene, ATP10C, has been shown to display predominantly maternal expression in brain and lymphocytes. The UBE3A gene is almost exclusively expressed in the brain, contains 16 exons, and encodes an E3 ubiquitin ligase involved in the ubiquitination pathway for degradation of a diverse range of protein substrates. The lack of ubiquitination could result in the inability to degrade or functionally alter targeted proteins.

AS may arise by several mechanisms (Table 9-1). Similar to PWS, the most common change in AS (in 70% of patients) is a deletion of the critical 15q11-q13 region. However, unlike PWS, in which the paternal allele is deleted, in AS the maternal allele is deleted. AS patients with a deletion have a more severe phenotype, possibly because of **haploinsufficiency.** In

haploinsufficiency, the amount of protein product is below normal. In 7% of AS individuals, phenotypic expression of the syndrome occurs as a result of uniparental disomy because of the inheritance of two copies of a paternal chromosome 15 in contrast to the normal inheritance of one paternal and one maternal allele. With both paternal UBE3A genes silenced, there is no functional UBE3A protein. In 3% of AS cases, an imprinting defect has been described. A cytogenetic rearrangement has been detected in about 1% of AS cases, and in 11% of cases, a mutation in the UBE3A gene itself has been reported. Although these mutations can arise de novo, they can be silently transmitted through several generations. For example, if a UBE3A mutation rose de novo on a paternal allele transmitted to a son, the son could transmit the mutation to a son or daughter to result in a normal phenotype. However, although this son could again transmit the silenced UBE3A mutation to his offspring, his sister could donate her mutated UBE3A paternally derived allele to her offspring, and the child would have AS. Lastly, in about 11% of AS individuals, the cause of the disease has not been established.

Diagnostic testing for AS or PWS involves a variety of methodologies (Table 9-1). Determining the genetic mechanism for the cause of the disease is important for determining recurrence risks for the family. Under most circumstances, initiating testing with methylation-specific PCR (mPCR) may be the most cost-effective approach (Figure 9-13). In mPCR genomic DNA is treated with sodium bisulfite before PCR to convert unmethylated cytosine residues to uracil without altering the methylated cytosine residues (those silenced in the 15q11-13 region). The subsequent PCR reactions use oligonucleotide primers specific to DNA strands that contain either uracil (unmethylated) or cytosine (methylated). mPCR provides a rapid and reliable diagnostic test to rule out PWS or AS. A positive result is present in >99% of PWS and about 80% of AS individuals. PWS individuals with a chromosomal rearrangement disrupting the genes in this area will not be identified by this test. Similarly, AS individuals with a UBE3A mutation, a chromosome rearrangement disrupting the genes in the region, or AS resulting from an unknown cause will not be diagnosed with this methodology. However, if the result is positive, FISH studies (to detect a deletion within 15q11-13) and/or uniparental disomy DNA testing should be done to determine the genetic mechanism of disease to support appropriate genetic counseling of the family.

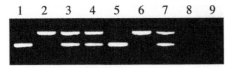

Figure 9-13

mPCR assay for the diagnosis of PWS and AS. Extracted DNA is treated with sodium bisulfate before amplification using multiplex PCR and oligonucleotide primers specific for modified DNA. Normal individuals show amplicons representing their methylated maternal allele and amplicons from their unmethylated paternal allele. PWS patients show only the maternal allele, and AS patients show only the paternal allele. Results observed following PCR amplification and gel electrophoresis of patients referred for PWS and AS testing. Patient DNA with patterns diagnostic of AS *(lanes 1 and 5)*, PWS *(lanes 2 and 6)*, and patients referred for AS or PWS but who have normal methylation patterns *(lanes 3 and 4)* are shown. Normal control DNA patterns and a negative control reaction in which no template DNA was added are indicated in *lanes 7 and 8*, respectively. No amplification products are observed in unmodified normal control DNA *(lane 9)*, illustrating the specificity of the PCR primers specifically for sodium bisulfate–modified DNA.

(Courtesy Jack Tarleton, Ph.D., Director of Genetics Laboratory, Fullerton Genetics Center, Mission Hospitals, Asheville, N.C.)

Complex Diseases

A complex or multifactorial inheritance pattern indicates interaction of one or more genes with one or more environmental factors. Multifactorial diseases are more prevalent in some families, with several affected family members, but the disease does not follow typical mendelian inheritance patterns. Disease may be present in multiple family members because of the sharing of similar disease-predisposing alleles and often the sharing of similar daily habits, routines, and diet. The degree of genetic and environmental contribution to a disease process varies among complex diseases, and identification of the causative genetic and environmental factors is challenging. Further, it is difficult to assess the relative importance of genetic and environmental influences in the development of a disease, though twin studies are often used. Among twins who were raised together, a greater concordance of disease among monozygotic (MZ) twins—who share all of their genes—than in dizygotic (DZ) twins—who share 50% of their genes—provides strong evidence of a genetic component to the disease. Conversely, disease concordance <100% in MZ twins is strong evidence that nongenetic factors play a role in the disease. Examples of largely adult-onset complex diseases include type 1 diabetes, multiple sclerosis, Parkinson disease, hypertension, alcoholism, and thrombophilia.

Thrombophilia

Deep vein thrombosis (DVT) occurs in about 1 per 1000 individuals, and complications from DVT, including pulmonary embolism, account for about 50,000 deaths per year. Venous thrombosis is caused by a disruption of normal hemostasis caused by the interaction of one or more genes and environmental factors and/or acquired conditions, including use of oral contraceptives, trauma, obesity, immobility, pregnancy, age, or surgery. Although the protein products of many genes are involved in the anticoagulation and coagulation pathway and are involved in the regulation of hemostasis, mutations in the factor V and prothrombin genes are associated with DVT,

represent the most common genetic cause of thrombophilia, and are common in the population.[6] Further, individuals with both mutations have a greater risk of a *recurrent* DVT than do those with just one, and may require different management. Despite the presence of these mutations and the same environmental and/or acquired factors as are present in other family members, it is impossible to predict an individual's clinical course. Thus venous thrombosis illustrates our lack of understanding in the interaction of known and uncharacterized risk factors in predisposition to a complex disease.

Activated protein C (APC) in conjunction with its cofactor, protein S, plays a key role in the anticoagulant system by inactivating membrane-bound factors Va and VIIIa. The inability to inactivate procoagulant factors Va or VIIIa could disturb hemostasis, heighten the coagulation pathway, increase the generation of thrombin, and promote clot formation. A G-to-A base substitution at nucleotide 1691 in exon 10 of the factor V gene is linked to the APC resistance phenotype. This nucleotide change results in an arginine-to-glutamine substitution at codon 506 (R506Q) in the factor V protein. Cleavage at the arginine residue at codon 506 by APC is the initial step of inactivation of the activated factor V protein, causing it to display a decreased affinity for factor Xa. As a result, there is reduced efficiency in catalyzing the activation of prothrombin to alpha-thrombin. However, substitution with a glutamine residue at this site prolongs inactivation of this molecule by APC by approximately tenfold, thereby shifting the balance of hemostasis to favor coagulation and increasing thrombin production. Interestingly, this mutation is quite common in the Caucasian population of Northern European descent, with a frequency of 3% to 5%, but is essentially absent in Asian, African, or Australian populations. This phenomenon is thought to result from the fact that the G-to-A mutation occurred as a single event approximately 21,000 to 34,000 years ago after the evolutionary divergence of non-Africans from Africans and of Caucasians from Mongoloids.

Heterozygous carriers have a 7.9-fold increased relative risk of thrombosis compared with a ninety-onefold increased risk for homozygotes. The risk for thrombosis is increased in the presence of other genetic or environmental and/or acquired factors. The mean age of onset of symptoms associated with thrombosis is 44 years in heterozygotes and 31 years in homozygotes. Further, although transmitted as a dominant trait—with carriers of this mutation possessing a lifelong risk—and because thrombophilia is a complex disease resulting from the interaction of both genetic and environmental and/or acquired factors, many heterozygote carriers remain asymptomatic.

In addition to the G1691A polymorphism in the FV gene, a G20210A variant in the 3′-untranslated region of the prothrombin gene is present in 18% of individuals with a documented family history of venous thrombosis. This common allele increases the risk of venous thrombosis 2.8-fold and is associated with increased plasma prothrombin (>1.15 kU/L). The risk of venous thrombosis is increased sixteenfold in G20210A carriers using oral contraceptives, and the risk of cerebral vein thrombosis increases 149-fold in G20210A carriers using oral contraceptives. In the Caucasian population, this base substitution is present in 6.2% of individuals with venous thrombosis compared with 2.3% of controls. This allele is mostly confined to the Caucasian population. Similar to the origin of factor V mutation G1691A, it is thought that the G20210A base substitution occurred as a single event after the divergence of Africans from non-Africans and of Caucasoid from Mongoloid subpopulations. Prothrombin, also referred to as factor II, is the precursor of thrombin and plays a primary role in fibrin production and clot formation. The G-to-A substitution increases the processing of the 3′ end of the pre-mRNA and thus functions as a gain-of-function mutation, culminating in increased mRNA accumulation and increased synthesis of protein. This aberration of RNA metabolism results in increased synthesis of prothrombin and thus fosters clot formation. Note that the substitution does not change the amino acid sequence of prothrombin.

Inheritance of both G1691A (factor V) and G20210A (factor II, prothrombin) together conveys at least a twentyfold increased risk for a venous thromboembolic event (VTE). They are commonly seen together in thrombophilic individuals thus supporting the additive genetic effect associated with complex diseases.[1]

DNA testing for G1691A and G20210A in clinical laboratories is performed by any one of several methodologies, with those most commonly reported being invasive cleavage of oligonucleotide probes (Invader assay), PCR coupled with restriction-endonuclease digestion and gel electrophoresis, and real-time PCR, usually with melting analysis (Chapter 5). Any testing platform is acceptable for clinical use as long as the procedure has been properly validated in the laboratory and follows appropriate quality assurance guidelines.[21]

DNA-based testing for factor V may be requested on an individual following an abnormal functional coagulation assay to confirm the diagnosis and to distinguish between heterozygotes and homozygotes. DNA testing may replace the functional assay for some individuals, such as those with lupus anticoagulant (which may interfere with the assay) and a markedly prolonged baseline aPTT or in family members of G1691A-positive individuals. Since there are multiple causes of thrombotic events, and several predisposing factors may be present in an individual, testing is especially recommended in individuals in whom a high clinical suspicion exists, such as individuals with: (1) venous thrombosis or pulmonary embolism and age under 50; (2) venous thrombosis at an unusual site (hepatic, mesenteric, portal, or cerebral veins); (3) recurrent VTE; (4) VTE and a strong family history of thrombotic disease; (5) VTE in pregnant women or women taking oral contraceptives; or (6) relatives who had VTE at age less than 50 years.

Benefits from DNA testing include the identification of individuals at risk for recurrent events, especially in situations that predispose to thrombosis, such as oral contraceptive use, management of pregnancy complications, or hormone replacement therapy. In addition, DNA testing enables the identification of at-risk family members. Screening is not recommended for populations or newborns nor is prenatal screening recommended. Although factor V R506Q represents the genetic factor in thrombophilia in greater than 50% of families with thrombosis, inherited defects in protein C, protein S, and antithrombin are detectable in approximately 10% to 15% of families with venous thrombosis. These latter, less common deficiencies are diagnosed by use of assays in the coagulation laboratory, and typically without DNA testing, because of the heterogeneity of mutations in these genes. Mutations at two other factor V arginine-cleavage sites have been reported, but

these mutations are rare and are not part of routine DNA testing.

Inherited Breast Cancer

Mutations in the two major breast cancer genes, BRCA1 and BRCA2, predispose individuals to breast and ovarian cancer and to prostate and colon cancer (BRCA1) or pancreatic cancer (BRCA2).[14] The incidence of mutations in these genes within the population is estimated to be between 1 in 500 and 1 in 1000. However, the combined frequency of three common mutations in the Ashkenazi Jewish population is as high as almost 3%. Breast carcinoma is second only to lung carcinoma as a cause of cancer-related death among women in the Western hemisphere, but familial breast cancer accounts for only 5% to 10% of all cases. BRCA1 and BRCA2 mutations are present in only about 20% of familial cases and are often associated with a younger age of onset. The progression rate of breast neoplasia appears to be accelerated in women who carry BRCA1 or BRCA2 mutations compared with other individuals who have breast carcinoma with or without a family history. In families in which breast cancer is segregating, but no BRCA1 or BRCA2 mutation has been detected, additional genes that predispose to breast cancer are likely, but have yet to be identified. The inability to identify breast cancer susceptibility genes in these families may reflect: (1) genetic heterogeneity in the family with mutations in several genes; (2) low penetrance of these mutations, making it difficult to distinguish family members without mutation from asymptomatic carriers in the studies; (3) an autosomal recessive mode of inheritance; or (4) breast cancer acting as a complex disease that results from the interaction of both several genes and environmental factors, thereby making it difficult to tease out the genetic component of the disease. Mutations in tumor-suppressor genes TP53 or ATM are also associated with "familial" cancer, including breast cancer in mutation-positive females. For the remaining families, gene-expression assays of tumor tissue may be instrumental for classification of families into subsets, aiding studies aimed at determining the genes involved in these familial cancers.

Mutations in BRCA1 and BRCA2 are inherited in an autosomal dominant fashion, with offspring of known carriers or of affected individuals possessing a 50% chance of inheriting the predisposing cancer gene mutation. Inheritance of the mutation does not convey a certainty of developing cancer nor indicate the type of cancer or the age of onset. The average cumulative risk of breast cancer for mutations in either BRCA1 or BRCA2 is about 27% to age 50 and 64% to age 70. Both environmental and genetic factors play a role in the development of breast or other cancers in mutation-positive individuals as does the type of DNA mutation in BRCA1 or BRCA2.

The BRCA1 gene is located on 17q21 (long arm of chromosome 17 banding region 21), spans 80 kb, and is composed of 24 exons, with 22 encoding the 7.8-kb mRNA that is translated into a protein of 1863 amino acids. The BRCA2 gene is located on 13q12-13 (long arm of chromosome 13 within banding region 12 and 13), spans 70 kb, contains 26 exons, encodes an 11.5-kb mRNA, and is translated into a protein of 3418 amino acids. BRCA1 and BRCA2 are considered tumor-suppressor genes requiring inactivation of both alleles for progression to neoplasm. In an individual with familial breast cancer, a mutant allele is inherited, and the second allele—the individual's wild-type allele—is inactivated through somatic mutation. BRCA1 and BRCA2 proteins are multifunctional, interacting with numerous other proteins in complex and separate systems involved in response to DNA damage, regulation of transcription, remodeling of chromatin, and regulation of cell growth.

Mutations in BRCA1 and BRCA2 are heterogeneous and located throughout each gene. More than 1000 mutations have been observed.

AC The range of mutations varies greatly among different populations, with some mutations unique to specific ethnic groups. In Ashkenazi Jewish breast and ovarian cancer families, mutations 185delAG and 5382insC are the ones primarily observed in BRCA1, and in families in whom these mutations are not present, the identification of other BRCA1 mutations is rare. In addition, BRCA2 mutation 6174delT has been observed in about 8% of Ashkenazi Jewish women diagnosed with breast cancer before age 42, but is rare in non-Jewish women diagnosed with breast cancer at the same age. BRCA1 mutation 943ins10 is an ancient mutation of West African origin, and mutation 2804delAA, estimated to have occurred about 32 generations ago, is seen in Dutch and Belgian families. The BRCA2 mutation 999del5 is common in the Icelandic population, whereas BRCA2 mutations S2835X and 5802del4 are common in Japanese breast cancer families. In contrast, BRCA1 and BRCA2 mutations are less commonly associated with familial breast cancer in Taiwanese and Chinese populations.

Testing for disease-associated mutations is made difficult by the heterogeneity of disease-causing mutations and the complexity of the BRCA1 and BRCA2 genes. Moreover, the clinical significance of some observed variants may be unknown, and some may be benign. The majority of BRCA1 and BRCA2 disease-associated mutations result in premature truncation of the protein and thus a loss of function. For this reason, the protein truncation test (PTT) is often employed as a screening method for mutation detection. In this methodology, multiple PCR primer pairs are designed to span the gene with each primer pair, including one primer that includes an RNA polymerase promoter and a translation initiation sequence. The resulting amplicons are incubated in an in vitro translation system, and the synthesized proteins are subjected to sodium dodecyl sulfate (SDS)-polyacrylamide gel electrophoresis for detection of truncated proteins.

In addition to PTT, various other screening techniques have been described to provide maximal sensitivity in mutation detection, yet high throughput of specimens. Other common screening assays include microarrays, denaturing high-performance liquid chromatography (DHPLC), single-strand conformation polymorphism (SSCP), denaturing gradient gel electrophoresis (DGGE), heteroduplex analysis (HA), and fluorescence-assisted mismatch analysis (FAMA). Other unique methods are used as well, including allele-specific gene expression analysis (AGE), multiplex ligation-dependent probe amplification (MLPA), and restriction endonuclease fingerprinting, SSCP coupled with capillary electrophoresis.

Although screening assays detect most DNA perturbations, DNA sequence (DS) analysis is required for precise identification of the base or bases involved. In many instances, a combination of screening methods is used, thereby reducing the region of the gene that requires DNA sequencing analysis. In addition, since unique mutations within various populations exist, information regarding the ethnicity of the patient may be valuable in determining the strategy for analysis, employing a method to detect those mutations most common in that population. An alternative approach is to eliminate screening of the gene and rather perform direct DS analysis of the BRCA1 and BRCA2 genes on each specimen.

Clinical testing for BRCA1 and BRCA2 is primarily performed on women with breast cancer and a strong family history of breast and/or ovarian cancer or on presymptomatic women with a strong family history of breast and/or ovarian cancer for which prior identification of a BRCA1 or BRCA2 mutation in the family may or may not have occurred. The likelihood of identifying a BRCA1 or BRCA2 mutation in a patient is increased to 10% or greater if: (1) breast cancer was diagnosed in two women in the family before the age of 50; (2) breast cancer was diagnosed in women in the family before age 50, and ovarian cancer was detected in one or more women in the family; (3) breast cancer was diagnosed after the age of 50 in one woman, and ovarian cancer was detected in two or more women in the family; (4) ovarian cancer is present in two or more family members; (5) male breast cancer is present, and breast or ovarian cancer is present in the family.

In presymptomatic cases, extensive genetic counseling addressing both the positive and possible negative aspects of genetic testing must be discussed with the patient before genetic testing is undertaken.[10] Counseling often involves participation of family members, usually spouses. Based on the family history, the genetic counselor should inform the patient of the likelihood that a BRCA1 or BRCA2 mutation could be segregating in the family, the risk of disease(s) associated with mutations, and an overview of prevention and surveillance options available for mutation carriers. Counseling may be needed for psychological issues, including the fear of cancer or medical procedures, past experiences involving loved ones with cancer, feelings of guilt about possibly transmitting a cancer-causing gene to children, and discrimination by employers or insurers if a positive test result is disclosed. The continued anxiety and uncertainty with some test results should be discussed as well. For example, in some instances when DNA from an affected family member is not available for testing, the presymptomatic individual must clearly understand that a negative result could imply the inability to detect the specific BRCA1 or BRCA2 gene mutation segregating in the family and would not exclude the possibility of a mutation in another breast cancer–susceptibility gene that may be present in the family. Further, the possibility of identifying a DNA alteration of unclear significance and the associated uncertainty and anxiety resulting from such a finding must also be discussed. A U.S. patent has resulted in clinical testing for BRCA1 and BRCA2 being available exclusively at one location within the United States; both false-negative test results and variants of uncertain significance are possible. The absolute control of diagnostic testing of these genes by one company for patient care is an issue of much debate.

Once an asymptomatic, mutation-positive woman has been identified, she may wish to undergo prophylactic bilateral mastectomy, oophorectomy, or specialized surveillance and prevention strategies for the early detection of both breast and ovarian cancer. The risk of breast cancer can be significantly lower in women choosing prophylactic surgery than in those opting for increased surveillance.

Inherited Colon Cancer

Colorectal cancer (CRC) is the second leading cause of cancer death in the United States, with about 5% of cases associated with inherited mutations linked to colon cancer syndromes.[16] The molecular basis of sporadic and inherited CRC involves two distinct pathways, one of chromosomal instability (CIN) and one associated with microsatellite instability (MSI).

The *CIN pathway* begins with the loss of function of the adenomatosis polyposis coli (APC) tumor-suppressor gene product, most often because of a somatic inactivating gene mutation on one allele followed by a chromosomal deletion encompassing the second APC allele and adjacent flanking DNA on chromosome 5q (Figure 9-14). APC is located on 5q21 (long arm of chromosome band 21), and since it is involved early in the tumorigenic process, it has been referred to as the

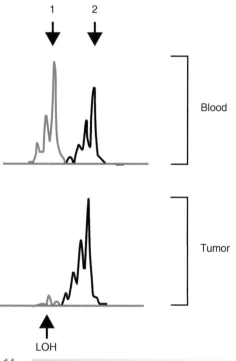

Figure 9-14

Electropherograms illustrating LOH in tumor DNA. Patient DNA is extracted from the peripheral blood and tumor tissue and amplified by PCR using an oligonucleotide primer pair specific for a polymorphic, microsatellite repeat locus contained within the chromosomal region thought to be deleted during tumorigenesis. One of the primers within the pair is labeled with a fluorescent dye. Amplicons are subjected to electrophoresis on a 5% denaturing polyacrylamide gel in an ABI DNA sequencer and analyzed using GeneScan software 3.1 b3. Constitutive DNA from the patient's blood illustrates heterozygosity for this marker with amplicons represented by alleles 1 and 2. In DNA from the tumor, a single peak representing a typical homozygous pattern is observed. Thus there is LOH in tumor DNA. This loss signifies the loss of the second allele and also indicates the loss of this region on the chromosome (see Color Plate 6).

"gatekeeper." The cascade of events proceeds with continued activation of the *KRAS* (Kirsten rat sarcoma virus, Chapter 14) proto-oncogene on 12p12.1 (short arm of chromosome 12 banding region 12.1) by somatic gene mutations (most frequently occurring in codons 12, 13, or 61), which in the presence of APC inactivation increases growth and proliferation of the cell. Further changes occur in the DNA in the tumor. Inactivation of the tumor-suppressor gene *DCC* (deleted in colon cancer) and frequent loss of adjacent tumor-suppressor genes on 18q (long arm of chromosome 18) including *SMAD4* and *SMAD* and the inactivation of tumor-suppressor gene *TP53* (Chapter 14, Box 14-2) on 17p (short arm of chromosome 17) are identified in late adenoma and carcinoma.

The *MSI pathway* in sporadic CRC arises from mutations or altered expression of genes involved in DNA mismatch repair (MMR) (Figure 9-15). As a result of an altered and thus dysfunctional MMR system, DNA replication errors, primarily within microsatellite repeats or repetitive sequences, remain uncorrected and accumulate. The changes in length of these sequences were recognized by early investigators. Although expansion or contraction of the microsatellite-repeat number is of little significance in much of the noncoding areas of the genome, some changes within coding regions of the genome and specifically within genes involved in cell growth and regulation alter the sequences of their protein products and thus affect their function.

Inherited CRC syndromes initiate as a result of an inherited mutation in one of the genes involved in the CIN or MSI pathway.[4] Although several CRC syndromes exist, the two most common are familial adenomatous polyposis (FAP) and hereditary nonpolyposis colorectal cancer (HNPCC). Most interestingly, tumors in FAP kindreds and tumors displaying CIN more frequently are found in the distal part of the colon, whereas tumors in HNPCC families and tumors displaying MSI more commonly occur in the proximal part of the colon.

Familial Adenomatous Polyposis

FAP has an incidence of 1 in 8000, is characterized by hundreds to thousands of adenomatous polyps throughout the large bowel, and is inherited in an autosomal dominant fashion. A person who inherits the mutation has an 80% to 100% chance of developing the disease. FAP accounts for less than 1% of CRC observed in the United States. In about 25% of cases no family history exists, indicating that these cases arise as a result of a new mutation; there is no tendency for paternal versus maternal origin of the mutated allele. Polyps first appear during the second decade of life. CRC ultimately develops approximately 10 to 15 years after the onset of polyposis, with the median age of CRC in untreated FAP individuals being about 40. Although an individual polyp in an FAP patient is no more likely to progress to cancer than a sporadic polyp, it is the sheer number of polyps in these individuals that increases the likelihood that one will progress to cancer. Further, individuals with FAP are at increased risk for developing cancer of the thyroid, small intestine, stomach, and brain. The gene responsible for FAP is the APC gene. The APC gene spans 8535 base pairs, contains 15 exons, and encodes a protein of 2843 amino acids with a molecular weight of about 312 kDa.

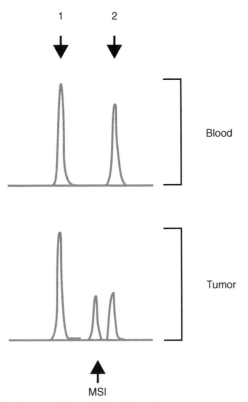

Figure 9-15

Electropherograms illustrating MSI in tumor DNA. Patient DNA is extracted from the peripheral blood and tumor tissue and amplified by PCR using an oligonucleotide primer pair specific for a microsatellite repeat locus. One of the primers within the pair is labeled with a fluorescent dye. Amplicons are subjected to electrophoresis on a 5% denaturing polyacrylamide gel in an ABI DNA sequencer and analyzed by GeneScan software 3.1 b3. Constitutive DNA from the patient's blood illustrates heterozygosity for this marker with amplicons represented by alleles 1 and 2. In DNA from the tumor, in addition to constitutive alleles 1 and 2, amplicons representing DNA fragments of a different size are present; these indicate a change in repeat number for one of the alleles. Because of dysfunctional MMR enzymes, mistakes occurring during the replication of microsatellite repeat sequences resulting in expansions or contractions of the repeat number remain unrepaired. In this case a contraction in the repeat number of allele 2 has occurred (see Color Plate 7).

AC   The APC protein is a multidomain, multifunctional protein, participating in several cellular processes, including cell adhesion and migration, signal transduction, microtubule assembly, and chromosome segregation. Best understood is the regulation of β-catenin levels through interaction with APC. β-catenin is required for binding with E-cadherin, a member of the calcium-dependent cell adhesion molecules, and is also involved in signal transduction pathways. Mutations altering the association of β-catenin with APC minimize degradation and increase cytoplasmic levels of β-catenin; this can affect cell-cell adhesion and the transcription of genes, promoting cell proliferation (specifically CMYC) or inhibition of cell death.

Studies on FAP families indicate that a wide variety of germline mutations exist; >95% result in truncated proteins, either because of a nonsense mutation (30%) or by a frameshift mutation, and most are contained within the 5′ half of the gene. In germline mutations, there are two hot spots at codons 1061 and 1309, with the most common mutation being an AAAAG deletion at codon 1309. These mutations leave the truncated APC protein unable to regulate β-catenin.

Genotype-phenotype correlations exist for some APC mutations. Individuals with truncating mutations at the extreme 5′ end of the gene (codons 1 to 163) or mutations at the carboxyl-terminal end of the gene (codons 1860 to 1987) have the attenuated form of the disease, developing a smaller number of polyps (<100). A severe phenotype is observed in individuals with mutations between codons 1250 and 1464, and individuals with truncating mutations between codons 1403 and 1578 are at an increased risk for extracolonic disease. Intrafamilial and interfamilial phenotypic variability exists even in the presence of an identical mutation and may be explained by a modifier gene or genes. The site of the inherited germline mutation appears to influence the type of somatic inactivating mutation occurring at their normal APC gene. If the germline mutation occurs between codons 1194 and 1392, the second hit to the normal allele is likely a deletion encompassing the APC allele. However, if the germline mutation is outside this region, the second hit will likely result in a truncating mutation within the mutation cluster region (MCR) between codons 1286 and 1513.

The PTT is most often used to test for mutations in a family because the majority of FAP mutations result in a truncated protein. Once a possible mutation has been detected, the region is sequenced to determine the precise identity of the mutation. When other screening or direct detection methodologies also are used, a sensitivity of about 87% is achieved. If the mutation within the family is identified, it is recommended that the family be referred for genetic counseling. DNA testing should be performed in at-risk family members as young as 10 to 12 years of age. Genetic testing results change the 50% pretest estimate of risk of disease to a risk of either 0% or 100%. Although DNA testing on an asymptomatic minor is typically not endorsed by the genetic community, in this scenario early identification of the mutation in these individuals will clearly impact their clinical management by initiating intense screening programs and possible prophylactic colectomy. Family members with a negative test result for the mutation do not have an increased risk of CRC and thus avoid intensive screening programs. Further, in some FAP mutation–positive families, preimplantation genetic diagnosis has been successfully employed to prevent the birth of a child with an inherited predisposition to FAP. If the mutation in the family cannot be identified, DNA linkage studies may be useful for presymptomatic identification of at-risk family members. If the mutation in the family cannot be identified and if DNA linkage studies are not informative or available, screening is recommended with yearly sigmoidoscopy as early as age 12. Further, when repeatedly negative sigmoidoscopy results are found, the recommended frequency of such exams decreases.

Hereditary Nonpolyposis Colon Cancer

The most common inherited CRC susceptibility syndrome is HNPCC, which represents about 2% to 3% of all CRC cases.

In contrast to FAP, HNPCC is characterized by a few polyps that possess an accelerated transformation potential to carcinoma in as little as 1 to 2 years. HNPCC is inherited as an autosomal dominant disorder with a penetrance of 80% to 85%. HNPCC individuals have a lifetime risk of 70% to 80% for developing CRC, thereby suggesting a role for other factors in this disease process.

To assist clinicians in identifying individuals in HNPCC kindreds and to help standardize the ascertainment and study of these families, the International Collaborative Group on HNPCC developed the Amsterdam criteria (AC). Basically the criteria for inclusion as an HNPCC family included at least three affected members spanning two successive generations with the diagnosis of colon cancer before the age of 50. In addition, one affected individual must be a first-degree relative of two other individuals, and because this mode of inheritance is consistent with autosomal dominant, the diagnosis of FAP must be excluded. Because some HNPCC families were excluded by these stringent criteria, and these criteria did not account for the risk to these individuals for cancers of other organs as well, the AC II were subsequently developed with a more inclusive set of criteria. The expanded definition would also include a kindred with multiple family members affected with HNPCC-associated cancers of the endometrium, ovary, stomach, hepatobiliary system, small bowel, ureter, or renal pelvis with a diagnosis before age 45 and demonstrating autosomal dominant transmission between two generations. In addition, if an individual has endometrial cancer or CRC before age 45 (which is about 30 years earlier than that seen in the general population) or a colorectal adenoma diagnosed before 40 years of age or if an individual has two HNPCC-related cancers, including two CRC at the same or different times (synchronous and metachronous CRC) or associated extracolonic cancer, the individual could meet the criteria as a possible HNPCC patient.

Although mutations in six MMR genes MSH2 (2p15-17), MSH6 (2p15-16), MLH1 (3p21), PMS1 (2q31), PMS2 (7p22), and MLH3 (14q24.3) have been linked to HNPCC, more than 90% of HNPCC mutations are observed in MSH2 and MLH1. HNPCC mutations are diverse and are located throughout these genes. Almost all errors made during DNA replication are repaired through the proofreading 3'- to 5'-exonuclease activity of DNA polymerase. Uncorrected errors of mismatched bases between the two strands are repaired before cell division through the MMR proteins. In addition to the repair of a mismatched base pair, the MMR system repairs "loop outs" from any unmatched bases that occur during the replication of a microsatellite or small repetitive sequences. In the case of HNPCC, a germline mutation in one of the six known MMR genes is inherited, causing one allele to be nonfunctional. In the tumor tissue of these individuals, the second allele has been rendered inactive through a second mutational hit. Uncorrected somatic replication errors thus accumulate within noncoding regions and insignificant locations throughout the genome and in coding regions of genes involved in cell growth and signaling and in DNA of other genes involved in DNA repair. Some targeted genes with repetitive sequences in their coding regions that have been shown to be altered in individuals with MSI include genes for transforming growth factor β type II receptor and insulin-like growth factor II receptor and the genes BAX (promotes apoptosis), MSH6, and MSH3.

MSI is identified in 90% of HNPCC-related CRC as opposed to only 15% to 20% of sporadic CRC. MSI in sporadic CRC is attributed to inactivation of gene expression of MLH1 through biallelic methylation rather than as somatic mutations or loss of heterozygosity (LOH) as seen in HNPCC-related CRC. Further, patients whose tumors demonstrate MSI have better survival and better response to chemotherapy than those whose tumors do not show MSI. No association between tumor MSI and survival was seen, however, in young patients under the age of 30.

Testing of tumor tissue for MSI (see Figure 9-15) is the initial laboratory step in investigation of HNPCC individuals because MSI is a measure of MMR deficiency and indicates probable defects in MMR genes through germline and somatic changes. International guidelines for analysis of MSI in CRC recommend a panel of five markers: BAT25, BAT26, D5S346, D2S123, and D17S250. MSI is characterized by the expansion or contraction of DNA sequences through the insertion or deletion of repeated sequences. If MSI is detected at two or more of the five loci, the tumor has a "high" frequency of MSI. If MSI is detected at one locus, the tumor has a "low" frequency of MSI. If MSI is not detected at any locus, the tumor is considered to be microsatellite stable.

If the family history supports the diagnosis of HNPCC and if MSI is confirmed in the tumor, DNA from the individual's blood can be referred for testing to identify the germline mutation that could be segregating in the family. Since most mutations occur in genes MLH1 or MSH2, DNA sequence analysis of these genes is most often used and is considered the gold standard, but it is expensive. Since many mutations result in prematurely truncated proteins, PTT is sometimes used as an initial screening tool. However, optimal mutation detection in HNPCC is achieved only by combining expert clinical selection of families with an extensive strategy to detect mutations.

If a mutation is identified, at-risk adult family members could pursue presymptomatic testing if desired and if appropriate genetic counseling is supplied. Similar to presymptomatic testing for other adult-onset disorders, the counseling session should include verification of the family history and discussion of the clinical course of the disease, including risks of developing the disease and issues in disease management. Discussions should be incorporated into the session, including how the individual will act upon both positive and negative results, feelings of survivor guilt or stigmatization, and the possibility of discrimination in insurance and employment. If a germline mutation is detected, a colonoscopy should be performed every 1 or 2 years starting at an age 5 years younger than the youngest age of diagnosis in the family. Further, because of the high incidence of endometrial cancer associated with HNPCC, at-risk women in the family should be screened for endometrial cancer annually with endometrial aspiration biopsy and transvaginal ultrasound beginning at age 25. Alternatively, if genetic testing is not pursued, relatives should begin an intensive screening program with a colonoscopy every 1 to 2 years starting between 20 and 30 years of age and then annually after age 40. If no mutation is detected in the proband, presymptomatic DNA testing for family members is not recommended. Some testing strategies may result in false-negative results caused by the inability of the assays employed to identify all mutations at these loci. However, some mutation-negative families may have germline mutations in other yet unknown MMR genes. Although detection of a mutation in a family that meets HNPCC criteria is not always possible, careful surveillance of at-risk family members in mutation-negative families is also considered critical.

REPORTING OF TEST RESULTS

As the preceding pages make clear, DNA testing for inherited diseases is complex, and it is most important to convey the results of a genetic test thoroughly. Results must be presented in a manner that is easily and accurately understood by a professional whose expertise is not genetics because, in many instances, primary caregivers will be communicating the test results to the patient. Unfortunately, however, with the increasing clinical demand for genetic testing and the increasing number of laboratories performing such tests, uniformity in communicating these complex results to referring clinicians does not exist.

A comprehensive genetic report should include the patient's name; medical record number and/or birth date; sex; ethnicity (if relevant); type of specimen and date received; specimen's laboratory identification number; laboratory test requested; name and address of laboratory performing the test; name and address of referring physician, hospital, or genetic counselor; date of report; brief interpretation of the results; and a descriptive comments section explaining the test results. Although preparation of the comments is labor intensive, the comments section is vital to a genetic report and should include the following: (1) brief clinical history of patient (indicating the reason for referral); (2) detailed explanation of the methodology (citing literature if possible); (3) description of the patient's results; (4) diagnostic accuracy of the assay (e.g., number of mutations detected by the test, percentage of mutations that would not be detected, possibility of genetic heterogeneity, and chance of genetic recombination); (5) clinical significance of the results (e.g., recurrence risk, genotype-phenotype correlation or penetrance, with citations of literature if possible); and (6) statement that genetic counseling for the patient is recommended to discuss the implications of the results for the health and management of the patient and, when mutations are identified, to inform the patient of the potential risk of the disease to other family members. (See also Chapter 7.)

Because many assays performed in clinical DNA laboratories have been developed by the laboratory or use commercially available "analyte specific reagents" (ASR) that are not approved by the U.S. Food and Drug Administration (FDA), reports in the United States often must include a disclaimer that states, "This test was developed and its performance characteristics determined by (laboratory name). It has not been cleared or approved by the U.S. Food and Drug Administration." In addition, the College of American Pathology recommends the additional statements: "The FDA has determined that such clearance or approval is not necessary. This test is used for clinical purposes. It should not be regarded as investigational or for research. This laboratory is certified under the Clinical Laboratory Improvement Amendments of 1988 (CLIA-88) as qualified to perform high complexity clinical laboratory testing." Lastly the report should be reviewed and signed by the laboratory director.

REFERENCES

1. Almawi WY, Tamim H, Kreidy R, Timson G, Rahal E, Nabulsi M, et al. A case control study on the contribution of factor V-Leiden, prothrombin G20210A, and MTHFR C677T mutations to the genetic susceptibility of deep venous thrombosis. J Thromb Thrombolysis 2005;19:189-96.
2. Bates GP. History of genetic disease: The molecular genetics of Huntington disease—a history. Nat Rev Genet 2005;6:766-73.
3. Bittel DC, Butler MG. Prader-Willi syndrome: clinical genetics, cytogenetics and molecular biology. Expert Rev Mol Med 2005;7:1-20.
4. Burt R, Neklason DE. Genetic testing for inherited colon cancer. Gastroenterology 2005;128:1696-716.
5. Chance PF. Genetic evaluation of inherited motor/sensory neuropathy. Suppl Clin Neurophysiol 2004;57:228-42.
6. Franchini M, Veneri D. Inherited thrombophilia: an update. Clin Lab 2005;51:357-65.
7. Gatchel JR, Zoghbi HY. Diseases of unstable repeat expansion: mechanism and common principles. Nat Rev Genet 2005;6:743-55.
8. Graw J, Brackmann HH, Oldenburg J, Schneppenheim R, Spannagl M, Schwaab R. Haemophilia A: from mutation analysis to new therapies. Nat Rev Genet 2005;6:488-501.
9. Hagerman PJ, Hagerman RJ. The fragile-X premutation: a maturing perspective. Am J Hum Genet 2004;74:805-16.
10. Henriksson K, Olsson H, Kristoffersson U. The need for oncogenetic counseling. Ten years' experience of a regional oncogenetic clinic. Acta Oncol 2004;43:637-49.
11. Horton WA, Lunstrum GP. Fibroblast growth factor receptor 3 mutations in achondroplasia and related forms of dwarfism. Rev Endcor Metab Disord 2002;3:381-5.
12. Hough C, Lillicrap D. Gene therapy for hemophilia: an imperative to succeed. J Thromb Haemost 2005;3:1195-205.
13. King LS, Singh RH, Rhead WJ, Smith W, Lee B, Summar ML. Genetic counseling issues in urea cycle disorders. Crit Care Clin 2005;21:S37-44.
14. Lux MP, Fasching PA, Beckmann MW. Hereditary breast and ovarian cancer: review and future perspectives. J Mol Med 2006;84:16-28.
15. McConkie-Rosell A, Finucane B, Cronister A, Abrams L, Bennett RL, Pettersen BJ. Genetic counseling for fragile x syndrome: updated recommendations of the national society of genetic counselors. J Genet Couns 2005;14:249-70.
16. Narayan S, Roy D. Role of APC and DNA mismatch repair genes in the development of colorectal cancers. Mol Cancer 2003;2:41.
17. Pietrangelo A. Hereditary hemochromatosis—a new look at an old disease. N Engl J Med 2004;350:2383-97.
18. Prior TW, Bridgeman SJ. Experience and strategy for the molecular testing of Duchenne muscular dystrophy. J Mol Diagn 2005;7:317-26.
19. Rowe SM, Miller S, Sorscher EJ. Cystic fibrosis. N Engl J Med 2005;352:1992-2001.
20. Smeitink J, van den Heuvel L, DiMauro S. The genetics and pathology of oxidative phosphorylation. Nat Rev Genet 2001;2:342-52.
21. Spector EB, Grody WW, Matteson CJ, Palomaki GE, Bellissimo DB, Wolff DJ, et al. Technical standards and guidelines: venous thromboembolism (Factor V Leiden and prothrombin 2021G>A testing): a disease-specific supplement to the standards and guidelines for clinical genetics laboratories. Genet Med 2005;7:444-53.
22. Taylor RW, Turnbull DM. Mitochondrial DNA mutations in human disease. Nat Rev Genet 2005;6:389-402.
23. Terracciano A, Chiurazzi P, Neri G. Fragile X syndrome. Am J Med Genet C Semin Med Genet 2005;137:32-7.
24. Watson MS, Cutting GR, Desnick RJ, Driscoll DA, Klinger K, Mennuti M, et al. Cystic fibrosis population carrier screening: 2004 revision of American College of Medical Genetics mutation panel. Genet Med 2004;6:387-91.
25. Williams CA. Neurological aspects of the Angelman syndrome. Brain Dev 2005;27:88-94.

REVIEW QUESTIONS

1. In the figure on the right, the inheritance pattern of the disease segregating in this family is most consistent with
   A. autosomal dominant.
   B. autosomal recessive.
   C. X-linked recessive.
   D. mitochondrial inheritance.

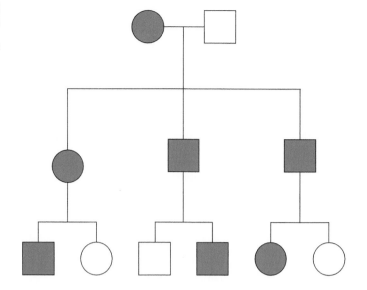

2. In the figure on the right, the inheritance pattern of the disease segregating in this family is most consistent with
   A. autosomal dominant.
   B. autosomal recessive.
   C. X-linked dominant.
   D. mitochondrial inheritance.

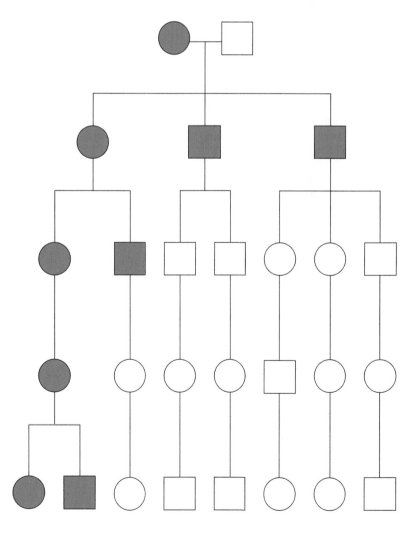

3. A 2-year-old African-American child has a past medical history of recurrent respiratory infections. His weight is in the lower 10th percentile. Repeat sweat chloride concentrations of 87 and 95 mmol/L are obtained and one copy of mutation 3120+1G>A is detected using the ACMG/ACOG recommended CF mutation screening panel. How do you explain these results?
   A. The child is a carrier of CF.
   B. The results are from erroneous sweat chloride concentrations caused by laboratory error.
   C. This child has classic CF with one mutation in CFTR and one mutation in another gene.
   D. This child is likely a compound heterozygote with two different CFTR mutations.

4. The 49-year-old younger brother of your patient has been given the diagnosis of HH. DNA testing revealed homozygosity for the C282Y allele. For this reason, your patient requested DNA testing. Homozygosity for the C282Y allele was observed. Your patient has no clinical findings associated with hemochromatosis. This is best explained by
   A. imprinting.
   B. incomplete penetrance.
   C. anticipation.
   D. allelic heterogeneity.

5. DNA linkage studies
   A. are useful for large genes when no common mutations exist.
   B. require participation from multiple family members.
   C. rely upon polymorphic DNA markers in close proximity to the disease gene.
   D. can yield erroneous results as a result of genetic recombination.
   E. all of the above.

6. In which of the following diseases is homozygosity for two mutant alleles not associated with a more severe clinical phenotype?

   A. Achondroplasia
   B. Charcot-Marie-Tooth
   C. Huntington
   D. Thrombophilia

7. Expansion of the CGG repeats in an *FMR1* premutation allele to a full mutation allele
   A. occurs during DNA replication.
   B. is less likely to occur with a CGG repeat length of 79 as compared with 59.
   C. is dependent on the sex of the fetus.
   D. is more likely to occur during male gametogenesis.

8. Prader-Willi syndrome
   A. is characterized by inappropriate bouts of laughter.
   B. can be caused by uniparental disomy with both alleles paternally derived.
   C. most often is caused by a de novo deletion of a paternal gene on 1 allele.
   D. is most efficiently confirmed using DNA sequencing.

9. Mutations in *BRCA1* and *BRCA2*
   A. are identified in most cases of breast cancer in women of the Western hemisphere.
   B. require additional environmental and genetic factors for the development of breast cancer in mutation-positive patients.
   C. are common in all ethnic populations.
   D. are most often missense mutations resulting in amino acid substitutions.

10. Microsatellite instability in colon cancer
   A. is associated with CIN.
   B. is associated with a worse prognosis in patients with no family history.
   C. arises from mutations or altered expression of DNA MMR genes.
   D. is observed in patients with familial adenomatous polyposis.

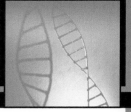

Chapter 10

Identity Assessment

Thomas M. Williams, M.D.
Victor W. Weedn, M.D., J.D.
Malek Kamoun, M.D., Ph.D.

OBJECTIVES

1. State how genetic variation is used in identity assessment, parentage testing, and engraftment studies.
2. Compare and contrast short tandem repeats (STRs) with variable numbers of tandem repeats (VNTRs).
3. List the assays that are used to assess identity, parentage, and engraftment.
4. Describe the HLA genes, their chromosomal locations, and other genetic features of these; state their significance in transplantation testing.
5. Determine, using methods for engraftment analysis, whether an engraftment has been successful.
6. State the role of exclusion testing in parentage assessment.
7. Design an assay using VNTRs for the purpose of identifying an individual and comparing him or her to suspect DNA.
8. Comply with chain of custody procedures in a legal case involving identity assessment.
9. Identify and resolve issues involving the ethical and social implications of identity testing.

KEY WORDS AND DEFINITIONS

Allele: One of a number of alternative forms of the same gene at a given locus (position) on a chromosome; except for X chromosome genes in males, each person inherits two alleles for each gene, one allele from each parent; these alleles may be the same or may be different from one another.

Amelogenin: A low molecular weight protein found in tooth enamel; the amelogenin gene is used for sex identification because the male version is longer than the female version.

Chain of Custody: A concept in jurisprudence that applies to the handling of evidence (such as a blood specimen) and its integrity; a process that tracks the movement of evidence through its collection, safeguarding, and analysis by documenting each person who handled the evidence, the date and time it was collected or transferred, and the purpose for the transfer.

Chimerism: The presence of more than one genetically distinct genome in a single individual, often the result of a bone marrow transplant.

Engraftment: In *hematopoietic cell transplantation*, the process of infused donor stem cells homing to the bone marrow of the recipient and producing blood cells of all types.

Exclusion: An outcome of an identity test that indicates that the tested individual was not the contributor of a tested sample.

Exon: Part of the coding region of a gene that codes for a gene product; region that specifies the amino acid sequence of a polypeptide during translation.

Forensics: A branch of science that deals with legal issues or criminalistics.

Hematopoietic Cell Transplantation (HCT): Transplantation of hematopoietic stem cells, usually from bone marrow, employed to treat some patients who have certain classes of disorders including leukemias and hereditary immune deficiencies.

Human Leukocyte Antigen (HLA): Classes of polymorphic genes located on chromosome 6p within the major histocompatibility complex that encode for the classic transplantation antigens found on the surface of nucleated cells; alleles of these genes are used for transplantation, forensic, parentage, and chimerism testing.

Inclusion: The opposite of *exclusion*; an outcome of an identity test that indicates that the tested individual may be the contributor of the tested sample; often accompanied by the probability that the tested individual contributed the tested sample.

Locus: The location of a gene on a chromosome; a locus is said to be polymorphic when the least common allele has a population frequency of at least 1 in 100.

Major Histocompatibility Complex (MHC): A large complex of genes located on chromosome 6p that contains the human leukocyte antigen region.

Microsatellite Locus (Plural: Loci): A locus with a *short tandem repeat* sequence of DNA of two base pairs up to five, six, or seven base pairs (according to differing definitions); typically the short sequences (e.g., AATG) are repeated 10 to 100 times (e.g., AATGAATGAATGAATGAATGA ATGAATGAATGAATGAATGAATG).

Minisatellite Locus (Plural: Loci): Locus containing *variable number of tandem repeats* of DNA sequences as short as 8 to 10 base pairs or as long as 50 to 100 base pairs.

Polymorphism: DNA sequence variations; differences in nucleotide sequences between two chromosomes at the same locus.

Restriction Fragment Length Polymorphism (RFLP— "riflip"): A subset of single nucleotide polymorphisms that are identified based on the ability of a restriction endonuclease to digest double-stranded DNA at the site of the variation.

Short Tandem Repeat (STR): Microsatellite sequence that contains a repeated nucleotide sequence of 2 to 7 base pairs; the number of repeats (copies) of the 2- to 7-bp sequence varies among individuals.

Single Nucleotide Polymorphism (SNP): A change in a single nucleotide.

Variable Numbers of Tandem Repeat (VNTR): Minisatellite repetitive sequences of, typically, 8 to 80 base pairs; found on DNA on both chromosomes and highly individualized; can be used to identify individuals and their offspring.

Identity testing exploits variations present within the human genome to distinguish among individuals. Identity assessment has five basic uses: (1) to confirm or refute that a sample is from a specific person in forensic testing; (2) to resolve questions regarding the identity of a clinical specimen; (3) to select donors for a planned transplant recipient to minimize the probability of rejection and improve graft survival via histocompatibility testing; (4) to assess whether hematopoietic cells are donor- or recipient-derived following hematopoietic cell transplantation; (5) to identify the parents of a child.

VARIATION IN THE HUMAN GENOME

Identity testing began with the use of serological methods to identify variations in proteins that differ among individuals. The discovery of the genetic basis for these protein differences and of genetic variability at loci not encoding proteins, coupled with technical advances, allowed the field to move to direct analysis of DNA. Genetic variation among individuals is extensive, with about 1 sequence difference for every 400 to 1000 nucleotides on autosomal chromosomes. Variants of a genetic **locus** in a population are referred to as **alleles.** A locus is said to be **polymorphic** when the least common allele has a frequency of ≥ 0.01 in a population. Although several alleles may be found in a population for an autosomal locus, an individual may have at most two alleles at that locus.

Genetic Variation Useful in Identity Testing

There are several classes of genetic variants in the genome; some are more useful than others for identity testing. Most of the variants used occur in the noncoding genetic regions, the *introns,* whereas some variants occur in the coding sequences, the **exons.** Highly repetitive sequence elements that contribute to the structure of centromeres and telomeres and hundreds of thousands of copies of transposable elements that move about the genome over time may vary among individuals. However, these repetitive sequence elements are generally not useful for identity testing. More than 1 million **single nucleotide polymorphisms (SNPs),** single point mutations, have been identified in the genome. A subset of SNPs can be identified based on the ability of a restriction endonuclease to digest double-stranded DNA at the site of the variation. These SNPs are referred to as **restriction fragment length polymorphisms (RFLPs).** SNPs and RFLPs have been important in genetic linkage analysis and the study of disease pathogenesis; however, they are less useful for identity testing because they usually have only two alleles.

Variable numbers of tandem repeat (VNTR) loci, also referred to as **minisatellite loci,** consist of repeated sequences of DNA. The core sequence is from 8 to 80 nucleotides long. The core is repeated from 4 to 40 times, thus forming 4 to 40 alleles. The allele size difference is detected as an RFLP if the locus containing the VNTR is digested with an appropriate restriction endonuclease and hybridized to a labeled DNA probe in Southern hybridization assays. The resulting DNA fragment lengths vary from 0.5 to >20 kb in different individuals. VNTRs are attractive for identity testing because the loci usually have a number of different alleles with relatively high allele frequencies. Minisatellite regions are commonly located near the telomeric end of chromosomes.

Short tandem repeat (STR) or **microsatellite loci** consist of DNA sequence motifs that have a core sequence of two to seven base pairs that is repeated in tandem several times.[4,11] Examples include the dinucleotide repeated four times, 5′ CACACACA 3′ and the tetranucleotide repeated three times, 5′ TTTATTTATTTA 3′. Thousands of STRs are scattered throughout the genome. Because they are flanked by unique sequences, each can be specifically amplified with the polymerase chain reaction (PCR) for analysis. In populations of individuals, multiple alleles may be present based on differences in the number of repeated motifs at the locus. STRs have many characteristics that make them ideal for identity testing:

(1) automated fluorescence analysis is available; (2) alleles can be assigned in a definitive manner following analysis; (3) STR loci are almost always transmitted in families in a mendelian fashion; (4) the loci may have 10 or more alleles, often with substantial allele frequencies, making them highly informative; and (5) extensive information is available about allele frequencies in many human populations for STRs commonly used in identity testing.[5]

Commercially available STR systems employ tetrameric and pentameric repeat loci, which produce fewer artifactual bands and are characterized by roughly equal amplification of both alleles in an individual (Figure 10-1). Fragments are labeled during the PCR amplification with fluorescently tagged primers that facilitate multiplexing.

Two special genetic regions with sufficient sequence variability for identity testing include the **human leukocyte antigen**

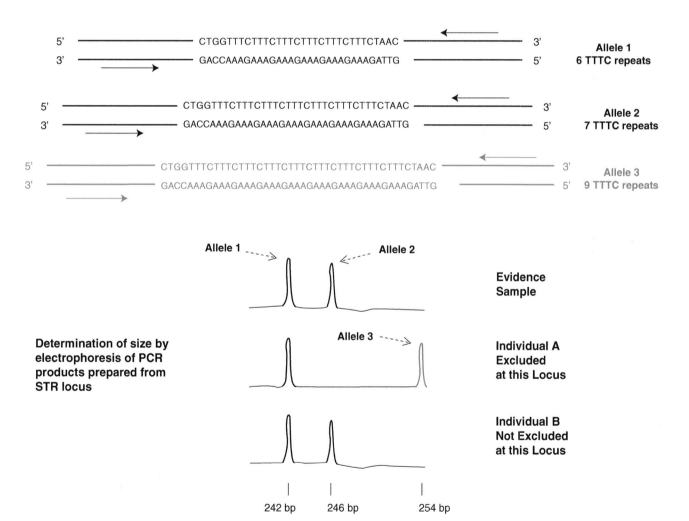

Figure 10-1

Identity testing via STR analysis. An STR locus is specifically amplified with the PCR using primers binding to unique sequences adjacent to the repeat motif in the genome. In the example shown, the polymorphic repeat is the tetramer TTTC. Three example alleles with 6, 7, and 9 repeats at this locus are shown. The genotype for an individual or evidence sample is determined by performing the PCR with a fluorescently labeled primer and sizing the products on a high-resolution gel with laser detection. The PCR products should differ in size from each other by multiples of four nucleotides. The use of several fluorescent dyes and different-sized PCR products allows multiplexing for assessment of a number of independently segregating STR loci simultaneously.

(HLA) loci within the **major histocompatibility complex (MHC)** and the mitochondrial DNA (mtDNA). The HLA loci described in the HLA Typing section later in this chapter are interesting in that the polymorphisms are densely packed and preferentially located in the exons rather than the introns of these genes on chromosome 6. Mitochondrial genome variation is useful in forensic identity testing and is described in that section.

Exclusion of Tested Individuals

Identity testing frequently excludes the tested person. **Exclusion** results can indicate that a suspect did not commit a murder or rape or that an alleged man did not father a child. The exclusion is based on the presence of alleles at a locus that make it impossible for him or her to be a contributor to the tested sample. For example, if the person has the alleles j and k at the autosomal locus L, then in the absence of mutations, it is not possible for him to be the major contributor to an evidence sample with the alleles m and n at L or to be the father of a child with the alleles m and p at L. In practice, laboratory protocols require that exclusion be based on incompatible results for at least two loci to rule out mutation events or other sources of error. In this context, "impossible" implies a situation in which samples have been collected correctly and have not been mislabeled, testing has been performed accurately, and results have been interpreted and reported appropriately.

Likelihood of Inclusion of Tested Individuals

If a tested individual has genotypes at several loci that are identical to the genotypes found in an evidence sample, then that person is not excluded as the contributor to the sample. The **inclusion** of a tested individual in identity testing is based on a probability calculation relying upon knowledge of the allele frequencies in human populations for the tested loci. For each locus, the likelihood that a random person of relevant ethnicity has a genotype identical to that found in the evidence sample is calculated. If the tested loci independently segregate during meiosis, the overall probability that a random person rather than the accused is responsible is calculated by multiplying the likelihoods for each locus. When several loci are tested and each has many possible alleles, it becomes extremely likely that an individual whose genotypes match those found in the evidence sample is the person who contributed the DNA to the sample.

Discriminatory power is the ability of an identity testing system to distinguish an individual or group from the rest of the population. The power of discrimination of a locus or testing system should not be confused with accuracy. ABO blood group typing is accurate but poorly discriminating, since this locus results in only a few phenotypes of generally high frequency in populations. Current identity test systems that employ a number of highly polymorphic loci may have powers of discrimination that exceed 1×10^{-10}, making it very unlikely that any unrelated individual on earth other than a nonexcluded suspect could be the source of an evidence sample. However, likelihoods of this magnitude should be viewed with knowledge that a variety of potential problems extraneous to the testing technology, involving sample collection and labeling and test interpretation and reporting, may lead to an erroneous result.

Parentage calculations are often performed using methods[1,9] that consider the prior probability that an individual is the father of a child. It is obvious, for example, that the prior probability of a man living in Boston being the father of a coworker's child is much greater than that of a Beijing inhabitant with no overt connection to the mother. Most crime laboratories in the United States do not report calculations using analyses that make assumptions about prior probability, but instead report the population phenotypic frequencies for Caucasian, African-American, and Hispanic populations and sometimes a likelihood ratio that an individual is the source of a DNA specimen. When questions arise regarding assumptions that must be made during the calculation of inclusion probabilities, laboratories generally choose the conservative option that favors the accused individual.

Samples Employed for Identity Testing

Samples for identity testing can be any specimen that contains DNA. Samples obtained from an individual for parentage testing or as a reference sample to be compared with DNA prepared from evidence are usually peripheral blood, buccal mucosa, or objects contaminated with human cellular remains or body fluids. Samples useful for testing may range from plucked hairs to bone marrow aspirates to paraffin-embedded tissue. Although subject to degradation over time in the presence of enzymes, acidic or basic conditions, or high temperature, DNA is a remarkably stable molecule that can be recovered and successfully analyzed from solutions, surfaces, and cells.

FORENSIC DNA TYPING

Forensics is the branch of science that deals with criminalistics. DNA testing has revolutionized this field.[13,24] Only fingerprint evidence can rival the ability of DNA as trace evidence left at a scene to identify a perpetrator. As a general rule, other trace evidence merely links an article, instrument, or material to a scene. The origin of DNA-based identity testing is generally traced to a 1985 article in *Nature* by Alec Jeffreys.[12] He coined the term "DNA fingerprint" and suggested that the hybridization of DNA probes to polymorphic genetic loci could be exploited for forensic purposes. Jeffreys first applied his techniques to civil and criminal cases in England. In the United States, DNA-based identity testing was introduced via commercial laboratories and later the Federal Bureau of Investigation (FBI). Today there are approximately 200 forensic DNA typing laboratories in the United States and many other DNA laboratories around the globe.

Forensic Applications

Forensic testing differs from clinical laboratory testing in several ways. (1) The forensic question is usually one of identity rather than one of presence or absence of a trait, character of a blot or gel, or analyte quantification as in most clinical laboratory analysis. (2) Specimens received by forensic laboratories are much more diverse than the typical blood, fluid, and tissue samples handled by clinical laboratories. (3) Clinical samples are collected under controlled circumstances, whereas evidence from which DNA must be isolated may be exposed to the environment in a variety of ways. Experiments may be necessary to validate testing for a particular case. (4) Evidentiary material cannot be replenished and may be present in only trace amounts. Testing may consume the sample and thus complete or repeat testing may be impossible. (5) Forensic

TABLE 10-1   DNA Typing Systems and Their Characteristics

Genetic Systems	Timeframe	PCR-Based	Discrimination	Comments
RFLP analysis of VNTRs	1980s-1990s	−	++++	Labor intensive
PCR dot-blots	1980s-1990s	+	+	Limited discrimination
STRs	Late 1990s to present	+	++++	Current mainstay
mtDNA	Mid 1990s to present	+	++	Used in hairs, skeletons
Y-markers	Beginning use	+	++	Male DNA
Alu repeats	Not yet in use	+	++	Population marker
SNPs	Not yet in use	+	+++	Useful for samples with highly degraded DNA

identity testing is scrutinized in a judicial environment requiring complete accounting for the **chain of custody** following its collection and strict validation of procedures. Most other laboratorians perform routine analyses of samples collected in defined ways. Forensic identity testing must contend with much more variability in samples and testing conditions.

Genetic Systems Used in Forensic Identification
Numerous genetic systems that are employed by forensic laboratories are summarized in Table 10-1.[3,20]

VNTR Analysis by RFLP
Jeffreys described a method to create a bar code–like DNA fingerprint based upon VNTRs. Because the probes Jeffreys used bind to several loci in Southern hybridization experiments and produce numerous bands per probe, they are termed "multi-locus probes." In the United States, laboratories prefer single locus probe (SLP) systems that hybridize to only a single genetic locus. SLPs generally yield one or two bands on an autoradiogram per probe. SLP genetic systems are more robust than multilocus probes: generating readily interpretable bands, having more precise allele frequency statistics, and are less sensitive to fragmentation of high molecular weight DNA.

RFLP VNTR testing with SLPs was the preponderant method of DNA typing in most forensic laboratories throughout most of the 1990s. RFLP VNTR testing commonly employed six genetic loci: D1S7, D2S44, D4S139, D10S28, D14S13, and D17S79. The resulting average discrimination for Caucasian Americans is approximately 1 in $1.2 \times 10.^9$ However, Southern hybridization–based RFLP analysis is expensive, labor intensive, difficult to automate, and less sensitive than PCR-based methods. Furthermore, RFLP tests suffer from allele sizing imprecision, requiring that the results be binned and statistical measures of confidence employed for interpretation. Finally, RFLP is sensitive to DNA degradation—an important issue with environmentally exposed forensic specimens. RFLP tests have been largely abandoned in favor of the more efficient PCR-based assays discussed below.[3]

Short Tandem Repeats
Most identity testing performed today relies on the PCR to amplify STR for size analysis. PCR testing is inherently sensitive, allowing routine analysis of nanogram quantities of genomic DNA and often successful testing of picogram quantities (one cell contains 5 to 10 pg of DNA). The PCR underlies the characterization of STR and other loci for forensic identity testing loci described in this and later sections.

STR testing is quick, less expensive, more forgiving with respect to technical skills needed, less sensitive to DNA degradation, and more amenable to automation when compared with the Southern hybridization methods described above. Although less discriminating than RFLP genetic markers, STR analysis can be made as powerful as Southern RFLP analysis through the use of large numbers of informative loci.

The National Institute of Justice provided funding for the initial application of STRs in forensics. STRs were used in forensic casework during the first Persian Gulf War and were widely adopted for testing by forensic laboratories in the United Kingdom and the United States in the mid to late 1990s.

The FBI laboratory's combined DNA index system (CODIS) blends forensic science and computer technology into an effective tool for investigating violent crimes. CODIS enables federal, state, and local crime labs to exchange and compare DNA profiles electronically, thereby linking crimes to each other and to convicted offenders. The FBI convened a panel of forensic scientists in 1998 that chose a panel of 13 CODIS core STR loci for use in the national DNA index system (NDIS). These "13 core loci" have become the standard for casework and data banking for most forensic laboratories around the world (Table 10-2). They have been commercialized as kits by several companies in a variety of formats. STRs are now routinely used in crime labs globally and typically yield discriminatory values of one in trillions to quadrillions.

Sex Markers and Y-Chromosome Markers
Amelogenin is a low molecular weight protein found in tooth enamel. The amelogenin gene is useful as a sex marker. The X chromosome amelogenin gene is shorter than its homologue on chromosome Y by a six–base pair polymorphism, allowing the distinction between individuals with 46,XY and 46,XX karyotypes. Males will display amelogenin genetic heterozygosity; females will exhibit homozygosity. Reagents for assessing the amelogenin locus are incorporated in commercially available STR kits.

Y-chromosome polymorphic loci are used as identifying loci found only in males. Before the use of these loci, the male-specific DNA obtained from a vaginal swab had to be "differentially extracted"—the DNA from spermatozoa was released after the female fraction from epithelial cells. This extraction step is unnecessary when using Y-chromosome loci. These loci include STRs or SNPs (described later in this chapter). Laboratories typically employ commercially available panels

TABLE 10-2	List of Short Tandem Repeats Core Loci

CURRENTLY AVAILABLE COMMERCIAL STR KITS				
Core Loci	Profiler	Cofiler	Identifiler	Powerplex 16
D3S1358	D3S1358	D3S1358	D3S1358	D3S1358
D5S818	D5S818		D5S818	D5S818
D7S820	D7S820	D7S820	D7S820	D7S820
D8S1170	D8S1170		D8S1170	D8S1170
D13S317	D13S317		D13S317	D13S317
D16S539		D16S539	D16S539	D16S539
D18S51	D18S51		D18S51	D18S51
D21S11	D21S11		D21S11	D21S11
CSF1PO		CSF1PO	CSF1PO	CSF1PO
FGA	FGA		FGA	FGA
THO1		THO1	THO1	THO1
TPOX		TPOX	TPOX	TPOX
vWA	vWA		vWA	vWA
			D2S1338	Penta D
			D19S433	Penta E
	Amelogenin	Amelogenin	Amelogenin	Amelogenin

The 13 STR core loci are listed against the STR systems present in the currently available commercial STR kits. Profiler, Cofiler, and Identifiler are available from commercial companies.

TABLE 10-3	Y-Chromosome Markers

European Minimal Haplotype	European Extended Haplotype	U.S. Haplotype
DYS19	DYS19	DYS19
DYS385a/b	DYS385a/b	DYS385a/b
DYS389 I/II	DYS389 I/II	DYS389 I/II
DYS390	DYS390	DYS390
DYS391	DYS391	DYS391
DYS392	DYS392	DYS392
DYS393	DYS393	DYS393
	YCAIIa/b	
		DYS348
		DYS349

Y-chromosome markers are listed in their major haplotype groups.

of 6 to 20 Y-chromosome STRs for analyses (Table 10-3). Y-chromosome SNPs are in development.

Y-chromosome polymorphic loci are linked, resulting in discriminatory power significantly less than a panel of independently segregating somatic STR loci. Discriminatory values are increased by using a large panel of Y-chromosome markers in conjunction with a large database of typed individuals. Note that fathers, sons, brothers, uncles, and paternal male cousins cannot be distinguished from one another when using Y-chromosome STRs.

Mitochondrial DNA

Mitochondrial genomes are circular double-stranded DNA molecules that are 16,569 base pairs long and are present as one or more copies within the mitochondria of a cell. Thus mitochondrial DNA (mtDNA) is present in hundreds to thousands of copies per cell. By contrast, only one copy of each nuclear DNA locus is present in each cell. mtDNA, unlike chromosomal DNA, does not undergo meiosis and does not participate in genetic recombination events. mtDNA remains stable over generations, except for the acquisition of mutations at a rate 10 to 20 times that of nuclear DNA.

mtDNA is transmitted to children via oocytes. Although it is generally thought that mtDNA is exclusively derived from the mother, a minor contribution from the father is occasionally present, particularly in disease states. The normal state of mitochondria is generally thought to be one of "homoplasmy," in which all the mtDNA has the same sequence. However, because of mutational events, a state of "heteroplasmy" in which more than one mtDNA sequence is present in the same tissue may exist. High-level heteroplasmy is generally of the order of 30% of the mtDNA sequence before it is reported. Unrecognized low-level heteroplasmy is common. Heteroplasmy appears to be somewhat tissue specific rather than uniform throughout the body. Thus two shed hairs may show discrepant mtDNA sequences. As a result of heteroplasmy, one or two nucleotide mismatches between two individuals is not an absolute basis for exclusion of a tested individual.

In the human mitochondrial genome, only approximately 1200 bases in the region of transcription origin, known as the "displacement loop" (D-loop) or "control region," are noncoding. This D-loop contains two hypervariable regions that contain the majority of polymorphisms useful for identity testing. mtDNA polymorphisms typically identified for forensics are useful for identity testing via DNA sequencing.[11] This method is expensive, labor intensive, and highly sensitive to contamination. A limited number of laboratories offer this service. However, more convenient hybridization technology for mtDNA testing has recently been introduced as a "linear array," which could be used for screening.

The mtDNA sequence obtained from a specimen is compared with a reference sequence (revised Cambridge sequence: www.mitomap.org/mitoseq.html, accessed December 14, 2006). Because mtDNA polymorphisms are linked, the individual polymorphism frequencies cannot be multiplied together to generate a likelihood of identity, such as independently segregating chromosomal locus allele frequencies. Instead the mtDNA haplotype identified in a sample is compared with those deposited in a database to derive a frequency statistic. Most mitochondrial haplotypes in the database are unique.

mtDNA is primarily useful in identity testing in three contexts. First, a sample may be available that contains mitochondrial but not nuclear DNA. For example, in shed hairs that do not have roots, generally only mtDNA is detected. Second, when the DNA within a specimen, such as skeletal remains, is substantially degraded, the high copy number of mtDNA makes it more likely to yield a result than nuclear DNA. Third, mtDNA analysis may become essential when only a distant relative is available for a reference specimen. In this example, nuclear DNA requires samples from multiple close members of the kindred, but mtDNA matching would require only a distant maternal relative.

Single Nucleotide Polymorphisms

A DNA locus whose polymorphism extends over a short region is generally preferable for identity testing because it may remain intact and available for analysis in the face of extensive levels of DNA degradation. Loci for which a single base pair varies in a population of individuals are referred to as SNPs. These are the most common type of polymorphisms in the human genome. Their analysis is particularly amenable to automation and DNA microarray technology using hybridization, polymerase extension, or ligation reaction assays. Despite a four-base possibility, most are biallelic with a dominant and nondominant allele. A large set of SNPs must be used to obtain significant discriminatory values. SNPs are not used in forensic laboratories at this time, but are likely to be used in the near future. SNP analysis is expected to be particularly useful in identifying individuals for whom only severely degraded DNA samples are available.

Instrumentation Used in Forensic Laboratories

Most forensic DNA testing is performed using capillary array electrophoretic (CE) systems. These systems have substantially faster run times and higher resolutions than slab gels. High-throughput capillary instruments are used as "batch" instruments for DNA data banking operations.

Instrumentation under development for forensic testing generally focuses on a goal of miniaturization yielding ultrafast and portable assays that would be useful for field testing. These new instruments use various types of chip technology. In 2005 the United Kingdom began sending vans with portable DNA testing capability to scenes of crimes.

Statistical Interpretation

In the early days of DNA-based identity testing, significant challenges were launched regarding the interpretation of DNA typing results. Questions included whether loci exhibit Hardy-Weinberg equilibrium* and whether allele frequencies vary significantly among ethnic groups.[6,9,14,25] Current forensic genetic systems have not demonstrated significant deviation from Hardy-Weinberg equilibrium. The systems also show greater intragroup allelic diversity than between-group diversity. A National Research Council panel was created to address these issues.[17] The resultant report (so-called "NRC I") introduced a "ceiling principle" to ensure the conservativism of the frequency estimates, which itself generated considerable controversy. This led to NRC II, which articulated the current standards of statistical analysis.[18] Statistical formulas are routinely applied to Caucasian, African-American, and Hispanic population databases. Specialized databases also exist for Native American Indian and for Pacific and African populations.

Convicted Offender Databases

All 50 states now have convicted offender databases. Initially, most databases exclusively contained sexual offenders, but the

recent trend is to expand the databases to include all felons. States have begun to consider collecting DNA evidence in connection with lesser crimes, such as burglaries, to help solve these cases, to potentially interdict the progression to more serious future offenses, and to identify "hits" in the databases linked to past serious crimes. Three states (Louisiana, Texas, and Virginia) have recently adopted legislation allowing collection of DNA specimens on arrest.

DNA profiles are placed in the NDIS. If a "hit" is determined, the local crime laboratories of the involved states are put in contact to discuss details. Identifying information other than the DNA profile is not entered into the system. Uploading of DNA profiles triggers quality assurance requirements and legal constraints on the use of the DNA specimens and profiles.

The use of identity testing and linked databases in crime investigation has been aggressively pursued in the United Kingdom. U.K. forensic scientists claim that approximately 50% of biological specimens from crime scenes result in hits in their databases, suggesting that a relatively small group of professional criminals perpetrate most crimes. They believe that DNA-based testing may be a more efficient tool for investigating crimes than traditional methods, such as canvassing neighborhoods.

Legal Issues

Early challenges to the practice and interpretation of DNA-based forensic identification have faded as the public, attorneys, and judges have become more knowledgeable about this technology. The most common challenges today involve issues regarding sample collection, preservation of the evidence, chain-of-custody documentation, and validation studies. New methods of DNA-based testing, such as to assess ethnicity or infer phenotypic features, or new applications, such as to identify an assailant from very small samples,[23] are likely to cause controversy in the future.

U.S. regulatory laws currently exist with the intention of providing some protection against genetic discrimination. In addition, many states have explicit laws on genetic discrimination. Through common law, the courts have also fashioned some privacy rights. In the specific case of DNA databases for law enforcement purposes, the FBI has all states sign agreements that pertain to privacy of the specimens and profiles. Nonetheless, many commentators believe that stronger laws should be enacted. The National Academy of Sciences is considering these issues in a project entitled "Identifying the Needs of the Forensic Science Community" impaneled in 2006. Population genomics has only superficially addressed issues of power and political process (see Ethics Box 10-1).

USE OF DNA TESTING FOR THE IDENTIFICATION OF CLINICAL SPECIMENS

Identity testing can also be used to confirm the identity of a clinical or anatomic pathology laboratory patient specimen.[22] Occasionally, questions arise regarding the identity of specimens in the clinical laboratory. In one approach to such questions, DNA prepared from a peripheral blood or buccal mucosa specimen is compared with DNA in the pathological specimen to confirm that it is derived from the patient. The authors have

---

*In a population containing the genotypes of AA, Aa, and aa, where p is the frequency of A and q is the frequency of a, the loci are at "Hardy-Weinberg equilibrium" if the frequency of AA is p^2, the frequency of Aa is $2pq$. If the population has no selection pressures, a randomly-mating population will display these frequencies.

ETHICS Box 10-1   Ethical and Social Implications

The ethical and social implications of genomic research in humans have been debated during the past decades, and this debate is likely to continue (reviewed in reference 15). Fear of genetic discrimination, particularly in the workplace and in health insurance, is often expressed over the prospect of DNA specimen or DNA typing information collection and storage.

Collection of human DNA is widespread, and the potential for increased collection is vast. Blood samples are collected in every hospital and clinic on a daily basis. Perhaps more disturbing is the DNA that remains as abandoned residues on drinking glasses, cigarette butts, toothbrushes, clothing, and handled objects. Of course not all DNA specimens are stored, but most states keep Guthrie spots (PKU cards) from newborns for years. Also, DNA can be retrieved from clinical cytology slides and biopsies embedded in paraffin blocks from pathology storerooms. Research, both genetic and nongenetic, frequently involves storage of blood or other specimens. Guidelines for human tissue repositories have been published (http://www.nhlbi.nih.gov/funding/policies/repos-gl.htm, accessed December 21, 2006).

The U.S. military mandates the collection of DNA specimens of all service members for use in identification of remains, but they are not tested unless needed. Law enforcement agencies in all fifty states collect and test DNA from convicted offenders (and some states permit collection on arrest), specifically for personal identification. Most often these collections are of felonies and sexual misdemeanors, but the categories of offenses continue to grow. The information is entered into local databases and often into the federal database. In most jurisdictions, the specimens are not destroyed, but retained. Although the databases of law enforcement agencies have greater oversight and legal protections than do other databases, the uses of "DNA dragnets" and of familial searches through low stringency matching are areas of current debate over law enforcement uses.

Protections against genetic discrimination are provided in the United States by legislation, executive order, common law, and administrative regulations of the executive branch of government. Protection is provided by laws including the Americans with Disabilities Act of 1990 (ADA), the Health Insurance Portability and Accountability Act of 1996 (HIPAA), and Title VII of the Civil Rights Act of 1964. A presidential executive order (2000) prohibited federal agencies from using genetic information in hiring and promotion decisions. Many states have explicit laws on genetic discrimination. The courts have fashioned some privacy rights through common law (i.e., the law that has grown up through court cases over centuries rather than through acts of legislatures). Finally, administrative regulations of the FBI require states to sign agreements regarding privacy of the specimens and profiles in DNA databases that are constructed for law enforcement purposes. Despite these protections, many commentators believe that stronger laws should be enacted.

Genetic privacy laws generally prohibit collection of specimens or information or prohibit misuse of specimens or related information. Requirements for anonymity or informed consent may enter in as well. Most privacy advocates prefer to prevent collection of specimens in the first place because of the potential for later misuse of the specimens once they are collected. Collected specimens act as "honey pots" for those looking for information, and there is potential for "mission creep" in which the specimens or information begin to be used for purposes beyond those for which they were collected. Advocates of preventing collection of specimens also invoke general "slippery slope" arguments and warn of the development of public complacency and cavalier attitudes by the keepers of the databases. On the other hand, advocates of achieving the utilitarian goals of genetic studies often cite the requirement to collect specimens and thus focus their efforts on attempts to maintain privacy through administrative security and by confidentiality policies and procedures.

Despite the strong genetic discrimination rhetoric, cases of actual genetic discrimination are rare. Perhaps the most notorious case involves the Burlington Northern Santa Fe (BNSF) for secretly testing workers for a rare genetic disorder associated with carpal tunnel syndrome. However, as the number of genetic tests increases and electronic databases grow, genetic discrimination cases are bound to appear.

---

encountered a variety of requests for this specialized identity service. (1) A patient lost confidence that her breast biopsy results were hers following a series of reporting errors involving the spelling of her name and her birth date. (2) A colon biopsy revealed a malignant tumor, but following surgery, the removed specimen was devoid of a tumor. (3) A stomach surgery was performed after a biopsy diagnosis of malignant tumor; no tumor was seen in the surgical specimen. (4) Multiple tissue blocks from two breast lumpectomy procedures were processed. Because of labeling errors, it was unclear to which patient the various paraffin-embedded blocks belonged. (5) A young male fractured his femur and developed osteomyelitis. A biopsy from the fracture site demonstrated acute inflammation but also a fragment of tissue that appeared to be a malignant tumor.

In cases 1-4, identity testing with STRs demonstrated that all the specimens in question truly belonged to the involved patients. In case 5, testing following microdissection of the tissue fragments revealed that the squamous carcinoma "floater" was derived from another individual. The availability of identity testing in situations such as these is a significant benefit to the involved patients and health providers.

In prenatal testing for inherited disorders, chorionic villus sampling (CVS) performed early in pregnancy is sometimes employed as a source of fetal DNA for testing. Testing for a disorder such as cystic fibrosis may reveal that the genotypes for the mother and the fetus are identical (e.g., that they are both heterozygous carriers of a cystic fibrosis mutation). This result is entirely consistent with the usual segregation of chromosomes during meiosis. However, there is a risk that the CVS material was not derived largely from the fetus but was decidual cells primarily from the mother. If the father is a carrier of a cystic fibrosis mutation, this may result in the failure to diagnose cystic fibrosis in a fetus. Identity testing is employed to confirm that the tested cells have a genotype distinct from those of the mother and are a valid sample from the fetus.

HLA TYPING

Obtaining well-matched tissue enhances transplanted organ and bone marrow survival. The human leukocyte antigen (HLA) alleles determine the tissue compatibility for the acceptance of transplanted grafts donated from another person (allografts). HLA genes encode highly polymorphic cell surface molecules that are strong alloantigens, permitting the body to recognize foreign tissue. A kidney allograft is rejected as a result of an immune response directed against HLA alloantigens, which are expressed on the graft but are absent from the host.

Genetic Features of HLA Genes

The HLA genes are located within a genetic complex designated as the major histocompatibility complex (MHC). The MHC includes about 4 Mb on the short arm of chromosome 6

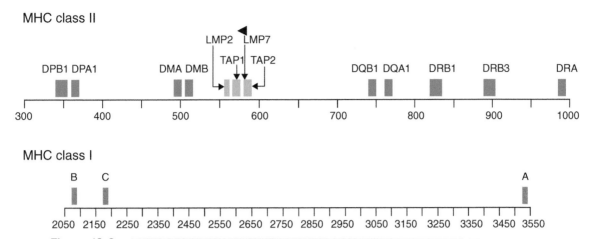

Figure 10-2

Map of the human MHC region. The organization of the most important class I and class II genes of the MHC is shown, with approximate genetic distances given in thousands of base pairs (kb). Genes are ordered from telomere to centromere. Not shown are MHC class III genes, which map between class I and class II genes (see Color Plate 8).

(6p21.3). Many of the more than 200 genes in the MHC are involved in the regulation of the immune response.[19] The genes encoding the HLA class I (A, B, and C) and the class II (DR, DQ, and DP) molecules are the most polymorphic loci in the human genome (Figure 10-2 and Table 10-4). These polymorphisms made the HLA loci an attractive and powerful early resource for identity testing.

HLA genes are codominantly expressed, and most individuals are heterozygous at the HLA class I and class II loci. Most of the sequence diversity for the HLA class I loci is located in the second and third exons and, for the class II loci, the second exon. These domains encode the peptide-binding regions of the HLA molecules. The pattern of allelic sequence diversity for both the class I and class II loci is unusual; most alleles differ from their closest neighbor by multiple substitutions, with some alleles differing in the second and third exons by as much as 15%. This pattern is suggestive of segmental exchange of nucleotide motifs between alleles of the same locus. As a result, different HLA alleles are mosaic-like combinations of a subset of all polymorphisms.[8,16]

Although many alleles (e.g., >400 for HLA-B and HLA-DRB1) are found in the worldwide population, a much smaller number (e.g., 30 to 50 for HLA-DRB1) is present in most individual populations. Importantly, different populations tend to have different frequency distributions of alleles and exhibit different patterns of linkage disequilibrium. This variability exists among both racial and ethnic groups.

The HLA genes exist in linkage disequilibrium, also referred to as gametic association. Gametic associations are regularly found between certain HLA alleles of A and B, C and B, B and DRB1, and DRB1 and DQB1 loci. The HLA genes are transmitted in families as haplotypes. The number of possible haplotypes is vast. However, because of linkage disequilibrium, the number of haplotypes found in a population is more limited.[16] Genetic recombination or crossing over in the HLA region is a relatively rare event, occurring for the most part no more than 1% per meiosis between A and B and between B and DRB1. Recombination can also occur between A and C and between B and C (0.6% and 0.2%, respectively).

TABLE 10-4	Names of the Most Important HLA Class I and Class II Genes and Their Encoded Polypeptide Ordered from Telomere to Centromere

Name	Encoded Polypeptide
HLA-A	Class I α-chain
HLA-C	Class I α-chain
HLA-B	Class I α-chain
HLA-DRA	DR α-chain
HLA-DRB3	DR β3-chain determining DR52 specificities
HLA-DRB1	DR β1-chain determining specificities DR1, DR2, DR3, DR4, DR5, etc.
HLA-DQA1	DQ α-chain
HLA-DQB1	DQ β-chain
TAP2	ABC (ATP binding cassette) transporter (associated with antigen presentation)
LMP7	Proteasome-related sequence (role in loading class I molecules with peptides)
TAP1	ABC (ATP binding cassette) transporter (associated with antigen presentation)
LMP2	Proteasome-related sequence (role in loading class I molecules with peptides)
HLA-DMB	DM β-chain (control peptide loading by class II molecules)
HLA-DMA	DM α-chain (control peptide loading by class II molecules)
HLA-DPA1	DP α-chain
HLA-DPB1	DP β-chain

Applications of HLA Typing

HLA allele identification has been used for transplantation, forensic, parentage, and chimerism testing. The latter three are of historical interest and are discussed elsewhere in this section.

Transplantation

Matching the HLA alleles of donors and recipients for renal transplantation improves long-term graft survival of kidneys from living related and unrelated donors and from deceased donors. For example, the half-life survival for a graft from an HLA-identical sibling is 23 years compared with a one haplo-type–related donor with a half-life of 12.8 years.[8] The effect of HLA matching on the survival of heart and lung transplants is also statistically significant. In contrast, the effect of HLA matching for liver transplants is uncertain.

Hematopoietic cell transplantation (HCT) is employed to treat several classes of disorders, such as leukemia and heredi-tary immune deficiencies. **Engraftment** occurs when infused donor cells replicate to produce new blood cells. HLA compat-ibility between donor and recipient in HCT affects not only the ability to achieve sustained engraftment of donor cells but also the risk of developing acute and chronic graft-versus-host disease (GVHD). Post-transplant risk of graft failure, GVHD, and mortality are affected by quantitative and qualitative char-acteristics of donor-recipient HLA allele mismatching. In allo-geneic stem cell transplantation, the donor is an individual who is genetically nonidentical and either related or unrelated to the recipient. Three different categories of donors are usually considered in the following order of preference: HLA geno-typically identical siblings, HLA-mismatched relatives, and unrelated donors, matched or mismatched. The goal when screening for an HLA-matched sibling donor is to identify which of any siblings have inherited the same HLA haplotypes from their parents.

HLA typing within families for transplantation sometimes leads to the discovery that the father is not the biological father of some or all of the children. There are a variety of opinions among healthcare providers about whether this pos-sibility should be discussed with the family before testing and how or whether "false paternity" should be reported to the family.

When a matched sibling donor does not exist for a patient requiring allogeneic HCT (70% of cases), searching for extended family members or donors from an unrelated bone marrow registry would be the next option. Registries of volunteer bone marrow donors and cord blood exist in most developed coun-tries (http://www.marrow.org, accessed December 21, 2006). Currently, approximately 65% of patients can find an accept-able donor among more than 4 million individuals registered in the U.S.-based national marrow donor program (NMDP). However, patients belonging to racial groups that are not well represented in the registries have a considerably decreased probability of finding a donor.

DNA-Based HLA Allele Identification

Most commonly used molecular diagnostic methods have been used to identify HLA alleles. Strategies based on oligonucle-otide probe hybridization, DNA sequencing, and allele-specific DNA amplification (see Chapter 5) have become the most common ones used currently for HLA typing. Each of these methods relies on amplification with PCR of genomic DNA of relevant regions of an HLA gene from the tested individual.[8] Samples for testing are usually peripheral blood, but may be any tissue containing nucleated cells.

Typing methods involve the design of primer pairs that are able to amplify all alleles at the target HLA locus with the polymorphic sequence motifs situated between the primer sites. Laboratories usually amplify at least exons 2 and 3 of class I genes and exon 2 of class II genes. Some prepare larger ampli-fication products for class I genes that include exon 1, exon 4, or both. Amplification primers may be located within exons or introns. Primers positioned in introns allow complete analysis of exons and inspection of exon-intron junctions for splice site polymorphisms. Primers must be carefully chosen to attain locus-specific amplification since the HLA loci are the products of gene duplication and divergence and retain substantial homology. Further, many HLA loci have closely related pseu-dogenes that do not encode functional polypeptides, but may result in nonspecific PCR products.[8]

The PCR products prepared are subsequently analyzed by a variety of methods. They can be hybridized to oligonucleotide probes in reverse or forward dot-blot assays. The panel of probes is chosen to cover critical polymorphic positions in the HLA gene tested. The pattern of reactivity of the panel can then be analyzed to assign allele identities.[8]

Alternatively, PCR products can be directly sequenced via dideoxynucleotide chain termination methods (see Chapter 5). This approach is increasingly attractive for allele level typing because of the large numbers of alleles known to exist at the HLA loci. The homozygous or heterozygous sequences obtained are compared with a library of known sequences of alleles for allele assignment.

A third commonly employed method, sequence-specific primer PCR (SSP-PCR), employs pairs of PCR primers chosen so that their 3′-most nucleotide or nucleotides are complemen-tary to a polymorphic position that distinguishes an allele or an allele group from other alleles. If the individual possesses the allele(s) of interest, the PCR will lead to a product whose size and presence are typically identified by agarose gel electro-phoresis or detected with real-time methods. A typing is per-formed by choosing many pairs of primers in independent reactions to cover all allele groups.[8]

Commercial reagents and software for analysis of results are available for each of these three methods. Laboratories tailor HLA typing assays to the specific applications discussed above. Choice of methods depends upon typing volume, turnaround requirements, and the resolution needed.

Interpretation of HLA Test Results

The number of alleles at the HLA class I and class II loci, and a listing of serologically defined specificities and their allele equivalents, are available online at several Web sites (http://www.anthonynolan.com/HIG, accessed December 21, 2006 or http://www.ebi.ac.uk/imgt/hla, accessed December 21, 2006). The alleles of each of the HLA antigens are numbered based on the original serological nomenclature. HLA alleles are now designated by a superscripted asterisk after the locus of origin and a number corresponding to the particular allele (e.g., HLA-A*0201). Parallel testing using serological and DNA genotyping of HLA alleles has led to the use of one nomencla-ture for the description of low-resolution typing in which the HLA assignment might include more than one possible related allele (e.g., HLA-A A*02) and a nomenclature reflecting the high-resolution allelic typing. Thus different HLA allele sub-types (e.g., for A*02) can appear indistinguishable when tested by serology or with a limited panel of nucleic acid probes so a generic or low-resolution typing is obtained. New HLA alleles are named by an international nomenclature committee. Annual HLA nomenclature reports with frequent updates are available at the Web sites listed above.

CHIMERISM AND HEMATOPOIETIC CELL ENGRAFTMENT ANALYSIS

Chimerism is defined as mosaicism with coexistence of cells derived from two different individuals. Successful HCT effectively results in chimerism with the recipient's hematopoietic cells derived from the donor. With the exception of monozygotic twins, it is possible to use polymorphic loci on chromosomes to distinguish between DNA prepared from cells derived from the recipient and cells from the donor. This is true even for siblings if enough loci are studied. Suppose the father and mother of two siblings have alleles j and k and s and t, respectively, at a locus. The likelihood that the two siblings will inherit an identical genotype such as js or jt at this locus is 1 in 4. The likelihood that the siblings will be identical for other studied loci for which the parents are similarly heterozygous is also 1 in 4. In this particular example of complete parental heterozygosity, the risk that no locus will be found at which the two siblings can be distinguished is 1 in 4^N where N is the number of independently segregating loci tested. Commercial engraftment testing reagents that include 9 to 16 independently segregating loci will virtually always reveal at least a single locus at which donor and recipient cells can be distinguished.

Methods for Performing Engraftment Analysis

Sources of DNA for engraftment testing are typically peripheral white blood cells or bone marrow aspirates. It is crucial to obtain genomic DNA samples from the recipient before the transplant to determine his or her native genotypes at the tested loci. Then post-transplant samples are compared with "pure" specimens from the donor and from the pre-transplant recipient. If a pre-transplant sample from the recipient is not available, another sample such as buccal cells, may be obtained. Care should be taken in interpreting results from these alternate sources, however, since donor-derived inflammatory cells may be present.

Testing can be performed on genomic DNA isolated from the entire cell population of the specimen. Alternatively, subsets of cells can be used to assess engraftment of specific cell lineages.[10] For example, engraftment of the T-cell versus non–T-cell components can be assessed based on expression of the CD3 surface molecule, a T-cell marker.

DNA typing methods used in engraftment analysis are summarized in Table 10-5. These methods have evolved similar to those used for identity testing in general. Initial methods relied on Southern blotting to detect RFLPs or VNTRs. These labor-intensive hybridization assays have been largely replaced by PCR-based methods.

One PCR-based strategy is to amplify a series of VNTR loci with subsequent separation of the DNA fragments on polyacrylamide gels.[21] Alleles are assigned via comparison with size standards after staining with ethidium bromide. The method will detect a small admixture of donor or recipient DNA of roughly 10%. Detection is enhanced to the <1% to 1% range with silver staining of the amplification products.

As described earlier in this chapter for forensic identification, fluorescent detection of PCR products derived from STR, or microsatellite loci, has been adopted by many laboratories for engraftment assays. This method is attractive because of the ability to automate the assay, the extensive characterization of these loci in a variety of populations, and their high degree of polymorphism. Surveys from the proficiency testing programs described below indicate that the majority of laboratories providing clinical engraftment testing currently analyze STR loci.

When the donor and recipient are of different genders, analysis of the sex chromosomes in post-transplant hematopoietic cells is useful in engraftment testing. Cytogenetic analysis of chromosomes in interphase cells with X- and Y-specific probes may be performed with fluorescent in situ hybridization assays. The percent donor or recipient cells is determined by assessing the ratio of cells with XX signals to those with XY signals. Alternatively, PCR-based analysis of X- and Y-chromosome loci can be carried out. For example, the reappearance of Y-specific amplification products in a male whose donor was his sister may indicate relapse of a malignancy. Polymorphic loci on chromosome X can be studied similar to the autosomal STR discussed above.

Selection and Interpretation of Short Tandem Repeat Loci

Engraftment testing is accomplished by preparing genomic DNA from donor and pre-transplant and post-transplant recipient specimens followed by PCR amplification of the selected STR loci. Amplification reactions are typically multiplexed using fluorescently labeled commercially available reagents as described above for forensic identity testing. Products are then separated via high-resolution slab or CE on an automated genetic analyzer. Comparison of DNA fragment sizes with a reference ladder allows software to assign alleles for each locus.

The analysis of a donor sample and a pre-transplant recipient sample allows the laboratory to identify which STR loci are informative (nonidentical genotypes) for the pair. A post-transplant sample can then be studied. If only fluorescent peaks from the donor are observed, then the cells studied are donor

TABLE 10-5	DNA Typing Methods Used in Engraftment Testing	
Method	**Description**	**Comment**
RFLP analysis of VNTR loci	Digest genomic DNA with restriction endonuclease and detect polymorphic VNTR loci by Southern blotting	Highly informative identity testing method also used in early forensics, now discarded because of its labor-intensive nature
PCR analysis of VNTR loci	Amplify VNTR loci and size by gel electrophoresis	Quite sensitive when bands are detected by silver staining
STR analysis	Multiplex amplification of several STR loci with sizing by fluorescent detection	Becoming the standard method in the field because of the efficiency and partial automation
Cytogenetics	Interphase analysis of X and Y chromosomes with fluorescent in situ hybridization	May be useful when donor and recipient are of different genders

in origin. Rarely, only recipient peaks will be seen, consistent with recipient origin of the cells. These assays can detect admixtures of cell populations down to approximately 3%. Therefore results indicating that a sample is exclusively from the donor are often reported as >97% donor. If fluorescent peaks derived from both the donor and the recipient are seen, the sample must be a mixture of cells from the two individuals.

The percent recipient in a mixed sample is calculated by summing the intensities of the informative recipient peaks and dividing by the sum of the intensities of the informative recipient and donor peaks. Many laboratories then average the percent recipient for each locus to arrive at a final result. Some laboratories run a calibration curve of artificial mixtures of donor and recipient DNA for each tested pair. Other laboratories validate the assay with calibration curves for a number of control "donor" and "recipient" mixtures and do not run new calibration curves for each new donor-recipient pair.

Applications of Microsatellite Locus Testing to Engraftment Analysis

Several clinical questions can be answered with engraftment testing. Is engraftment of donor cells proceeding well in the weeks following a stem cell transplant? In the setting of a history of successful engraftment, do subsequent studies demonstrate a resurgence of recipient-derived hematopoietic cells indicating a relapse? Has stable chimerism developed following transplantation with the production of hematopoietic cells derived from both the donor and recipient?

The correlation of engraftment testing results with the clinical history is crucial for interpretation of results. Thus appropriate communication between the engraftment testing laboratory and the transplantation team is essential. Consultation with a hematopathologist may be helpful in interpreting results in complex cases.

A result indicating 85% donor cells and 15% recipient cells might be equally consistent with an engrafting marrow 3 weeks after transplantation or with relapse 6 months following transplantation. The date of the transplant in relation to sample collection, the conditioning regimen used before transplant, and evidence from peripheral smear or bone marrow aspirate examination may be helpful in interpreting results. Unusual history if unknown can cause considerable confusion. For example, some recipients may have received more than one stem cell transplant or may have had a donor who is an identical twin.

The interpretation of an engraftment result from a single sample can be difficult. Multiple samples collected at intervals after transplantation may reveal changes in the fraction of donor and recipient over time that can be correlated with the evolving clinical picture.

PARENTAGE TESTING

Questions regarding the parentage of minor and adult children arise frequently in modern society. Generally at issue is whether a particular man is the father of a child. The same methods are applied to a search of a mother, a situation that sometimes arises when an adopted person is trying to find his or her biological parents. As discussed in the chapter introduction, parentage testing allows an individual to be excluded or not excluded as the parent of a child. If not excluded, the likelihood that the individual is the parent is calculated. Court-ordered and privately sought parentage testing is usually performed to facilitate decisions regarding responsibility for the financial support of a child. However, there are other reasons individuals may wish to establish parentage; an example is the settlement of an estate. As discussed earlier, laboratories performing other types of identification tests for purposes unrelated to parentage (e.g., HLA typing for transplantation) should be aware of the possibility of inadvertently uncovering "false paternity."

Methods, Instrumentation, and Sample Requirements

Methods for parentage testing have evolved considerably over time similar to other human identification applications. Initial methods relied on serological techniques to identify red cell antigens, such as the ABO and the MNS groups, and the highly polymorphic HLA antigens found on most cells. Since 1990 there has been a substantial migration of parentage laboratories to DNA-based methods, especially to those based on analysis of STR alleles. The significant advantages of these PCR-based assays with detection of fluorescently labeled DNA fragments on automated genetic analyzers are discussed in the section on forensic identification. Recently SNPs have also been introduced in commercial parentage laboratories.

Selection and validation of testing methods are key issues in parentage testing. Specific requirements for parentage testing may be mandated by local laws and agreements. Thus the choice of methods and genetic systems should be based on an agreement between the client(s) and the laboratory.

Nonstandardized methods should not be used as the sole methods within a parentage testing laboratory. In addition, a nonstandard method should be used only if it is documented that the method is used in at least one other laboratory, thus making it possible to obtain a second opinion based on repeated testing.

Like other forms of identity testing, samples for parentage testing may be any specimen containing chromosomal DNA. In practice, programs generally perform testing on peripheral blood samples or buccal smears. Buccal smears are increasingly preferred because they offer a noninvasive means of sample collection, which is especially convenient when testing minors.

Reporting of Test Results

In addition to the usual parentage test reports, laboratories are occasionally asked to provide interpretative reports when less than complete information is available. The usual report is discussed next, and the interpretive reports are discussed afterwards.

Test Reports

The results should include all the information requested by the client and necessary for the interpretation of the test results and all information required by the method used. If the weight of evidence is calculated, it must be based on likelihood ratio principles, such as the paternity index.[2,7]

Exclusion of a Tested Individual

The most common parentage testing involves genotyping several polymorphic loci in samples from a trio consisting of the mother, child, and presumed father. Inspection of the alleles found in the mother and the child at the genetic loci analyzed reveals alleles that must have been contributed by the child's biological father. If the presumed father does not have an obligatory allele at one of the tested loci, he is excluded as the biological father. Laboratories require the absence of an obligatory allele for at least *two* loci in a tested man to exclude him as the father. The requirement of multiple loci reduces the possibility of making an error caused by a technical problem or caused by a rare mutation at one of the examined loci.

The power of an analyzed locus to exclude a tested man depends upon the number of alleles found at the locus and their allele frequencies in human populations. ABO typing can exclude a tested man, but has a relatively poor probability of exclusion of about 15%. The HLA and VNTR loci have many alleles, and a single locus may have greater than 90% probability of excluding a falsely accused man. The STR loci have an intermediate number of alleles. A single STR locus typically has a 30% to 60% likelihood of excluding an incorrectly presumed man. The ease of STR analysis makes these loci attractive for parentage testing even with their lower exclusion power. If a number of STRs that independently segregate during meiosis are studied, a cumulative probability of exclusion can be calculated based on the product of exclusion power for each tested locus. The use of 9 to 16 unlinked, and therefore independent, STRs provided in commercially available human identity reagents generally results in at least a 99% probability of exclusion of an incorrectly presumed man.

Inclusion of a Tested Individual
The alleles found at the analyzed loci may be entirely consistent with the presumed man being the biological father of the child. In this case, the likelihood that he is truly the father, rather than a random individual who is not excluded, is calculated. A number of assumptions underlie accurate calculations of the likeliness of parentage. Tested individuals must be properly identified, testing must be accurate, and allele frequencies in relevant populations must be well characterized.

The probability of parentage (W) and the paternity index (PI) are two closely related values that express the likelihood that the tested man is truly the father, rather than another man who by chance shares alleles at a tested locus. Calculation of the PI takes into account allele frequencies at the locus in relevant populations. If multiple independent loci are analyzed, a cumulative PI based on the products of the individual loci is calculated. Government entities typically require that the paternity index be >100:1 and the probability of parentage be >99% for inclusion of a man. Other evidence bearing on the probability that a man is the father before testing is performed can be integrated with test results to calculate a posterior probability of parentage. The prior probability that a presumed man is the father is typically set at 50%, but a range of likelihoods given different prior probabilities (e.g., 10% to 50%) can be calculated for comparison.

Opinions, Interpretations, and Problems
Standard parentage testing requires samples from the trio described above. However, there are many cases in which the mother, child, and putative father may not all be available for testing. If a sample cannot be obtained from the mother, it may still be possible to exclude a tested man or to calculate his probability of paternity. For example, the finding of locus L

genotypes 1,3 for the child and 4,5 for the tested man is inconsistent with the hypothesis that he is the father, whether or not we know the mother's genotype. Similarly, when the presumed man is not available, testing performed for individuals related to him may be used to calculate the likelihood that he is the biological father of the child in question.

Whereas STRs and VNTRs are usually transmitted in a faithful mendelian fashion, mutations can occur. A child and tested man may be encountered who share an allele at all but one of the tested loci. The possibility that the man is truly the father and that a mutation has occurred at the mismatched locus should then be entertained. If additional loci are tested with no additional genetic inconsistencies discovered, the likelihood of paternity can be calculated by considering the frequency of mutations at the mismatched locus. Alternatively, additional genotyping may reveal more exclusions, making it unlikely that the tested man is truly the father. Laboratories should apply procedures for estimating uncertainty of measurement. The measurement of uncertainty of tests should be known and should be included in the interpretation of test results.

QUALITY ASSURANCE, PROFICIENCY TESTING, AND ACCREDITATION
Quality programs for identity laboratories differ based on the type of testing performed: forensic, HLA, chimerism, or parentage. Each will be discussed deparately.

Forensic DNA Analysis
Crime labs are unregulated, except in the case of submission of DNA results to the NDIS through the CODIS software. The DNA Identification Act of 1994 gave the FBI regulatory oversight of DNA profiles entered into the national database. The legislation called for a DNA advisory board that produced recommended standards, based largely on guidelines of the FBI's technical working group on DNA analysis methods (TWGDAM). The scientific working group on DNA analysis methods, which has replaced the TWGDAM, now advises the FBI director to create standards revisions.

The FBI's standards for forensic DNA testing laboratories require accreditation. Forensic Quality Services and the American Society of Crime Laboratory Directors/Laboratory Accreditation Board (ASCLD/LAB) accredit crime laboratories based upon ISO/IEC 17025 standards. Forensic community requirements include minimal educational credits and experience, proficiency testing twice a year per analyst, and annual audits. All testing requires a technical and an administrative review. An additional NDIS audit is required by the FBI. Judicial scrutiny provides another layer of critical review of those cases heard in court. Defense review and challenge, however, vary greatly.

Proficiency test providers for forensic laboratories include the Collaborative Testing Service, the College of American Pathologists (CAP), Cellmark Diagnostics, and Quality Forensics.

Standard reference materials from the National Institute of Standards and Technology (NIST) are available for RFLP Profiling (SRM 2390), PCR-based profiling DNA standard (SRM 2391b), Y-chromosome testing (SRM 2395), and mtDNA testing. Standards require annual NIST-traceable comparisons.

HLA Testing

Quality control and assurance programs for HLA testing should be similar to those for other types of PCR-based testing. The NMDP and the American Society for Histocompatibility and Immunogenetics (ASHI) maintain a cell repository of a subset of known alleles (http://www.ashi-hla.org, accessed December 21, 2006). As in other PCR-based testing, strict measures to prevent contamination of pre-PCR areas with genomic DNA and PCR products are essential. Importantly, testing for contamination arising from products prepared in SSP PCR is challenging because the many PCR reactions necessary to type an individual often result in products varying in size and composition. Measures to prevent contamination in PCR-based testing are widely described; such information is available online at the ASHI Web site.

Several proficiency-testing programs are available in the United States. These include the CAP, the ASHI, and the Southeastern Organ Procurement Foundation. Each offers comprehensive programs to assess laboratories' ability to correctly identify HLA alleles. The University of California at Los Angeles has offered an international cell exchange program for many years. Laboratories are challenged to correctly type samples that often include unusual or recently described alleles.

Clinical histocompatibility laboratories are high complexity laboratories that must have a Clinical Laboratory Improvement Amendments (CLIA) license in the United States. Laboratories may be inspected and accredited by the CAP or the ASHI. The United Network for Organ Sharing, NMDP, and CLIA have all designated ASHI with deemed status for purposes of HLA laboratory accreditation. Laboratories are generally directed by individuals with Ph.D., M.D., or both degrees. ASHI administers a program to assess the qualifications of doctoral level individuals to direct ASHI-accredited laboratories. Directors can take a certifying examination administered by the American Board of Histocompatibility and Immunogenetics (ABHI). The ABHI also certifies laboratory staff as histocompatibility technologists and specialists. Information is available on the ASHI Web site.

Chimerism and Hematopoietic Cell Engraftment

Proficiency testing programs for engraftment testing are offered by the CAP and the ASHI. Challenge specimens are typically artificial mixtures of genomic DNA from two related or unrelated individuals. In both surveys, participant laboratories have demonstrated a high degree of agreement for challenge samples. The standard deviation of participant results testing a 50%-50% mixture of "donor" and "recipient" cells is typically 2 to 4%. For mixtures that approach the sensitivity threshold of the assay (for example 6% recipient, 94% donor), somewhat broader standard deviations are typical.

Quality control and assurance programs for engraftment testing should be similar to those for other types of identity testing. Assays may require as little as 1 ng of genomic DNA. Thus strict measures to prevent contamination of pre-PCR areas with genomic DNA and PCR products are important.

Accreditation of programs may be through the ASHI or the CAP. Since engraftment testing is a variant of identity testing, the standards used are often those written for parentage and other forms of identity testing. However, because engraftment testing deals with subpopulations of cells and the relative proportions of cells, organizations such as the ASHI have developed accreditation standards specifically for engraftment testing.

Parentage Testing

The quality control and assurance measures for parentage testing are similar to those for other types of human identity testing. Positive identification of samples, prevention of DNA contamination, the use of control alleles of known size, and the validation of software employed for genetic analysis and calculation are among measures common to identity testing programs. Population distribution data for the systems used must be documented. In addition, mutation frequencies of the systems used must be documented and used appropriately.

The laboratory should have a policy and procedure for the resolution of complaints received from clients or other parties. Parentage testing programs involving knowledge of sensitive family information results may be employed in legal proceedings. Samples and records including information stored electronically must be handled carefully to ensure their privacy, confidentiality, and security. Laboratory procedures for documentation of the identity of individuals contributing samples for study and the chain of custody of specimens should be very detailed.

Recommendations and standards for parentage testing are formulated by government agencies or professional organizations (e.g., the Standards for Parentage Testing Laboratories of the American Association of Blood Banks [AABB]). The AABB administers a laboratory inspection and accreditation program.[1] The ASHI and the CAP also publish relevant standards. The CAP and the AABB jointly offer a proficiency testing survey.

REFERENCES

1. American Association of Blood Banks. Standards for Parentage Testing Laboratories, 5th Edition. 2001;1-57.
2. Baur MP, Elston RC, Gurtler H, Henningsen K, Hummel K, Matsumoto H, et al. No fallacies in the formulation of the paternity index. Am J Human Genet 1986;39:528-36.
3. Budowle B, Moretti T, Smith J. DNA typing protocols: molecular biology and forensic analysis, Eaton Publishing Co., Natick, MA, 2000.
4. Butler JM. Forensic DNA typing: biology and technology behind STR markers, Academic Press, London, 2000.
5. Butler JM, Reeder DJ. STR DNA Internet Database. http://www.cstl.nist.gov/div831/strbase (accessed December 21, 2006).
6. Chakraborty R, Kidd KK. The utility of DNA typing in forensic casework. Science 1991;254:1735-9.
7. Elston RC. Probability and paternity testing. Am J Human Genet 1986;39:112-22.
8. Erlich HA, Opelz G, Hansen J. HLA DNA typing and transplantation. Immunology 2001;14:347-56.
9. Evett IW, Weir B. Interpreting DNA evidence. In: Statistical genetics for forensic scientists, Sinauer Associates, Inc., Sunderland, MA, 1998.
10. Fernandez-Aviles F, Urbano-Ispizua A, Aymerich M, Colomer D, Rovira M, Martinez C, Nadal E, Talarn C, Carreras E, Montserrat E. Serial quantification of lymphoid and myeloid mixed chimerism using multiplex PCR amplification of short tandem repeat-markers predicts graft rejection and relapse, respectively, after allogeneic transplantation of CD34 selected cells from peripheral blood. Leukemia 2003;17:613-20.
11. Holland MM, Parsons TJ. Mitochondrial DNA sequence analysis—validation and use for forensic casework. Forensic Science Review 1999;11:21-50.
12. Jeffreys AJ, Wilson V, Thein SL. Hypervariable "minisatellite" regions in human DNA. Nature 1985;314:67-73.

13. Jeffreys AJ, Wilson V, Thein SL. Individual specific "fingerprints" of human DNA. Nature 1985;316:76-9.
14. Lander ES, Budowle B. DNA Fingerprinting dispute laid to rest. Nature 1994;371:735-8.
15. Langfelder EJ, Juengst ET. Ethical, Legal, and Social Implications (ELSI) Program: National Center for Human Genome Research, National Institutes of Health. Politics Life Sciences 1993;(2):273-5.
16. Little AM, Parham P. Polymorphism and evolution of HLA class I and II genes and molecules. Rev Immunogenet 1999;1:105-23.
17. National Research Council. DNA technology in forensic science. National Academy Press, Washington, D.C., 1992.
18. National Research Council. The evaluation of forensic DNA evidence. National Academy Press, Washington, D.C., 1996.
19. Rhodes DA, Trowsdale J. Genetics and molecular genetics of the MHC. Rev Immunogenet 1999;1:21-31.
20. Rudin N, Inman K. An introduction to forensic DNA analysis, second edition, CRC Press, Boca Raton, FL, 2001.
21. Schichman SA, Suess P, Vertino AM, Gray PS. Comparison of short tandem repeat and variable number tandem repeat genetic markers for quantitative determination of allogeneic bone marrow transplant engraftment. Bone Marrow Transplant 2002;29:243-8.
22. Shibata D. Identification of mismatched fixed specimens with a commercially available kit based on the polymerase chain reaction. Am J Clin Pathol 1993;100:666-70.
23. Van Oorschot RAH, Jones MK. DNA fingerprints from fingerprints. Nature 1997;387:767.
24. Weedn VW, Hicks JW. The unrealized potential of DNA testing, Research in Action, National Institute of Justice, Washington, D.C., 1998.
25. Wooley J, Harmon RP. The forensic brouhaha: science or debate? Am J Human Genet 1992;51:1164-5.

INTERNET SITES

www.anthonynolan.com/HIG—The Anthony Nolan Trust, HLA Informatics page
www.ashi-hla.org—American Society for Histocompatibility and Immunogenetics
www.cstl.nist.gov/div831/strbase—National Institute of Standards and Technology, Short Tandem Repeat DNA Internet Database
www.ebi.ac.uk/imgt/hla—European Bioinformatics Institute, IMGT/HLA Sequence Database
www.marrow.org—National Marrow Donor Program
www.mitomap.org/mitoseq.html—Human Mitochondrial DNA Revised Cambridge Reference Sequence

REVIEW QUESTIONS

1. The type of testing performed routinely in crime labs around the world is
    A. RFLP.
    B. dot-blots.
    C. STRs.
    D. SNPs.
    E. mtDNA.
2. Depending upon the jurisdiction, DNA may be collected for law enforcement purposes from all EXCEPT
    A. all newborns.
    B. convicted felons.
    C. sexual misdemeanor offenders.
    D. arrestees.
    E. burglars.
3. Forensic DNA identity testing dates back to
    A. 1965.
    B. 1975.
    C. 1985.
    D. 1995.
    E. 2000.

4. Which of the following DNA tests would most likely be used by a crime lab in 2007 to successfully yield a result from a degraded DNA specimen?
    A. STRs
    B. RFLP
    C. SNPs
    D. mtDNA
    E. ALU repeats
5. A 23-year-old male with acute myelogenous leukemia received a hematopoietic stem cell transplant from his HLA-matched brother. Eight months post-transplant, relapse of his leukemia is suspected. Analysis of which one of the following genetic systems would be most effective in evaluating the identity of the recipient's hematopoietic cells?
    A. X and Y chromosome identification by fluorescent in situ hybridization
    B. mtDNA analysis
    C. STR locus allele identification
    D. HLA typing
    E. ABO testing
6. A 2-year-old with acute lymphoblastic leukemia received a hematopoietic stem cell transplant from an unrelated donor. One month following the transplant, engraftment testing of the patient's peripheral blood mononuclear cells revealed that 20% are recipient in origin and 80% are donor derived. Which one of the following statements best interprets these data?
    A. There is failure of the donor stem cells to completely engraft.
    B. Relapse of the acute lymphoblastic leukemia is occurring.
    C. Stable chimerism of recipient and donor stem cells has developed.
    D. A nonmyeloablative conditioning regimen was used before the transplant.
    E. Additional clinical information is needed for appropriate interpretation of the results.
7. Nucleic acid–based testing to identify an inherited disorder in a fetus was performed. Results demonstrated that the mother and the fetus shared identical genotypes at the relevant genetic locus. For which of the following samples would it be most important to prove with identity testing that the fetal sample was not contaminated with maternal cells?
    A. A chorionic villus sample obtained at 11 weeks gestation
    B. Amniotic cells obtained at 15 weeks gestation
    C. Amniotic cells obtained at 26 weeks gestation
    D. Umbilical cord blood cells obtained at delivery
    E. All of the above
8. An STR locus was genotyped using genomic DNA from a 3-year-old and from a man suspected to be her biological father. Results are shown below:
STR locus genotype:
    Suspected man: **a** and **c** alleles
    3-year-old: **a** and **d** alleles
Given these results, which of the following statements is most likely to be true?
    A. The tested man is excluded as the biological father.

B. The 3-year-old's d allele was contributed by her biological mother.

C. The 3-year-old's a allele was contributed by her biological father.

D. The tested man may be the biological father of the 3-year-old.

E. The results suggest that a laboratory error has been made.

9. An STR locus on chromosome 4 was assessed using genomic DNA obtained from a man for paternity testing. Analysis showed homozygosity for allele q at the tested locus. The allele frequency for allele q in a relevant population is 0.2. Which of the following best approximates the likelihood that a random man in the population would be homozygous for allele q at this locus?

A. 0

B. 0.01

C. 0.04

D. 0.1

E. 0.4

10. A 35-year-old man requires a bone marrow transplant for treatment of severe aplastic anemia. The odds that any one of his siblings will be an exact allele-level match at the HLA-A, B, C and DR loci are

A. less than 1 in 4.

B. 1 in 4.

C. 1 in 2.

D. 1 in 8.

E. less than 1 in 8.

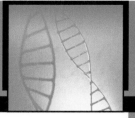

Molecular Methods in Diagnosis and Monitoring of Infectious Diseases

Andrea Ferreira-Gonzalez, Ph.D.
James Versalovic, M.D., Ph.D.
Sultan Habeebu, M.D., Ph.D.
Angela M. Caliendo, M.D., Ph.D.

OBJECTIVES

1. List three applications of molecular microbiological testing in addition to its use in diagnosis of an infection.
2. List five types of organisms for which the use of molecular testing is often required in the clinical laboratory.
3. Discuss the advantages and limitations of molecular testing for infectious disease including analytical and clinical sensitivity and specificity, rapidity of testing, cost, throughput, and technical skill required.
4. Compare the traditional methods of diagnosis of *Chlamydia trachomatis* (CT) and *Neisseria gonorrhoeae* (GC) infections with molecular methods; list the advantages and limitations of molecular testing over conventional methods for these infectious agents.

5. Contrast low- and high-risk types of human papillomavirus (HPV) and explain the outcomes of each type; name two high-risk types of HPV.

6. Describe two methodologies for detection and classification of HPV.

7. Discuss HIV-1 including its replication, genetic groups, molecular tests used to monitor therapies, current standard of treatment, and issues with the use of viral-load testing as a diagnostic tool.

8. State the clinical utility of antiviral resistance testing for HIV-1.

9. Compare and contrast genotypic and phenotypic tests for resistance of HIV to antiviral drugs.

10. Describe herpes simplex virus (HSV) including routes of infection, symptoms, and possible outcomes of the two types, and state the clinical utility of polymerase chain reaction (PCR) to diagnose central nervous system (CNS) and neonatal infections with the virus.

11. List and explain two methods for the detection of enterovirus RNA in clinical specimens; state the clinical utility of both.

12. Describe cytomegalovirus (CMV) including routes of infections, symptoms, diagnosis in an immunocompromised individual, traditional and molecular detection methods for both latent and active CMV, and the clinical utility of assessing the risk of CMV infection in individuals with acquired immunodeficiency syndrome (AIDS).

13. Describe *Mycobacterium tuberculosis* (MTb) including routes of infection, symptoms, traditional and molecular detection methods, and the clinical utility of molecular testing for extrapulmonary MTb infections.

14. State the importance of controlling for amplification inhibition in molecular assays, particularly in assessment of MTb infection.

15. Describe hepatitis C virus (HCV) including routes of infection, symptoms, qualitative and quantitative RNA analysis of the virus, genotypic heterogeneity, and genotyping assays.

16. List four applications for HCV RNA testing.

17. State the clinical utility of a molecular assay to identify methicillin-resistant *staphylococcus aureus* (MRSA); list two types of identification assays and their principles.

18. Describe the use of pulsed-field gel electrophoresis in the assessment of vancomycin-resistant enterococci (VRE).

19. State the differences among the three categories in the Centers for Disease Control and Prevention's (CDC's) classification of bioterrorism agents, and categorize a given agent based on its ability to be disseminated, its mortality rates, and its ability to cause panic in the public.

20. Identify the types of samples that are appropriate for analyzing for the presence of a bioterrorism agent.

21. State the utility of quantitative real-time PCR for the detection and identification of bioterrorist agents.

22. Design a nucleic-acid–based test for a given infectious disease, including specimen processing, nucleic acid amplification, and product detection; choose appropriate target sequences, include internal controls, and perform analytical and clinical verification.

23. State the necessity for quality control and assurance in the process of infectious disease molecular testing; discuss the types of controls needed, the need for proficiency testing, result interpretation, and reporting.

KEY WORDS AND DEFINITIONS

Analyte-Specific Reagent: Reagent(s), usually purchased, that are used in *laboratory-developed tests (LDTs)* that confer specificity for detecting a particular analyte; ASRs include antibodies, specific receptor proteins, ligands, and oligonucleotides.

Bioterrorism: The use of pathogenic organisms or biological toxins to produce disease and/or death in humans for the purpose of spreading fear and terror in the community.

Inhibition: In regard to amplification, "inhibition refers to the lack of formation of amplified gene products, which may be due to substances like hemoglobin, that inhibit the DNA polymerase enzyme used in PCR that makes copies of the DNA target sequence; in many assays, an 'inhibition control' must be added to the sample to determine whether an interfering substance has caused inhibition of the enzymatic reaction".

Laboratory-Developed Test (LDT): A test developed by a laboratory; in molecular microbiology, this usually refers to an assay for an infectious agent for which there are no FDA-cleared commercially available assay methods or systems.

Molecular Test: Tests or assays involving the extraction, purification, and processing of DNA or RNA (nucleic acids) in various ways to obtain specific information in the investigation of a given condition; often used for the diagnosis and monitoring of an infectious disease.

Multiplex Assay: The use of different probes, chromogens, PCR primers, etc. in a single assay to detect or quantify more than one target; in molecular microbiology, the targets are the DNA or RNA of infectious agents.

Pathogen: An infectious agent that causes a disease.

Preemptive Therapy: Therapy administered to an identified high-risk group before development of symptoms in an attempt to prevent the development of active disease.

Prophylactic Therapy: Therapy administered to all patients in a group of individuals that are treated without stratification of risk, thus involving treatment of a greater number of patients than in *preemptive therapy*.

Resistance: The lack of response of an infectious agent to a therapy, such as an antibiotic, antiviral agent, or other therapeutic drug.

Resistance Testing: In molecular microbiology, genotypic assays that identify specific mutations or nucleotide changes that are associated with an increased *resistance* to a specific drug such as antiviral drug; phenotypic resistance assays do not identify the mutations; rather they measure the ability of the bacteria or virus to grow in the presence of drug.

Sensitivity: There are two broad types of sensitivity of an assay, analytical sensitivity and diagnostic or clinical sensitivity; analytical sensitivity is defined by analysts as the change in assay signal for a unit change in concentration of analyte; it is often used by microbiologists to mean the minimum concentration or amount of RNA or DNA that can reliably be detected in an assay; the high sensitivity (by either definition of analytical sensitivity) of PCR assays for pathogens is achieved through the several million–fold amplification of the pathogen's nucleic acid; **diagnostic or clinical sensitivity** (Chapter 8) **refers to the ablity of an assay to identify individuals with a specific infection or disease state**.

Specificity: There are two broad types of specificity of an assay, analytical and clinical; analytical specificity (or "selectivity," which is the preferred term of analysts) of a test refers to the extent to which a test can determine particular analyte(s) in a complex mixture without interference or cross-reactivity from other components in the mixture; in molecular microbiology, this term often refers to the ability of an assay to amplify and/or detect only the unique regions of the pathogen's genome that avoid cross-reactivity with related species; **clinical specificity** (Chapter 8) of a test refers to the ability of an assay to identify those individuals without the specific infection or disease state; it is the proportion of individuals free of the target condition (usually infection, for the purposes of this chapter) whose test results are negative; see Chapter 8.

Viral-Load Testing: Quantification of the genomic viral nucleic acid in blood (e.g., copies per mL of plasma), which is usually used to assess disease prognosis and/or response to therapy; for example, with HIV, testing is done (1) to determine when to initiate antiretroviral therapy, (2) to monitor response to therapy, and (3) to predict time to progression to AIDS.

In laboratory medicine, the term "molecular" is often applied to tests or assays of DNA and RNA from clinical specimens to obtain specific information in the investigation of a given condition. Since their introduction, **molecular tests** have profoundly affected the management of infectious diseases. In contrast to microbial culture methods, molecular methods are rapid, thus allowing early decisions about treatment to be based on data about the pathogen(s) in an individual patient. Molecular methods have provided a means to detect pathogens that could not be easily detected by traditional methods, such as culture, antigen detection, or serology. Molecular methods can not only quantify the nucleic acids of pathogens in clinical samples but also determine the genetic makeup of the pathogen and thus predict, for example, its response to antimicrobial drugs. The methods have thus transformed the approaches to predicting and monitoring the response to therapy, assessing the risk of disease development, and determining the prognosis of disease. It is not surprising that the range of pathogens for which molecular testing is used is large and growing. For reference, lists of Food and Drug Administration (FDA)-cleared or FDA-approved molecular tests that are available for bacterial and viral pathogens are provided in Tables 14-2 and 14-3, respectively.

The first part of this chapter reviews the indications for molecular testing in the management of infectious diseases and the advantages and limitations of molecular tests. Because the field is expanding rapidly, we provide links throughout the chapter to Web sites where recent developments can be monitored. The next section describes nucleic acid testing for specific pathogens, with a section heading for each pathogen or pair of related pathogens. These sections include discussion of the clinical utility of the testing and are focused on those pathogens for which molecular testing is considered the standard of care. The third section addresses molecular testing for agents of **bioterrorism.** The final section describes the steps in the development and implementation of molecular microbiological assays in the clinical laboratory.

INDICATIONS FOR MOLECULAR TESTING

The range of clinical uses for molecular microbiology is broad and extends beyond detection of specific pathogens to arrive at a diagnosis. The breadth of applications can be appreciated

to some extent by simply considering three prominent examples:

- *Monitoring of response of viral infections to therapy:* Monitoring is achieved by quantitative measurement of the concentration of viral nucleic acid ("viral load") in blood. Molecular monitoring of the viral load has become the standard of care for managing individuals with human immunodeficiency virus–1 (HIV-1) infections and/or acquired immunodeficiency syndrome (AIDS), hepatitis C virus (HCV) infections, and cytomegalovirus (CMV) infections.
- *Providing a prognosis:* A mutation profile or genotype of an organism is used to predict the response pattern of the particular strain to available drugs. Genotyping may be performed before the initiation of therapy, as in infants born with (HIV-1) from their infected mothers, or performed following the development of resistance to ongoing therapy to find drugs to which the virus is susceptible. For HCV infections, the genotype determines the duration of therapy and also predicts the likelihood of its success.
- *Tracing an outbreak of infection to its source:* Molecular methods provide the fastest and most accurate means of tracing an outbreak of infection to its source. Nucleic acid sequencing allows detailed "strain typing" of the organism following outbreaks of infection in a hospital or in the community. Conventional methods may not be able to type the pathogen beyond the species level or may require several days to achieve strain typing. In addition to fast turnaround time, molecular methods also provide high-throughput approaches to handling large numbers of cases.

Molecular testing methods have a variety of advantages in clinical microbiology over traditional culture and microscopic methods and immunochemical tests. In some cases, traditional methods do not even exist, or they suffer serious drawbacks for clinical use. When conventional methods are available, the advantages and limitations of molecular methods must be understood and weighed in deciding on the role if any of a molecular method in current testing for infectious diseases.

When Are Molecular Methods Necessary?

Molecular methods are often necessary in the clinical laboratory for the diagnosis of diseases caused by certain organisms. Such organisms fall into five groups:

1. *Organisms for which culture methods are not available:* Culture methods are not available for the identification of all organisms. Common examples include the hepatitis viruses and the syphilis agent *Treponema pallidum.*
2. *Fastidious organisms:* These are pathogens with special requirements for their growth in the laboratory. The most demanding of this group are again the viruses, some of which require cultured mammalian cells for their growth (such as the herpesviruses). Rickettsiae are also obligate intracellular organisms and require cultured cells for their culture. Some bacteria also fall into this group of fastidious pathogens (for example, *Helicobacter pylori*).
3. *Slow-growing organisms:* A major indication for molecular testing in this group is the need to achieve a

reasonable turnaround time and thereby enable the early institution of the appropriate drug therapy for the patient and early isolation of the patient where the diagnosis requires such action to prevent spread of disease. Common examples of this group of pathogens are mycobacteria (which cause tuberculosis and related illnesses) and Bartonella species.

4. *Pathogens for which culture methods are insensitive:* Culture is unable to detect some pathogens in certain clinical specimens. For example, HSV, the cause of herpes encephalitis and herpes meningitis, is difficult to culture in cerebrospinal fluid. Culture of Lyme disease–causing Borrelia species is slow, requires special culture media, and lacks sensitivity, making Borrelia prime candidates for molecular diagnosis. PCR of skin biopsy is currently the most sensitive and specific test for Lyme disease in the early (erythema migrans) phase.

5. *Organisms that cannot be fully characterized by culture:* These organisms cannot be identified by culture methods; they are fully identified by molecular testing using polymerase chain reaction (PCR) primers targeted at 16S ribosomal gene sequences conserved among all bacteria or fungi as the case may be. The amplification product is identified by sequencing.

Advantages of Molecular Tests

Sensitivity

In general, molecular methods are the most sensitive techniques available for the detection and identification of pathogens. The correspondingly low detection limit is particularly useful when dealing with specimens that contain very low concentrations of the pathogen. The high **sensitivity** of the methods is often achieved by amplification of the **pathogen's** nucleic acid several million–fold (Chapter 5). The high sensitivity of molecular techniques demands great care to prevent contamination of specimens with organisms from the environment during collection, transport, and processing of the specimen (Chapter 3) and to prevent contamination of specimens, samples, and reagents with amplified DNA in the laboratory (Chapter 7).

Specificity

Molecular techniques are designed to achieve high **specificity** for the organism that the test is designed to detect. This minimizes falsely positive results. High specificity is achieved through targeting of primers and probes to unique regions of the pathogen's genome. The degree of specificity required in a test is controllable (for example, primers can be designed to be not only genus- or species-specific but strain-specific). At the other extreme are primers for nucleic acid amplification designed to be "group-specific" rather than pathogen-specific; thus primers may be designed to amplify all fungi by targeting ribosomal DNA sequences conserved among fungi. The fungus responsible for a particular infection is then identified by sequencing the amplification product.

Rapidity

PCR-based molecular tests are very rapid. Some tests are capable of detecting and identifying the infective agent in less than 2 hours after receipt of the specimen in the laboratory.

High Throughput

Molecular assays are amenable to very high throughput via automation. Hundreds of samples can be assayed in one run using PCR devices capable of using 384-well plates. All steps of the assay may be automated using robotics. With each run lasting less than 3 hours on average, several runs may be made per day, further increasing the throughput rate. This is a major advantage for molecular techniques in the investigation of large outbreaks of infectious diseases. The combination of high sensitivity, specificity, rapidity, and high throughput of molecular techniques is difficult to approach let alone match by any other currently available technology or technique.

Applicability to Archival Material

Molecular tests do not require viability of the pathogen for pathogen detection and identification. This characteristic of molecular assays makes it possible to identify the cause(s) of infection from archival material. A case in point is the recent identification of *Rothia mucilaginosa* from paraffin blocks of bone marrow, brain, and choroid plexus. The archival material could be frozen tissue, frozen nucleic acid, embalmed tissue (such as Egyptian mummies), or fixed tissue (as in archived frozen or paraffin-embedded pathology, autopsy and cadaver specimens).

Drug Targeting of Specific Mutations/Proteins

The use of molecular techniques has shed some light on the genes and specific mutations responsible for virulence and/or drug **resistance** in many organisms. This information may be used to design drugs that target the specific products (proteins) of the genes. Such drugs may be designed to inactivate the protein by binding to an important region (domain) of the protein; important examples are several drugs, such as the nucleoside transcriptase inhibitors, that are used to treat AIDS.

Better Understanding of Resistance Mechanisms

Molecular testing has enabled the development of databases containing genotypic and phenotypic specific mutation information known to contribute to drug resistance in certain infections. This is the basis of the molecular assays (genotyping) used to investigate drug resistance in HIV-1 infected patients.

Limitations of Molecular Tests for Pathogens

Inability to Distinguish Live from Dead Pathogens

Most molecular tests, being assays for a nucleic acid sequence, cannot distinguish dead from live pathogens. This is important clinically in deciding between current or active infection and past infection or exposure. Though not a common problem, persistence of DNA can confound patient management decisions.

Cost

The cost of molecular tests varies widely depending on the test. Currently, molecular tests are generally more expensive than conventional assays. It is expected that this will change as more molecular assays become available and the use of molecular tests becomes more widespread.

Requirement for Technical Skills

Another disadvantage of molecular testing is the technical skill required. As the need for molecular testing grows and becomes recognized by more and more laboratories, molecular training of medical technologists will be given higher priority, and it is hoped that trained technologists and technicians will eventually be available to meet the needs of all laboratories.

Limited Availability

Along with the training of more technical personnel will come the availability of molecular testing in routine laboratories rather than the current situation in which most molecular tests are performed in reference laboratories and academic medical centers.

Lack of National and International Standardization of Assays

Standardization is especially important in quantitative assays, such as **viral-load testing.** Without standardization it is difficult to compare, for example, treatment results between two medical centers because the viral-load assays of the two laboratories may not be standardized.

SPECIFIC PATHOGENS

This section will review nucleic acid testing as it applies to specific pathogens with a focus on those pathogens for which nucleic acid testing is considered the standard of care.

Chlamydia trachomatis and Neisseria gonorrhoeae

The organisms *Chlamydia trachomatis* (CT) and *Neisseria gonorrhoeae* (GC) will be discussed together because several of the available nucleic acid tests for these pathogens are **multiplex assays,** reflecting the common clinical desire to test for both pathogens in a single specimen. Though CT and GC can each cause a variety of clinical infections, we will focus on genital infections.

Detection of CT is a challenging and important public health issue. CT is a major cause of genital infections, with an estimated 1 million cases occurring annually among sexually active adolescents and young adults in the United States. The need for testing is increased by several facts. Many of the infections are asymptomatic and untreated and thus are passed to others. Even when symptoms are present they are not specific for CT, so a test is needed. Moreover, in women, 10% to 40% of infections progress to pelvic inflammatory disease (PID) if untreated; CT infection thus is a likely cause of secondary infertility in women in the United States. In pregnant women, there is the additional risk of transmitting the infection to the newborn during labor and delivery, leading to pneumonia or conjunctivitis in the newborn. GC also may present in various ways, and the clinical presentations overlap those of CT.

The traditional methods for the diagnosis of CT infections include cell culture, immunofluorescent antigen detection, enzyme immunoassay, and, more recently, nonamplified nucleic acid detection. These traditional methods have been replaced in many laboratories with amplified nucleic acid tests because of their greater sensitivity in detecting CT from genital specimens. For GC, which was traditionally diagnosed based on culture methods that rely on selective media, nucleic acid testing does not offer a significant improvement in sensitivity when culture is performed under ideal conditions. However, GC is a fastidious organism, which can lead to a decreased sensitivity of culture, particularly when specimen transport is required before culturing. Nucleic acid testing for GC offers a sensitive and reliable alternative to culture.

In addition to a high sensitivity and specificity, nucleic acid testing offers several advantages over conventional culture and antigen-detection methods for the diagnosis of CT and GC. Testing for both pathogens can be done on a single specimen, and for some multiplex assays, testing is performed in a single reaction. The DNA and RNA of GC and CT are much more stable than the infectious organisms, which accounts for some of the improved sensitivity of molecular assays. The stability of nucleic acid avoids the necessity of immediate transport to the laboratory, and specimens may be stored refrigerated or at room temperature before transport. The transport and storage requirements vary among tests, so it is important to refer to the package insert for specific details. An additional advantage of nucleic acid testing is the use of urine specimens, which for women allows testing to be done without the need for a pelvic examination. In males, urine offers a convenient and sensitive alternative to collection with a urethral swab and increases the likelihood that asymptomatic males will agree to be tested.

FDA-cleared tests for the detection of CT and GC (see Table 14-2) from clinical specimens can use a variety of specimens, including cervical swabs, urethral swabs, and urine from both asymptomatic and symptomatic individuals. Not all assays are approved for all conditions, and the current assays are not FDA-cleared for oral, rectal, respiratory, or conjunctival specimens. The performance characteristics of the assays vary (details are available in the package inserts); however, some general comments can be made concerning all of the tests. The diagnostic sensitivity of the tests varies depending on the specimen type and whether the patient is asymptomatic or symptomatic. For males, the sensitivity of testing urine specimens is nearly equivalent to testing urethral swabs.[25] A limited volume (20 mL to 50 mL) of first-passed urine is preferred because larger volumes will lead to a decreased concentration of organisms in the sample and thus reduced sensitivity. With proper specimen collection, male urethral swabs and urine specimens have a sensitivity of nearly 100% for the detection of GC or CT. For women, cervical swab specimens provide the highest sensitivity for the detection of GC and CT, with many studies showing a sensitivity of 90% to 95%.[25] Urine specimens can be used, but they generally result in a lower sensitivity than cervical swabs (75% to 85%). An alternative to urine testing in women is the use of self-collected vaginal swabs, which have shown in some studies a sensitivity that is equal to that obtained with cervical swabs.

Nucleic acid testing is not the standard of care for diagnosing CT and GC in cases of sexual abuse. Some have suggested its use in cases of sexual abuse of adults if testing is done using two assays, each of which targets a different region of the genome. This is not practical for clinical laboratories because most use only one assay, and no single transport medium can be used for all of the FDA-cleared CT and GC molecular assays. For cases of sexual abuse in children, culture is still recommended for the detection of GC and CT.

Nucleic acid testing for the detection of CT or GC cannot be used as a test of cure because DNA can be detected in urine samples for up to 3 weeks after completion of therapy. If DNA testing must be used, sample collection should be delayed for at least 3 weeks after initiation of therapy.

For several GC assays, there is a reduced specificity because of cross-hybridization of primers with nongonococcal *Neisseria* species. The ProbeTec test has been reported to produce false-positive results with *Neisseria flavescens*, *Neisseria lactamica*, *Neisseria subflava*, and *Neisseria cinerea*, and the Amplicor assay can produce false-positive results with *N. flavescens*, *N. lactamica*, and *Neisseria sicca*. Because of cross-reactivity with these nongonococcal species of *Neisseria*, there is concern about generating false-positive results with pharyngeal specimens.[23] However, *N. cinerea*, *N. lactamica*, *N. subflava*, and *N. sicca* have also been isolated not only from the pharynx but also from genital mucosa, so it is also possible to generate false-positive results from genital specimens as well.

Other sources of false-positive results include carryover contamination of amplified product and cross-contamination during specimen collection, transport, or processing. Concerns over these issues have led to a discussion of confirmatory testing for CT and GC since false-positive results can have psychosocial or medicolegal ramifications. False-positive results in a low-prevalence population can significantly reduce the predictive value of a positive result. For example, though the specificity of nucleic acid testing for GC or CT generally ranges from 98% to 99%, the positive predictive value may be as low as 60% to 70% in a population with a low prevalence. CDC Guidelines for sexually transmitted disease (STD) testing provide recommendations to clinical laboratories on the use of confirmatory testing for CT and GC.

False-negative results from **inhibition** of amplification are a concern for both GC and CT testing and have been reported for both cervical swabs and urine specimens. Inhibition rates may vary considerably depending on the amplification method and are related in part to the method used for nucleic acid extraction. For tests that use a crude lysate in testing (such as the Amplicor and ProbeTec tests), inhibition rates tend to be higher than those seen with the Aptima combo test, which uses a target capture method to purify nucleic acid. For the assays that test a crude lysate, it is useful to add an internal control or amplification control to each sample to test for inhibition of amplification. Results are not reported as negative for GC or CT unless the internal control is amplified in the sample. There are no clear guidelines concerning when it is appropriate to discontinue use of an internal control. However, to contain costs, some laboratories discontinue the use of the internal control if inhibition rates are less than 1%.

There is interest in performing CT and GC testing for liquid cytology specimens because a single specimen can be used for cervical cytology (Pap smear), HPV testing, and CT and/or GC testing. The CT and GC testing would be performed on the liquid specimen that remained after completion of the Pap smear and HPV testing. Though this simplifies sample collection for the clinician, there are several drawbacks to this approach that must be considered. The instruments used to prepare the liquid Pap smears were not designed to control for cross-contamination during processing, which may lead to false-positive results. CT and GC testing may not be performed until after the Pap smear results and HPV testing are complete, which could delay diagnosis and treatment of CT or GC infections. Moreover, there may be inadequate specimen remaining to complete CT and GC testing, thus requiring the patient to make a return visit for collection of an additional sample. For these reasons, many laboratories require separate specimens for CT and GC testing.

Decisions regarding the choice of a specific amplification test for the detection of CT and GC should not be based solely on the cost of reagents. Other key factors to consider include test performance characteristics, such as diagnostic sensitivity and specificity, and whether the test has been cleared for urine and swab specimens in both symptomatic and asymptomatic individuals. Ideally the test should include an internal control, particularly if a crude lysate is used in the assay. Other factors to consider are degree of automation, ease of use, work flow issues, and space and equipment needs.

Human Papillomavirus

Anogenital human papillomavirus (HPV) infections are common in both men and women. It is estimated that more than 24 million men and women in the United States are currently infected with HPV. HPV is a sexually transmitted infection; it is most common among sexually active young women ages 15 through 25 years. In one study, cervicovaginal HPV was found in 43% of sexually active college women during a 3-year period.

The types of HPV that are spread through sexual contact are classified as either low risk or high risk for progression to malignancy. There are multiple types of both low-risk and high-risk HPV. Infections with HPV can lead to a variety of outcomes, ranging from benign genital warts to penile or cervical cancer. The outcome is driven by the type of HPV. Genital warts or condylomata acuminata are caused by low-risk HPV types and have a low likelihood of progressing to malignancy. Conversely, penile cancer in men and cervical cancer in women are associated with high-risk HPV infections. Infections can, however, be transient and progression to cancer occurs over decades.

Until recently the sole standard method of screening for cervical cancer was to search for abnormal cells by cervical cytology (Pap smear). A common morphological change associated with HPV infection includes atypical squamous cells of undetermined significance (ASCUS). (Less common and more troubling are low-grade squamous intraepithelial lesion [LSIL] and high-grade squamous intraepithelial lesion [HSIL]). The prevalence of ASCUS on Pap smears is approximately 5% to 10%, with rates as high as 20% reported in sexually active women. Not all women with ASCUS progress to cervical cancer. HPV testing now plays an important role in assessing which women with ASCUS are at the highest risk of developing cervical cancer. Current recommendations are to test all women with ASCUS for the presence of high-risk HPV. Those women with positive test results for high-risk HPV DNA should undergo further clinical and pathological examination (colposcopy), whereas those patients with negative test results for HPV DNA can be followed according to routine practice.

Testing for high-risk HPV has been considered as a primary screening tool for women 30 years of age and older,[19] regardless of whether they have ASCUS detected on a Pap smear. This is based on the observation that women more than age 30 who have persistent infection with high-risk types of HPV are at the greatest risk of developing cervical cancer. Women who have a normal Pap smear and a negative HPV screening result are at very low risk of developing cervical cancer and would require less frequent screening than those with either an abnormal Pap smear or a positive HPV screening result.

Proper use of HPV testing requires not only detection of the virus or viral DNA, but also classifying it as either low risk or high risk. Currently the only available FDA-cleared test for the detection and classification of HPV DNA is the Hybrid Capture 2 (HC2) test (Digene Corp. Gaithersburg, Md.). The test relies on signal amplification technology and probe hybridization. The test uses two separate pools of RNA probes, one for detecting high-risk HPV DNA and another for low-risk HPV DNA. The high-risk pool contains RNA probes specific for 13 HPV types (16, 18, 31, 33, 35, 39, 45, 51, 52, 56, 58, 59, and 68), and the low-risk pool of RNA probes detects five others (types 6, 11, 42, 43, and 44). The test results are reported as high-risk or low-risk HPV DNA detected. There is no identification of the specific high-risk type or low-risk type. PCR-based assays for the detection and typing of HPV are mainly used in research laboratories; PCR-based methods are in commercial development for use in the clinical laboratory. There are three commercial kits currently available outside the United States. GenoID's kit, called GenoID Reveal HPV Real-Time HPV Detection Kit, is claimed to be the first commercially available real-time detection kit for HPV for clinical diagnostic use. The kit was announced in November 2005 by the Hungarian company GenoID. The PCR assay can be performed on a number of platforms (LightCycler, ABI 7700, etc.) and it detects all high-risk and low-risk HPV genotypes. BioCore, a South Korean company, produces two kits for PCR-based detection of HPV; one kit detects all clinically important HPV types, whereas the other is targeted specifically at the prevalent, clearly high-risk HPV types 16 and 18.

The hybrid capture 2 (HC2) test has been FDA-cleared for three indications: (1) aiding in the diagnosis of sexually transmitted HPV infections (high-risk and low-risk test), (2) testing of specimens from patients with ASCUS-grade cytology results to determine the need for colposcopy (high-risk test only), and (3) primary screening of women age 30 and older (high-risk test only). The recommended specimen types for HPV DNA testing include cervical swabs, liquid-based cytology specimens, and cervical biopsy specimens.

Several new approaches to HPV testing are under investigation that may provide more insight into identifying those women at highest risk of progressing to cervical cancer. These include assessing if there is prognostic value in determining HPV viral load and evaluating expression of HPV E6 and E7 messenger RNA (mRNA) as markers for viral persistence and disease progression.

Human Immunodeficiency Virus Type 1

HIV-1, the causative agent of AIDS, is an RNA virus belonging to the genus lentivirus of the family Retroviridae (retroviruses; in retroviruses, the genomic nucleic acid is RNA, which is copied to make DNA, which is the reverse of the usual direction). The replication of the virus is complex and involves reverse transcription of the RNA genome into a double-stranded DNA molecule, which is subsequently integrated into the host genome. The reverse-transcriptase enzyme does not have proofreading capabilities, leading to errors in making the copies and thus to the marked genetic diversity of HIV-1. There are three distinct genetic groups: the (1) major (M) group, (2) outlier (O) group, and (3) N (non-M, non-O) group. Viruses in the M group are further divided into subtypes or clades, designated A to D, F to H, J, and K based on the sequence diversity

within the HIV-1 *gag* and *env* genes. Group M virus is found worldwide, with clade B the predominant subtype in Europe and North America.

Complex replication cycles (involving RNA and DNA) and the high genetic diversity are two important factors that influence the design and interpretation of HIV-1 molecular assays.

Viral-Load Testing

The management of persons infected with human HIV-1 has been revolutionized by both viral-load and **resistance testing.** With these tools, it is possible to maximize the effectiveness of antiretroviral therapy for an individual. Viral-load testing became the standard of care around 1996, followed more recently by resistance testing. The clinical utility of viral-load testing (which refers to quantifying HIV-1 RNA, usually from plasma) has been well established. Testing is used to predict time to progression to AIDS, to determine when to initiate antiretroviral therapy, and to monitor response to therapy. Higher viral loads are associated with a more rapid progression to AIDS and death. Viral-load testing is used more routinely in decisions regarding when to initiate antiretroviral therapy and in monitoring response to therapy. Treatment guidelines are updated regularly (see http://www.aidsinfo.nih.gov [accessed March 12, 2007]) and recommend initiating therapy for individuals based on several factors, including CD4 cell count, viral loads, and symptoms.

The current standard for treating HIV-1–infected individuals is to use combinations of protease inhibitors (PIs) or nonnucleoside reverse-transcriptase inhibitors (NNRTIs) with nucleoside analogs. This combination therapy is often referred to as highly active antiretroviral therapy or HAART. Initial use of these effective drug combinations in individuals who have not been treated with them before ("naïve" individuals) is expected to decrease viral-load values by at least 2 $\log_{10}$ copies/mL (that is, to 1/100th of the starting load). The goal of therapy is to achieve viral-load values below the limit of detection of currently available assays (50 copies/mL). Achieving this goal is not always possible, particularly in individuals with very high pretreatment viral-load values or in those who have failed in prior therapeutic regimens. Guidelines for the use of HIV-1 RNA concentrations in clinical practice have been published and are frequently updated (http://www.aidsinfo.nih.gov/ [accessed March 12, 2007] and http://www.iasusa.org [accessed March 12, 2007]). In general, a plasma HIV-1 viral load should be measured before beginning therapy (baseline) and then again at 2 to 8 weeks after the initiation of therapy to determine the response to therapy. Testing is then repeated at 3- to 4-month intervals to evaluate continued effectiveness of the regimen. Any increase in viral load should be confirmed with repeat testing because a variety of other illnesses can transiently increase viral load. When a significant increase in viral load has been documented, HIV-1 resistance testing should be considered (see below).

Molecular assays are also useful in the diagnosis of acute HIV-1 infection in neonates in whom serological test results for anti-HIV antibodies may be misleadingly positive because of maternal IgG that crossed the placenta. Such seropositivity of an uninfected newborn of an HIV-positive mother may persist into the second year of life. Both qualitative proviral DNA tests and viral-load assays are useful for the diagnosis of HIV-1 infection in newborns, but viral-load assays are not FDA-approved for diagnosis, and there are no FDA-approved proviral DNA assays. The diagnosis of HIV-1 infection in a newborn requires testing at several different time points, usually shortly after birth and then again at 6 weeks to several months of age.

The use of HIV-1 viral-load testing for *diagnosing* acute HIV-1 infection in adults is more controversial. The currently available viral-load assays are approved only for use in patients known to be infected with HIV-1, but they have clear utility in the diagnosis of acute infection, which is defined as the period after exposure to the virus but before seroconversion. In this "window period," the enzyme-linked immunosorbent assay (ELISA) and Western blot assays are, by definition, negative or indeterminate, so additional testing is necessary. Individuals with acute infection are often symptomatic with a syndrome that resembles mononucleosis and may include fever, fatigue, rash, lymphadenopathy, and oral ulcers. During this acute infection, the plasma concentration of viral RNA is very high, usually 10^5 to 10^7 copies/mL, and viral-load measurements are a useful diagnostic tool. Acute HIV-1 infection should be suspected in an individual with appropriate symptoms and risk factors. In these individuals, testing for acute HIV-1 infection would include an ELISA and a viral-load assay. Care must be taken to correctly interpret these test results because individuals with acute HIV-1 infection would be expected to have a negative or indeterminate ELISA and/or Western blot result and a very high viral load (greater than 100,000 copies/mL). The concern with using viral-load testing to diagnose acute HIV infection is that false-positive results have been reported. In one study, the false-positive results were usually lower than 2000 copies/mL. Before diagnosing acute HIV infection, individuals must be educated regarding the limitations of these tests and must give informed consent to testing. To minimize the likelihood of reporting a false-positive result, repeat testing should be done on all specimens with a detectable viral load and HIV-1/2 ELISA should be obtained at the time of viral-load testing. It is critical to remember that patients with the acute retroviral syndrome should have very high concentrations of HIV-1 RNA. Recently, a qualitative HIV RNA assay has been approved by the FDA (APTIMA HIV-1 RNA, Gen-Probe), which may also be useful in the diagnosis of acute HIV infection.

Characteristics of HIV-1 viral-load assays that are currently FDA-approved are listed in Table 11-1. The lower limit of quantification differs among the three assays. The reportable concentration range of each of the Amplicor assays is limited, so both an ultrasensitive and a standard version of the test are needed to cover the clinically important range of viral-load values. Viral-load assays must be able to accurately quantify the various viral subtypes. In the United States and Europe, subtype B is the most common, though infections with non-B subtypes are becoming more common and are certainly an important cause of HIV-1 infection globally. The Versant bDNA assay will accurately quantify HIV-1 subtypes A thru G, and the Amplicor RT-PCR version 1.5 will accurately quantify subtypes A through H. The earlier Amplicor assay (version 1.0) underquantified non-B subtypes and has been replaced by the 1.5 assay version. The NucliSens nucleic acid sequence-based amplification (NASBA) assay underestimates concentrations of subtype G. None of the currently available assays is recommended for the quantification of group O virus. Viral-load values obtained with the different assays may not always agree, so it is recommended to choose one assay when monitoring patients over time.

TABLE 11-1	Characteristics of Quantitative HIV (Viral-Load) Assays Approved by the FDA*	
Test	**Amplification Method**	**Reportable Range**
Amplicor HIV Monitor v1.5 Test (Roche Diagnostics, Indianapolis, IN)	RT-PCR	Ultrasensitive: 50-100,000 copies/mL Standard: 400-750,000 copies/mL
Versant HIV-1 RNA 3.0 Assay (Bayer Diagnostics, Tarrytown, N.Y.)	bDNA	75-500,000 copies/mL
NucliSens HIV-1 QT Assay (bioMerieux, Durham, N.C.)	NASBA	176-3,470,000 copies/mL

RT-PCR, *Reverse transcriptase-polymerase chain reaction*; bDNA, *branched DNA*; NASBA, *nucleic acid sequence-based amplification.*
For FDA listings of these and any newer tests, visit http://www.accessdata.fda.gov/scripts/cdrh/cfdocs/cfRL/listing.cfm (accessed December 23, 2006) and use test code MTL.

The available viral-load assays have an intraassay imprecision (standard deviation) of approximately 0.18 $\log_{10}$ copies of HIV-1 RNA per mL at a concentration of 1500 copies/mL.[2] Based on this degree of analytical variation and on the typical day-to-day biological variation in a patient, changes in viral load should exceed 0.5 $\log_{10}$ (threefold change in number of copies/mL) to represent a biologically relevant change in viral replication. Reporting viral-load results as $\log_{10}$ copies/mL is recommended and will assist in preventing clinicians from overinterpreting small changes in viral load. This is particularly important for values near the limit of quantification, in which assay variability is the greatest. A variety of acute and opportunistic infections and vaccinations can transiently increase HIV-1 RNA in plasma, so it is recommended not to measure viral load for monitoring of individuals who are acutely ill and those who have been recently vaccinated.

Viral-load testing is routinely performed on plasma specimens, and ethylenediaminetetraacetic acid (EDTA) is the anticoagulant of choice. Acid citrate dextrose is also an acceptable anticoagulant, but for the Amplicor and Versant assays blood anticoagulated in heparin is unacceptable because heparin inhibits the reactions. It is critical to handle clinical specimens properly to minimize the risk of RNA degradation during specimen collection and transport. Plasma should be separated within 6 hours of collection and ideally stored at −20 °C, although plasma viral RNA is stable at 4 °C for several days. For laboratories performing testing from specimens collected at remote sites, VACUTAINER Plasma Preparation Tubes (PPTs) can be useful. The tube is centrifuged at the collection site (opalescent white; see Table 3-2). A gel provides a physical barrier between the plasma and cells, and tubes can be shipped without the need to transfer the plasma into a separate tube.

Resistance Testing

Four general classes of antiretroviral drugs are used in clinical care: (1) nucleoside reverse-transcriptase inhibitors (NRTIs),

NNRTIs, (3) PIs, and (4) a new class of drug, fusion inhibitors. Viral resistance can occur with each of these classes of drug, particularly when viral replication is not maximally suppressed during therapy. The current standard of care is to use regimens that contain a combination of drugs, usually a PI or NNRTIs with several NRTIs, because resistance is less likely to occur on the complex regimens than on monotherapy.

A variety of studies have evaluated the clinical utility of antiviral resistance testing in HIV-1–infected individuals, and most though not all have shown clinical utility of resistance testing compared with choosing therapy based on previously used drugs. Guidelines for the appropriate use of HIV-1 resistance testing in adults have been established by an International AIDS Society-USA panel of experts.[16] Resistance testing is recommended in patients who are failing on an initial antiretroviral regimen and in those failing after numerous regimens. In addition, resistance testing is recommended before initiating therapy for patients who have been infected within the previous 2 years. Resistance testing is also recommended in pregnant women to optimize treatment and in hopes of minimizing transmission of HIV-1 infection to the neonate. As it is possible to transmit drug-resistant virus, it is also recommended that resistance testing be done on patients who first come to medical attention with acute or recent (within 12 months) HIV-1 infection, particularly if the person from whom HIV-1 was acquired ("source patient") is known and is receiving antiretroviral therapy.

Genotypic assays identify specific mutations or nucleotide changes that are associated with a decreased susceptibility to an antiviral drug and are performed in clinical laboratories by automated sequencing techniques. The effective use of genotypic resistance testing requires an extensive understanding of the genetics of antiretroviral resistance. The currently available assays will detect mutations in the reverse-transcriptase and protease genes; modifications of existing assays are under way to detect the resistance mutations associated with fusion inhibitors.

The initial step in genotypic assays is the isolation of HIV-1 RNA from plasma, followed by RT-PCR amplification and sequencing of the reverse-transcriptase and protease genes. The analysis of the results involves sequence alignment and editing, mutation identification by comparison with a wild-type sequence, and interpretation of the clinical significance of the mutations identified. Most clinical laboratories performing genotypic resistance testing rely on commercial assays that provide reagents and software programs to assist with the interpretation of the results. Two assays have been cleared by the FDA, the Trugene HIV-1 Genotyping Kit and OpenGene DNA Sequencing System (Bayer Diagnostics Corp., Tarrytown, N.Y.) and the ViroSeq HIV-1 Genotyping System (Celera Diagnostics/Abbott Molecular, Des Plaines, Ill.). In addition to these commercial assays, several laboratories have developed automated-cycle sequencing assays for HIV-1 resistance testing.

The interpretation of genotypic resistance testing is complex. The interpretation of resistance mutations uses "rules-based" software that takes into account cross-resistance and interactions of mutations. The commercially available systems generate a summary report that lists the various mutations that have been identified in the reverse-transcriptase and protease genes, and each drug is reported as resistant, pos-

sibly resistant, no evidence of resistance, or insufficient evidence. A comprehensive discussion of the specific mutations associated with each antiretroviral drug and the interactions of mutations is beyond the scope of this chapter, but is available from a variety of sources[16] including the following Web sites: http://hiv.lanl.gov/content/index (accessed March 12, 2007) and http://www.iasusa.org (accessed March 12, 2007).

Phenotypic resistance assays measure viral replication in the presence of antiretroviral drugs. Results of phenotypic assays are typically reported as the inhibitory concentration of a drug that reduces in vitro HIV-1 replication by 50% (IC_{50}). The IC_{50} is usually reported as the fold change in IC_{50} relative to a wild-type strain. Initially, phenotypic assays required the isolation of infectious HIV-1 from a blood specimen. Newer phenotypic assays use high-throughput automated assays based on recombinant DNA technology. For these assays, HIV-1 RNA is amplified from a plasma specimen, eliminating the need for a viral isolate. The RNA is inserted into a virus that is grown in the presence and absence of each tested antiviral drug. This testing is not performed in clinical laboratories, and the technology is available from only two commercial laboratories (Monogram Biosciences, San Francisco, Calif. and Antivirogram, Virco, Mechelen, Belgium). Results are reported as a fold change in IC_{50} for the patient specimen compared with wild-type virus. A "virtual phenotype" is also available commercially for assessing HIV-1 drug resistance. With a virtual phenotype, rather than performing a phenotypic assay directly, the information is inferred from the genotypic assay. The results of the genotypic assay are entered into a database containing matching genotypic and phenotypic results from thousands of clinical specimens, and the closest matching phenotypic results are averaged and reported as the virtual phenotype.

Both phenotypic and genotypic assays are used in clinical care: some clinicians prefer phenotypic testing because it is a direct measure of viral susceptibility, whereas others prefer genotypic testing because the development of a mutation may precede phenotypic expression of resistance. Other advantages of genotypic testing include relatively rapid turnaround time (a few days), easier availability, and lower cost than phenotypic testing. Providers often use genotypic testing routinely and rely on phenotypic testing for patients who have failed multiple regimens and have very complex genotypic results. If both assays are used, it is key to remember that the results of the two assays may not agree because the presence of a resistance mutation does not ensure its expression in a phenotypic assay.

A limitation of the currently used genotypic and phenotypic assays is that they can detect only those mutants that make up at least 20% of the total viral population. Regimens chosen based on resistance testing may not always be effective because, when the drug acts on the sensitive majority population of virus, a minority viral population that was not detected and was not sensitive to the drug will quickly become the majority population. Drug selection pressure is also needed for some resistance mutations to persist at detectable concentrations in the viral population. When the drug therapy is discontinued, the wild-type virus may quickly predominate. For this reason, it is recommended that specimens for resistance testing be obtained while the patient is on antiretroviral therapy.

The minimum viral load required for reliable resistance testing is approximately 1000 copies/mL. Because genotyping assays are especially sensitive to RNA degradation, care must be taken to properly handle the specimen after collection. Guidelines outlined for collection and transport of specimens for testing in viral-load assays should be followed for resistance testing.

Herpes Simplex Virus

Herpes simplex virus (HSV), a member of the herpesvirus family, is a double-stranded DNA virus. Following primary infection, the virus remains latent in sensory neurons and can be reactivated under a variety of situations, including stress, trauma, sun exposure, and various immunocompromised states. HSV types 1 and 2 produce various clinical syndromes involving the skin, eye, central nervous system (CNS), and genital tract. Although nucleic acid testing has been used to detect HSV DNA in all of these clinical manifestations, this discussion will focus on the use of HSV PCR for the diagnosis of CNS infections since nucleic acid amplification testing is widely viewed as the standard of care for the diagnosis of these infections.

HSV causes both encephalitis and meningitis[26]; in adults, HSV encephalitis is usually caused by infection with HSV type 1, and HSV meningitis is most commonly caused by HSV type 2. HSV encephalitis is a severe infection with a high morbidity and mortality; treatment with acyclovir reduces the mortality from approximately 70% in untreated infections to 19% to 28%. Neurological impairment, however, is common (about 50%) in those who survive.[26] HSV encephalitis may reflect primary infection or reactivation of latent infection. HSV meningitis is usually a self-limited disease that resolves during the course of several days without therapy. In some patients, the disease may recur as a lymphocytic meningitis over a period of years.

Neonatal HSV infection occurs in 1:3500 to 1:5000 deliveries in the United States.[26] It is most commonly acquired by intrapartum contact with infected maternal genital secretions and is usually caused by HSV type 2. In the newborn, there are three general presentations of the disease: (1) skin, eye, and mouth disease accounts for approximately 45% of infections, (2) encephalitis accounts for 35%, and (3) disseminated disease accounts for 20%. As disseminated disease is often associated with neurological disease, CNS disease occurs in about 50% of newborns with neonatal HSV infection.

HSV encephalitis cannot be distinguished clinically from encephalitis caused by other viruses, such as West Nile virus, St. Louis encephalitis virus, and eastern equine encephalitis virus. Historically the gold standard for the diagnosis of HSV encephalitis required brain biopsy with identification of HSV by cell culture or immunohistochemical staining. This approach provided high diagnostic sensitivity (estimated to be 99%) and diagnostic specificity (approximately 100%), but it required an invasive procedure, and several days elapsed before results were available. Cell culture of cerebrospinal fluid (CSF) has a diagnostic sensitivity of less than 10% for the diagnosis of HSV encephalitis in adults. Tests that measure HSV antigen or antibody in CSF have diagnostic sensitivities of 75% to 85% and diagnostic specificities of 60% to 90%.[26] Because of the limitations of conventional methods, there was interest in assessing the clinical utility of PCR for the detection of HSV DNA from the CSF of patients with encephalitis.

A key study compared HSV PCR on CSF specimens with a brain biopsy[20] in patients with suspected HSV encephalitis. The diagnostic sensitivity and specificity of PCR were greater than 95%, and the diagnostic sensitivity of HSV PCR did not decrease significantly until 5 to 7 days after start of therapy. PCR is positive early in the course of illness, usually within the first 24 hours of symptoms, and in some individuals, HSV DNA can persist in the CSF for weeks after initiating therapy.[20]

The clinical utility of HSV PCR has also been established for the diagnosis of neonatal HSV infection. In one study,[17] HSV DNA was detected in the CSF of 76% (26 of 34) of infants with CNS disease, 94% (13 of 14) with disseminated infection, and 24% (7 of 29) with skin, eye, or mouth disease. The persistence of HSV DNA in the CSF of newborns for greater than 1 week after initiating therapy is associated with a poor outcome.

Detection of HSV DNA in CSF by PCR has become the standard of care for the diagnosis of HSV encephalitis and neonatal HSV infection. In newborns with disseminated disease, HSV DNA may be detected in serum or plasma specimens and can be a useful diagnostic tool in newborns if it is not possible to do a lumbar puncture. Though the diagnostic sensitivity of HSV PCR is high, it is not 100%, so a negative PCR test result may not rule out HSV as the cause of disease, particularly if the pretest probability is high. In this situation, it is important to consider repeat testing.

As with HSV encephalitis, HSV meningitis cannot be distinguished clinically from other viral meningitides, although recurrence of viral meningitis is a strong clue that HSV may be the etiological agent. Unlike HSV encephalitis, HSV meningitis has not been the subject of large studies evaluating the clinical utility of PCR for diagnosis. Nonetheless, because the diagnostic sensitivity of cell culture of CSF specimens is only approximately 50%, HSV PCR of CSF is commonly used in the evaluation of meningitis and considered the gold standard.

Currently there are no FDA-cleared assays for the detection of HSV DNA from clinical specimens, and the performance characteristics of existing assays may vary. There are analyte-specific reagents (ASRs) available, including the LightCycler assay (Roche Diagnostics, Indianapolis), which is designed for the detection of HSV DNA types 1 and 2. Distinguishing between HSV types 1 and 2 may not be necessary because the clinical management is the same for both infections. Primers used for the detection of HSV DNA commonly target the polymerase, glycoprotein B, glycoprotein D, or thymidine kinase genes. It is important that the primers not amplify DNA from other herpesviruses that are associated with neurological disease; these include cytomegalovirus (CMV), varicella zoster virus, human herpesvirus type 6, and Epstein-Barr virus.

HSV PCR assays need low detection limits (several hundred copies per milliliter of specimen) to be useful in evaluation of neurological disease. This is particularly true for the diagnosis of meningitis in which CSF concentrations of DNA tend to be lower than those seen with encephalitis. HSV neurological disease rarely occurs without an increased CSF white blood cell count or protein concentration.[24] Caution should be exercised in applying this generalization to immunocompromised individuals, however, because they may not mount a typical inflammatory response to HSV infection. Although PCR of CSF specimens is clearly the gold standard for the diagnosis of HSV-related neurological disease, results should be interpreted with caution since neither diagnostic sensitivity nor diagnostic specificity is 100%. Test results should always be interpreted within the context of the clinical presentation of the patient. If results do not correlate with the clinical impression, repeat testing should be performed.

Enteroviruses

Enteroviruses are a diverse group of single-stranded RNA viruses belonging to the Picornaviridae family. The group includes polioviruses, enteroviruses types A through D, and parechovirus (human echovirus). Numerous clinical presentations are seen with the nonpolioviruses, including acute aseptic meningitis, encephalitis, exanthems, conjunctivitis, acute respiratory disease, gastrointestinal disease, myopericarditis, and a sepsislike syndrome in neonates. Diagnoses have been based on clinical presentation or culture methods or both. Cell culture methods have several drawbacks, including (1) the requirement to inoculate multiple cell lines because no single cell line is optimal for all enterovirus types; (2) the inability to grow some enterovirus types in cell culture; (3) the limited diagnostic sensitivity of cell culture (65% to 75%); and (4) the long turnaround time of 3 to 8 days for those enteroviruses that do grow in a cell culture. The long turnaround time for the culture means that results are rarely available in a time frame to influence clinical management. Nucleic acid testing offers several important advantages over cell culture, including improved analytical and diagnostic sensitivity and shorter turnaround time. As a result, nucleic acid testing is considered the new gold standard for the diagnosis of aseptic meningitis and neonatal sepsis syndrome caused by the enteroviruses.

Two methods are used for the detection of enteroviral RNA from clinical specimens: RT-PCR and NASBA (see Chapter 5). The primers used in clinical testing most commonly target the highly conserved 5'-untranslated region of the gene (5'UTR) and will detect polioviruses and enteroviruses. These primers will not detect echovirus types 22 and 23, which have been reclassified as parechoviruses, although these viruses can cause aseptic meningitis. In general, molecular assays are very sensitive and quite specific, although sequence similarities may allow amplification of some types of rhinoviruses. As with HSV, there is no FDA-cleared assay for the detection of enterovirus RNA from clinical specimens. Several ASRs are available for detection of enterovirus RNA from CSF specimens to assist laboratorians in assay development.

The clinical utility of nucleic acid testing for the diagnosis of enteroviral infections has been documented in a variety of clinical studies, with the testing showing a diagnostic sensitivity equal to or greater than that of cell culture, a high diagnostic specificity, and faster turnaround time than cell culture. Several studies have suggested that the introduction of molecular methods for the diagnosis of enteroviral infections in infants and pediatric patients can lead to cost savings in other parts of the hospital because of the decreased length of hospital stay, reduction in the use of antibiotics, and reduction in imaging studies. The cost savings may be small, however, because the durations of hospital stay and antibiotic use are limited, with or without enterovirus testing, for patients with viral meningitis. To maximize the benefit to patient care and cost savings, testing should be available daily.

As mentioned above, many molecular assays detect rhinoviruses, and most will detect polioviruses. These two factors can lead to unexpected and misleading positive results when testing respiratory or stool specimens. The diagnosis of enterovirus meningitis should be based on testing of CSF specimens, whereas investigation of suspected sepsis syndrome in the neonate is best made by testing serum, plasma, or CSF samples.

Perinatal Group B Streptococcal Disease

In the 1970s Group B streptococcal (GBS) disease was the leading infectious cause of neonatal morbidity and mortality, with case rates of 2 to 3 per 1000 live births and case-fatality rates as high as 50%.[9] In 1996, consensus guidelines from the CDC, the American Academy of Pediatrics, and the American College of Obstetrics and Gynecology were issued in an effort to reduce the rate of GBS disease in newborns.[9] The guidelines called for use of intrapartum prophylactic antibiotics for GBS using either a risk-based or screening-based approach. In the risk-based approach, antibiotics were administered based on the identification of one of the following risk factors: intrapartum fever, prolonged rupture of membranes, or imminent preterm delivery. For the screening-based approach, vaginal and/or rectal cultures were collected at 35 to 37 weeks of gestation, and those women with positive cultures received intrapartum antibiotics. Since the widespread implementation of these guidelines, the number of cases of GBS disease has decreased, but GBS remains a serious cause of neonatal infection. GBS disease in the newborn is classified as either early disease, which occurs within 1 week of life and usually presents as a sepsis syndrome or pneumonia, or late disease, which is defined as that presenting at greater than 1 week of life and presenting most commonly as sepsis or meningitis.

GBS colonization of pregnant women is common, with a prevalence of 10% to 30%; colonization may be transient, chronic, or intermittent.[9] Those women who are colonized are 25 times more likely to deliver infants with early onset GBS disease.[9] The effectiveness of the 1996 guidelines for the prevention of neonatal GBS was recently reevaluated, and it was determined that the screening approach to GBS prevention was greater than 50% more effective than the risk-based approach. Based on these findings, in 2002 the CDC issued updated guidelines recommending that vaginal and/or rectal GBS screening cultures be done on all pregnant women. The exceptions included women with a previous infant that had GBS disease or those with GBS bacteriuria during pregnancy because these women require intrapartum antibiotics. The risk-based approach is to be used only for women with unknown GBS status at the time of labor and delivery. See the CDC guidelines[9] for a more detailed description and refer to the CDC Web site for updates (http://www.cdc.gov/, accessed March 12, 2007).

Methods for GBS screening cultures have been standardized and include collection of a vaginal and/or rectal swab and transport to the laboratory in either Amies or Stuart media. The specimen is then inoculated into an enrichment broth (LIM broth), incubated for 18 to 24 hours, and then subcultured onto a sheep's-blood agar plate. GBS is then identified based on colony morphology, hemolysis, and latex agglutination testing. This two-step method ensures maximal sensitivity for GBS detection. GBS cultures usually require 2 to 3 days to complete. Since GBS is universally susceptible to penicillin and ampicillin, antimicrobial susceptibility testing is not routinely performed, but is needed for women with a serious allergy to penicillin.

A recent study evaluated the clinical utility of using a real-time PCR assay for the detection of GBS in pregnant women.[1] A real-time PCR assay was compared with cultures in 112 pregnant women and was found to have a diagnostic sensitivity of 97%, a diagnostic specificity of 100%, and negative and positive predictive values of 98.8% and 100%, respectively. Testing results were available within 45 minutes of the time the specimen arrived in the laboratory, which raised the possibility of offering real-time testing to women who are in labor. This could be especially useful for women who are seen with an unknown GBS status; based on current guidelines, these women would receive intrapartum antibiotics based on risk factors. Because women without risk factors are still at risk of delivering newborns with GBS disease, PCR testing would undoubtedly offer a more sensitive method for GBS detection than one based on risk factors alone. In addition, intrapartum testing would be useful in identifying women whose GBS status changes in the interval between screening culture (weeks 35 to 37 of gestation) and the time of delivery.

Recently a real-time PCR assay was cleared by the FDA (IDI-Strep B using the Cepheid SmartCycler, Infection Diagnostic Inc., Quebec) for the detection of GBS from vaginal and/or rectal swabs in pregnant women. In a multicenter clinical trial, the IDI-Strep B test demonstrated a diagnostic sensitivity of 94% and a diagnostic specificity of 96% compared with intrapartum culture (IDI-Strep B package insert). The assay requires a few simple hands-on steps to prepare the specimen. The testing cartridge is then inserted into the SmartCycler, and testing is complete in less than 1 hour. The test also includes an internal control to monitor for inhibition of amplification. The IDI-Strep B test offers a rapid and sensitive alternative to GBS culture. More recently another real-time assay for the detection of GBS has been cleared by the FDA (Cepheid, Sunnyvale, CA). The advantages of these molecular assays need to be balanced with the challenge of providing intrapartum test results to clinicians within 1 to 2 hours at any time of day or night, and the cost of nucleic acid testing must be compared with the cost of culture. If intrapartum testing is done, there will not be adequate time for erythromycin and clindamycin susceptibility testing, so women with severe penicillin allergies will require therapy with vancomycin. An alternative approach is to replace antepartum culture at 35 to 37 weeks of gestation with the real-time PCR assay. With the availability of an FDA-cleared test, there will be more discussion on the use of GBS PCR testing of pregnant women.

Cytomegalovirus

CMV, a member of the herpesvirus family, is a double-stranded enveloped DNA virus. CMV causes a clinically minor infection in immunocompetent individuals, but remains an important pathogen in immunocompromised individuals, including persons with AIDS, transplant recipients, and those on immune-modulating drugs. Primary infection is usually asymptomatic in immunocompetent persons, though a small percentage of individuals with CMV infection may develop a mononucleosis type of syndrome. Following the primary infection, a lifelong latent infection is established, which does not cause clinical symptoms. However, if an infected individual becomes immunocompromised, the virus can reactivate, leading to a wide variety of clinical syndromes.

The most severe CMV infections are seen in those individuals who acquire their primary infection while immunocompromised. In persons with AIDS, CMV disease rarely occurs when the CD4 cell count is above 100 cells/mm; the most common clinical presentations are retinitis, esophagitis, and colitis. In transplant recipients, the occurrence and severity of CMV disease are related to the CMV serostatus of the organ donor and recipient, the type of organ transplanted, and the overall degree of immunosuppression. For example, CMV disease tends to be more severe in lung transplant recipients than in renal transplant recipients. For all types of organ recipients, the most severe disease occurs when a CMV-seronegative recipient receives an organ from a CMV-seropositive donor, and the primary CMV infection occurs while the person is immunosuppressed. CMV disease can also occur in seropositive individuals whether they receive an organ from a seropositive or seronegative donor. The clinical findings associated with CMV disease in transplant recipients are diverse and include interstitial pneumonitis, esophagitis and colitis, fever, leukopenia, and less commonly, retinitis and encephalitis.

The diagnosis of CMV disease represents a challenge because of the presence of the latent infection. Immunocompromised individuals can have an asymptomatic, clinically insignificant, low-level, persistent infection that must be distinguished from clinically important active CMV disease. The distinction can be challenging when using sensitive molecular assays that can detect small amounts of CMV DNA in clinical specimens.

Traditionally the diagnosis of CMV disease relied on the detection of CMV from clinical specimens by use of cell culture techniques in human diploid fibroblasts. Though considered the gold standard, these conventional culture methods are labor intensive and have a long turnaround time of 1 to 3 weeks. In addition, the assays lack adequate analytical sensitivity for detecting CMV present in blood specimens. The rapid shell-vial culture method can provide results in 1 to 2 days and is useful for detection of CMV in tissue, respiratory, and urine specimens. However, this assay may also fail to detect CMV in blood. Many laboratories rely on the antigenemia assay, which detects the matrix protein pp65 in polymorphonuclear cells. This semiquantitative assay is rapid, and the number of CMV antigen-positive cells correlates with the likelihood of CMV disease, but the assay is labor intensive, and CMV antigen is not stable in whole blood specimens for periods of greater than 24 hours.

In light of the limitations of culture and antigen-detection methods, there has been great interest in using nucleic acid testing for the detection and quantification of CMV DNA from plasma and blood specimens. The two qualitative assays that have been cleared by the FDA for detection of CMV from blood specimens are the Hybrid Capture System CMV DNA test (version 2) (Digene Corp., Gaithersburg, Md.) and the NucliSens CMV test (bioMerieux, Durham, N.C.). The Hybrid Capture assay (Chapter 5) is a signal-amplification assay that detects CMV DNA in whole blood specimens. The NucliSens assay uses NASBA technology (Chapter 5) to detect pp67 late mRNA in whole blood specimens. The isothermal NASBA assay detects pp67 RNA but not CMV DNA, eliminating concerns about detection of DNA in latent infection. Quantitative molecular CMV assays that are available include the Hybrid Capture assay mentioned above and the Amplicor CMV MONITOR test (Roche Diagnostics, Indianapolis), a DNA PCR assay (neither of which has been cleared by the FDA). In addition to using commercially available assays, many laboratories have developed assays, so-called **laboratory-developed tests** (LDTs), that use standard and real-time PCR methods for CMV. These LDTs use various specimen types, nucleic acid extraction methods, target genes, calibrators, and detection methods. As a result, viral-load values obtained with the different assays may not always agree. This makes it difficult to compare results among clinical studies that use these assays and to establish concentrations of CMV DNA that correlate with clinical disease.

The analytical performances have been evaluated for the Amplicor PCR and Hybrid Capture assays. The imprecision (expressed as standard deviations) of the assays ranges from 0.11 to 0.48 $\log_{10}$, with greater variability seen below 1000 copies/mL (3.0 $\log_{10}$ copies/mL).[4,7] In general, the Amplicor assay is more reproducible than the Hybrid Capture assay. Based on these data, changes in viral load (copies per milliliter) less than threefold to fivefold may represent assay variability rather than clinically relevant changes in viral replication.

An unsettled issue for CMV molecular assays is the appropriate specimen type for testing. Almost all assays use either plasma or whole blood, with concentrations of CMV DNA measured in whole blood higher than those measured in plasma. Because pp67 RNA is intracellular, the NucliSens assay uses whole blood samples. Likewise the Hybrid Capture assay has been designed to measure CMV DNA in whole blood specimens. The Amplicor PCR assay can accommodate blood or plasma specimens. CMV DNA may be detected in whole blood or leukocytes of individuals without active CMV disease. Some studies have shown a good association between high CMV DNA concentrations in plasma and active CMV disease[6] and suggest that detecting CMV DNA in plasma rather than in leukocytes may provide a better correlation with clinical disease because the detection of CMV DNA in plasma suggests active viral replication. However, it is clear that CMV DNA can also be detected in the plasma of patients without active CMV disease.[5,6] In addition to specimen type, assay format may be useful in distinguishing active disease from asymptomatic infection. For example, the pp67 mRNA detected in the NucliSens assay is expressed in high concentrations in patients with active disease and is not expressed during latent infection. This has been supported in studies that have shown that the NucliSens assay is positive less frequently than assays that detect CMV DNA. For CMV DNA-based assays, correlation with clinical disease requires quantifying CMV DNA to establish a concentration of CMV DNA that correlates with the likelihood of disease. The concentration of DNA that predicts disease will be higher in assays that use whole blood specimens than in those that test plasma specimens.

The clinical uses of CMV molecular assays are diverse and include assisting in decisions regarding initiating preemptive therapy, diagnosis of active CMV disease, and monitoring response to therapy. **Preemptive therapy** refers to the use of a laboratory test to identify a group of individuals at higher risk for developing CMV disease. For example, all members of the group would be tested for the presence of CMV DNA in their blood or plasma, and only those testing positive would be treated. Therapy is administered before development of symptoms in an attempt to prevent the development of active disease. By contrast, with **prophylactic therapy**, all patients in the group are treated, without further stratification of risk, thus involving treatment of a greater number of patients.

Molecular assays have utility for the diagnosis of active CMV disease because CMV DNA concentrations are higher in patients with active CMV disease than in those with asymptomatic infection. A study in liver transplant recipients using the Amplicor PCR assay showed that the median peak viral load in patients with asymptomatic infection was 1850 copies/mL compared with 55,000 copies/mL for those with active disease. The viral-load cutoff that was most predictive of the development of active disease was between 2000 and 5000 copies/mL of plasma.[16a] A similar study in renal transplant recipients using the Hybrid Capture assay showed that the risk of developing CMV disease increased from 1.5% with a viral load of 10,000 copies/mL of blood to 73% when the viral load was 1 million copies/mL of blood. It is important to note that the viral-load cutoffs differed in the two studies because of the use of different assays and differences in specimen type (plasma versus whole blood).

Once active CMV disease has been diagnosed, molecular assays are useful in monitoring response to therapy. Viral-load values decrease rapidly after beginning appropriate antiviral therapy, and several studies have reported that CMV DNA is cleared from the plasma within several weeks of initiating therapy.[5,6] Failure of viral loads to decrease promptly should raise concerns of possible treatment failure because persistently elevated concentrations of CMV DNA during therapy have been seen in patients with documented resistance of CMV to the therapy.[5] Molecular assays also have clinical utility in identifying patients at risk of relapsing CMV infection. In solid-organ transplant recipients, patients with a detectable viral load after completing 14 days of ganciclovir therapy for CMV infection are at increased risk of relapse. Similarly, an increased risk of relapse has been shown for patients with persistent pp67 mRNA after completing a course of therapy. The rate of decline in CMV DNA after initiating therapy can be used to predict risk of relapse of CMV infection. In one study, CMV DNA was cleared from the plasma in 17 days for patients without recurrent CMV disease compared with 34 days for those with evidence of recurrent disease.[16b] By following viral-load concentrations weekly after initiating antiviral therapy, it may be possible to identify those at risk of recurrent disease and thus intensify therapy and possibly prevent recurrent disease.

CMV DNA concentrations are also useful in assessing the risk of developing CMV disease in persons with AIDS. Detection of CMV DNA in plasma has been associated with an increased risk of developing CMV disease and an increased risk of death. In addition, each $\log_{10}$ increase in viral load (i.e., each tenfold increase in concentration) has been associated with a threefold increase in the risk of developing CMV disease. The clinical importance of CMV viral load in patients was further established in patients with advanced AIDS in whom the CMV DNA load was found to be more predictive of developing CMV disease or death than HIV-1 viral load. Individuals with a CD4 cell count of less than 50 cells/mm and an HIV-1 viral load of greater than 10,000 copies/mL of plasma are at greatest risk of developing end-organ CMV disease. In this group of individuals, a rise in CMV DNA above the limit of detection of either the Hybrid Capture or Amplicor PCR assays was associated with the development of CMV end-organ disease. This study identifies a group of HIV-1–infected individuals that may benefit from monitoring CMV viral load and preemptive therapy for the prevention of CMV end-organ disease.

A major challenge that remains for laboratories offering these assays is the difference in results among assays. A well-characterized CMV DNA standard reference material for use in calibrating the assays could greatly assist in achieving agreement of viral-load values among different tests, thus facilitating the determination of CMV concentrations that predict or correspond to clinical events.

Mycobacterium tuberculosis

Mycobacterium tuberculosis (MTb) causes a wide range of clinical infections, including pulmonary disease, miliary tuberculosis, meningitis, pleurisy, pericarditis, peritonitis, gastrointestinal disease, genitourinary disease, and lymphadenitis. MTb infection was in steady decline in the United States until the late 1980s into the early 1990s, when the number of reported cases began to increase. This resurgence in the number of infections was related to the AIDS epidemic, homelessness, and a decreased focus on tuberculosis control programs. By the late 1990s, the infection rate had declined to an all time low. One group in which the infection rate continues to rise is foreign-born persons; the rise is due to immigration from countries with a high prevalence of MTb infections. This increase in MTb infections focused considerable attention on the development of assays for the rapid diagnosis of MTb infections, and molecular methods were at the center of this effort. The goal was to design very sensitive assays that would allow for the direct detection of MTb from clinical specimens. However, this goal has proven to be more difficult to reach than originally anticipated.

The standard methods for detection of MTb include acid-fast bacilli (AFB) smear and conventional and liquid culture methods. The AFB smear is rapid, but has a poor diagnostic sensitivity of 20% to 80%. Another challenge with the AFB smear is that it cannot distinguish MTb from nontuberculous mycobacteria (NTM), such as *Mycobacterium avium*-complex (MAC). This distinction is important because disseminated MAC and MTb are both common infections in persons with AIDS. Culture methods for the detection of MTb are sensitive, but growth detectable by standard methods may require 6 to 8 weeks in a culture. Growth often occurs more quickly in liquid culture than with conventional methods, but can still require 1 to 3 weeks. With these limitations of culture methods, there was great enthusiasm for nucleic acid testing as a rapid, sensitive method for detection of MTb, especially given the needs to rapidly isolate patients with active, untreated disease and to initiate prompt therapy, particularly in immunocompromised hosts.

Two nucleic acid amplification tests have been approved by the FDA for detection of MTb from clinical specimens: the Amplified (MTD® *Mycobacterium tuberculosis* Direct) Test (Gen-Probe, Inc., San Diego), and the Amplicor *Mycobacterium tuberculosis* Test (Roche Diagnostics, Indianapolis). The MTD test is based on transcription-mediated amplification of ribosomal RNA. The Amplicor test is based on PCR technology and the target is the 16S ribosomal RNA gene. The MTD test

has broader clinical applications because it can be used to test both AFB smear–positive and smear-negative respiratory specimens. The Amplicor test is approved only for AFB smear–positive respiratory specimens. Neither assay has been approved for nonrespiratory specimens, which limits their clinical utility for diagnosis of extrapulmonary MTb infections. This is unfortunate because diagnosis of some of these infections is often difficult. In addition to these commercially available assays, LDTs are widely used, and a key advantage of these assays is the ability to test respiratory and nonrespiratory specimens.

Both the MTD test and the Amplicor test have a diagnostic sensitivity of 95% to 98% when using AFB smear–positive respiratory specimens, and the specificity ranges from 99% to 100%. However, early studies showed that the diagnostic sensitivity for AFB smear–negative specimens was ~50%. Based on these data, it was clear that the test could not be used to rule out MTb infection on smear-negative respiratory specimens. This further limited the clinical utility of these tests because it became clear that the nucleic acid testing would be used to supplement the AFB smear and culture rather than replace these testing modalities. Another limitation of the currently available nucleic acid assays is that they can be used only on specimens from patients who had not received antituberculosis therapy within the past 12 months. This limitation was included because DNA can persist in respiratory secretions (and other body fluids) for months after the mycobacteria are no longer viable.

The MTD test was subsequently reformulated and evaluated in a clinical trial comparing this test with a culture and to the probability of MTb infection as determined by a panel of experts. The diagnostic sensitivity and specificity of the test were 86% and 98%, respectively. The positive and negative predictive values were 91% and 97%, respectively. Based on this study, the reformulated MTD test was approved by the FDA for use on both AFB smear–positive and AFB smear–negative specimens. The CDC has established guidelines for the use of nucleic acid testing on respiratory specimens.[8,11] Patients with a positive AFB smear and a positive nucleic acid testing result should be presumed to have MTb infection, and there is no need for additional nucleic acid testing. If the sputum smear is AFB positive, if two or three specimens are negative by nucleic acid testing, and if inhibition of amplification has been ruled out, then the patient can be presumed to have NTM infection. If the sputum specimen is AFB smear–negative and repeatedly positive by the MTD test (Note: the Amplicor test is not approved for use with smear-negative samples), then the patient can be presumed to have MTb infection. For patients with an AFB-negative smear, a negative nucleic acid test result does not rule out MTb infection.

A key consideration with molecular assays is controlling for inhibition of amplification. This is particularly critical for the detection of MTb nucleic acid from respiratory specimens because these specimen types often contain blood or glycoprotein, which can inhibit amplification. The Amplicor assay contains an internal control, and a negative result can be reported only if the internal control is detected. The MTD test does not contain an inhibition control, though many laboratories include such a control by adding a positive control material to a second aliquot of the clinical specimen.

An important role for molecular assays is in the diagnosis of extrapulmonary MTb infections, such as meningitis, pleuritis, pericarditis, or peritonitis, because these infections can be very difficult to diagnose by traditional methods. The MTD and Amplicor tests have been used on CSF specimens for the diagnosis of MTb meningitis, although the tests have not been approved by the FDA for this indication. In addition, PCR LDTs have been developed with the flexibility needed to test a variety of clinical specimens. As mentioned for respiratory specimens, it is critical to remember that a negative nucleic acid test result does not rule out extrapulmonary MTb infection, and molecular assays using these complex body fluids should include an inhibition control.

Though there are considerable limitations to the currently available nucleic acid tests for the detection of MTb infection, they have a role in the clinical laboratory in that they can provide a rapid diagnosis. The goal would be to develop assays with a higher diagnostic sensitivity (>99%) for AFB smear–negative specimens because this may eliminate the need to culture specimens that are negative when tested in nucleic acid assays.

Hepatitis C Virus

HCV, an RNA virus, is a major cause of chronic liver disease. According to the National Health and Nutrition Examination Survey (NHANES) of 1988–1994, approximately 4 million Americans were infected with HCV, and 2.7 million were estimated to have chronic infection. After acute infection, 80% to 85% of individuals develop a chronic infection, and 2% to 4% of these individuals develop cirrhosis and end-stage liver disease, making end-stage liver disease secondary to HCV the most common indication for liver transplantation in the United States. The development of molecular testing for HCV infection has been a major advance in the clinical care of infected individuals because the virus cannot be grown in a culture.

Detection and Quantification of HCV RNA

The applications of HCV RNA testing include assisting in the diagnosis of HCV infection, excluding HCV infection as the etiological agent of symptoms, screening the blood supply, and monitoring response to therapy and determining the duration of therapy. Qualitative molecular assays are used to confirm the diagnosis of HCV infection, which is particularly important in distinguishing seropositive individuals who have cleared the infection from seropositive persons who have chronic infection. Individuals who have cleared the infection will not have detectable RNA, whereas those with persistent infection will have detectable RNA. Recent data from the CDC have shown that 95% of positive results of screening ELISA that have a high signal-to-cutoff ratio (s/co) are confirmed as true positives. For these specimens, confirmation testing is not routinely needed. For specimens with a low s/co, confirmation testing should be done with either a recombinant immunoblot assay (RIBA) or by detection of HCV RNA. If HCV RNA detection is used as the confirmatory test, then RNA-negative specimens should be tested in the RIBA. This is to distinguish a false-positive ELISA result from true infection. Alternatively, repeat testing for HCV RNA should be done because viremia may be intermittent, and HCV infection should not be ruled out based on a single negative HCV RNA test result. Qualitative molecular assays are also used to diagnose HCV infection in infants born to HCV-infected mothers. Since maternal IgG antibody

can cross the placenta, these infants can be seropositive into the second year of life. Detection of HCV RNA in the plasma or serum of the newborn shortly after birth would be diagnostic of infection. Detection of HCV RNA in plasma or serum can be a useful diagnostic test in immunocompromised individuals, such as those with end-stage HIV-1 infection, because they may not mount a normal immune response to the virus and may not be seropositive.

Qualitative HCV RNA testing is also used to define a treatment response to therapy for HCV infection because these assays are very sensitive, with lower limits of detection between 5 and 50 IU/mL plasma. Virologic response to therapy is defined as an undetectable HCV RNA after completion of therapy, whereas a sustained virologic response is defined as an undetectable viral load 24 weeks after completion of therapy. More recently, qualitative HCV RNA assays have been developed for screening the blood supply. HCV RNA is detectable in serum during the "window period" between infection and seroconversion (when test results for HCV antibodies are negative). Because most individuals with recently acquired HCV infection are asymptomatic, testing of blood donors for HCV RNA allows identification of individuals at risk for transmitting HCV infection who would have been missed if testing were done with only serological assays. Nucleic acid–based testing for HCV RNA has reduced the window period by an average of 26 days.[18] By screening the blood supply with HCV antibody testing alone, it was estimated that 1 in 100,000 units contained HCV RNA, but with the addition of testing by nucleic acid amplification technology (often called NAT) for HCV, the risk is projected to be reduced to 1 in 367,000 units.[18]

Several large clinical trials have established the benefit of treatment of chronic HCV infection with ribavirin and pegylated interferon-α (interferon-α with addition of polyethylene glycol [PEG]). Overall, sustained virological response rates (SVRs) of 54% to 56% are obtained; patients who have the genotypes 1, 4, or 6 have SVRs of only 42% to 46%, compared with 76% to 82% for those with genotype 2 or 3 infections. In addition, there was no additional benefit to treating genotype 2 and 3 infections for 48 weeks compared with 24 weeks, thus allowing for a shorter course of therapy for genotype 2 and 3 infections.

Although genotype is a stronger predictor of response to therapy than viral load (see below), recent studies have shown the utility of determining the viral load after 12 weeks of therapy. Patients who fail to have a 2 $\log_{10}$ drop in HCV RNA concentrations (i.e., concentrations are one one hundredth the initial concentrations) at 12 weeks after initiating combination therapy have a 3% likelihood of responding to therapy compared with 65% for patients who do achieve a 2 $\log_{10}$ drop in viral load. By determining HCV viral load at baseline and again after 12 weeks of therapy, patients who are very unlikely to respond to therapy can be identified earlier in the course of therapy. This will allow for discontinuation of potentially toxic drugs and a reduction in the cost of therapy. On the other hand, individuals with a 2 $\log_{10}$ drop in viral load will have therapy continued for either 24 or 48 weeks depending on the HCV genotype and other risk factors.

Several qualitative assays have been approved by the FDA for the detection of HCV RNA in plasma or serum specimens. The Amplicor HCV test and the COBAS Amplicor HCV test (Roche Diagnostics, Indianapolis) are based on RT-PCR technology; the COBAS test allows for automation of the amplification and detection steps. Both versions of the Amplicor test have a lower limit of detection of 50 international units (IU)/mL (50 international units per liter, or 50 IU/L). The Versant HCV RNA Qualitative Assay (Bayer Diagnostics, Tarrytown, N.Y.) uses transcription-mediated amplification (TMA) and can detect as few as 5 IU/mL of HCV RNA. In addition to these tests, RT-PCR LDTs are also used in some laboratories. Two additional qualitative assays are available only for screening the blood supply: the Procleix HIV-1/HCV assay (Gen-Probe, Inc., San Diego) based on TMA technology (Jackson, Smith, Knott, Korpela, Simmons, Piwowar-Manning, McDonough, Mimms, Vargo, 2002) and the AMPLISCREEN HCV Test v2.0 (Roche Diagnostics, Indianapolis), which is an RT-PCR assay. Both assays report a lower limit of detection of less than 50 IU/mL.

Various tests are available for the quantification of HCV RNA. The Versant HCV RNA 3.0 assay (Bayer Diagnostics Corp., Tarrytown, N.Y.) is the only currently FDA-approved assay for HCV viral-load testing. The assay is based on bDNA technology and has a broad dynamic range and a lower limit of quantification of 615 IU/mL. The Amplicor HCV MONITOR test (Roche Diagnostics, Indianapolis) has a similar limit of quantification (600 IU/mL), but a much more limited linear range. Dilution of the clinical specimen is needed to measure viral loads greater than 500,000 IU/mL. Several large clinical studies evaluating the efficacy of interferon-ribavirin therapy have used an RT-PCR assay developed by the National Genetics Institute (NGI) (SuperQuant). A recent advance in HCV testing has been the availability of several real-time RT-PCR assays. These assays have a lower limit of detection similar to those seen for the qualitative HCV assays (10 to 50 IU/mL) and a broad dynamic that allows for the accurate quantification of HCV concentrations up to 10 to 100 million IU/mL. The availability of these real-time assays could allow laboratories to replace both their current qualitative and quantitative tests. At this time, real-time tests are available as ASRs from Roche Diagnostics and Abbott Molecular (Des Plaines, Ill.).

Earlier versions of the Amplicor RT-PCR and bDNA assays did not accurately quantify all genotypes of HCV and usually underestimated the concentrations of genotypes 2 and 3. However, the current versions of the Amplicor RT-PCR (version 2.0), Versant bDNA (version 3.0), and real-time assays accurately quantify all HCV genotypes.[15,21] The availability of an established World Health Organization (WHO) international standard has allowed standardization of HCV assays with reporting of results as international units per milliliter.

The intraassay imprecision (SDs) of the HCV Versant bDNA and Amplicor RT-PCR assays ranges from 0.05 to 0.3 log_{10}; the Versant bDNA assay is slightly more precise. The biological variation of HCV viral load (as SD) ranges from 0.5 log_{10} to 0.75 log_{10}. Based on these data, changes in HCV viral load need to exceed 1 log_{10} (i.e., a tenfold change in concentration) to represent significant changes in viral replication.

HCV Genotyping

A hallmark of HCV infection is genetic heterogeneity, resulting from the low fidelity of the RNA-dependent RNA polymerase, which frequently introduces random nucleotide errors during viral replication. These replication errors could yield 10 to 100 nucleotide changes per position per year, giving rise to many genetic variants (quasispecies) of the virus in a single patient. Based on the identification of these genomic differences, HCV has been classified into six major genotypes (numbered 1 through 6), additional less common genotypes, and multiple subtypes (designated by letters) within each major genotype. Interestingly, the HCV genotype and subtype do not change during the course of the chronic infection. There are geographical differences in the distribution of HCV types. In the United States, approximately two thirds of the infections are type 1, with the remaining being mostly types 2 and 3.

The HCV genome contains well-defined 5'- and 3'-untranslated regions (5'UTR and 3'UTR). The 5'UTR is the most conserved portion of the genome and is frequently used as the target for molecular assays, including genotyping assays. The HCV genome is divided into seven areas: the core region that encodes the capsid C protein, the E1 and E2 regions that encode the envelope proteins (gp33 and gp72), and several nonstructural protein regions (NS2, NS3, NS4, and NS5). The NS5B region shows less sequence homology than the 5'UTR, and sequencing of NS5B has been successfully used for genotyping HCV.

HCV genotyping, along with pretreatment viral load, age, gender, and the presence of hepatic fibrosis, can be used to determine the duration of antiviral therapy, with genotype being the strongest predictor of a sustained virological response.

Several methods have been developed for genotyping and/or subtyping HCV (see Table 14-3), but most clinical laboratories use either the reverse hybridization-based line probe assay (INNO-LiPA HCV II, manufactured in Belgium for Bayer Corp., Norwood, Mass.) or direct DNA sequencing. The INNO-LiPA assay is based on reverse hybridization of 5'UTR amplified products with genotype-specific probes. This assay is convenient to use for many clinical laboratories because genotyping can be done directly from the amplicons generated in the Amplicor HCV Test (Roche Diagnostics, Indianapolis) and the Amplicor HCV Monitor tests. The INNO-LiPA HCV II discriminates and identifies the six major HCV genotypes and associated subtypes. The INNO-LiPA is accurate in typing HCV, but cannot reliably distinguish some of the subtypes of HCV. There is not sufficient sequence variation in the 5'UTR to allow distinction between subtypes 2a and 2c, and reverse hybridization data of subtypes 1a and 1b may be discordant with NS5B in ~10% of cases. Currently, this is not a significant limitation of the assay because treatment decisions are based on viral genotype not subtype. In addition, the INNO-LiPA method is user friendly and well suited for routine use in clinical laboratories that perform HCV genotyping.

Automated sequencing assays, developed both commercially and in the laboratory, are available to genotype HCV, and the genomic regions commonly used include 5'UTR, NS5B, and core. Sequencing methods require sequence alignment and comparison with reference sequences to determine the genotype and subtype. An HCV genotyping kit based on automated sequencing (Trugene HCV 5'NC, Bayer Diagnostics, Tarrytown, N.Y.) targets the 5'NC region. Though this assay can accurately type HCV, like the INNO-LiPA assay it is unable to accurately subtype the virus.[22] When more variable regions of the virus are sequenced, such as NS5B, it is possible to determine both viral type and subtype.

A 2002 study reported on the use of real-time PCR with melting curve analysis as a method to genotype HCV.[3] Using a single pair of fluorescence resonance energy transfer (FRET) probes, it was possible to distinguish types 1a/b, 2a/c, 2b, 3a, and 4 on the basis of differences in melting temperatures. This method showed good concordance with INNO-LiPA. Real-time PCR with melting curve analysis is a reliable method for typing HCV. As with other methods using the 5'UTR of the virus, it will not accurately subtype all samples. Other methods using real-time PCR technology for genotyping HCV are also under development.

Methicillin-Resistant *Staphylococcus aureus*

Staphylococcus aureus (S. aureus) is the leading cause of hospital-acquired infections in the United States and worldwide. The organism is carried in the skin or nose of healthy people, and an estimated 25% to 30% of the American population carries the organism in their nose. This gram-positive coccus is responsible for a wide clinical spectrum of infections, including folliculitis (furuncles) and carbuncles (the common boil), impetigo, cellulitis, food poisoning, toxic shock syndrome, osteomyelitis, pneumonia, endocarditis, scalded skin syndrome, and meningitis. Furuncles, carbuncles, and cellulitis commonly occur in diabetics with poor blood glucose control. In severe cases, infection may spread via the blood (hematogenous spread) from these skin infections, leading to complications such as endocarditis (especially in cardiac valves with congenital or acquired defects), osteomyelitis, orbital cellulitis (especially from boils in the face), and leptomeningitis. Meningitis may also occur following head injury with open skull fracture or after otitis media in children or, rarely, as an iatrogenic infection following brain surgery.

S. aureus strains that are resistant to methicillin and oxacillin are called methicillin-resistant *Staphylococcus aureus* (MRSA) and sometimes oxacillin-resistant *Staphylococcus aureus* (ORSA). MRSA is mostly acquired in the hospital and is then termed hospital-acquired MRSA (HA-MRSA). MRSA infections in individuals who have not been hospitalized within the previous year and have not undergone an invasive medical procedure including catheterization are termed community-acquired MRSA (CA-MRSA). In the past few years, there has been a dramatic increase in the number of cases of CA-MRSA, which often occur in otherwise healthy individuals. MRSA is usually resistant to all β-lactam agents, including cephalosporins and carbapenems. Unlike CA-MRSA, HA-MRSA is usually multidrug resistant, including resistance to erythromycin and clindamycin. Vancomycin has been the mainstay for the treatment of MRSA, which explains why the recent emergence of vancomycin-intermediate MRSA (VISA) and vancomycin-resistant MRSA (VRSA) is particularly disturbing. There have been few cases of infection by VRSA reported in the United States, and in each case, vancomycin resistance has been attributed to the transfer of a plasmid carrying the vanA operon to the S. aureus.[12]

MRSA produces a protein called penicillin-binding protein, PBP2a. This protein is encoded by the gene *mecA*. Alterations in PBP2a result in reduced binding of the protein to β-lactam agents, resulting in drug resistance. Some coagulase-negative *Staphylococcus* (CoNS) strains also have the *mecA* gene, but are not included in the term MRSA. The *mecA* gene is carried on a staphylococcal chromosomal cassette (SCC*mec*) element. HA-MRSA carries SCC*mec* types I, II, or III, which confers the multidrug resistance phenotype. CA-MRSA carries SCC*mec* types IV or V and is usually susceptible to many non–β-lactam drugs.

Clinical laboratories still rely on culture and phenotypic assays for the identification of pathogens and resistance testing. The identification of S. aureus by phenotypic methods requires culture for 24 to 48 hours and an additional 24 hours for resistance testing to confirm MRSA. There are many phenotypic methods for distinguishing S. aureus from CoNS. The tube coagulase test is the standard routine method for identifying S. aureus. Other tests include the slide coagulase test, latex agglutination tests, DNase and heat-stable nuclease tests, and many commercial biochemical tests using kits and automated systems.

Molecular Tests for MRSA

Molecular tests can identify MRSA in a few hours or a day rather than the current 3 to 4 days that are needed for culture methods. Timeliness can not only reduce healthcare costs to the patient, but also reduce the risk of transmitting the MRSA to healthcare workers and other patients, a crucial step for infection control. Molecular tests are also sensitive and thus can increase the detection rate of MRSA, especially in cases of heteroresistance in which the resistant subpopulation is a very small minority and in cases of mixed infections in which other members of the mixed infection may outgrow the MRSA in culture. The high analytical sensitivity of molecular assays and their excellent lower limits of detection permit direct detection of MRSA from clinical samples (e.g., nasal swabs) without the need for culture. Molecular assays are also highly specific and thus able to distinguish, for example, *mecA*-carrying CoNS from true MRSA. Finally, on rare occasions, phenotypic tests for S. aureus give equivocal results, creating a need for alternative methods. Testing for susceptibility to oxacillin also sometimes gives equivocal results, again highlighting the need for alternative methods.

Molecular methods for pathogen identification and susceptibility testing are becoming popular in academic and reference laboratory settings, and they are slowly making inroads in most routine laboratories where they would have the greatest impact on patient care and infection control. Numerous molecular methods are in use or under development; most are based on PCR. Species-specific primers have been designed, targeting such genes as *nuc* (nuclease), *coa* (coagulase), *spa* (protein A), *femA*, *femB*, *Sa442*, 16sRNA, and surface-associated fibrinogen-binding protein genes. Assays have been developed for real-time PCR on such platforms as the LightCycler, SmartCycler, COBAS TaqMan, Rotorgene, and Stratagene.

At least four methods are available commercially for MRSA detection and identification.

1. The Hy-Labs method, Hy-MRSA, is based on multiplex PCR and is applied to bacterial colonies or samples from blood culture bottles. Detection is by UV light after gel electrophoresis. A limitation of multiplex PCR is the possibility of false-positive results in mixed cultures of S. aureus and CoNS as a result of simultaneous detection of the *mecA* gene and an S. aureus–specific sequence from two separate organisms.

2. The Roche LightCycler MRSA kit is based on PCR. It uses the same primers to amplify the *mecA* gene and an internal control, but the latter is detected by fluorescence from a different dye than that for the *mecA* gene. Using the MagNA Pure for automated DNA extraction, results are ready within 3 hours from specimen receipt in the laboratory. Of note, the *mecA* gene can be present in both *S. aureus* and CoNS, so an assay targeting only the *mecA* gene cannot distinguish these organisms.

3. The EVIGENE MRSA kit from AdvanDx is a gene probe colorimetric assay based on signal amplification following sandwich hybridization of *mecA* and *nuc* probes to targets in a blood culture sample in a microtiter plate. It is claimed to provide positive identification directly from blood culture samples in about $3^{1}/_{2}$ hours. The results may be read visually or by an ELISA plate reader. The reagent set includes a positive control that detects the 16S rRNA present in all staphylococci.

4. The IDI-MRSA from GeneOhm Sciences is the only method currently approved by the FDA for the direct detection of MRSA in nasal swabs. It uses real-time PCR to amplify part of the staphylococcal cassette chromosome *mec* (SCC*mec*) and the *orfX*. Results are claimed to be ready 1 hour after collection of a nasal swab. An evaluation of the IDI-MRSA kit using 1657 isolates of MRSA found a diagnostic sensitivity of 98.7% and a diagnostic specificity of 98.4%.

A fifth company, MultiGen Diagnostics, Inc. provides commercial DNA sequencing-based diagnostic services for the identification of MRSA from most clinical samples. Results are available the same day that the sample is received by the company. The service involves the use of "syndrome driven panels" to simultaneously screen for and identify multiple organisms in the same test, regardless of whether they are bacterial, viral, fungal, parasitic, or any combination thereof.

Vancomycin-Resistant Enterococci

Enterococci are gram-positive organisms and are part of the normal flora of the human colon and urinary tract. They were previously classified as Group D streptococci. Enterococci are fastidious organisms and are mostly facultative anaerobes. Although generally considered less virulent than the other gram-positive cocci, such as *S. aureus* and *Streptococcus pneumoniae*, they have emerged as significant causes of hospital-acquired infections where they rank as the second most common cause of urinary tract infections and the third most common cause of bacteremia and of skin and soft tissue infections. Other infections by enterococci include wound infections, intraabdominal abscesses, subacute bacterial endocarditis, and meningitis. The genus *Enterococcus* includes 14 species, but the overwhelming majority of infections are due to *Enterococcus faecalis* (80% to 90%) and *Enterococcus faecium* (5% to 10%). Most infections originate from an intestinal or urinary site, and the risk factors include urinary or intravascular catheterization, prolonged hospitalization, use of multiple antibiotics, renal insufficiency, immunosuppression, recent intraabdominal or cardiothoracic surgery, and severe underlying disease.

Enterococci resistant to vancomycin are called vancomycin-resistant enterococci (VRE). Drug resistance in enterococci is of two types: intrinsic and acquired. Intrinsic resistance to vancomycin is usually a low-level drug resistance and is found in isolates of *Enterococcus gallinarium*, *Enterococcus casseliflavus*, and *Enterococcus flavescens*. The latter is the most common non*faecalis* and non*faecium* enterococcus isolated in hospital patients. In contrast, acquired resistance is usually a high-level resistance and is found in *E. faecalis* and *E. faecium*, the two most pathogenic members of the genus *Enterococcus*. Acquired resistance has also been demonstrated in *Enterococcus raffinosus*, *Enterococcus avium*, and *Enterococcus durans*. Acquired resistance is transmitted via R-plasmids, which are "promiscuously" passaged between enterococci. The genes responsible for vancomycin resistance include *vanA*, *vanB*, *vanC*, *vanD*, and *vanE*. The *vanA* and *vanB* genes are responsible for acquired resistance and are spread from organism to organism. By contrast, *vanC* is responsible for intrinsic resistance, is not spread between organisms, and has not been associated with serious infections. It is therefore important for clinical laboratories to distinguish *vanC* enterococci (*E. gallinarium* and *E. casseliflavus/E. flavescens*) from *vanA* and *vanB* enterococci.

The reservoirs for VRE are colonized and infected patients and colonized healthcare workers. VRE is a major infection-control problem in hospitals and nursing homes; preventive measures are effective in limiting the spread of infection. Toward this goal, the Hospital Infection Control Practices Advisory Committee (HICPAC) of the CDC has issued a number of recommendations covering the prudent use of vancomycin, educational programs, role of the clinical laboratory, and other hospital measures.[10] HICPAC has declared the microbiology laboratory as the first line of defense against the spread of VRE in the hospital.

VRE are normally detected in one of three ways: (1) aerobic culture of a normally sterile site, (2) VRE culture screen, or (3) as an incidental finding in stool culture. Presumptive identification of enterococci is based on the morphology of bacterial colonies, a Gram stain (gram positive), and a positive pyrrolidonyl arylamidase (PYR) test. For identification to species level, pigment and motility tests are applied, followed by determination of the drug susceptibility profile to ascertain whether the organism carries the *vanA*, *vanB*, or *vanC* gene. Determination of the type of resistance gene carried by the isolates is critical for infection-control purposes.

The main molecular approach currently routinely used for the subtyping of VRE is by use of gel electrophoresis with pulsed electrical fields (see section on Electrophoresis in Chapter 5). The banding patterns of different isolates are compared and combined with available epidemiological data to determine the relatedness of the isolated VRE strains. PCR-based assays have been developed for the diagnosis of enterococcal infections. Assays aimed at detecting all clinically relevant enterococci at the genus level are targeted at the *tuf* gene, which encodes the elongation factor EF-Tu. PCR assays that identify the individual resistance genes (*vanA*, *vanB*, etc.) use primers that hybridize to genotype-specific conserved DNA sequences. A multiplex PCR assay has been developed that simultaneously detects resistance genes and identifies the clinically relevant enterococcus at the species level. Sequencing techniques have mainly targeted the 16S ribosomal RNA genes and include chain termination sequencing and pyrosequencing techniques. Sequencing allows estimation of the genetic diversity within each resistance gene type. Other available molecular methods include ribotyping or ARDRA (amplified ribosomal DNA restriction assay), REP-PCR (repetitive extragenic palindromic PCR), and RAPD (random amplified polymorphic DNA).

Two methods are commercially available for the molecular diagnosis of VRE. A real-time PCR-based VRE detection method (Roche Diagnostics, Indianapolis, IN) provides identification and differentiation of the resistance genes of VRE (*vanA*, *vanB*, and *vanB2/3*). It includes an internal control, which is amplified by the same primers that amplify the resistance genes. The VRE and internal control amplicons are detected separately by use of specific probes that carry different-colored fluorescent dyes; these molecules are detected by their characteristic fluorescence at different wavelengths (in different "channels" of the instrument) (see Detection under Real-Time PCR in Chapter 5). Results are available within 3 hours of receiving the clinical specimen in the laboratory. These reagents do not detect the *vanC*, *vanD*, and *vanE* resistance genes. The EVIGENE VRE method is similar to the EVIGENE MRSA method in that it uses the same gene probe technology, and results are ready in $3\frac{1}{2}$ hours. The method detects *vanA* and *vanB* genes and the 16S rRNA gene (positive control) present in all enterococci. The two methods show high concordance for isolates of enterococci. As with MRSA, MultiGen Diagnostics, Inc. provides commercial DNA sequencing-based diagnostic services for the identification of VRE from most clinical samples. Results are available the same day that the sample is received by the company.

BIOTERRORISM AND BIOWARFARE

Bioterrorism refers to the use of pathogenic organisms or biological toxins to produce death and disease in humans for the purpose of spreading fear and terror in the community. Use of the same agents in conventional warfare is termed biowarfare. "Bioterrorism" will be used for the rest of this text and should be understood to mean bioterrorism or biowarfare or both depending on the context. Bioterrorism is not a new development; as far back as the 6th century BC the Assyrians are recorded to have poisoned the wells of their enemies with the fungus rye ergot; the Romans used the corpses of diseased animals for the same purpose. In the 14th century AD, the invading Mongols (Tartars) reportedly catapulted the bodies of dead and dying plague victims into the city of Kaffa, today's Feodosiya, in the Ukraine. This resulted in the unanticipated spread of the disease beyond the city limits and is thought to be responsible for the pandemic of bubonic plague ("Black Death") that spread across Europe in the Middle Ages. In 1763 the Native American population was decimated by British soldiers who systematically spread smallpox in the population using smallpox-infested blankets as gifts to the Indians. More recent bioterrorist attacks include the poisoning of several salad bars in Oregon with *Salmonella* by followers of Bhagwan Shree Rajneesh in 1984; the Aum Shinrikyo cult released aerosolized anthrax and botulinum toxin in Japan between 1990 and 1995; and the dissemination of *Bacillus anthracis* spores through the United States Postal Service in 2001.

The technological advancements of the 20th century coupled with the many international wars led many countries to research and stockpile biological weapons, including the United States, the Soviet Union, Germany, Japan, and most recently, Iraq. These stockpiles have mostly been destroyed following ratification of the 1972 Geneva Convention on the Prohibition of the Development, Production, and Stockpiling of Bacteriological and Toxin Weapons and on Their Destruction. The heightened concern today about bioterrorism is the fear that terrorist groups and rogue nations will acquire the technology to develop and stockpile biological weapons of mass destruction.

Agents of Bioterrorism

Bioterrorism agents are typically naturally occurring pathogens, but they may be modified to enhance their virulence, to make them resistant to available vaccines and drugs, or to make it easy to disseminate them widely in the environment in a short time. The CDC has classified bioterrorism agents into categories A, B, and C based on their ability to be disseminated, their mortality rates, their ability to cause panic in the public or disrupt society, and the actions required for public health preparedness.[13] Category A agents pose the highest risk to national security and include pathogens that are easily disseminated or spread from person to person, cause high mortality rates, can cause panic in the public, and require special preparedness measures. Category A agents include variola major (smallpox), *Bacillus anthracis* (anthrax), *Yersinia pestis* (plague), *Clostridium botulinum* toxin (botulism), *Francisella tularensis* (tularemia), the hemorrhagic fever viruses Filoviruses (Ebola, Marburg, etc.), and Arenaviruses (Lassa, Junin, etc.). Category B agents pose the next highest risk to national security and include pathogens that are moderately easy to disseminate, cause low mortality rates, are less likely to cause public panic, and require only enhancement of currently available diagnostic and surveillance techniques. Category B agents include *Coxiella burnetii* (Q fever), *Brucella* species (brucellosis), *Burkholderia mallei* (glanders), *Burkholderia pseudomallei* (melioidosis), alphaviruses (Venezuelan encephalomyelitis and western and eastern equine encephalomyelitis), *Rickettsia prowazekii* (typhus fever), *Chlamydia psittaci* (psittacosis), ricin toxin (from *Ricinus communis*, i.e., castor beans), staphylococcal enterotoxin B, epsilon toxin of *Clostridium perfringens*, food safety threats (*Salmonella* species, *Escherichia coli* O157:H7, and *Shigella dysenteriae*), and water safety threats (*Vibrio cholerae* and *Cryptosporidium parvum*). Category C agents pose the least risk to national security and include pathogens that could be engineered for widespread dissemination because of their availability, ease of production, and potential for high mortality rates. Category C agents include Nipah virus (encephalitis), hantaviruses (Hanta pulmonary virus syndrome), tick-borne hemorrhagic fever viruses (e.g., Crimean-Congo hemorrhagic fever), tick-borne encephalitis viruses, yellow fever virus, severe acute respiratory syndrome virus, rabies virus, and multidrug-resistant MTb.

Bacillus anthracis

Bacillus anthracis is a gram-positive, large nonmotile bacillus with central-to-subterminal spores. The pathogen causes the disease anthrax. Anthrax occurs in three different forms, namely (1) cutaneous anthrax, (2) gastrointestinal anthrax, and (3) inhalational or pulmonary anthrax. Inhalational anthrax is rare in humans as a natural infection, but it is the most dangerous form of anthrax and the most likely route of a bioterrorist attack (dissemination of aerosolized or powdery anthrax spores). Specimens containing natural *B. anthracis* can be handled by most laboratories, but aerosolized specimens or powders require specialized handling. There are many PCR-based methods for the detection of *B. anthracis*. These target genes, such as the lethal factor (*lef*), protective antigen gene A (*pagA*), and capsular protein genes A, B, and C (*capA*, *capB*, and *capC*), are located on plasmids, and the small acid-soluble protein gene (SASP) is located on the bacterial chromosome. The presence of the plasmids is essential for *B. anthracis* to be pathogenic.

Yersinia pestis

Yersinia pestis is a member of the Enterobacteriaceae family and is a poorly-staining gram-negative coccobacillus. It is the cause of plague, which occurs in three forms; (1) bubonic plague (lymph nodes infected), (2) pneumonic plague (lungs infected), and (3) septicemic plague (spread to the circulation). Pneumonic plague is the deadliest of the three and is essentially uniformly fatal if untreated. Plague is most likely to occur in the pneumonic form in a bioterrorist attack. PCR-based assays for the detection of *Y. pestis* include targets such as the plasminogen activator gene (*pla*), the murine toxin gene (*mlt*), and the fraction 1 antigen gene (*f1a*).

Francisella tularensis

Francisella tularensis is a fastidious, extremely tiny, gram-negative coccobacillus that causes a potentially severe or fatal illness called tularemia. There are four types of tularemia: (1) ulceroglandular tularemia (sores on hands and fingers, with swollen lymph nodes on the same side); (2) oculoglandular tularemia (eyes infected along with swollen lymph nodes); (3) glandular tularemia (swollen lymph nodes but no sores); and (4) typhoidal tularemia (high fever, abdominal pain, and fatigue). A pneumonic form can occur if the bacteria are inhaled; this is the form most likely to occur in a terrorist attack. At least three types of tularemia biological weapons are known to have been developed: (1) liquid and dry weapons based on the natural strains, (2) antibiotic-resistant strains, and (3) vaccine-subverting strains. PCR assays for *F. tularensis* target genes such as the Francisella outer protein A (*fopA*) and a major membrane protein precursor, *tul4*.

Brucella abortus

Brucella abortus, like *F. tularensis*, is an extremely small, gram-negative coccobacillus. It is the causative agent of brucellosis, an infection with protean manifestations, including flulike symptoms such as fever, headaches, cough, chest pains, backache, sweats, and weakness, or severe infections involving the heart, CNS, joints, and other organs. The best clinical specimens are blood and bone marrow. There are PCR assays for the detection of *Brucella* species, and a major target of these assays is the genus-specific perosamine synthetase gene (*per*).

Variola Virus (Smallpox)

Smallpox is a highly contagious infection caused by the variola virus, with two variants called variola major (the more virulent variant) and variola minor. Variola is a member of the *Orthopoxvirus* genus, the largest animal viruses, some of which are larger than some bacteria. Smallpox was officially eradicated in 1980 as declared by the WHO. Only two laboratories in the world continue to keep samples of the virus: the CDC in Atlanta, Ga., and the State Research Center of Virology and Biotechnology in Koltsovo, Russia. Vaccination against small-

pox was discontinued following its eradication. However, after the 2001 anthrax attacks in the United States, there have been concerns that smallpox virus might be used as a terrorist agent. Suspicion of smallpox in a patient must be immediately reported to the Emergency Response Office at the CDC and to state public health authorities. Variola virus specimens must be handled only by a national laboratory, not a reference or sentinel laboratory. Commercial PCR assays have been developed for the detection of smallpox virus.

Responses to Bioterrorism

In 1999 the CDC established a network of laboratories that have the capacity to respond to biological and chemical terrorism. This network is called the laboratory response network (LRN). The LRN is a national network of approximately 140 laboratories and includes federal laboratories (at the CDC, FDA, U.S. Department of Agriculture [USDA], etc.), state and local public health laboratories, military laboratories (operated by the Department of Defense), food testing laboratories (FDA, USDA, etc.), environmental laboratories (to test water samples), veterinary laboratories (USDA, animal testing), and international laboratories (located in Canada, the United Kingdom and Australia).[14] LRN laboratories are categorized into national, reference, and sentinel laboratories depending on the level of testing the laboratory is capable of and the level of infectivity of agents the laboratory can handle without exposing workers to the agent. National laboratories are the best equipped and have the resources to handle highly infectious agents and type agents to the subspecies or strain level. Reference laboratories have the capacity to detect and confirm the presence of a bioterrorism agent, thereby enabling a timely response in the event of an actual bioterrorist attack. Sentinel laboratories are the hospital-based or private laboratories that perform routine diagnostic testing and have contact with the patient. The sentinel laboratory's duty is to refer suspicious clinical samples to the appropriate reference laboratory.

Recent threats of bioterrorism and the ongoing war on terrorism have highlighted the need to have in place the ability to rapidly detect and identify bioterrorism agents in the event of a terrorist outbreak of infectious diseases. The ideal method (combination of technology and platform or instrument) should be rapid, sensitive, specific, reproducible, and capable of detecting and identifying agents in complex clinical, environmental, or industrial samples. The method should be simple (user friendly), portable, require minimal sample processing, be capable of detecting multiple agents simultaneously in a single reaction, and amenable to high throughput analyses. It should also be capable of detecting altered agents (genetic, antigenic, or chemical modification) and uncommon variants of typical pathogens. No single method meets all these criteria. Currently available methods span the spectrum of technologies and platforms used in clinical and environmental microbial testing. Routine culture, staining, and biochemical typing (manual and automated) remain the gold standard for the detection and identification of agents of bioterrorism. These require several days and may not be versatile enough to detect new or modified agents. Faster approaches generally involve immunological and molecular techniques.

A wide variety of samples may need to be processed for testing agents of bioterrorism. Human blood contains heme, which inhibits *Taq* DNA polymerase in as low a concentration as 0.004%. Stool contains many substances (bile salts, etc.) that inhibit PCR and numerous bacteria that may act as contaminants in a molecular assay. It is critical to concentrate urine by centrifugation, followed by DNA extraction to achieve success with molecular techniques. Nasal and throat swab specimens are the mainstay for the detection of aerosolized agents, such as the recent anthrax spores attacks. Food and water supplies could also be used as routes of bioterrorist attacks. Food contains many substances that inhibit PCR, including lipids and complex carbohydrates. The level of pathogens in water is usually so low that extensive concentration of the pathogen is required before it can be detected by any currently available technique, including PCR. Environmental samples include soil, air, and surfaces. The air is currently monitored in more than 30 undisclosed major cities in the United States by the BioWatch program, a program that uses air samplers to test for biological and chemical threat agents 24 hours a day, 7 days a week in the designated cities. BioWatch uses PCR-based techniques because of the sensitivity and rapidity with which the techniques are able to detect nucleic acids. In the attacks of 2001, the Brentwood Mail Processing and Distribution Center in Washington, DC was severely contaminated by *B. anthracis* spores. Contaminated surfaces at the facility were investigated using several techniques of sample collection (such as wipes and vacuuming), and the best approaches were defined.

Most molecular techniques available for the detection and identification of bioterrorist agents are based on quantitative real-time PCR using agent-specific primers and probes. Many types of probes are used, including TaqMan probes, dual FRET probes, molecular beacons, scorpion probes, and many instruments. Various approaches have been taken to make systems that are small, portable, and rugged to facilitate their use in the field in rapid response to bioterrorism. Methods are commercially available for the detection and identification of bioterrorism agents including *B. anthracis*, *Y. pestis*, *F. tularensis*, smallpox virus, and *E. coli* O157:H7.

A different approach is to use PCR and 16S rDNA gene sequencing. The sequence obtained is used to query GenBank and other databases for the sequence with the best match. This method is able to rapidly detect pathogens and identify them to the strain level. It has been applied to the identification of *B. anthracis*, *Y. pestis*, *F. tularensis*, *B. mallei*, *B. pseudomallei*, and *Brucella species*. The technique sometimes fails to differentiate between strains of a given species. For example, many *B. anthracis* strains have identical 16S rDNA sequences. Various other techniques are under evaluation, including multiplex PCR microarray assays that detect multiple pathogens in a single reaction.

DEVELOPMENT OF MOLECULAR ASSAYS FOR INFECTIOUS DISEASES

Nucleic–acid-based testing for infectious diseases, as for other clinical conditions, involves three major steps: (1) specimen processing, (2) nucleic acid amplification, and (3) product detection. Several systems automate one or two steps, and automation of all three steps in a single analyzer is expected from manufacturers in the near future.

Molecular infectious disease laboratories use both commercial and laboratory-developed assays. Commercially available kits usually contain complete reagent sets, which provide quality-controlled reagents that have been manufactured under good manufacturing practices (GMP). The manufacturer has determined the performance characteristics of the entire molecular test for a particular performance claim. Many clinical laboratories find it necessary to develop their own methods (LDTs) to detect infectious agents for which there are no commercial FDA-cleared tests.

Analyte-Specific Reagents

Laboratories developing LDTs need to be aware of rules concerning **analyte-specific reagents** (ASRs). The FDA introduced the term ASR to refer to such reagent(s) used in LDTs that confer specificity for detecting a particular analyte. In the United States, the jurisdiction of the FDA includes reagents used in diagnosis or treatment of disease. ASRs include antibodies, specific receptor proteins, ligands, and oligonucleotides. The FDA has mandated that laboratories using ASRs must label their reports with the statement, "This test was developed and its performance characteristics determined by (laboratory name). It has not been cleared or approved by the U.S. Food and Drug Administration." LDTs that use primers and probes made in the laboratory are not covered by this rule.

Test Development

After a clinical need has been identified, a careful literature search should be undertaken to determine the best target and specimen type for a given clinical condition. Target sequences must be chosen to prevent cross-hybridization with other known sequences. A preliminary evaluation of published protocols or use of generic default concentrations for PCR components can be a useful starting point. The next step is to optimize the different steps of the analytical process together, including nucleic acid extraction, amplification, detection, and quantification. For amplification procedures, variables to be optimized may include buffer pH, nucleotide concentration, $MgCl_2$ concentration, type of polymerase, primer concentration, and annealing temperature.

As part of the process of test evaluation, the laboratory needs to evaluate the need for internal controls. Internal controls, which are added to the clinical specimen before processing, are often used to determine if nucleic acid degradation occurred during specimen processing and/or to detect the presence of inhibitors of amplification. The more widely used internal controls are synthetic segments of nucleic acid that use the same primer sequence as the target molecule, with a portion of the sequence internal to the primer binding sites that is unique to the internal control. This allows simultaneous amplification of the internal control and target, but they can each be identified by using sequence-specific probes or physical separation of the two products by size or melting point.

In quantitative methods for DNA and RNA (as in viral-load assays), the concentration of an organism's nucleic acid is calculated by comparison of the signal from the sample and that from calibrators of known concentration. Calibrators may be external or internal. External calibrators avoid competition with the target sequence for reaction components, such as enzyme and nucleotides, and can be naturally occurring. The major disadvantage of external calibrators is that, unlike internal controls, they are not subject to the same reaction efficiencies or inhibition as the target sequence in the patient specimen.

TABLE 11-2	Guidelines and Standards for Molecular Infectious Disease Testing	
Organization	**Guideline**	**Internet Address**
Clinical and Laboratory Standards Institute	MM-3-A Molecular Diagnostic Methods for Infectious Diseases MM-6-A Quantitative Molecular Diagnostics for Infectious Diseases MM-9-A Nucleic Acid Sequencing Methods in Diagnostic Laboratory Medicine MM-10-A Genotyping for Infectious Diseases: Identification and Characterization	www.nccls.org (accessed 12/23/06) or www.clsi.org (accessed 12/23/06)
FDA	Guidance for industry in the manufacture and clinical evaluation of in vitro tests	http://www.fda.gov/(accessed 12/23/06)
ASM	Cumitech 31: February 1997. Verification and Validation of Procedures in the Clinical Microbiology Laboratory; ASM Press.	www.asm.org (accessed 12/23/06)
ASTM	Guide E1873-97: Standard Guide for Detection of Nucleic Acid Sequences by the Polymerase Chain Reaction Technique Guide E2048-99: Standard Guide for Detection of Nucleic Acids of the *Mycobacterium tuberculosis* Complex and Other Pathogenic Mycobacteria by the Polymerase Chain Reaction Technique	www.astm.org (accessed 12/23/06)

FDA, *Food and Drug Administration;* ASM, *American Society of Microbiology;* ASTM, *American Society for Testing and Materials.*

Test Verification

Verification of molecular infectious tests is an involved process that can be divided into two phases: analytical and clinical verification. The first phase is the analytical verification, which provides critical information about the performance of the test. The second phase is the clinical verification, which provides information regarding the clinical indications for the test, such as information about the appropriate settings, including disease states and populations for which the test can be used. Listed in Table 11-2 are guidelines that can be useful for development of validation programs. Table 11-3 outlines a checklist to assist in the verification process for a molecular assay.

Analytical Verification

As noted above, laboratories must assess each LDT's analytical sensitivity and specificity, precision, and linear or reportable range. Control materials, obtained from commercial suppliers, can be used for quality control. Assessment of analytical performance characteristics should use materials that are similar to the intended patient specimen and are carried through the entire testing process.

The linear range of an assay is the span of analyte concentrations for which the final value output is directly proportional to the analyte concentration, with acceptable error. Evaluating multiple aliquots of at least four different concentrations of the analyte may assess the linearity of a quantitative assay.

Analytical sensitivity can be determined by performing serial dilutions of an appropriate number of samples containing known amounts of the analyte.

Every assay has an upper and lower limit of quantification (LOQ) and a limit of detection (LOD). The LOQ is higher than the LOD. The LOQ is the lowest concentration of analyte that can be measured with a defined uncertainty (such as imprecision with a coefficient of variation less than 20%). The LOD is usually defined as the lowest concentration of analyte that produces a signal that from the analytical signal from a sample that is free of analyte (a "blank"). This is also referred to as the limit of the blank. A newer definition of LOD is the lowest concentration that will, with an agreed probability (such

TABLE 11-3	Checklist for Verification of Molecular Infectious Disease LDT
Name of Test	Name should identify the particular organism and/or disease and/or condition to be tested.
Intended use	Identify the particular microorganism and parameter(s) tested and indicate the use of the test (e.g., diagnosis, prognosis, monitoring response to treatment, guiding therapy, etc.).
Indications for use	Provide clinical condition(s) and specific patient population(s).
Method category	Methodology used for the test
Testing procedure	Specimen types, specimen handling and transport procedures, nucleic acid isolation and storage, description of the test procedure, reports, expected results and technical interpretation
Test results	Mock representative examples of results
Analytical verification	Analytical sensitivity, analytical specificity, precision, and linear dynamic range for quantitative assays
Quality control and quality assurance	QC and QA program. Register for proficiency program and identify informal proficiency program if no HHS-approved program exists.
Assay limitations	Delineate and discuss potential limitations.
Clinical data	Clinical condition evaluated, patient population, demographics, sample size estimate. Peer-reviewed literature is accepted as a means to evaluate the clinical condition.
Clinical verification	Clinical sensitivity, clinical specificity, positive predictive value, negative predictive value
Reporting of test results	Examples of different reports and clinical interpretation
Clinical utility	Potential clinical benefit to patient

as 90%), produce a signal that is above the limit of the blank. (For details, see *Tietz Textbook of Clinical Chemistry and Molecular Diagnostics*, 4th edition.)

Analytical specificity is the ability of an analytical method to detect and/or quantify what the method is intended to measure. For infectious disease testing, it is particularly important to ensure that primers and probes do not hybridize with nucleic acid from organisms present in the normal flora or those that cause similar clinical syndromes.

Clinical Verification

The proposed indications for use of the test should be defined before starting the clinical verification. As for any tests, the indication for use of an assay could involve (Chapter 8) (1) the making of a diagnosis, (2) the ruling out of a diagnosis, (3) the provision of prognostic information, or (4) the monitoring of disease, which includes, especially in infectious diseases, establishing resolution of the disease. The first step is to formulate a clinical question (Chapter 8), which should take into account the management decision that needs to be made, the role of the test in decision making, and the target population in which the test will be applied. Known analytical limitations (e.g., precision and linear range) should be taken into consideration when determining the clinical indication for each assay.

Determination of diagnostic accuracy requires attention to both the population and the type of sample used. This is important because the results for a method in a given population using a specified sample type may not apply to another population or to another sample type in the same population. Investigation of the diagnostic specificity should include samples from patients with diseases that should be ruled out using the test (Chapter 8). Specimens from healthy donors are specifically useful for those tests intended for screening of asymptomatic populations. The clinical utility of an infectious disease test can also be affected by factors such as microbial-host interactions; microbial dynamics, variants, and mutations; and replicative fitness of the microbial agent.

Quality Control and Quality Assurance

A quality assurance program (Chapter 7) addresses all aspects of the testing process from test selection to interpretation and use of results. In the United States, the extent of quality assurance and quality control performed for any molecular assay depends on whether the test is FDA cleared, is "for research use only," is being used "off-label" (for nonapproved uses), or is an LDT. In general, LDTs require more extensive quality control because the analytical performance must be established and maintained by the laboratory. Establishment of critical control values for every critical reagent, such as composition, concentration, and purity of critical reagents, should be developed during the validation process. Tolerance limits should be established for each of these reagents, and quantitative criteria should be developed whenever possible to prevent subjective evaluation of the quality of the critical reagent.

Controls

Careful selection of control material and types of controls is vital for the interpretation of test results. For molecular assays, internal controls may be required to detect inhibition of amplification, to assess adequacy of extraction of nucleic acid from the clinical specimens, or to identify degradation of nucleic acid during the extraction procedure. Negative and positive controls are needed as required by CLIA'88 regulations, and all must be processed in every clinical test run. The positive control should be present at or near the limit of detection of the assay for qualitative methods. By contrast, a control near the limit of quantification is needed for quantitative methods because quantitative results cannot be generated for samples with lower concentrations. The January 2003 CLIA'88 final rule included for quantitative assays the use of a negative and two concentrations of positive control in every run. Positive controls should be at a clinically relevant concentration of the nucleic acid target sequence in a background of nucleic acid lacking the target sequence.

To check for inhibitors, an internal control can be added to the sample. If this is not possible, two aliquots of the specimen can be tested, with one of them containing added target. For a specimen to be considered negative, the test result for the specimen amplified directly must be negative, and the specimen with added target nucleic acid must be positive. The amount of target nucleic acid added to the patient specimen should be close to the limit of detection of the assay, so that low levels of inhibition can be detected. This practice is much more labor intensive and costly than using an internal control. The use of these controls can be discontinued if the inhibition rate is determined to be less than 1%.

Proficiency Testing

Laboratories performing molecular infectious disease testing should subscribe to appropriate proficiency testing programs. For those analytes for which there is no Department of Health and Human Services–approved proficiency program or survey, it is the responsibility of the laboratory to develop an informal proficiency program such as sample exchange with another laboratory performing the test for the same analyte or by retesting already characterized patient specimens. The concepts of proficiency testing are described in Chapter 7.

Interpretation of Results

Interpretation of the results of molecular assays for infectious diseases requires an understanding of the target organism's biology and the pathogenesis of the related infectious disease(s), and advantages and limitations of the technology used. Some of the challenges in interpreting these tests are unique to molecular tests, such as correlating nucleic acid detection with the presence of the disease.

Interpretation of a negative result requires consideration of the assay's analytical and diagnostic sensitivities and the efficiencies of nucleic acid extraction and amplification. A false-negative result may be due to inhibition of or decreased efficiency of amplification. Insufficient sample, inappropriate specimen type, inappropriate timing of sample collection, and degradation of nucleic acid during transport and handling are other sources of false-negative results.

The factors that need to be considered when interpreting a positive result include assay specificity and contamination. Specificity of molecular infectious disease assays is related to the primers and probes used during amplification and detection and/or quantification steps. False-positive results can also occur as the result of cross-contamination with template target from other specimens and/or carry-over contamination of amplified products. This is not a problem with signal amplification methods, but can be of significant concern for target amplification methods, such as PCR, NASBA, TMA, and SDA. The use of real-time assays, which do not require postamplification handling of the product, greatly reduces the risk of carry-over contamination. Cross-contamination of clinical specimens with target DNA during specimen collection, transport, and processing can occur with any method.

Molecular tests for infectious diseases do not provide information regarding the viability of an organism. Nucleic acid for certain microorganisms can be found for a period of time after treatment is initiated. HSV DNA can be detected in CSF of patients with encephalitis for 2 weeks or longer after initiation of acyclovir therapy. Monitoring of response to therapy is best done using quantitative methods. One exception is the use of a qualitative RT-PCR method to monitor response to treatment to interferon and ribavirin in HCV-positive patients. In this instance, the absence of detectable HCV RNA from plasma or serum specimen is used to define the virological response to treatment.

Detection of nucleic acid of a pathogen does not ensure that the organism is the cause of the disease. The organism might be forming part of the normal flora, colonizing a specific area, or causing infection but not disease. One of the primary uses of molecular assays for CMV is for distinguishing active CMV disease from clinically insignificant CMV infection. Early studies evaluating the clinical utility of CMV DNA assays were very sensitive, and as a result, CMV DNA was detected in immunocompromised patients with disease and those without CMV disease and even in healthy donors. Development of quantitative molecular methods, use of plasma as the specimen, and detection of CMV mRNA rather than DNA have been used to overcome this shortfall. Cutoff values have been proposed as a means to discriminate infection from clinically relevant disease.

A common application for quantitative molecular assays is in monitoring of disease progression or response to therapy over time. To determine if changes in the quantitative values are clinically significant or caused by expected fluctuations of the measurement, one must consider analytical and biological variability. For example, for the current HIV-1 viral-load assays, to allow for both assay and biological variability, changes in the viral load must exceed $0.5 \log_{10}$ (a threefold change in concentration) to represent a biologically significant change in viral replication.

Reporting of Qualitative and Quantitative Results

Reporting of molecular qualitative tests is simple because the nucleic acid is either present or "not detected" in the patient specimen. It is important to emphasize the use of "undetectable" or "not detected" rather than "negative" because the organism might be present in the patient specimen but below the detection limit of the test. It is important to include in the report the detection limit and specificity of the test.

Reporting of results for quantitative molecular infectious disease assays is more complex and requires understanding of intrinsic analytical variables that might affect the test results. Various units are use to express values for quantitative molecular assay results. The reporting unit could be copies, genome equivalents, or international units of the target nucleic acid per

unit (usually volume) of specimen. The unit of volume typically used for specimens such as plasma is the milliliter, but concentrations may also be related to a number of leukocytes (e.g., 10,000). Results of quantitative assays are usually reported as either copies/mL or $\log_{10}$ copies/mL. (This is not in compliance with international agreements to use the liter as the unit of volume.) As with all assays, results above the dynamic range should be reported as greater than the upper limit (such as "greater than 100,000 copies/mL"), and samples in which quantification was not possible should be reported as less than the lower limit of the assay (e.g., "less than 400 copies/mL").

Communication of Results to Patients and Confidentiality of Results

Because of the power of molecular methods in microbiology, test results carry critical information about an individual's health and even about his or her future well-being. As with testing for inherited disorders (Chapter 9), learning of a positive result of a molecular test for a serious infectious disease may be devastating. Thus it has generally been believed that communication of results is best done by trained individuals, and in some situations, the decision to test may be best made in consultation with a physician.

Confidentiality of patient results has long been a concern in microbiology laboratories, in part because of mandatory reporting of results of some tests to state health departments. The molecular diagnostics laboratory is subject to such reporting, and it is thus essential that the laboratory know the regulations in the state or states it serves. In all cases, laboratorians have an obligation to respect the privacy of individuals whose samples they test. Some considerations are included in Ethics Box 11-1.

ETHICS Box 11-1 — **Ethical Considerations in Molecular Microbiology**

The results of molecular tests for many infectious diseases have important implications beyond their immediate medical utility in guiding treatment and judging prognosis. A health insurance company, for example, may wish to use an old report of a positive test result as evidence of a "preexisting condition" and thus deny coverage for treatment. Such concerns raise important questions about confidentiality of test results. Some examples of issues that have generated concern are given below; not all have been resolved.

- How can confidentiality of the HIV testing results best be maintained? Should the results be in the patient's medical record? What if the "patient" was tested as a blood donor, not as a patient?
- Should sexual partners of patients ever be given access to results of tests for sexually transmitted disease? Should a spouse of a person who died? If so, who should decide?
- When a healthcare worker is exposed to blood from a patient, rapid testing of that patient is done to determine if he or she has a blood-borne pathogen, such as HCV or HIV. This information is important for medical management of the healthcare worker's exposure. In this situation, how is the patient's privacy best maintained?

Maintaining confidentiality of medical records has always been an important part of the job of all medical professionals. It has become even more important now that powerful, diagnostically accurate tests are available that carry clear implications for a person's future.

This ethical note was prepared by D.E. Bruns.

REFERENCES

1. Bergeron MG, Ke D, Menard C, Picard FJ, Gagnon M, Bernier M et al. Rapid detection of group B streptococci in pregnant women at delivery. N Engl J Med 2000;343:175-9.
2. Brambilla D, Leung S, Lew J, et al. Absolute copy number and relative change in determinations of human immunodeficiency virus type 1 RNA in plasma: effect of an external standard on kit comparisons. J Clin Microbiol 1998;36:311-14.
3. Bullock GC, Bruns DE, Haverstick DM. Hepatitis C genotype determination by melting curve analysis with a single set of fluorescence resonance energy transfer probes. Clin Chem 2002;48:2147-54.
4. Caliendo AM, Schuurman R, Yen-Lieberman B, Spector SA, Andersen J, Manjiry R et al. Comparison of quantitative and qualitative PCR assays for cytomegalovirus DNA in plasma. J Clin Microbiol 2001;39:1334-8.
5. Caliendo AM, St George K, Kao SY, Allega J, Tan BH, LaFontaine R et al. Comparison of quantitative cytomegalovirus (CMV) PCR in plasma and CMV antigenemia assay: clinical utility of the prototype AMPLICOR CMV MONITOR test in transplant recipients. J Clin Microbiol 2000;38:2122-7.
6. Caliendo AM, St. George K, Allega J, Bullotta AC, Gilbane L, Rinaldo CR. Distinguishing cytomegalovirus (CMV) infection and disease with CMV nucleic acid assays. J Clin Microbiol 2002;40:1581-6.
7. Caliendo AM, Yen-Lieberman B, Baptista J, Andersen J, Crumpacker C, Schuurman R et al. Comparison of molecular tests for detection and quantification of cell-associated cytomegalovirus DNA. J Clin Microbiol 2003;41:3509-13.
8. Centers for Disease Control and Prevention. Nucleic acid amplification tests for tuberculosis. MMWR Morb Mortal Wkly Rep 1996;45:950-2.
9. Centers for Disease Control and Prevention. Prevention of Perinatal Group B streptococcal disease. MMWR Morb Mortal Wkly Rep August 16 2002:1-26.
10. Centers for Disease Control and Prevention. Recommendations for preventing the spread of vancomycin resistance. Recommendations of the Hospital Infection Control Practices Advisory Committee (HICPAC). MMWR Recomm Rep. Sep 22 1995;44(RR-12):1-13.
11. Centers for Disease Control and Prevention. Update: Nucleic acid amplification tests for tuberculosis. MMWR Morb Mortal Wkly Rep 2000;49:593-4.
12. Centers for Disease Control for Prevention. Brief report: vancomycin-resistant *Staphylococcus aureus*. MMWR Morb Mortal Wkly Rep 2004;53:322-3.
13. Centers for Disease Control for Prevention. Department of Molecular Virology and Micrology, Baylor College of Medicine. Potential Bioterrorism Agents. http://www.bcm.edu/molvir/eidbt/eidbt-mvm-pbt.htm, accessed March 12, 2007.
14. Centers for Disease Control and Prevention. The laboratory response network: partners in preparedness. http://www.bt.cdc.gov/lrn/, accessed March 12, 2007.
15. Detmer J, Lagier R, Flynn J, Zayati C, Kolberg J, Collins M et al. Accurate quantification of hepatitis C virus (HCV) RNA from all HCV genotypes by using branched-DNA technology. J Clin Microbiol 1996;34:901-7.
16. Hirsch MS, Brun-Vezinet F, Clotet B, Conway B, Kuritzkes DR, D'Aquila RT et al. Antiretroviral drug resistance testing in adults with human immunodeficiency virus type 1: 2003 recommendations of an international AIDS Society-USA panel. Clin Infect Dis July 1 2003;37:113-28.
16a. Humar A, Gregson D, Caliendo AM, McGeer A, Malkan G, Krajden M, Corey P, Greig P, Walmsley S, Levy G, Mazzulli T. Clinical utility of quantitative cytomegalovirus viral load determination for predicting cytomegalovirus disease in liver transplant recipients. Transplantation 1999;68:1305-11.
16b. Humar A, Kumar D, Boivin G, Caliendo AM. Cytomegalovirus (CMV) viral load kinetics to predict recurrent disease in solid organ transplant patients with CMV disease. J Infect Dis 2002;186:829-33.
17. Kimberlin DW, Lakeman FD, Arvin AM, Prober CG, Corey L, Powell DA et al. Application of the polymerase chain reaction to the diagnosis and management of neonatal herpes simplex virus disease. National

Institute of Allergy and Infectious Diseases Collaborative Antiviral Study Group. J Infect Dis 1996;174:1162-7.
18. Kolk DP, Dockter J, Linnen J, Ho-Sing-Loy M, Gillotte-Taylor K, McDonough SH et al. Significant closure of the human immunodeficiency virus type 1 and hepatitis C virus preseroconversion detection windows with a transcription-mediated-amplification-driven assay. J Clin Microbiol 2002;40:1761-6.
19. Kulasingam SL, Hughes JP, Kiviat NB, Mao C, Weiss NS, Kuypers JM, Koutsky LA. Evaluation of human papillomavirus testing in primary screening for cervical abnormalities: comparison of sensitivity, specificity, and frequency of referral. JAMA 2002;288:1749-57.
20. Lakeman F, Whitley RJ. Diagnosis of herpes simplex encephalitis: Application of polymerase chain reaction to cerebrospinal fluid from brain-biopsied patients and correlation with disease. National Institute of Allergy and Infectious Diseases Collaborative Antiviral Study Group. J Infect Dis 1995;171:857-63.
21. Martinot-Peignoux M, Boyer N, Le Breton V, Le Guludec G, Castelnau C, Akremi R, Marcellin P et al. A new step toward standardization of serum hepatitis C virus-RNA quantification in patients with chronic hepatitis C. Hepatology 2000;31:726-9.
22. Nolte FS, Green AM, Fiebelkorn KR, Caliendo AM, Sturchio C, Grunwald A, Healy M. Clinical evaluation of two methods for genotyping hepatitis C virus based on analysis of the 5' noncoding region. J Clin Microbiol 2003;41:1558-64.
23. Palmer HM, Mallinson H, Wood RL, Herring AJ. Evaluation of the specificities of five DNA amplification methods for the detection of *Neisseria gonorrhoeae*. J Clin Microbiol 2003;41:835-7.
24. Simko JP, Caliendo AM, Hogle K, Versalovic J. Differences in laboratory findings for cerebrospinal fluid specimens obtained from patients with meningitis or encephalitis due to herpes simplex virus (HSV) documented by detection of HSV DNA. Clin Infect Dis 2002;35:414-19.
25. Van Der Pol B, Ferrero DV, Buck-Barrington L, Hook E 3rd, Lenderman C, Quinn T et al. Multicenter evaluation of the BDProbeTec ET System for detection of *Chlamydia trachomatis* and *Neisseria gonorrhoeae* in urine specimens, female endocervical swabs, and male urethral swabs. J Clin Microbiol 2001;39:1008-16.
26. Whitley R, Lakeman F. Herpes simplex virus infections of the central nervous system: therapeutic and diagnostic considerations. Clin Infect Dis 1995;20:414-20.

REVIEW QUESTIONS

1. All of the following are advantages of molecular assays EXCEPT
    A. improved analytical and clinical sensitivity compared with conventional methods.
    B. more rapid turnaround time compared with culture.
    C. inability to distinguish live from dead organisms.
    D. amenability to high throughput testing.
    E. high specificity caused by use of primers and probes.
2. Which of the following statements concerning testing for *C. trachomatis* is correct?
    A. Culture is more specific and sensitive than PCR.
    B. PCR is the test of choice in cases of suspected sexual abuse of adult women.
    C. For women, PCR testing is more sensitive using urine than vaginal swabs.
    D. For men, PCR testing of urine and urethral swabs are equal in diagnostic sensitivity.
    E. Diagnostic sensitivity of PCR is increased by collecting a large (>50 mL) volume of urine.

3. When monitoring HIV-1–infected patients with viral-load assays, what change in viral load represents a biologically relevant change in viral replication?
   A. Twofold
   B. $0.2 \log_{10}$
   C. Fivefold
   D. $0.5 \log_{10}$ (threefold)
   E. $1.0 \log_{10}$

4. The current FDA-cleared HIV-1 genotyping assays detect mutations that confer resistance to all of the following classes of drugs EXCEPT
   A. nucleoside reverse transcriptase inhibitors
   B. nonnucleoside reverse transcriptase inhibitors
   C. protease inhibitors
   D. fusion inhibitors

5. Which HIV-1 subtype is most common in the United States?
   A. A
   B. B
   C. C
   D. D
   E. F

6. Compared with brain biopsy as the gold standard, the diagnostic sensitivity of PCR using CSF specimens for the diagnosis of HSV encephalitis is
   A. 50%.
   B. 65%.
   C. 75%.
   D. 95%.
   E. 100%.

7. Which of the following statements regarding CMV is correct?
   A. Persons with AIDS develop disease when their CD4 cell count is approximately 200 cells/mm^3.
   B. Detection of DNA in blood is diagnostic of active disease.
   C. The concentration of DNA in plasma is higher than in whole blood.
   D. A preemptive therapy approach will treat more individuals than a prophylactic therapy approach.
   E. Detection of DNA in plasma after completing therapy represents a risk factor for relapsing infection.

8. What decrease in HCV viral load is needed after 12 weeks of therapy to predict a treatment response?
   A. $0.5 \log_{10}$
   B. $1.0 \log_{10}$
   C. $1.5 \log_{10}$
   D. $2.0 \log_{10}$
   E. $2.5 \log_{10}$

9. An assay designed to detect vancomycin resistance in *E. faecium* should target which of the following genes?
   A. *vanA*
   B. *vanC*
   C. *mecA*
   D. *orfX*
   E. *capA*

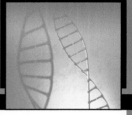

Chapter 12

Pharmacogenetics

Gwendolyn A. McMillin, Ph.D., D.A.B.C.C.

OUTLINE

OBJECTIVES

1. State the specific actions that phase I and phase II enzymes have on substrates and give examples of these enzymes.
2. Compare and contrast genotyping and phenotyping in regard to pharmacogenetic assessment.
3. Describe genotyping strategies for assessing allelic variants of a given drug metabolizing enzyme.
4. Characterize the molecular diagnostic tests that are used to detect allelic variants of drug metabolizing enzymes.
5. List the specific drugs that CYP2D6, CYP2C19, and CYP2C9 metabolize.
6. List the specific drugs that thiopurine S-methyltransferase (TPMT) metabolizes.
7. List the specific drugs that N-acetyltransferases (NAT1 and NAT2) metabolize.
8. Discuss possible future directions that the field of pharmacogenetics will take, including genotyping tests for new drugs, optimizing therapeutic drug dosing, and reducing drug toxicity.

KEY WORDS AND DEFINITIONS

Adverse Drug Reactions (ADRs): Any undesirable side effect or toxic reaction that is caused by the administration of a drug; ADRs are a leading cause of morbidity and mortality in the United States.

Cytochrome P-450 (CYP): A large family of drug metabolizing enzymes that are also important in metabolism of steroid hormones, fatty acids, and other substances; these isozymes are involved in metabolism of more than 50% of all drugs; many CYPs are polymorphic and may account for variation among individuals in their response to drugs; phenotypes associated with genotypes range from poor to rapid metabolizers.

Drug Metabolism: The process by which drugs are chemically modified in the body; most often metabolism involves one or more enzymes; although the primary purpose of drug metabolism is to promote inactivation and elimination of the drug, some drug metabolites possess pharmacological activity and may persist in the body longer than the parent drug.

Genotyping: Detection of specific genetic variants; some correlate with drug response phenotypes.

Metabolizer: A description of the drug metabolism phenotype. Specifically, an individual's rate of metabolism as it relates to a specific therapeutic drug; poor metabolizers (PMs) metabolize a drug slowly if at all, whereas an ultrarapid metabolizer (UM) converts a drug to its metabolite(s) very quickly, as compared with the "normal" so-called extensive metabolizer (EM).

N-Acetyltransferase (NAT): A family of metabolic enzymes that acetylate drugs, such as procainamide (cardiac medication) and sulfonamides (antibiotics), in addition to a number of environmental toxins; slow and fast acetylator phenotypes are well characterized in several populations.

Pharmacogenetics: The variations in a single gene or small group of related genes that affect the pharmacology of a drug; the study of human genetic variation as revealed by various reactions to a drug.

Pharmacogenomics: The variations in several genes, or the genome, that influence drug handling; the use of human genetic information for the design of new pharmaceuticals.

Phenotyping: The observable reaction or response of an individual (such as to a specific drug); the phenotype is based upon that individual's genes, but also influenced by factors such as concomitant medications, liver function, and renal function.

Prodrug: An inactive or less active drug that must be first metabolized to the active form of the drug to elicit the desired therapeutic effect.

Thiopurine S-Methyltransferase (TPMT): A metabolic enzyme that methylates and thereby inactivates 6-mercaptopurine (6-MP) and azathioprine, drugs used to treat several conditions, such as cancer and immune-mediated disease; individuals either lacking this enzyme or that possess enzyme with compromised function may require lower doses of the drugs to prevent toxicity.

UDP-Glucuronyltransferase (UGT): A family of metabolic enzymes that glucuronate, and thereby inactivate, drugs such as irinotecan (cancer therapeutic); genetic variants of UGT1A1, such as those in its promoter region, are associated with phenotypes that require dose reductions as a result of higher risk of toxicity.

The term **pharmacogenetics** has been pieced together from the words pharmacology (the study of drugs, drug action, and metabolism) and genetics (the study of how traits are inherited). Pharmacogenetic testing in a clinical setting links patients' genetics (genotype and/or haplotype) with the metabolism and clearance of drugs (pharmacokinetics) or with the actions and effects of drugs (pharmacodynamics). Whereas the terms pharmacogenetics and *pharmacogenomics* are frequently used interchangeably, pharmacogenetics as used in this chapter considers how variation in a single gene or small group of related genes affects the pharmacology of a drug. In contrast, **pharmacogenomics** considers how variation in several genes, or the genome, influences drug handling. Pharmacogenomics may lead to development of new drugs and future clinical laboratory tests. Clinical pharmacogenetic test results today may be useful for guiding the selection of specific medications and for optimizing dosing, but do not include all genes that may be involved in drug pharmacokinetics or pharmacodynamics. Thus no single test will predict the best drug or best dose for all patients. However, specific dosing guidelines based on pharmacogenetic information are being developed to support the application of these test results for therapeutic drug management in several clinical settings. Such individualized pharmacotherapy is anticipated to reduce the number of **adverse drug reactions (ADRs),** a leading cause of morbidity and mortality in the United States (Table 12-1), and also to maximize drug efficacy.

TABLE 12-1	Estimated Occurrence of Adverse Drug Reactions in the USA in 1994, in Thousands (95% Confidence Interval)		
	ADRs in Patients While in Hospital	ADRs Responsible for Patient Admission to a Hospital	Total ADRs
All severities	3670 (2618-4596)	1547 (1033-2060)	4987 (3976-5995)
Serious	702 (635-770)	1547 (1033-2060)	2216 (1721-2711)
Fatal	63 (41-85)	43 (15-71)	106 (76-137)

Modified from Lazarou J, Pomeranz BH, Corey PN. Incidence of adverse drug reactions in hospitalized patients: a meta-analysis of prospective studies. JAMA 1998;279:1200-5. Reproduced with the permission of the American Medical Association.

The goal of this chapter is to familiarize the reader with pharmacogenetic testing. This chapter begins with a discussion of general issues, including potential tests to offer in the clinical laboratory, choosing appropriate testing strategies, characteristics of a gene that make it a good candidate for pharmacogenetic testing, and characteristics of medications or other xenobiotics that support the need for pharmacogenetic testing. In the following sections, detailed information for seven well-characterized and polymorphic genes (*TPMT, CYP2D6, CYP2C19, CYP2C9, UGT1A1, NAT1,* and *NAT2*) is described. Variation in these genes contributes to intersubject variation in enzyme activity, kinetics, substrate specificity, and/or stability. Such variation is reflected in the ability of an individual to appropriately respond to medications that are substrates of these enzymes. This alteration in response to the medication defines the phenotype. The correlation of phenotypes and genotypes for these and several other proposed genetic targets is discussed in this chapter as well.

DEFINING PHARMACOGENETIC TARGETS AND WHAT TESTING TO CONSIDER

The response to drugs and other xenobiotics (foreign compounds absorbed by the human body) depends on many processes, such as route of administration, amount absorbed, any biotransformation (metabolism) that occurs, affinity of the parent compound and metabolite(s) for endogenous receptor(s) or other target(s) responsible for drug action, and the process of elimination. For the sake of simplicity, the term "drug(s)" will be used throughout this chapter with the understanding that many principles of pharmacogenetics that apply to medications may also apply to other xenobiotics. Each process mentioned above involves several proteins that are coded from corresponding genes. Consequently, pharmacogenetic targets include any polymorphic gene that encodes for the many different proteins involved in these processes. To date the best-studied pharmacogenetic targets are those involved in **drug metabolism.** Common features of pharmacogenetic tests of proven usefulness include: (1) the enzyme of interest is the primary pathway for metabolism of the drug or the pathway that displays the greatest variance; (2) changes in metabolic enzyme activity resulting from genetic polymorphism have a significant effect on the relationship between dose and plasma concentration; (3) the efficacy and/or toxicity of the drug correlate with changes in plasma drug concentration; and (4) the drugs affected by the pharmacogenetic variability possess a narrow therapeutic index. Further, pharmacogenetic testing is of particular usefulness for those drugs that require a long period of time to establish efficacy or to optimize dose. Advocates of pharmacogenetics anticipate that future testing opportunities will include the ability to identify a population of nonresponders for a particular drug. Examples of drug classes that may benefit from pharmacogenetic testing include cancer chemotherapy, immunosuppressants, antidepressants, antipsychotics, anticoagulants, antihypertensives, and lipid-lowering therapies.

In general, *drug metabolism* serves to do one or more of the following: inactivate a substrate and increase water solubility of the substrate for excretion; bioactivate a substrate to an active, toxic, or mutagenic principle; or less commonly, extend the elimination half-life of a pharmacologically active or potentially toxic metabolite. A **prodrug** is a drug that is inactive in the parent form, but is metabolized to an active compound. Codeine, for example, is an inactive drug that is converted to the active drug morphine and is therefore described as a prodrug. Metabolic reactions are often divided into phase I and phase II categories, as depicted in Figure 12-1.

Phase I reactions are functionalization reactions and, as such, convert the parent compound into a more polar metabolite by introducing or removing a single functional group. Examples include oxidation, reduction, and hydrolysis. Most phase I reactions are oxidative and are mediated by cytochrome P-450 (CYP) isozymes. CYPs are heme-containing enzymes that are synthesized from a superfamily of CYP genes and are classi-

fied into families, and further into subfamilies, based on amino acid homology. The primary *CYPs* that are believed to contribute to drug metabolism are *CYP1A2, CYP2B6, CYP2C9, CYP2C19, CYP2D6, CYP2E1,* and the *CYP3A* family. All of these *CYP* families exhibit genetic variation that has been associated with clinically significant phenotypic differences caused by changes in enzyme activity, stability, and/or substrate affinity. Most CYP isoenzymes are also susceptible to dramatic differences in expression (>1000-fold), caused by genetic variation, and by induction or inhibition mediated by endogenous and exogenous compounds, including enzyme substrates. Products of phase I reactions may be eliminated or undergo additional modification, such as through phase II reactions. Phase II reactions may occur independent of or before phase I reactions.

Phase II enzymes are generally transferases involving enzyme-mediated conjugation with acetyl, glucuronyl, amino acid, or sulfate groups. These enzymes are not typically induced or inhibited to the same degree as CYPs. However, exhausting the substrates or cofactors for transfer, such as glutathione or acetyl CoA, will prevent the corresponding transferase reactions from occurring.

APPROACHES TO PHARMACOGENETIC TESTING

Pharmacogenetics is important to patient care because for many drugs there are differences in drug metabolism and drug response among individuals. These differences significantly alter the safety and success of therapy. Pharmacogenetic testing allows the physician to predict if a patient is likely to fail therapy or suffer an ADR before initiating therapy. This knowledge can lead to a change in drug dosage or drug selection, thus preventing an undesired outcome.

Two major approaches are available to predict how well an individual will metabolize a medication: **phenotyping** and **genotyping.** *Phenotyping* is accomplished by testing metabolic activity—either by administering to the patient a safe drug, often called a probe drug, that is known to be metabolized by the same enzyme or pathway as the intended therapeutic drug or alternatively, by measuring the drug metabolizing enzyme activity using peripheral blood cells as a surrogate to the metabolism of the whole patient. Examples of probe drugs include dextromethorphan for assessing CYP2D6 activity and caffeine for NAT2. Examples of enzyme-based phenotyping tests that have been successfully implemented include pseudocholinesterase for detecting individuals with susceptibility to prolonged apnea when given succinylcholine or other similar medications; TPMT for detecting individuals with susceptibility to hematological toxicity with azathioprine (AZA) or 6-mercaptopurine (6-MP); and glucose-6-phosphate dehydrogenase (G6PD) for detecting susceptibility to hemolysis in response to drugs such as primaquine, sulfonamides, chloramphenicol, and vitamin K. These techniques directly measure drug metabolism phenotype and, under highly controlled circumstances, provide the most meaningful information. There are, however, several limitations to the phenotypical approach. For example, the probe compound must be easy to administer in the target population, be relatively inexpensive, and exhibit pharmacokinetics that support convenient collection of specimens from the patient. Even with these variables controlled, phenotyping may be difficult to accomplish because of other potentially confounding

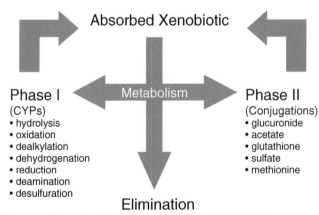

Figure 12-1

Simplified scheme of the primary metabolic reactions associated with xenobiotic handling in humans. Absorbed xenobiotics (drugs or other exogenous compounds) may be eliminated without biotransformation or be transformed into a metabolite through phase I and/or phase II reactions. The metabolite may be further metabolized by phase I or phase II reactions before elimination. Phase I reactions are primarily oxidative and are most commonly mediated by CYP isozymes. Phase II reactions involve conjugations to form glucuronides, acetates, and other adducts.

factors, such as diet, comedications, recent blood transfusion, hormone fluctuations, consumption of alcohol or over-the-counter medications, and disease status. Thus phenotyping illustrates the "state" rather than the "trait."

Pharmacogenetic testing, determining genotypes and/or haplotypes, is the second major approach to predicting drug metabolism and drug response. Pharmacogenetics may be useful for predicting pharmacodynamic response by identifying inherited genetic characteristics that either account for differences in phenotype from a structural basis or are clearly associated with phenotype through rigorous clinical studies. Phenotypes may be related to single nucleotide polymorphisms (SNPs), an array of SNPs on one allele (intragene haplotype), a combination of SNPs between two alleles (haplotype), complete gene deletions, or gene replications. Variants may occur in coding, noncoding, and promoter regions of a gene. Neither phenotyping nor pharmacogenetic testing is intended to replace clinical assessments of drug response or replace the need for therapeutic drug monitoring. Several considerations of these two testing approaches are summarized in Table 12-2. Examples of both approaches will be given throughout this chapter; however, more emphasis is given to the pharmacogenetic approaches because of the growing evidence supporting genotyping as a superior means of classifying enzymatic capacity. That evidence includes the facts that genotyping assays are less expensive, are more reproducible between laboratories, are not subject to intraindividual variability because of a specific set of clinical conditions or biological variations that complicate phenotyping assays, and are less invasive (i.e., a single blood sample for genotyping; several samples for phenotyping).

Although genotyping has many advantages over phenotyping, there are limitations to genotyping that must be recognized. For example, some of the assays using target amplification are prone to false-negative results because they rely on the presence or absence of a polymerase chain reaction (PCR) product. Short of sequencing the entire gene, currently available genotyping techniques cannot detect all possible variants. Because of the large amount of variation in many genes, suites of variants are screened, potentially missing some important genetic variations because the patient possesses a rare or novel polymorphism that is not detected by the screen. Further, polymorphisms with unknown clinical significance may also be identified by some techniques. Extreme care must be taken to ensure that these data are not misinterpreted.

Another disadvantage of genotyping is that it may not accurately predict function of the expressed protein. Using CYP2D6

as an example, it has been shown that patients of a single common genotype have metabolic ratios (a ratio of parent to metabolite concentrations often used to describe the metabolic phenotype) that span a 1000- to 10,000-fold range. The precise reason for this broad range is unknown, but it is probably related to individual differences in expression of the CYP2D6 gene, inherent alternative metabolic pathways, significant interlaboratory and intraindividual variability in phenotype measurements, and possible combinations of other minor undetected genetic polymorphisms in the CYP2D6 gene.

Finally, specific interactions between the target enzyme or protein and other drugs, chemicals, or some foods can change the phenotype, such as by converting a "normal" or extensive **metabolizer** (EM) phenotype to a poor metabolizer (PM) phenotype. For example, grapefruit juice has been shown to inhibit CYP3A4, and many antidepressant medications (e.g., tricyclics and selective serotonin reuptake inhibitors) are known to act as both substrates and inhibitors of CYP2D6.[16] Such drug and food interactions can have extremely important consequences for patients and can be difficult to both recognize and monitor.

CLINICAL APPLICATION OF PHARMACOGENETIC TESTING

Pharmacogenetic testing is only clinically useful when there is sufficient information to interpret the results. This information must be derived from in vivo, human studies demonstrating a clear phenotype. Many examples of this type of information can be found in the peer-reviewed literature, but most data are based on retrospective studies, and there is no single printed source in which all of this information has been collated. The Pharmacogenetics and Pharmacogenomics Knowledge Base (www.pharmgkb.org) is a publicly available internet research tool developed by Stanford University with funding from the National Institutes of Health (NIH) and is part of the NIH Pharmacogenetics Research Network (PGRN), a nationwide collaborative research consortium. Its aim is to aid researchers in understanding how genetic variation among individuals contributes to differences in reactions to drugs. This regularly updated database provides genetic and clinical information derived from research studies at various medical centers in the PGRN.

Currently, published dosing guidelines relate to specific combinations of pharmacogenetic markers and drugs. For example, Kirchheiner et al have published dose recommendations for 20 antidepressant medications based on single versus

TABLE 12-2	Comparing Phenotype and Genotype Testing Strategies	
	Phenotype	**Genotype**
Represent	"State," represents current response; may not represent inheritance	"Trait," represents inheritance; may not be consistent with the phenotype
Sensitive to gene expression	Yes	No
Sensitive to protein function	Yes	No
Requires collection of multiple specimens	Commonly	No
Requires administration of a probe drug	Commonly	No
Other limitations	Specimen instability for enzyme or other protein of interest may lead to inaccurate results	May not include all clinically relevant genes and/or alleles
	May not be appropriate for a patient who recently received a blood transfusion	Genotype to phenotype relationship (interpretation) may not be known

chronic maintenance therapy and genotypes for both *CYP2D6* and *CYP2C19*.[11] Average recommended adjustments of "standard" doses vary from 20% of the usual dose for PMs using venlafaxine, paroxetine, or desipramine to 300% of the usual dose for ultrarapid metabolizers (UM) using mianserin. Similar work suggesting specific dose ranges or adjustments based on phenotype-genotype relationships has been conducted with other substrates of these CYP isoenzymes (see CYP2D6 and CYP2C19 sections later in this chapter), AZA and 6-MP (see TPMT section of this chapter), warfarin (see CYP2C9 section of this chapter), and antipsychotics.

Many ongoing clinical trials for efficacy and toxicity of new pharmaceutical products or new indications for previously developed pharmaceuticals have employed pharmacogenetic or pharmacogenomic testing. Thus it is anticipated that pharmacogenetic guidelines and possibly companion tests will be simultaneously released to market with the pharmaceutical.

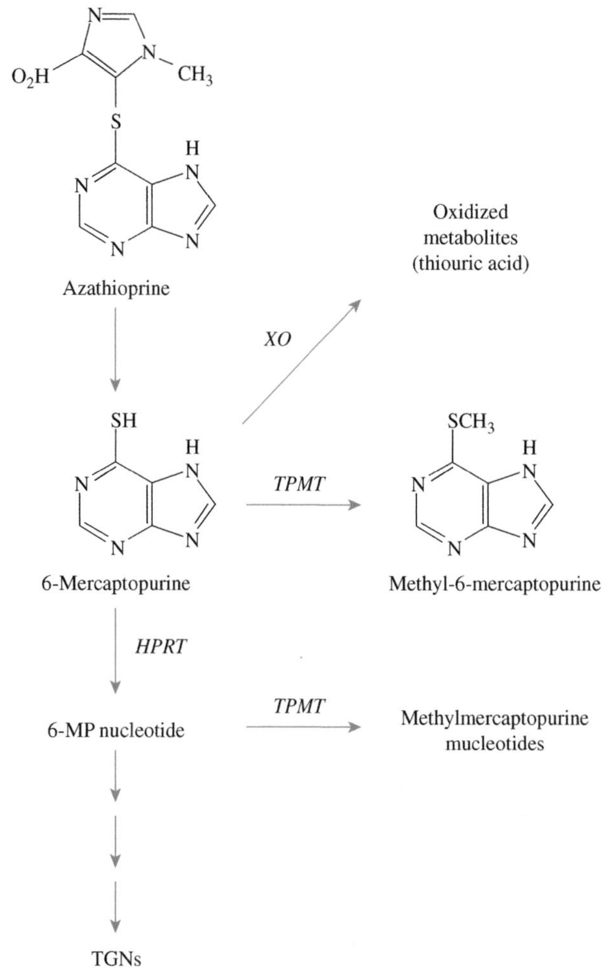

BEST EXAMPLES OF CLINICALLY RELEVANT PHARMACOGENETIC TARGETS

For each of seven genes, *TPMT*, *CYP2D6*, *CYP2C19*, *CYP2C9*, *UGT1A1*, *NAT1*, and *NAT2*, this chapter provides an overview of background information, the relationship between genotype and phenotype, unique testing methods, and clinical applications of testing.

Thiopurine S-Methyltransferase

Thiopurine S-methyltransferase (TPMT) is a phase II metabolic enzyme that catalyzes the inactivation of 6-MP by S-methylation, thus preventing it from forming thioguanine nucleotides (TGN). TPMT also affects AZA, which is a prodrug metabolized to 6-MP, as shown in Figure 12-2. Endogenous substrates for TPMT are currently unknown. AZA and 6-MP are used in the therapeutic management of a diverse range of conditions, including leukemia, rheumatic diseases, inflammatory bowel disease, and solid organ transplantation. These agents are cytotoxic, acting via incorporation of TGN into DNA. Outside of the bone marrow, these agents can be oxidatively inactivated by xanthine oxidase or methylated by TPMT. In hematopoietic tissue, however, the effect of xanthine oxidase is negligible, leaving TPMT as the only significant inactivation pathway. Thus hematopoietic tissues are susceptible to damage in cases in which TPMT activity is very low. TPMT activity is highly variable in all large populations studied to date; approximately 90% of individuals have high activity, 10% have intermediate activity, and 0.3% have low or undetectable enzyme activity. This trimodal activity is a direct result of enhanced proteasomal degradation of TPMT.[20] Numerous studies have shown that TPMT-deficient patients are at high risk for severe, and sometimes fatal, hematological toxicity.

Genotype to Phenotype

The molecular basis for variable TPMT activity has now been defined for the majority of patients. TPMT activity is inherited as an autosomal codominant trait,[24] exhibiting genetic polymorphism in all populations studied to date. Eleven variant *TPMT* alleles have been identified, including nine SNPs leading to amino acid substitutions, *TPMT*2*, **3A*, **3B*, **3C*, **3D*, **5*, **6*, **7*, and **8*; one change leading to the formation of a stop codon, *TPMT*3D*; and a change that destroys a splice site: *TPMT*4*. Three alleles, *TPMT*2*, **3A*, and **3C*, account for

Figure 12-2
Simplified scheme of the metabolism of azathioprine and 6-MP to TGNs. *TPMT*, Thiopurine S-methyltransferase; *XO*, xanthine oxidase; *HPRT*, hypoxanthine phosphoribosyltransferase.
(Redrawn from Clunie GP, Lennard L. Relevance of thiopurine methyltransferase status in rheumatology patients receiving azathioprine. Rheumatology (Oxford) 2004;43:13-8. Reproduced by permission from Oxford University Press.)

about 95% of intermediate or low enzyme activity cases (Figure 12-3). All three alleles associated with lower enzyme activity have enhanced rates of proteolysis of the alloenzymes (protein products of the variant alleles). The presence of a *TPMT* variant allele is 90% sensitive and 99% specific for predicting TPMT phenotype; patients with one wild-type allele and one of these variant alleles (i.e., heterozygous) have intermediate activity, and patients inheriting two variant alleles are TPMT deficient (see Figure 12-4). Genotyping tests, however, may not detect TPMT deficiency in all patients, particularly those with a rare or unknown but clinically significant variant. Other genes also influence the disposition of and response to mercaptopurines. For example, an inosine triphosphate (ITPA)–deficient phenotype may provide an additional mechanism for thiopurine-related toxicity.[3] This phenotype, like TPMT deficiency, is clinically benign until a patient is exposed to a thiopurine therapeutic, such as 6-MP or AZA. The ITPA deficiency phenotype is associated with a 94C>A polymorphism of *ITPA* and

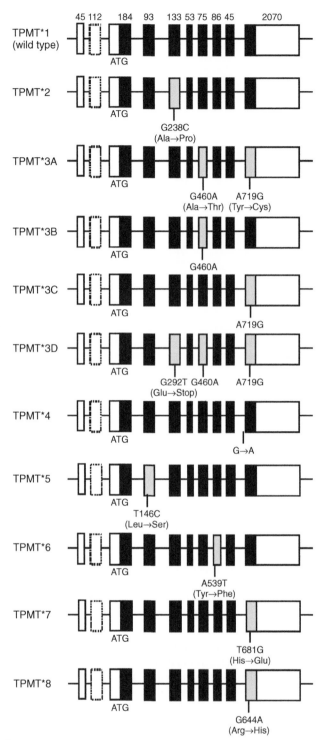

Figure 12-3

TPMT allele variants. Blue boxes represent mutations that result in amino acid changes. TPMT*4 is a 5′ splice site mutation for exon 10 that does not alter an amino acid. White boxes represent untranslated regions. Black boxes represent exons in the open reading frame. The dashed box represents exon 2, which was detected in 6.25% of human liver cDNAs during initial evaluation.

(From McLeod HL, Siva C. The thiopurine S-methyltransferase gene locus—implications for clinical pharmacogenomics. Pharmacogenomics 2002;3:89-98. Reproduced by permission from Future Medicine Ltd [London].)

approximately 25% residual red cell ITPase activity. Consequently the metabolite 6-thio-ITP accumulates and may contribute to toxicities previously associated only with TPMT deficiency. Although currently not well characterized, determination of genotypes for *TPMT*, *ITPA*, and potentially other genes may form the best strategy for predicting risk of adverse reactions associated with AZA and 6-MP therapy.

Testing

TPMT testing may occur via at least three routes: biochemical phenotyping by determining TPMT activity within erythrocytes from the patient; metabolic phenotyping by determining concentrations of 6-MP and thioguanine; or genotyping. Biochemical phenotyping depends on stable enzyme activity between the times of blood collection and analytical testing. This approach is also limited to patients who have not received a blood transfusion over the weeks previous to TPMT testing. Metabolic phenotyping requires that AZA or 6-MP be administered before testing. This approach is therefore most useful for patients who have experienced an adverse event or for monitoring therapy in those for whom TPMT activity is known to be impaired. *TPMT* genotype correlates well with TPMT activity in leukemia cells, as would be expected for germline mutations. By using PCR-based assays to detect the three signature mutations in these alleles, a rapid and relatively inexpensive assay may identify >90% of all variant alleles. In Caucasian populations, *TPMT*3A* is the most common variant *TPMT* allele. Studies in Caucasian, African, and Asian populations have revealed that the frequency of these variant *TPMT* alleles differs among various ethnic populations. East and West African populations have a frequency of variant alleles similar to that of Caucasians, but the variant alleles in the African populations were preponderantly *TPMT*3C*. Among African Americans, *TPMT*3C* is the most prevalent allele, but *TPMT*2* and *TPMT*3A* are also found. In Japanese and Chinese populations, *TPMT*3C* is almost exclusively the causative variant allele. In other Asian populations, the *TPMT*3C* is also preponderant, but the *3A and *6 alleles have also been observed in Indian and Malay children, respectively.[5] Detailed descriptions of relevant methods are found in Chapter 5.

Clinical Application

TPMT was the first widely used pharmacogenetic marker for individualizing drug therapy based on a patient's biochemical phenotype (erythrocyte enzyme activity) or genotype. Patients with a "low methylator" status (homozygous variant or compound heterozygote) may tolerate standard doses, but are at significantly greater risk of toxicity, often necessitating a lower dose of these medications (as low as 5% of standard doses). Prospective determination of functional TPMT status is useful for preventing mercaptopurine toxicity. Whether TPMT testing is based on phenotype or genotype, the goal is individualized dosing and controlled systemic exposure.

An analysis of mercaptopurine therapy for childhood acute lymphocytic leukemia (ALL) found that TPMT-deficient patients tolerated full doses of mercaptopurines for only a brief period (7% of the scheduled weeks of therapy), whereas heterozygous and homozygous wild-type patients tolerated full doses for 65% and 84% of scheduled weeks of therapy during the $2\frac{1}{2}$ years of treatment, respectively. The percentage of weeks in which mercaptopurine dosage had to be decreased to prevent

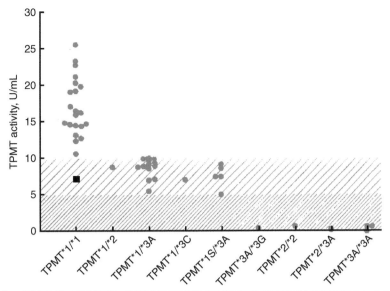

Figure 12-4
TPMT activity as related to genotypes determined by mutation-specific PCR methods. The heavily shaded area depicts the range of TPMT activity in erythrocytes that defines TPMT deficiency (<5 U/mL of packed red blood cells); the lightly shaded area depicts intermediate activity that defines TPMT heterozygous phenotypes (5 to 10 U/mL of packed red blood cells); and the nonshaded area depicts the range of TPMT activity in patients who have homozygous wild-type phenotypes. Blue circles indicate patients with concordant genotype and phenotype; the square indicates one patient with discordant genotype and phenotype (TPMT*1/*1).
(From Yates CR, Krynetski EY, Loennechen T, Fessing MY, Tai HL, Pui CH, et al. Molecular diagnosis of thiopurine S-methyltransferase deficiency: genetic basis for azathioprine and mercaptopurine intolerance. Ann Intern Med 1997;126:608-14. Reproduced by permission from the American College of Physicians.)

toxicity was 2%, 16%, and 76% in wild-type, heterozygous, and homozygous variant individuals. Collectively, these studies demonstrate that the influence of *TPMT* genotype on hematopoietic toxicity is most dramatic for homozygous variant patients, but is also of clinical relevance for heterozygous individuals, who represent about 10% of patients treated with these medications.

A potentially valuable role for TPMT status testing is before intravenous AZA loading, a strategy shown to be safe in the management of Crohn's disease. Dose-related toxicities resulted in AZA discontinuation in 10% to 20% of cases, and it was estimated that over 6 months 20% of patients would need TPMT analysis to prevent one serious adverse event. TPMT status testing before taking AZA has been modeled to be cost-effective in a variety of theoretical situations. Analysis of some recent studies suggests that by optimizing the maximum AZA dose between 0.75 and 3 mg/kg/day, depending on TPMT status testing (with a drastic reduction in dosage for patients homozygous for variant *TPMT* alleles), considerable cost savings can be made by preventing hospitalization and rescue therapy for leukopenic events. Furthermore, one study reported that the median dose reduction required for TPMT-deficient patients was 90.8% (range, 50% to 94%), with a median dose reduction in *TPMT* heterozygotes of 67% (range, 0% to 93%). This study included only patients referred for hematopoietic toxicity. However, previous studies have reported that heterozygous patients needed only 15% to 30% dose reduction to prevent serious side effects.[6,12]

Cytochrome P-450 2D6 (CYP2D6)

Cytochrome P-450 (CYP) 2D6 (CYP2D6), originally named debrisoquine 4-hydroxylase, is a phase I enzyme known to metabolize more than 100 drugs and environmental toxins as substrates. Examples of drugs and drug classes metabolized by CYP2D6 are shown in Table 12-3. CYP2D6 is also inhibited by several compounds, some of which are substrates. More than 80 genetic variants have been described in the *CYP2D6* gene. In general, the variants can be grouped according to the resulting alterations in protein function. These groupings correlate well with the four major phenotypes described historically for CYP2D6: EMs, PMs, intermediate metabolizers (IMs), and UMs. The major coding sequence variants described result in decreased function with the exception of gene duplication, which results in increased metabolic capacity if a functional gene has been duplicated. Of Caucasians, approximately 5% are UM, and 5% to 10% are PM. Only 1% to 3% of African Americans and Asians are PM, but many are IM. The frequency of UM in East Africans and Spaniards is reported to be much higher than in Caucasians, from 7% to 29%.[16]

Genotype to Phenotype

The relationship between the CYP2D6 enzyme function (phenotype) and the *CYP2D6* genotype has been extensively characterized. Genetic variability accounts for the tetramodal distribution of CYP2D6 activity that is described historically by the phenotypes. The rank order of metabolic capacity is UM > EM > IM > PM, representing approximately 5% to 7%,

TABLE 12-3	Examples of Drug Substrates for CYP2C19, CYP2C9, and CYP2D6		
2C19	**2C9**	**2D6**	
Amitriptyline	Amitriptyline	Alprenolol	Minaprine
Carisoprodol	Celecoxib	Amitriptyline	Nebivolol
Citalopram	Diclofenac	Amphetamine	Nortriptyline
Clomipramine	Fluoxetine	Aripiprazole	Ondansetron
Cyclophosphamide	Fluvastatin glyburide	Atomoxetine	Paroxetine
Hexobarbital	Glibenclamide	Bufuralol	Perhexiline
Imipramine	Glimepiride	Carvedilol	Perphenazine
Indomethacin	Glipizide	Chlorpheniramine	Phenacetin
Lansoprazole	Glyburide	Chlorpromazine	Phenformin
Moclobemide	Ibuprofen	Clomipramine	Promethazine
Nelfinavir	Irbesartan	Codeine	Propafenone
Nilutamide	Lornoxicam	Debrisoquine	Propranolol
Omeprazole	Losartan	Desipramine	Risperidone
Pantoprazole	Meloxicam	Dexfenfluramine	S-metoprolol
Phenobarbitone	Nateglinide	Dextromethorphan	Sparteine
Phenytoin	Phenytoin	Duloxetine	Tamoxifen
Primidone	Piroxicam	Encainide	Thioridazine
Progesterone	Rosiglitazone	Flecainide	Timolol
Proguanil	S-naproxen	Fluoxetine	Tramadol
Propranolol	Suprofen	Fluvoxamine	Venlafaxine
Rabeprazole	Tamoxifen	Haloperidol	
R-mephobarbital	Tolbutamide	Imipramine	
S-mephenytoin	Torsemide	Lidocaine	
Teniposide	S-warfarin	Methoxyamphetamine	
R-warfarin		Metoclopramide	
		Mexiletine	

From Flockhart DA. Clinically relevant drug interaction table. This table is updated frequently. http://medicine.iupui.edu/flockhart/table.htm (Accessed August 30, 2004). Reproduced with the permission of David A. Flockhart, M.D., Ph.D.

60%, 25%, and 10% of most populations, respectively. A summary of *CYP2D6* alleles and consequences is shown in Figure 12-5.

CYP2D6 phenotypes have historically been determined through the use of probe drugs. Urine collected at a specified time after administration of the probe drug (e.g., 8 hours) is analyzed for the parent drug and a metabolite that is primarily generated via CYP2D6. The ratio of parent and metabolite concentrations is referred to as the metabolic ratio (MR). Example parent-metabolite pairs used commonly as probe drugs for CYP2D6 include debrisoquine/4-hydroxydebrisoquine (Figure 12-6), dextromethorphan/dextrorphan, and nortriptyline/10-hydroxynortriptyline. The need to administer a probe drug and to collect urine over several hours has limited the practical utility of patient phenotyping. Although the MR is theoretically a good indicator of enzyme expression and function at the time of the test, marked variation has been demonstrated in this phenotypical characteristic for nearly every CYP2D6 genotype. Interpretation of MRs must consider the specificity of the probe drug for the CYP2D6 and also the elimination kinetics of the parent and metabolite.[4,14]

Testing

The *CYP2D6* gene, like other CYP genes, is relatively challenging to genotype because of the presence of pseudogenes and also because of the need for identification of gene dose, specifically duplications and deletions of the gene. Because duplicated genes can be either functional (*CYP2D6*1*, *CYP2D6*2*, or *CYP2D6*35*) or nonfunctional (e.g., *CYP2D6*4*), it is

important that the testing method identify what allele has been duplicated. To separate *CYP2D6* from structurally similar pseudogenes, *CYP2D6* genotyping protocols often employ long-PCR or nested PCR strategies with a first PCR step designed to amplify a large *CYP2D6*-specific region. Small nucleotide changes within this region, including SNPs and smaller insertions and/or deletions of one or a few bases, are then detected in a second amplification step either designed as a PCR-restriction fragment length polymorphism (RFLP) assay or as an allele-specific PCR without subsequent digestion. By evaluating the entire gene, both known and unknown mutations can be detected. Other technologies used for genotyping include real-time PCR methods and microarrays. *CYP2D6* and other CYP pharmacogenetic screening protocols may detect only the most common variants.[4] Detailed descriptions of relevant methods are found in Chapter 5.

Clinical Applications

CYP2D6 metabolic status can be applied to prescribing of medications that are known to be transformed by this enzyme. Such medications may be avoided entirely, or the dose can be optimized based on how CYP2D6 affects the drug. For example, many therapeutic drugs are administered as prodrugs. Prodrugs must be metabolized to the active principle to elicit the desired therapeutic effect. An example is codeine, an alkaloid obtained from opium or prepared from morphine by methylation. Codeine must be activated, through metabolism mediated primarily by CYP2D6, to morphine to produce analgesia. Therefore a CYP2D6 PM could not activate codeine like an

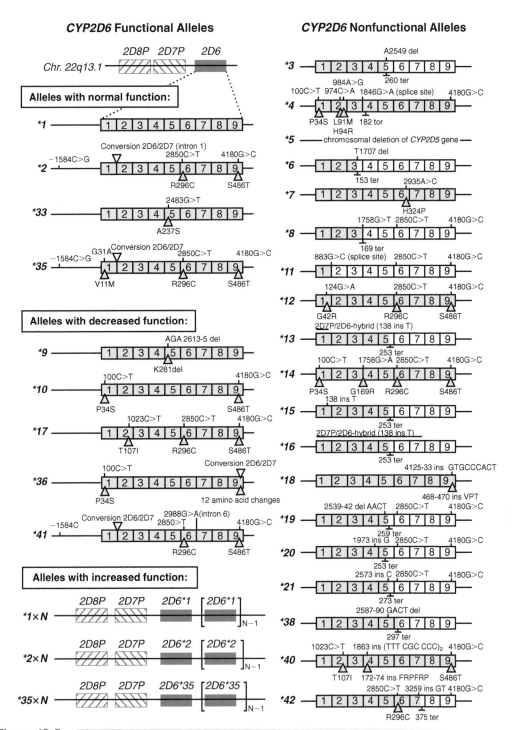

Figure 12-5
Structure of functional and nonfunctional *CYP2D6* alleles. Only alleles with available phenotypical information are shown. The nine exons are indicated by numbered boxes with DNA polymorphisms indicated on top (*del*, deletion, *ins*, insertion). Predicted amino acid changes and translation termination (*ter*) codons are indicated below. Open reading frames are indicated by blue shaded boxes. Silent mutations and some promoter and intronic polymorphisms and alleles with uncertain function are not shown.
(From Zanger UM, Raimundo S, Eichelbaum M. Cytochrome P450 2D6: overview and update on pharmacology, genetics, biochemistry. Naunyn Schmiedebergs Arch Pharmacol 2004;369:23-37. Reproduced by permission from Springer.)

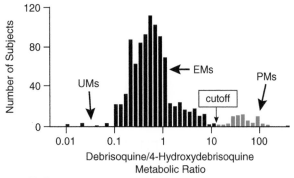

Figure 12-6

Histogram of the "debrisoquine metabolic ratio" in a typical Caucasian population. Metabolic ratios were determined from the concentrations of debrisoquine and 4-hydroxydebrisoquine (metabolite) in a urine specimen collected 8 hours after a 10-mg dose of debrisoquine. The data demonstrate a clear distinction between PM (*blue*), EM, and UM phenotypes.
(From Caldwell J. Pharmacogenetics and individual variation in the range of amino acid adequacy: the biological aspects. J Nutr 2004;134:1600S-4S; discussion 30S-32S, 67S-72S. Reproduced by permission from the American Society for Nutritional Sciences.)

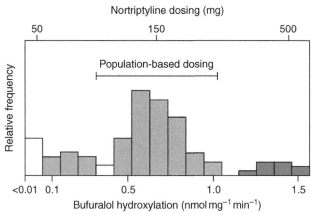

Figure 12-7

Variation in drug metabolism and NT dosing in the European population, based on cytochrome P-450 CYP2D6 activity (hydroxylation of bufuralol). Within the population four phenotypes can be identified: PMs, who lack the functional enzyme; IMs, who are heterozygous for one functional allele or have two partially defective alleles encoding the enzyme; EMs, who have two normal alleles; and UMs, who carry duplicated or multiduplicated functional *CYP2D6* genes. The relative frequency of these phenotypes refers to the European population as a whole. The doses of NT that are required to achieve therapeutic levels in all phenotypes are given. Despite this variation in metabolizing capability, population-based dosing is used today and is based on the average plasma levels obtained in a given population for a given dose.
(From Ingelman-Sundberg M. Pharmacogenetics of cytochrome P450 and its applications in drug therapy: the past, present and future. Trends Pharmacol Sci 2004;25:193-200. Reproduced by permission from Elsevier.)

EM would and may not experience analgesia with standard doses. A PM may be best served clinically by selecting a different analgesic agent. An IM is likely to require higher doses of codeine than an EM, and a UM may require lower doses of codeine than an EM. Indeed, the UM phenotype can lead to excessive, possibly toxic concentrations of active drug, such as excessive morphine generated after a dose of codeine is administered to a UM.

A similar example relates to tamoxifen, an estrogen receptor antagonist used for breast cancer. Tamoxifen is converted by CYP2D6 to endoxifen, the compound thought to be responsible for the clinical effects of tamoxifen. Women with impaired CYP2D6 do not respond well to tamoxifen therapy, and in fact have higher rates of relapse. In this situation, pre-therapeutic evaluation of women considering tamoxifen therapy may be important.

Most drugs, however, are inactivated by CYP2D6. For example, nortriptyline (NT) and other antidepressant medications are inactivated by CYP2D6. A CYP2D6 PM requires lower doses of NT than an EM to produce similar serum concentrations of active drug (see Figure 12-7). For the purpose of applying a *CYP2D6* genotype to clinical practice, homozygosity or compound heterozygosity for *CYP2D6* PM alleles is consistent with a PM phenotype. The presence of a single PM allele may lead to either an EM or an IM phenotype. Individuals with a PM phenotype have been successfully treated by reducing the dose of antidepressant medications that are inactivated by CYP2D6 by 40% to 80%.[11] Another example is provided by metoprolol succinate, used as a treatment for hypertension and angina pectoris. The therapeutic effect of this agent is proportional to serum concentrations, and striking differences in serum levels are observed with CYP2D6 PM and EM individuals following a single dose of metoprolol.

The accelerated rate of metabolism seen with UM phenotypes may lead to accelerated inactivation of active parent drug substrates. The consequences of a UM phenotype may include subtherapeutic concentrations of active drug at standard dosages. To compensate for increased metabolism, UM subjects have been successfully treated with megadoses (twofold to twelvefold greater than the standard dose) of some drugs that are inactivated by CYP2D6 to obtain therapeutic efficacy. Because most drugs act through multiple mechanisms that may or may not relate to the concentration of parent and/or metabolites, high-dose therapy may be associated with unrecognized risks, such as ADRs. Thus individuals with UM phenotypes may be best served by selecting therapeutic medications that are metabolized by an alternate (non-CYP2D6) route.

Cytochrome P-450 2C19 (CYP2C19)

CYP2C19 is a member of the CYP2C family, which includes CYP2C8, CYP2C9, CYP2C18, and CYP2C19 of which only *CYP2C9* and *CYP2C19* exhibit substantial genetic variability. Although substrate overlap between the family members exists, CYP2C19 is specifically associated with the 4'-hydroxylation of the S-enantiomer of the anticonvulsant mephenytoin and was originally named mephenytoin hydroxylase. CYP2C19 is a phase I enzyme for the metabolism of a number of other therapeutic drugs, including citalopram, diazepam, omeprazole, propranolol, and proguanil (see Table 12-3). Like the CYP2D6 isoenzyme, specific genetic variants of *CYP2C19* lead to PM and IM phenotypes with respect to a number of common therapeutic drugs. In contrast to the debrisoquine polymorphism, the UM phenotype has not been characterized for this enzyme.[14,16]

Genotype to Phenotype

At least 20 allelic variants of *CYP2C19* have been described. The EM phenotype has historically been composed of both the homozygous and heterozygous genotypes. The PM phenotype is inherited in an autosomal recessive manner. Like the *CYP2D6* polymorphisms, there are significant interethnic differences in the prevalence of the CYP2C19 PM phenotype. The PM phenotype occurs in 2% to 5% of Caucasian and black Zimbabwean Shona populations and 10% to 23% of Asian populations.[2]

Table 12-4 lists the most common *CYP2C19* polymorphisms with the nucleotide change, amino acid changes, and associated enzyme activity phenotype. The principal genetic variant in PMs of S-mephenytoin is *CYP2C19*2*, arising from a 681G>A, which results in a splicing defect and essentially no enzyme activity. The second most common *CYP2C19* allele (*CYP2C19*3*) associated with the PM phenotype results from a single nucleotide substitution 636G>A, which produces a premature stop codon and no active enzyme product. The allele frequency of *CYP2C19*2* is reported as 32% in East Asians and 71% in Polynesians (Vanuatu) and is approximately 15% in Caucasians and African Americans. The allele frequency of *CYP2C19*3* is reported as 6% to 10% in East Asians, 13.3% in Polynesians, and <1% among Caucasians. Additional alleles, such as *CYP2C19*4*, **5*, **6*, **8*, **9*, **10*, and **12* may also contribute to the CYP2C19 PM phenotype.[4,14]

Testing

Genotyping tests for detection of polymorphic *CYP2C19* variant alleles are similar to those described for *CYP2D6*.

Clinical Applications

The proton pump inhibitor omeprazole is primarily inactivated by the CYP2C19 enzyme, and thus its metabolism is subject to this genetic polymorphism (see Figure 12-8). The homozygous variant subjects had 100% cure of upper gastrointestinal ulcers after omeprazole-based therapy versus 65% and 25% for heterozygous and homozygous wild-type patients, respectively. No dose adjustments have been proposed for treating *Helicobacter pylori* infections.

The antimalarial prodrugs proguanil and chlorproguanil require CYP2C19-dependent bioactivation for therapeutic efficacy. A clear gene-dose effect has been observed for the oxidation of proguanil to cycloguanil and 4-chlorophenylbiguanide. Clinical response has been shown to be affected in CYP2C19 PM individuals.

Currently the most common reason for genotyping *CYP2C19* is to explain inappropriate response to antidepressant medications. For example, CYP2C19 is the primary enzyme responsible for converting amitriptyline (AT) to its active metabolite NT. Monitoring serum or plasma concentrations of both AT and NT as a sum is used to guide AT therapy. However, the utility of *CYP2C19* genotyping for this application is somewhat controversial. Using a quantitative gene dose model, it was found that *CYP2D6* but not *CYP2C19* genotyping is most useful in AT therapy based on the fact that *CYP2C19* polymorphisms alter the ratio of AT to NT, but not the sum of the two. The model was derived in a Caucasian population, whereas *CYP2C19* PMs are much more common in Asian populations. CYP2D6 is also thought to be more important than CYP2C19 for newer antidepressants. However, genotyping *CYP2C19* becomes very important for a CYP2D6 PM, when CYP2C19 shifts from a minor to a major route of metabolism. A second example is phenytoin, for which CYP2C19 is considered a minor route of metabolism and CYP2C9 the major route of metabolism. If CYP2C9 is impaired or deficient, CYP2C19 becomes a major route of metabolism.[10,18]

TABLE 12-4	Common CYP2C19 and CYP2C9 Alleles Associated with a Poor Metabolizer Phenotype			
Allele	**Nucleotide Changes**	**Effect**	**ENZYME ACTIVITY**	
			In vivo	**In vitro**
CYP2C19*2A	99C>T; **681G>A;** 990C>T; 991A>G	Splicing defect	None	
CYP2C19*2B	99C>T; 276G>C; **681G>A;** 990C>T; 991A>G	Splicing defect; E92D	None	
CYP2C19*3	**636G>A;** 991A>G; 1251A>C	Stop codon	None	
CYP2C9*2	430C>T	R144C		Decr
CYP2C9*3	1075A>C	I359L	Decr	Decr

From Human Cytochrome P450 (CYP) Allele Nomenclature Committee. CYP allele nomenclature. http://www.imm.ki.se/CYPalleles (Accessed December 5, 2004). Reproduced with the permission of Sarah C. Sim, Web master.

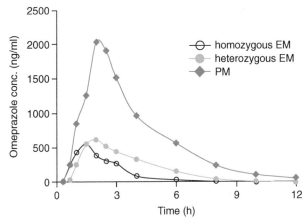

Figure 12-8

Mean plasma concentration-time profile of omeprazole after oral administration of 40 mg omeprazole (in the form of two 20-mg Losec capsules) to 27 male Chinese subjects phenotyped for CYP2C19 activity with mephenytoin. Plasma concentrations of omeprazole were significantly higher in PMs than in homozygous EMs or heterozygous EMs. In addition, the elimination half-life for omeprazole was 2.3-fold greater in PMs than in EMs (p < 0.001).

(From Yin OQ, Tomlinson B, Chow AH, Waye MM, Chow MS. Omeprazole as a CYP2C19 marker in Chinese subjects: assessment of its gene-dose effect and intrasubject variability. J Clin Pharmacol 2004;44:582-9. Reproduced by permission from Sage Publications, Inc.)

Cytochrome P-450 2C9 (CYP2C9)

CYP2C9, like CYP2C19, is a member of the CYP2C family and exhibits substantial genetic variability. Although substrate overlap between the family members exists (see Table 12-3), CYP2C9 is specifically associated with metabolism of the sulfonylurea hypoglycemic agent tolbutamide. CYP2C9 is also thought to be responsible for 90% of phenytoin metabolism and is very important to the metabolism of S-warfarin. Like the CYP2C19 isoenzyme, specific genetic variants of CYP2C9 lead to PM and IM phenotypes with respect to a number of common therapeutic drugs. In contrast to the debrisoquine polymorphism, the UM phenotype has not been characterized for this enzyme.[16,17]

Genotype to Phenotype

At least 12 allelic variants have been described in this gene, the most common of which are shown in Table 12-4. Two variant alleles of CYP2C9 (CYP2C9*2 and CYP2C9*3) account for most CYP2C9 PM phenotypes.[14] The allelic frequency of CYP2C9*2 has been reported as 8% to 19% in Caucasians and 1% to 4% in African Americans and Canadian Native Indians. This allele has not been detected in Asians. The allelic frequency of CYP2C9*3 has been reported as 6% to 10% in Caucasians, 1.7% to 5% in Asians, and 0.5% to 1.5% in African Americans. Studies in vitro have shown that the protein produced by the CYP2C9*3 variant is less than 5% as efficient as the CYP2C9*1 allozyme, whereas CYP2C9*2 shows about 12% of CYP2C9*1 allozyme activity in most assays.

CYP2C9*2 and CYP2C9*3 alleles result in PM phenotypes in the homozygous state, and IM phenotypes when heterozygous. Two additional alleles, found in African Americans, have been described, CYP2C9*5 and CYP2C9*6. The CYP2C9*6 in a homozygous individual was shown to contribute to an extremely long phenytoin elimination, with a half-life approximately 5.8 times longer than CYP2C9 EMs. The CYP2C9*8 allele has been shown in vitro to have greater activity than the wild-type enzyme, demonstrating 175% tolbutamide hydroxylase activity of recombinant wild type (see Figure 12-9). It was previously believed that no UM phenotypes existed for the CYP2C9 gene; however, CYP2C9*8 may dispel that notion.

Testing

Genotyping tests for detection of polymorphic CYP2C9 variant alleles are similar to those described for CYP2D6.

Clinical Applications

Examples of therapeutic compounds metabolized by CYP2C9 include nonsteroidal antiinflammatory drugs (NSAIDs), irbesartan, naproxen, and fluvastatin (see Table 12-3). Proposed dose adjustments based on phenotype have been published for CYP2C9 drug substrates, such as warfarin, glipizide, tolbutamide, and phenytoin.[9]

A multigene application of pharmacogenetics to address variable pharmacokinetics and pharmacodynamics is the warfarin application, with CYP2C9 and VKORC1. Warfarin is the most widely prescribed anticoagulant medication in the

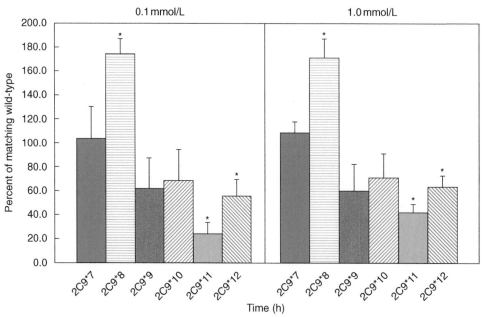

Figure 12-9

Tolbutamide hydroxylase activity of recombinant wild-type (CYP2C9*1) and new variant CYP2C9 alleles. CYP2C9 alleles were expressed in Escherichia coli and partially purified. For each variant allele, three individual preparations (two preparations for CYP2C9*7) were purified from bacteria simultaneously with wild type. Each preparation was assayed in triplicate at high (1 mmol/L) and low (0.1 mmol/L) substrate concentrations on the same day. Values are given as a percentage of enzymatic activity of the wild-type allele. *Significantly different from CYP2C9*1 protein activity (p < 0.05).

(From Blaisdell J, Jorge-Nebert LF, Coulter S, Ferguson SS, Lee SJ, Chanas B, et al. Discovery of new potentially defective alleles of human CYP2C9. Pharmacogenetics 2004;14:527-37. Reproduced by permission from Lippincott Williams & Wilkins.)

world. It is difficult to predict the appropriate dose of the drug because individuals differ widely in their responses to it. Weekly maintenance doses vary twentyfold. The consequences of inappropriate dosing are life threatening. A number of algorithms for predicting dose are available. Variables often considered include age, body weight, diet, and concomitant medications. Recent data demonstrate that individuals with the CYP2C9*2 and CYP2C9*3 polymorphisms have impaired metabolism of warfarin and thus increased plasma concentrations of the drug with standard dosing. As illustrated in Figure 12-10, standard 5 mg/day maintenance dosing of warfarin in subjects with CYP2C9 variants can lead to an excessive warfarin exposure, resulting in an exaggerated anticoagulant response. The clinical impact of CYP2C9 polymorphism includes increased risk of serious or life-threatening bleeding complications and increased time to achieve a stable INR if the dosages are not lowered to accommodate their reduced metabolizer phenotype. Other genes that may impact warfarin dosing have also been studied. Variation in VKORC1, the gene encoding for vitamin K epoxide reductase complex subunit 1, has been shown to significantly affect warfarin dosing as well. The combination of genotypes for CYP2C9 and VKORC1 is thought to account for approximately 40% of the variability in warfarin dose.[23] Combining genetic information with physical data such as height and age can account for additional variability in dosing and has the potential to substantially reduce the risk of overdosing warfarin. Inherited impairment of CYP2C9 activity may also increase the risk for severe ADRs after NSAID use.

UDP-Glucuronosyltransferase 1A1 (UGT1A1)

The **UDP-glucuronyltransferase (UGT)** superfamily of enzymes is responsible for glucuronidation of many xenobiotics, resulting in compounds with greater water solubility. Impairment of this enzyme system leads to accumulation of compounds that would otherwise be eliminated. The mammalian UGT family is composed of 117 members that can be divided among UGT1, UGT2, UGT3, and UGT4. The UGT1 and UGT2 families are most efficient at glucuronidation in humans, and the UGT1 family is of most interest clinically. The human UGT1 genes are approximately 200 kb and are found on chromosome 2q37. The 5-exon genes of the UGT1 family each contain a unique first exon, plus four exons that are shared between the genes; the exon 1 may have evolved by a process of duplication, leading to the synthesis of proteins with identical carboxyl-terminal and variable amino-terminal domains. The hepatic isoforms include UGT1A1, 3, 4, 6, and 9, whereas UGT1A7, 8, and 10 have been localized to extrahepatic tissues, such as the mouth, esophagus, intestine, pancreas, and colon. Of these, the clinical consequences of genetic variations have been best studied for the UGT1A1 family.

An important substrate for the UGT1A1 family is bilirubin. This isoform is the only efficient route for metabolism of bilirubin in humans. Mutations in UGT1A1 that lead to complete absence of UGT1A1 activity have been associated with the severe hyperbilirubinemia seen with Crigler-Najjar syndrome. More than 30 SNPs that lead to nonfunctional UGT1A1 have been identified. Variation in the number of TA repeats within the TATA box region of the UGT1A1 promoter has been associated with Gilbert-Meulengracht disease, a clinically benign, mild hyperbilirubinemia.[15]

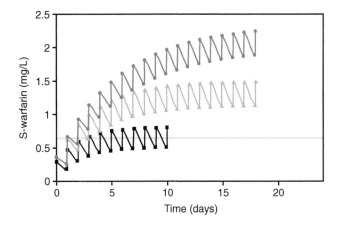

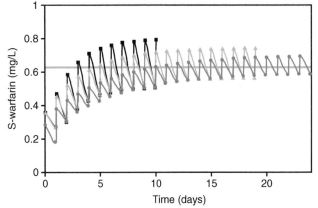

Figure 12-10

Model of warfarin dosing based on CYP2C9 genetics. In both panels, the conventional therapeutic S-warfarin target level is shown (horizontal line) for reference. The top panel depicts a model for warfarin therapy in patients using the standard 5-mg/day dose with all genotypes. CYP2C9*1/*1 individuals (j, shown with black squares) on 5 mg, twice per day would attain stable and therapeutic serum S-warfarin levels (0.68 µg/mL) in approximately 4 days. CYP2C9*1/*2 (m, shown with blue triangles) and CYP2C9*1/*3 (d, shown with blue circles) individuals on the same 5-mg dose are modeled to attain S-warfarin serum levels that are both too high by the second day and, if not adjusted, would lead to overanticoagulation. CYP2C9*1/*2 patients would stabilize at twice therapeutic serum levels after 10 to 12 days, but CYP2C9*1/*3, if not adjusted, would continue to rise. The bottom panel depicts serum S-warfarin level outcomes for a dosing regimen modified for genotype. All patients would be given the standard 5-mg dose twice, then switched to a CYP2C9 genotype adjusted dose for maintenance, CYP2C9*1/*2 receiving 3 mg and CYP2C9*1/*3 receiving 1.5 mg. This genotype-adjusted dosing could result in CYP2C9*1/*2 and CYP2C9*1/*3 achieving stable, therapeutic S-warfarin levels in 10 days, thereby preventing overanticoagulation in these individuals.

(Adapted from Linder MW, Looney S, Adams JE III, Johnson N, Antonino-Green D, Lacefield N, et al. Warfarin dose adjustments based on CYP2C9 genetic polymorphisms. J Thromb Thrombolysis 2002;14:227-32. With kind permission of Springer Science and Business Media.)

Genotype to Phenotype

Variations in the number of TA repeats are known collectively as UGT1A1*28. This allele is further described by the number of repeats, 5 to 8. The A(TA)$_7$TAA variant contains an additional TA from the wild-type sequence of A(TA)$_6$TAA and leads to a 30% reduction in the promoter activity of the UGT1A1. Other variants include A(TA)₅TAA and A(TA)₈TAA. The expression efficiency is inversely proportional to the number of repeats so that the TA5 variant confers increased expression over the TA6, and the TA7 and TA8 variants confer reduced expression. The frequency of the A(TA)₇TAA, the most common variant that adversely impacts expression, is approximately 40% in Caucasian and African-American individuals and approximately 16% of Asians.

Testing

Tests for detection of *UGT1A1*28* are commercially available. Methods for detection of other UGT variants include standard techniques, such as those described in Chapter 5.

Clinical Applications

The best studied example of a pharmacogenetic application for *UGT1A1*28* genotyping is with irinotecan. Irinotecan is widely used in metastatic colorectal cancer and also in other tumors, such as lung and liver. Irinotecan is a prodrug, converted by carboxylesterases to produce the active, cytotoxic metabolite SN-38. This metabolite is a topoisomerase inhibitor that is inactivated by UGT1A1. Individuals possessing variant TA repeats are susceptible to dose-limiting toxicity with irinotecan, including severe diarrhea and/or neutropenia. It is proposed that the risk of toxicity is near 0% for patients with the TA6/6 genotype, approximately 12.5% for patients with the TA6/7 genotype, and approximately 50% for patients with the TA7/7 genotype. It is recommended that patients with the TA7/7 genotype receive a reduced dose of irinotecan as compared with the dose given to patients with a TA6/6 genotype.[1]

UGTs are known to be induced by aryl hydrocarbons and phenobarbital. The flavonoid chrysin has been studied for its ability to induce UGT1A1 specifically in the gastrointestinal tract because it is not well absorbed and would therefore stay within the gastrointestinal tract and promote elimination of irinotecan, potentially minimizing the opportunity for drug-induced diarrhea. Coadministration of other drugs, such as loperamide, may also prevent or alleviate the diarrhea associated with irinotecan. Similarly, coadministration of erythropoietin, granulocyte-colony stimulating factor, or other agents may minimize or shorten the duration of the neutropenic effects of irinotecan.[21] Because other UGTs, the CYP3A family, and drug transporters, such as the ABCB1, ABCC2, and ABCG2, are also involved in the disposition of irinotecan, additional study will be required to determine the most effective strategy for identification and management of individual susceptible to the toxicity of irinotecan. As data accumulate, the utility of genotype-based dose optimization versus co-administration of compounds that counteract or relieve the associated toxicities will be better characterized.

N-Acetyltransferases (NAT1 and NAT2)

The **N-acetyltransferase (NAT)** polymorphism is one of the earliest pharmacogenetic targets recognized and characterized. NATs are phase II enzymes that catalyze the transfer of an acetyl moiety from acetyl CoA to homocyclic and heterocyclic arylamines and hydrazines. Substrates include drugs, carcinogens, toxicants, and possibly endogenous compounds. Slow metabolizer phenotypes, which may affect up to 90% of some populations, are manifested by changes in protein expression, protein stability, and enzyme kinetics.

Genotype to Phenotype

The first NAT polymorphism, attributed to an enzyme originally called "isoniazid transacetylase," was recognized in the 1950s with isoniazid (L-isonicotinyl hydrazide), a drug used to treat tuberculosis. Population studies revealed a bimodal distribution in plasma and urine levels of the N-acetylated isoniazid metabolite. Concentration of the parent drug was highly correlated with the prevalence of toxic symptoms, including hepatotoxicity and a painful and progressive peripheral neuropathy that affected up to one third of Caucasian and African-American patients. From this initial work, patients were phenotypically described as "fast acetylators" or "slow acetylators." Slow acetylators excrete large amounts of the parent drug relative to the acetylated metabolite when compared with fast acetylators. Family studies identified a strong genetic linkage of this phenotype and suggested that the phenotype was inherited as an autosomal recessive trait.

Studies with additional substrates for NAT demonstrated that the phenotype was not relevant to all substrates. For example, the NAT phenotype was clearly recognized for arylamines, such as isoniazid, some sulfonamides, amrinone, dapsone, procainamide, caffeine, and clonazepam. The phenotype was not observed with other arylamine substrates, such as p-aminobenzoate (PABA) and p-aminosalicylate (PAS). A folate catabolite, p-aminobenzoylglutamate, is the only endogenous NAT substrate proposed. However, *NAT2* knock-out and *NAT1* and *NAT2* double knock-out mice do not express phenotypical abnormalities, suggesting that these enzymes are not required for development or function.[19]

In 1965 it was proposed that two isoforms of NAT, later named NAT1 and NAT2, were responsible for the differences in phenotypes observed previously. Of the two proposed isoforms, NAT2 correlated best with the isoniazid (polymorphic) phenotype. It was also suggested that the fast and slow acetylator phenotypes were caused by differences in expression or protein stability, rather than in the enzyme kinetics. Subsequently, it was found that although most substrates exhibit higher specificity for either NAT1 or NAT2, most substrates have affinity for both NAT1 and NAT2 (see Chapter 14 for Table of NAT substrates).

Nonetheless, substrates were commonly classified as monomorphic (substrates of NAT1) or polymorphic (substrates of NAT2) until the mid-1990s.

NAT1, which is now recognized to be polymorphic, is extremely unstable and therefore more difficult to study than NAT2. Because of stability differences and overlapping substrate specificity, tissue localization studies for the NATs have been challenging. It is now recognized that both NAT1 and NAT2 are expressed throughout the gastrointestinal tract and in the lung, bladder, ureter, and liver.[25]

There are three human NAT genes that are mapped to chromosome 8p22. The *NAT1* and *NAT2* genes share 87% nucleotide sequence identity and 81% amino acid sequence identity. The third gene, *NATP*, is thought to be a noncoding pseudogene. Each of the NAT genes has an intronless open reading frame exon of 870 bp and codes for 290 amino acids.[22] Many variant alleles have been described for both NAT1 and NAT2. (See Chapter 14 for table of Common NAT1 and NAT2 Alleles Associated with a Slow Acetylator Phenotype.)

The wild-type alleles, although the term is somewhat arbitrary because of high population frequencies of multiple alleles, are NAT1*3 and NAT2*4. For NAT2, former common nomenclature included M1 for NAT2*5A, M2 for NAT2*6A, and M3 for NAT2*7A. The NAT2*5, *6, *7, *13, and *14 alleles are thought to account for more than 99% of slow acetylator phenotypes. NAT2 slow acetylators are common in many populations: approximately 83% of Egyptians; 40% to 60% of Caucasians, Europeans, and African Americans; 10% to 30% of Asians; and 5% of Canadian Eskimos. The NAT1*10 is the most common variant NAT1 allele in many human populations, but the phenotype-genotype relationship is not well defined. NAT1*10 allele frequency is reported high in a Japanese population (62.3%) compared with a European population (29%). Other NAT1 alleles that appear rare in humans produce enzymes with definitively reduced activity, and potential clinical implications include NAT1*14, 15, 17, 19, and 22.[7,13]

The three-dimensional crystal structures of the two NAT isoenzymes have been determined. Structural studies suggest that the active catalytic site of the NATs involves three amino acids, a cysteine residue juxtaposed with histidine, and aspartate residues. The C-terminus is responsible for substrate specificity. The acetylation reaction occurs through a classical two-step mechanism, where an acetyl moiety is transferred from acetyl CoA to NAT and then from NAT to the arylamine to form an arylamide. As shown in Figure 12-11, N-acetylation, thought to primarily generate nontoxic stable products, is mediated by both NAT1 and NAT2. O-Acetylation is also mediated by both NAT1 and NAT2 and is thought to generate reactive products that may spontaneously decompose to form nitrenium ions. Nitrenium ions are electrophiles that may subsequently bind covalently to intracellular nucleophiles, such as DNA or proteins, and be responsible for cell death, mutagenesis, or other toxicities. An intramolecular N,O-acetyltransfer reaction is mediated primarily by NAT1 and also may lead to reactive products. Other enzymes that may interrupt or contribute to these reactions include CYP1A2, prostaglandin H synthase, UDP-glucuronosyltransferase, and sulfotransferase.

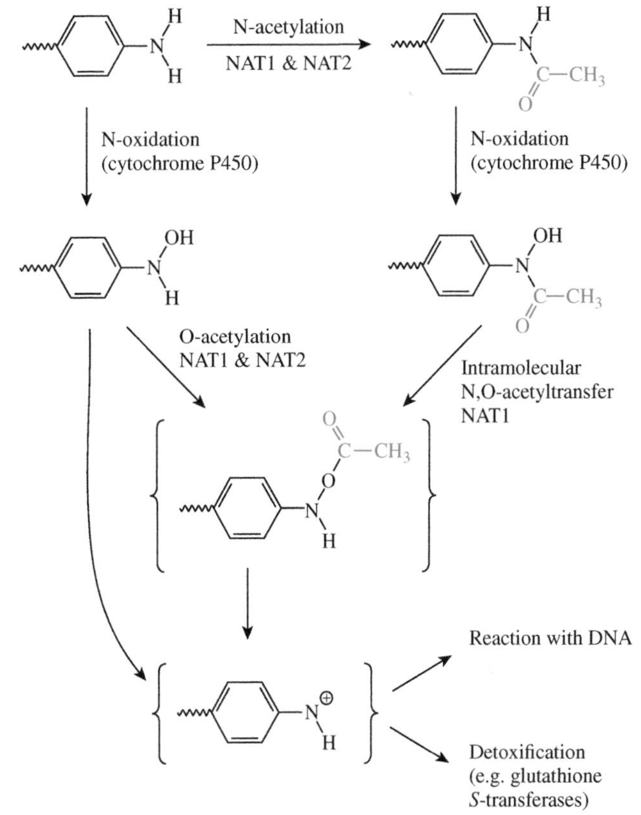

Testing

Variables that affect NAT phenotyping include the substrate or probe drug used, age and disease status of the individual, medications, dietary factors such as ingestion of well-cooked meat, and life-style factors such as cigarette smoking or occupational exposure to NAT substrates. The most common method of NAT1 phenotyping is to measure enzyme activity in isolated lymphocytes using PABA, PAS, or another relatively specific NAT1 substrate. However, phenotyping in vivo with a probe drug has also been performed. The most common phenotyping method for NAT2 is to administer a probe drug and evaluate ratios of parent/metabolite or metabolite-A/metabolite-B concentrations. Probe drugs may include any relatively specific NAT2 substrate, the most common and safe of which is caffeine. One published phenotyping method involves administration of 200 mg of caffeine following an overnight fast. Urine is collected 4 and 5 hours later. The 5-hour specimen is analyzed for caffeine metabolites 5-acetylamino-6-formylamino-3-methyluracil (AFMU) and 1-methylxanthine (1X). Cutoffs for acetylator phenotypes are based on the ratio of AFMU/1X. Considering a bimodal distribution of acetylators, a ratio of less than 0.66 is used to define slow acetylators. Because a trimodal distribution has been described and may be of interest, a ratio higher than 3.0 could define "ultrarapid"

Figure 12-11

Schematic view of the role of NAT enzymes in the metabolism of aromatic amines. N-acetylation might be a detoxification reaction in a number of cases; however, after N-hydroxylation of aromatic amines (e.g., by CYP enzymes), NAT enzymes can bioactivate these intermediates by either O-acetylation or intramolecular N,O-acetyltransfer, leading to the formation of nitrenium ions, which might react with DNA or alternatively be detoxified by, for example, GST enzymes. Importantly, it is shown that a number of other biotransformation enzymes are also involved in the metabolism of aromatic amines as well.

(Redrawn from Wormhoudt LW, Commandeur JNM, Vermeulen NPE. Genetic polymorphisms of human N-acetyltransferase, cytochrome P450, glutathione-S-transferase, and epoxide hydrolase enzymes: relevance to xenobiotic metabolism and toxicity. Crit Rev Toxicol 1999;29:59-124. Reproduced by permission from Taylor and Francis, Inc.)

acetylators; a ratio between 0.66 and 3.0 would define a classic rapid acetylator or in a trimodal distribution, an "intermediate" acetylator phenotype.[7]

Genotyping can predict NAT phenotype quite well, with concordance of 90% to 100% for NAT2. For NAT2, an example of the phenotype-genotype relationship published by Cascorbi et al in 1995 with a population of unrelated Germans is depicted by histogram (Figure 12-12). Only 6.7% of genotypes did not agree with the phenotypes in this study.[8,13]

Clinical Applications

NAT status has been implicated in propensity for experiencing ADRs and, unlike the CYPs and TPMT, NAT status has been associated with risk of disease, including immunological disorders—such as rheumatoid arthritis and systemic lupus

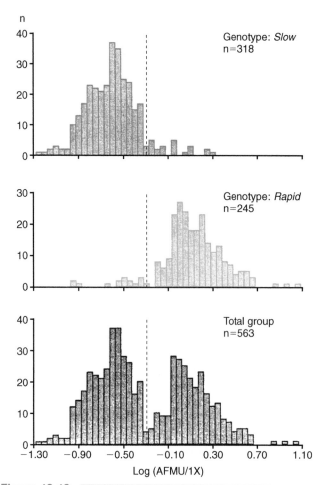

Figure 12-12

Histogram of NAT2 phenotypical activities as obtained by the caffeine test: 5-hour urine collection obtained after administration of caffeine and analyzed for caffeine metabolite concentrations. Values represent the logarithmically transformed ratio of metabolites AFMU and 1X. From the distinct bimodal distribution an antimode of $\log(0.50) = -0.30$ was obtained (*dotted line*).
(From Cascorbi I, Drakoulis N, Brockmoller J, Maurer A, Sperling K, Roots I. Arylamine N-acetyltransferase (NAT2) mutations and their allelic linkage in unrelated Caucasian individuals: correlation with phenotypical activity. Am J Hum Genet 1995;57:581-92. Reproduced by permission from the University of Chicago Press.)

erythematous—and several cancers, particularly bladder, lung, gastric, and colorectal. Exposure to NAT substrates can be related to cigarette smoking, some medications, occupational exposure (cooking, dye, and rubber industries), and several environmental toxicants (for more detail, see Chapter 14 for Table of NAT substrates). NAT testing may be important for individuals at high risk of exposure to NAT substrates or in whom adverse reactions to probable NAT substrates have been experienced.

Neither genotyping nor phenotyping methods are widely available for clinical testing. However, research involving the genotyping or phenotyping of NAT polymorphisms has significantly impacted pharmacotherapy with NAT substrates and drug development. With isoniazid, the recognition of distinct phenotypical differences that led to ADRs furthered research into the pathological mechanisms. For example, the neuro-

pathic consequences are linked to pyridoxine deficiency, which can be prevented by coadministration of pyridoxine to all patients. Because rapid acetylators are less likely to respond to the conventionally administered dose, the isoniazid dosing intervals are changed from once per week to twice per week. For procainamide, determining the acetylator status is accomplished through routine therapeutic drug monitoring of the parent and metabolite, N-acetylprocainamide (NAPA). The dose of procainamide is adjusted based on the parent/metabolite ratio. In the development of amonafide, a chemotherapeutic agent inactivated by NAT conjugation, acetylator-based dosing was defined through clinical trials. Although the drug is no longer in development, it is an example of how pharmacogenetic phenomena can support individualized therapy.

Other Pharmacogenetic Targets and Future Directions

As discussed previously in this chapter, any protein for which the related gene exhibits polymorphism has potential pharmacogenetic implications. With relationship to drug metabolism, additional CYPs including *CYP1A2*, *CYP2B6*, *CYP2E1*, *CYP3A4*, and *CYP3A5* have also been proposed as important pharmacogenetic targets. Other phase II enzymes that exhibit marked genetic variability among individuals, particularly the glutathione *S*-transferases, may be clinically important as well. In addition, genetic variation in alcohol dehydrogenase, catechol *O*-methyltransferase, and dihydropyrimidine dehydrogenase (DPYD) is important. The interrelationship of these various enzymes as major versus minor and dependent versus independent mechanisms of metabolism for a single compound will be important to determine the most clinically useful and cost-effective pharmacogenetic testing strategy. Also important will be to gain a better understanding of haplotype relationships and the possible implications of heterozygote variants for a single gene and combinations of related genes.

Beyond metabolism, pharmacogenetic targets that may become important to therapeutic drug monitoring (TDM) and pharmacotherapeutics in general include genes that encode for any protein associated with drug handling, such as drug transporters (e.g., p-glycoprotein and lipoproteins), drug receptors (e.g., dopamine, adrenergic, and serotonin receptors) or effectors (e.g., folate metabolism and catecholamine transporters). Genotyping both CYP2C9 and VKORC1 (discussed in the CYP2C9 section) provides an excellent example of a pharmacogenetic testing strategy that considers gene variants that affect both the pharmacokinetics and pharmacodynamics of warfarin. For examples of pharmacogenetic targets not explicitly discussed in this chapter for which some genotype-to-phenotype relationship has been demonstrated, see table of Additional Pharmacogenetic Targets in Chapter 14.

Additional studies, particularly prospective and outcome-related, are also required to apply pharmacogenetic findings to the clinic. From an interpretive perspective, more guidelines for dose adjustments need to be established, including consideration of how the dosing recommendations are affected by co-prescribed medications and/or environmental factors. Closer integration of pharmacy professionals with clinical laboratories and clinicians will improve success in pharmacogenetic applications. Commercially available and cost-effective methods for genotyping or phenotyping are also required. The future of pharmacogenetic testing is likely to be driven most by the consumer and by the pharmaceutical providers that promote pharmacogenetic testing, such as in package labeling recommendations. Clinical trials for new pharmaceutical agents are currently considering the benefits of pharmacogenetic testing for individual products. Theoretically, it is possible that individuals will someday carry something analogous to an ID card that contains personal genetic information that may guide drug and dose selection.

Cancer treatments are of particular interest to pharmacogenetics and pharmacogenomics research because ADRs are extremely common during chemotherapy and because the window of opportunity for treatment of the cancer is narrow. In addition to the role of drug metabolizing enzymes discussed previously in this chapter (TPMT, CYPs, UGT1A1, NAT1, and NAT2), DPYD and methylenetetrahydrofolate reductase (MTHFR) are known to play a role in predicting patients' susceptible to toxicity from cancer chemotherapy. DPYD is involved in the metabolism of 5-fluorouracil (5-FU), and MTHFR is involved in the metabolism of methotrexate. DPYD*2A, the most common variant allele of DPYD that leads to a nonfunctional DPYD protein, is caused by a G>A transition. The presence of this allele is correlated with severe toxicity and mortality following treatment with standard doses of 5-FU. The presence of C677T and A1298C variants in MTHFR affects the risk of toxicity and dosing requirements, respectively, of methotrexate.

Complementary to pharmacogenetics, "toxicogenetics" may apply similar concepts to risk stratification, such as for establishing risk of cancer thought to be triggered by environmental or dietary exposure to a wide variety of xenobiotics. This area is where ethics may slow availability of testing because most pharmacogenetic markers studied thus far have not been associated with disease or risk of disease. Shown in Table 12-5 are some of the genetic targets that have been studied with regard to risk of various cancers and also because of their role in the activation or inactivation of cancer chemotherapeutics. Genes that encode for drug metabolizing enzymes are of most interest for this application because it is through these enzymes that xenobiotics become activated or inactivated. The glutathione S-transferases (GSTs) are associated with risk of developing cancer caused by environmental triggers. At least 16 GSTs have been identified, which are divided into classes designated as alpha (A), kappa, mu (M), pi (P), sigma, theta (T), zeta, and omega. The GSTM1 deficient trait has, for example, been associated with higher risk of lung and bladder cancer. With additional study and validation of these and other genetic markers, preemployment testing to identify individuals with high susceptibility to chemical carcinogens may become important for occupational settings such as agriculture and manufacturing.

The field of pharmacogenetics is currently benefiting pharmacotherapeutics by improving dose optimization tools for a select group of medications. Studies suggest that pharmacogenetic tools are potentially useful for dose selection and optimization of many clinically important drugs, particularly those with a narrow therapeutic index (e.g., cancer chemotherapeutics), those that have a narrow opportunity to exert efficacy (e.g., immunosuppressants), those that require weeks or more to determine therapeutic efficacy (e.g., antidepressants), and those that are at high risk for adverse effects and are administered chronically (e.g., lipid lowering). Pharmacogenetics also

TABLE 12-5	Pharmacogenetic Targets Involved in Xenobiotic Metabolism and Important in Cancer		
Polymorphic Gene Important to Metabolism	**Chemotherapeutic Drug Substrates**	**Carcinogen Substrates**
CYP2B6	Cyclophosphamide Ifosfamide	
CYP2C9	Cyclophosphamide Ifosfamide	
CYP3A4	Teniposide Etoposide Ifosfamide Vindesine Vinblastine Vincristine Cyclophosphamide Paclitaxel Docetaxel	Aflatoxin B1 6-aminochrysene
DPYD, TYMS	5-Fluorouricil	
GSTA1, GSTA2 GSTM1	Cyclophosphamide	Cumene hydroperoxides Aflatoxin B1 epoxides Benzo[a]pyrene 4,5 oxide Trans-stilbene oxide 4-nitrochinolone 1-oxide
GSTP1	Thiotepa Cyclophosphamide Ethacrynic acid	
GSTT1		Ethylene oxide Methyl chloride Dichloromethane
MTHFR	Methotrexate	
NAT2	Amonafide	Aromatic amines Heterocyclic amines
TPMT	6-MP Azathioprine	
UGT1A1	Irinotecan	

Modified from Brockmoller J, Cascorbi I, Henning S, Meisel C, Roots I. Molecular genetics of cancer susceptibility. Pharmacology 2000;61:212-27; McLeod HL, Papageorgio C, Watters JW. Using genetic variations to optimize cancer chemotherapy. Clinical Advances in Haematology and Oncology 2003;1:107-11.

shows promise in the investigation of ADRs, including postmortem, and for assessing risk for xenobiotic-related conditions, including some cancers.

ETHICAL CONSIDERATIONS

Because a clear phenotype associated with most pharmacogenetic targets is relatively undefined, the implications and risks of possessing a genetic variant are not well understood. Defining the phenotype is even less clear for genes (and associated proteins) that are known to be affected by environmental, dietary, and endogenous factors. Commonly, an EM genotype is expressed as a PM phenotype as a result of concomitant medications. Another, more theoretical, scenario is that a patient may fail to respond to a medication because of genetic variants in the drug receptor that mediates the drug response. Yet a similar phenotype (change in receptor expression or function) may also result as a consequence of hormonal shifts that occur with stress, the onset of puberty, or pregnancy, for example. No test can predict patient management or life-style.

Even without well-defined genotype-phenotype relationships, many ethical questions surround pharmacogenetic testing, simply by virtue of the fact that genes are the analytical target. Such questions relate to how testing will affect a person's healthcare, employability, and ability to obtain health and life insurance, and how pharmacogenetic testing will affect future drug therapy. In addition, ethical issues surrounding pharmacogenetic testing may be based on whether or not the pharmacogenetic variant is associated with risk or severity of disease. Thus far, associations between most pharmacogenetic targets and disease are weak or are not known. This will likely change as the involvement of various genes and gene-xenobiotic relationships to pathogenesis are better understood. Genotype-phenotype relationships as they relate to pharmacotherapy and environmental exposures will continue to evolve as more experience accumulates and clinical studies are pursued.

Examples of ethical questions we are asking of pharmacogenetic testing are shown in Ethics Box 12-1.

ETHICS Box 12-1   Ethical Considerations

Among the many ethical issues facing the field of pharmacogenetics are the following:

- What are the implications to family members when a genetic variant is detected? Should family members be tested? Can nonpaternity be identified through pharmacogenetic testing?
- How will patients know if a genetic variant that is detected and thought to be of no clinical consequence is later shown to be associated with disease or other clinical concern?
- Will identification of pharmacogenetic variants affect insurability for patients?
- Will toxicogenetic testing lead to genetic-based discrimination in hiring practices?
- Will patients with pharmacogenetic variants be discriminated against in drug development efforts? That is, will drugs be developed and be available to specific genetically defined populations? If so, will genetically defined minority groups have fewer or no options for pharmacotherapy?
- Because of the potential benefits of pharmacogenetic testing in guiding drug and dose selection, should clinicians be ethically required to offer testing to all patients that may benefit from such testing? Should testing be denied for patients who do not require drugs that have pharmacogenetic testing associations?
- What role should government play in managing these issues?

Unanswered questions such as these raise critical issues that extend outside the laboratory and require thoughtful attention from patients, clinicians, payers, and lawmakers. Laboratorians will need to be active in these deliberations to ensure that the testing is understood.

REFERENCES

1. Ando Y, Ueoka H, Sugiyama T, Ichiki M, Shimokata K, Hasegawa Y. Polymorphisms of UDP glucuronosyltransferase and pharmacokinetics of irinotecan. Ther Drug Monit 2002;24:1116.
2. Brosen K, de Morais SM, Meyer UA, Goldstein JA. A multifamily study on the relationship between CYP2C19 genotype and s-mephenytoin oxidation phenotype. Pharmacogenetics 1995;5:312-7.
3. Cao H, Hegele RA. DNA polymorphisms in ITPA including basis of inosine triphosphatase deficiency. J Hum Genet 2002;47:620-2.
4. Chou WH, Yan FX, Robbins-Weilert DK, Ryder TB, Liu WW, Perbost C, et al. Comparison of two CYP2D6 genotyping methods and assessment of genotype-phenotype relationships. Clin Chem 2003;49:542-51.
5. Collie-Duguid ES, Pritchard SC, Powrie RH, Sludden J, Collier DA, Li T, McLeod HL. The frequency and distribution of thiopurine methyltransferase alleles in Caucasian and Asian populations. Pharmacogenetics 1999;9:37-42.
6. Evans WE, Hon YY, Bomgaars L, Coutre S, Holdsworth M, Janco R, et al. Preponderance of thiopurine S-methyltransferase deficiency and heterozygosity among patients intolerant to mercaptopurine or azathioprine. J Clin Oncol 2001;19:2293-301.
7. Gross M, Kruisselbrink T, Anderson K, Lang N, McGovern P, Delongchamp R, et al. Distribution and concordance of N-acetyltransferase genotype and phenotype in an American population. Cancer Epidemiol Biomarkers Prev 1999;8:683-92.
8. Hickman D, Sim E. N-acetyltransferase polymorphism. Comparison of phenotype and genotype in humans. Biochem Pharmacol 1991;42:1007-14.
9. Higashi MK, Veenstra DL, Kondo LM, Wittkowsky AK, Srinouanprachanh SL, Farin FM, Rettie AE. Association between CYP2C9 genetic variants and anticoagulation-related outcomes during warfarin therapy. JAMA 2002;287:1690-8.
10. Kerb R, Aynacioglu AS, Brockmoller J, Schlagenhaufer R, Bauer S, Szekeres T, et al. The predictive value of MDR1, CYP2C9, and CYP2C19 polymorphisms for phenytoin plasma levels. Pharmacogenomics J 2001;1:204-10.
11. Kirchheiner J, Brosen K, Dahl ML, Gram LF, Kasper S, Roots I, et al. CYP2D6 and CYP2C19 genotype-based dose recommendations for antidepressants: a first step toward subpopulation-specific dosages. Acta Psychiat Scand 2001;104:173-92.
12. Marra CA, Esdaile JM, Anis AH. Practical pharmacogenetics: the cost effectiveness of screening for thiopurine s-methyltransferase polymorphisms in patients with rheumatological conditions treated with azathioprine. J Rheumatol 2002;29:2507-12.
13. Meyer UA, Zanger UM. Molecular mechanisms of genetic polymorphisms of drug metabolism. Annu Rev Pharmacol Toxicol 1997;37:269-96.
14. Mizutani T. PM frequencies of major CYPs in Asians and Caucasians. Drug Metab Rev 2003;35:99-106.
15. Owens IS, Basu NK, Banerjee R. UDP-glucuronosyltransferases: gene structures of UGT1 and UGT2 families. Methods Enzymol 2005;400:1-22.
16. Rendic S, Di Carlo FJ. Human cytochrome P450 enzymes: a status report summarizing their reactions, substrates, inducers, and inhibitors. Drug Metab Rev 1997;29:413-580.
17. Schwarz UI. Clinical relevance of genetic polymorphisms in the human CYP2C9 gene. Eur J Clin Invest 2003;33 Suppl 2:23-30.
18. Steimer W, Zopf K, Von Amelunxen S, Pfeiffer H, Bachofer J, Popp J, et al. Allele-specific change of concentration and functional gene dose for the prediction of steady-state serum concentrations of amitriptyline and nortriptyline in CYP2C19 and CYP2D6 extensive and intermediate metabolizers. Clin Chem 2004;50:1623-33.
19. Summerscales JE, Josephy PD. Human acetyl CoA: arylamine N-acetyltransferase variants generated by random mutagenesis. Mol Pharmacol 2004;65:220-6.
20. Tai HL, Fessing MY, Bonten EJ, Yanishevsky Y, d'Azzo A, Krynetski EY, et al. Enhanced proteasomal degradation of mutant human thiopurine S-methyltransferase (TPMT) in mammalian cells: mechanism for TPMT protein deficiency inherited by TPMT*2, TPMT*3A, TPMT*3B or TPMT*3C. Pharmacogenetics 1999;9:641-50.
21. Tobin PJ, Beale P, Noney L, Liddell S, Rivory LP, Clarke S. A pilot study on the safety of combining chrysin, a non-absorbable inducer of UGT1A1, and irinotecan (CPT-11) to treat metastatic colorectal cancer. Cancer Chemother Pharmacol 2006;57:309-16.
22. Vatsis KP, Weber WW, Bell DA, Dupret JM, Evans DAP, Grant DM, et al. Nomenclature for N-acetyltransferases. Pharmacogenetics 1995;5:1-17.
23. Wadelius M, Chen LY, Downes K, Ghori J, Hunt S, Eriksson N, et al. Common VKORC1 and GGCX polymorphisms associated with warfarin dose. Pharmacogenomics J 2005;5:262-70.
24. Weinshilboum RM, Sladek SL. Mercaptopurine pharmacogenetics: monogenic inheritance of erythrocyte thiopurine methyltransferase activity. Am J Hum Genet 1980;32:651-62.
25. Windmill KF, Gaedigk A, Hall PM, Samaratunga H, Grant DM, McManus ME. Localization of N-acetyltransferases NAT1 and NAT2 in human tissues. Toxicol Sci 2000;54:19-29.

1. Pharmacogenetic testing will not
    A. identify drug-drug interactions.
    B. predict toxicity to a drug.
    C. predict response to a drug.
    D. distinguish rapid from slow metabolizers.
    E. guide drug and dose selection.
2. Results describing the phenotype or genotype of TPMT are useful for dosing the following drug:
    A. irinotecan.
    B. amitriptyline.
    C. azathioprine.
    D. atomoxetine.
    E. cisplatin.
3. Interpretation of CYP2D6 genotyping results depends on all of the following EXCEPT
    A. how the CYP2D6 variant(s) detected by the assay affects enzyme function.
    B. the age of the patient.
    C. the presence or absence of gene duplications.
    D. the specific variants detected by the genotyping assay.
    E. the number of variant alleles detected.
4. The pair of genes used to predict appropriate doses of warfarin is
    A. CYP2C9 and CYP2C19.
    B. CYP2D6 and CYP2C19.
    C. CYP2C19 and NAT2.
    D. UGT1A1 and CYP2C9.
    E. VKROC1 and CYP2C9.
5. The dosing of a prodrug may be affected by pharmacogenetic results because
    A. PMs may require lower doses of the prodrug than EMs.
    B. PMs may require a different drug than EMs.
    C. EMs may require higher doses of the prodrug than PMs.
    D. PMs may require lower doses of the prodrug than IMs.
    E. UMs may require higher doses of the prodrug than EMs.

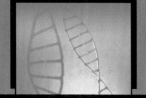

Chapter 13

Molecular Genetics in Diagnosis of Human Cancers

Kojo S. J. Elenitoba-Johnson, M.D.*

OUTLINE

OBJECTIVES

1. Contrast oncogenes with tumor-suppressor genes and list three of each.
2. Describe how genetic alterations lead to specific leukemias or lymphomas.
3. Compare and contrast (a) the chromosomal translocations that lead to hematological malignancies and (b) immunoglobulin gene rearrangements.
4. List the analytical tools that are available to assess gene rearrangements and chromosomal translocations.
5. List and describe two chronic non-*BCR-ABL* myeloproliferative disorders and the gene involved.
6. List two solid tumors, stating the name, a gene involved, and the type of genetic alteration that leads to the disorder.

The author gratefully acknowledges the original contribution of the following work, on which portions of this chapter were based: Chapter 23, Tumor Markers, by Daniel W. Chan, Ronald A. Booth, and Eleftherios P. Diamandis in Burtis CA, Ashwood ER, Bruns DE, editors: Tietz Textbook of Clincal Chemistry and Molecular Diagnostics, ed 4, St Louis, 2006, Saunders.

KEY WORDS AND DEFINITIONS

Apoptosis: A specialized form of cell death known as programmed cell death; it involves the activation of a specific group of proteins, known as caspases, with eventual nuclear fragmentation and formation of a characteristic ladder pattern on gel electrophoresis of the degraded DNA.

B Lymphocyte (B Cell): B lymphocytes are cells that are involved with the production of antibodies in the humoral immune response; the "B" in B cell represents the bursa of Fabricius, which is the organ where B cells mature in birds.

Breakpoint Cluster Region (BCR): BCR refers to a region of chromosome 22 that is a partner in a large proportion of chromosomal *translocations* involving the *ABL1* (also called *ABL*) gene on chromosome 9; the breakpoints in this chromosome are clustered within this BCR region, hence its name; the *BCR-ABL* fusion occurs as a consequence of the translocation involving chromosomes 9 and 22 and is characteristic of chronic myeloid (or "myelogenous") leukemia; see also Gene Rearrangement.

Carcinoma: Malignant new growth (*neoplasm*) of cells that arises from epithelium; found in skin or the lining of body organs, such as in breast, prostate, lung, stomach, or bowel; tend to infiltrate into adjacent tissue and to spread to distant organs.

Clonal: The term clonal refers to the origin of cells from a single progenitor (clone), which gives rise to progeny that are genetically identical to the original parental cell; the term is often used to encapsulate the concept that cancers arise from a single cancerous cell whose growth regulatory mechanisms have gone awry and that generates more tumor cells with cancerous growth characteristics.

Cytogenetics: The study of chromosome structure.

FAB: French-American-British classification system for certain types of leukemia.

Gene Rearrangement: Relocation of a segment of DNA within a gene.

Immunoglobulins: Immunoglobulins are antibody molecules produced by mature B cells or plasma cells.

Immunoglobulin Heavy and Light Chains: Immunoglobulins are proteins composed of two light chains and two heavy chains; there are two types of light chains, kappa (κ) and lambda (λ); the heavy chains in an immunoglobulin may be gamma (γ), alpha (α), mu (μ), delta (δ), or epsilon (ε) to produce, respectively, immunoglobulins G, A, M, D, and E (see Figure 13-1 for the corresponding gene structures); an immunoglobulin molecule contains only κ or λ light chains and only one type of heavy chain.

Leukemia: Leukemias are neoplastic proliferations of hematopoietic cells and are characteristically based in the bone marrow and peripheral blood, but may be found elsewhere.

Lymphoma: Lymphoma refers to malignant neoplasms that originate from lymphocytes in lymphatic tissues, such as lymph nodes, spleen, or tonsillar tissues; lymphomas are generally classified into Hodgkin or non-Hodgkin lymphoma; Hodgkin's lymphoma is a specific category first described by Thomas Hodgkin in 1832 and characterized by the presence of the Reed-Sternberg (RS) cell, which accounts for only a small proportion of the cellular infiltrate; non-Hodgkin lymphomas include all other types of lymphomas and may be of B-cell, T-cell, or natural killer (NK)-cell origin.

Malignant (Tumor or Cell): Having the potential to invade and destroy surrounding tissues and to spread to distant parts of the body.

Minimal Residual Disease (MRD): When used in relation to cancer, MRD refers to low-level residual disease after treatment, particularly chemotherapy; especially in the hematological malignancies, molecular markers have been used to identify and quantify very low levels of remaining tumor burden to establish disease persistence or relapse.

Monoclonal: Characterized by a single clone of cells. See description of clonal above.

Neoplasia/Neoplasm: Neoplasia ("new growth" in Latin) is used to refer to tumors and encompasses benign and malignant tumors, or *neoplasms*.

Oncogene: A deregulated gene that leads to uncontrolled cell growth and tumor formation; the normal cellular equivalent of the oncogene is known as a *proto-oncogene*.

Oncogenesis: The progression of genetic and cellular changes that lead to formation of a malignant tumor.

Sarcoma: A malignant tumor of tissues of mesodermal origin, such as bone and muscle.

T-Cell Receptor: These proteins are similar to immunoglobulins, but are found only on the surface of mature T lymphocytes; the T-cell receptors bind specific antigens.

T Lymphocyte (T Cell): T lymphocytes are cells that are involved in the immune response; types of T lymphocytes include cytotoxic T cells, helper T cells, and regulatory T cells (also called suppressor T cells); the "T" in T cell represents the thymus, which is the organ where these lymphocytes mature.

Translocation, Chromosomal: A chromosomal translocation occurs when a piece of a chromosome breaks off and fuses to another chromosome; this added piece of chromosomal material can produce specific disorders, such as chronic myeloid leukemia (CML).

Tumor-Suppressor Gene: A gene that reduces the propensity of a cell to become malignant; thus loss of the proteins encoded by the tumor-suppressor gene can favor the formation of carcinomas, sarcomas, leukemias, and lymphomas, depending on the cell in which the loss occurs.

Research over the last few decades has established that acquired genetic mutations underlie the pathogenesis of several forms of human cancer. **Malignant neoplasms** can be categorized into the hematological malignancies and solid tumors. The hematological malignancies include leukemias, lymphomas, myeloproliferative disorders, and plasma cell myeloma. The solid tumor malignancies include the **carcinomas, sarcomas,** and several other types of cancers that give rise to discrete tumor growths in various organs and tissues. The genetic aberrations that occur in tumor cells may affect single DNA bases, many bases, or even large pieces of chromosomes. Thus the changes may be (1) point mutations (replacements, deletions, or insertions of one or a few nucleotides) in DNA, (2) larger deletions or amplifications (making multiple copies) of DNA, (3) gains or losses of entire chromosomes, or (4) translocations of parts of a chromosome, usually to another chromosome. These genetic abnormalities involved in malignant neoplasm formation commonly lead to deregulation of the function of *proto-oncogenes*, **tumor-suppressor genes,** or genes involved in the regulation of **apoptosis.** Identification of the characteristic genetic abnormalities that lead to specific malignancies has permitted the development of tumor-specific therapies and of molecular tests for the malignancies. These tests are important in the diagnosis, monitoring, and management

TABLE 13-1	Oncogenes Found in Some Human Tumors		
Oncogene	**Function**	**Product**	**Type of Cancer**
Mutated *NRAS* (N-*ras*)	Signal transduction	Guanine diphosphate (GDP)/guanine triphosphate (GTP) binding protein	Acute myeloid leukemia, neuroblastoma
Mutated *KRAS* (K-*ras*)	Signal transduction	GDP/GTP binding protein	Leukemia, lymphoma
Translocated *MYC* (c-*myc*)	Transcription regulation	Binds to DNA	B- and T-cell lymphoma, small cell lung carcinoma
Amplified *CERBB2* (c-*erb* B-2, her-2/neu)	Growth factor receptor	Tyrosine kinase	Breast, ovarian, gastrointestinal
ABL/BCR (c-*abl/bcr*) translocation	Signal transduction	Tyrosine kinase	Chronic myelocytic leukemia
Amplified *MYCN* (N-*myc*)	Transcription regulation	Binds to DNA	Neuroendocrine
Overexpressed *BCL2* (*bcl-2* [e.g., in immunoglobulin fusion gene])	Blocks apoptosis	Mitochondrial membrane protein	Leukemia, lymphoma

of specific forms of cancer and selection of the most appropriate therapy for the patient's condition.

ONCOGENES AND TUMOR-SUPPRESSOR GENES[23]

The aberrantly regulated growth of tumor cells is thought to occur because of genetic mutations. Multiple genetic alterations may be necessary for the transformation of a cell from a normal to a cancerous state, a process called oncogenesis. Two important classes of genes are implicated in the development of cancer: **oncogenes** (genes that promote the transformation of cells into cancer cells) and *tumor-suppressor genes* (genes that suppress oncogenesis).

Oncogenes often are derived from proto-oncogenes, which are normal cellular genes. The proto-oncogenes become oncogenic when they have been altered by dominant mutations, such as *point mutations, insertions,* deletions, **translocations,** or *inversions* that alter the function of the gene. Certain genes in viruses also have the potential to be oncogenic. Most oncogenes code for proteins that function at some stage of activation of cells and promote cell division. Examples of oncogenes are given in Table 13-1.

Tumor-suppressor genes give rise to cancers when there is *loss* of function of the gene. Deletion of a tumor suppressor on one allele and a point mutation on the remaining allele is a common mechanism for inactivation of tumor-suppressor genes. The proteins encoded by many tumor-suppressor genes are involved in the regulation of progression through the cell division cycle or in the regulation of DNA repair.[23] Some examples of tumor-suppressor genes are listed in Table 13-2.

Oncogenes

Animal tumor viruses carry genes that change ("transform") otherwise normal cells into tumor cells. These genes are called viral oncogenes and represent some of the first-described oncogenes. Noninfected normal cells contain normal cellular genes called *proto-oncogenes* that are related in DNA sequence to viral oncogenes, but do not function as oncogenes in their normal state. These genes code for products that are involved in normal cellular processes, such as cellular mechanisms for growth (growth-factor signaling pathways). Activation of proto-oncogenes, usually by mutation, is frequently found to be associated with cancers (Table 13-1). In some types of cancer,

TABLE 13-2	Tumor-Suppressor Gene Mutations Associated With Some Human Tumors
Gene	**Tumor Type**
VHL	Kidney
APC (adenomatosis polyposis coli)	Colorectal
CDKN2A (p16)	Bladder, glioblastoma, melanoma
WT1	Wilms' tumor
BRCA2, RB1	Breast
RB1	Retinoblastoma, osteosarcoma, small cell lung
CDH1 (P16 E-cadherin)	Breast
BRCA1	Neurofibromatosis 1, melanoma, breast
TP53 (p53 protein)	Breast, colorectal, lung, liver, renal cell, bladder, sarcomas
DCC (deleted in colorectal carcinoma)	Colorectal
NF2	Neurofibromatosis 2, meningioma

mutations in certain proto-oncogenes are extremely common; for example, mutations in one of the *ras* genes are seen in about 90% of adenocarcinomas of the pancreas.[3] Overexpression or unregulated activation of the proto-oncogene leads to abnormal cell growth and increased risk of developing a malignancy.

An oncogene that has become especially important for clinical laboratories is *ERBB2* (also called *her-2/neu* or *c-erbB-2*). (For a note on gene names, see Box 13-1.) Breast cancers with increased expression of this gene can be treated with an antibody, Herceptin, raised against the HER-2/neu protein. Herceptin is intended for use in patients in whom the *ERBB2* oncogene is overexpressed, making assays for the gene or for its protein product mandatory before treatment. Immunohistochemistry has been used to identify tumors in which HER-2/*neu* protein is increased, and fluorescent in situ hybridization (FISH) has been used for detection of HER-2/*neu* gene amplification. The number of copies of the gene and the level of protein expression can be measured in extracts of the tumor tissue by real-time PCR and immunoassay, respectively. Serum immunoassays work by virtue of the fact that a fragment of the Her-2/*neu* protein is released into the bloodstream where it can be detected and its concentration measured.

A Note on Names and Symbols for Human Genes

Dealing with the multiple names and symbols for a given gene can be frustrating for students (and everyone else). Several names for a gene may appear because the gene was discovered by different research groups, and each group gave it a name. Clinical workers may prefer a name that describes the gene's association with disease (for example, "B-cell lymphoma 2"), but researchers may prefer a name that indicates the function associated with the gene, and others may prefer a name that indicates the organism in which the gene was first found.

A Web site (http://www.gene.ucl.ac.uk/nomenclature/) under the auspices of The Human Genome Organization (usually referred to as HUGO) lists HUGO-approved names and symbols for almost 24,000 human genes. Gene symbols are always in capital italics. For each gene name and symbol, the Web site lists aliases and previous symbols. The site is easily searched so that by entering any of these names or symbols, whether it is approved or not, you can find a listing that will provide other names and symbols.

The editors of this book have attempted to use the HUGO-approved names and symbols. We provide commonly used aliases in parentheses so that students will not be surprised by them when they are used by physicians or laboratory workers. It is not possible to list all 24,000 gene names in this book. The Web site of the HUGO Gene Nomenclature Committee can be a useful resource.

For further discussion of other specific oncogenes see reference information in Chapter 14, Box 14-1.

Tumor-Suppressor Genes

Evidence of the existence of tumor-suppressor genes arose when hybrid cells were made from normal and malignant cells. Surprisingly the hybrid cells did not take on the characteristics of the malignant cells, but behaved normally. It was concluded that normal cells contained a gene that suppressed the expression of the malignant phenotype. Reversion to malignancy occurred when the cultured cells lost normal chromosomes.

The clinical usefulness of detection of mutations in tumor-suppressor gene mutations lies not only in the diagnosis and prognosis of cancer, but also in the prediction of susceptibility when a mutation of a tumor-suppressor gene is carried in the germline (not just in the malignant cells), as with the breast cancer genes BRCA1 and BRCA2. As with oncogenes, assays for most tumor-suppressor genes are not routinely performed in molecular diagnostics laboratories at the present time. Descriptions of some specific tumor-suppressor genes are included for reference in Chapter 14, Box 14-2.

MOLECULAR DIAGNOSIS OF HEMATOPOIETIC NEOPLASIA

Hematopoietic neoplasms are divided into the leukemias and lymphomas. The **leukemias** are neoplastic proliferations of hematopoietic cells and are characteristically based in the bone marrow and peripheral blood. Thus the diagnostic material evaluated in these cases is typically bone marrow or peripheral blood. The leukemias are classified according to a putative lineage commitment (such as lymphocyte or myeloid cell lineage) or stage of differentiation (e.g., lympho*blastic*, lympho*cytic*, etc.) and clinicopathological characteristics, such as the manner of disease onset and the aggressiveness of clinical

course (acute versus chronic). The tumor cells in acute leukemias are immature cells with limited differentiation. By comparison, the neoplastic cells in chronic leukemias are mature and differentiated.

The **lymphomas** are neoplasms of B or T or NK lymphocytes. Lymphomas typically present as tumorous enlargements of peripheral lymphoid tissues or in tissues outside the lymphatic system (extranodal). As with the leukemias, the lymphomas are subclassified into distinct clinicopathological entities based on lineage and degree of differentiation. Despite their designation as primarily tissue-based neoplasms, malignant lymphomas may involve the bone marrow or peripheral blood. Conversely, acute leukemias may present as extramedullary (i.e., outside the bone marrow) tumors. Malignant lymphomas are categorized into Hodgkin and non-Hodgkin lymphomas. The neoplastic cell in Hodgkin lymphoma is a B cell with characteristic morphological features called the RS cell. The RS cell and its morphological variants typically account for only a small proportion of the cellular infiltrate in Hodgkin lymphomas. Hence, identification of genetic abnormalities in Hodgkin lymphomas has been challenging.

Clonality of Lymphomas

In malignancies the malignant cells typically have the property of *clonality*. Because the cells are clones, the DNA in each cell is essentially identical to that in each of the other malignant cells. Determination of clonality can be useful in determining if a collection of cells is malignant. This is especially true in lymphomas, which can be difficult to distinguish from benign proliferations of lymphocytes in which the cells are not clones. A property of DNA in lymphocytes allows testing for clonality.

B lymphocytes are able to change the arrangement of segments of DNA in the genes that code for **immunoglobulins** (Ig). Similarly, **T lymphocytes** can rearrange segments of genes that code for antigen-recognizing proteins called **T-cell receptors** (TCR) that reside on the surface of T cells. The rearrangements of DNA sequences are part of the mechanism by which these genes are able to code for the many Ig and TCR proteins that cells need to bind the vast variety of antigens that the body encounters from pathogens and toxins.

Each mature lymphocyte expresses a specific antigen-receptor protein and carries the corresponding rearranged antigen-receptor gene. The rearranged antigen-receptor gene represents a specific marker for each mature lymphocyte and its **clonal** progeny. Malignant lymphomas arise from clonal lymphoid proliferations that can be identified by the detection of a predominant antigen-receptor **gene rearrangement.** A table of such lymphomas is provided in Chapter 14 for reference.

The introduction of molecular biological techniques into hematopathology has refined lymphoma diagnostics and altered classification of the lymphomas.[12] Studies of clonality in lymphocytes have played an important role in this evolution.

ASSAYS TO DETERMINE CLONALITY

Initially, Southern blot hybridization (SBH) methodology was used to detect clonal antigen-receptor gene rearrangements. The Southern blot technique (Chapter 5) is still considered the gold standard for specificity for detection of clonality throughout a broad range of lymphoid malignancies. More recently, however, SBH has been complemented or completely replaced in most laboratories by polymerase chain reaction (PCR)-based strategies.

Immunology Review

Before discussing the specific clonality assays used currently, the molecular basis of B- and T-cell rearrangements is discussed, followed by brief discussions of the common issues of SBH and PCR methodologies.

Molecular Genetic Basis for Immunoglobulin Gene Rearrangements

Igs are produced exclusively by B lymphocytes and constitute the hallmark of the humoral immune response. Immunoglobulin G (IgG) molecules contain two identical 50 to 70 kDa **immunoglobulin heavy chains,** associated with two identical **immunoglobulin light chains** (κ or λ) of approximately 23 kDa. The IgG chains are linked by noncovalent forces and interchain disulfide bridges and together form a bilaterally symmetrical structure. Heavy chains contain one variable (V) and three constant (C) regions or "domains"; light chains contain one V domain and only one C domain. In both heavy and light chains, the V domain consists of four relatively invariable framework regions (FRs) of 15 to 30 amino acids. The FRs are separated by three short (9 to 12 amino acids) hypervariable or complementarity determining regions (CDR). In both heavy and light chains, the CDR3 region is the farthest away from the amino terminus and exhibits the greatest sequence variability among the three CDRs. The C-terminal region of secreted Ig molecules binds to complement components and Fc receptors. The Ig gene variable regions are the targets for DNA-based assessment of B-lymphocyte clonality.

To generate the large number of unique antibody molecules needed for immunity, B cells rely on the random recombination of Ig gene segments and postrecombination mutational events called somatic hypermutation. During somatic hypermutation, small mutations in the CDRs of the Ig genes are introduced. This process of hypermutation occurs when the B cell is in the germinal center of the lymph node and is driven by antigen exposure. Ig molecules with higher affinity (a better fit) for their antigenic targets result from somatic hypermutation. The three Ig genetic loci are located on chromosome 14q32 for the Ig heavy chain (IgH) gene, chromosome 2p12 for the Ig kappa light chain (Igκ) gene, and chromosome 22q11 for the Ig lambda light chain (Igλ) gene. In genes that form the Ig and other antigen receptors, four regions or components must be appropriately "brought together" for transcription to occur. The segments are referred to as: variable (V), diversity (D), joining (J), and constant (C) regions. Whereas both the Ig heavy and light chain genes contain V, J, and C regions, only the IgH genes contain D regions (Figure 13-1). The IgH gene contains approximately 87 V_H, 30 D_H, and 6 J_H segments. Through the random recombination of the Ig gene segments, the human immune system has the potential to create an enormously diverse set of ~10^9 unique primary Ig molecules (Figure 13-2). The C-region genes are initially uninvolved in the rearrangement process, but are subsequently juxtaposed to their respective VJ or VDJ complexes during RNA splicing. Incorporation of different C regions during IgH RNA splicing permits antibody class switching. Antibody (Ig) class switching is the process by which an antibody with the same antigen specificity is switched from an IgG to an IgA (a switch from a C_H gamma chain segment to a C_H alpha chain segment) or other class of antibody. The C_H segments determine the Ig class and provide various nonantigen recognition functions to the antibody (Ig) molecules. Thus a specific V(D)J rearrangement can be expressed as an IgG, IgA, or other Ig class. During B-lymphocyte development, IgH gene rearrangement occurs first followed by the kappa and then lambda gene rearrangements. Light chain loci undergo a similar but less complex recombination process involving the joining of V to J segments since there are no light chain D segments.

The process of Ig gene rearrangement has been exploited in molecular diagnostics for the identification of clonal lymphoid proliferations. In this regard, because the majority (~95%) of B-cell lymphomas or leukemias can be detected by an analysis of just the IgH locus, it has become customary to limit Ig clonality assays to the IgH locus.

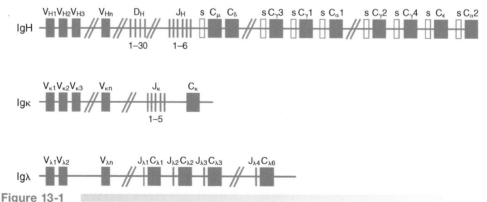

Figure 13-1

Schematic representation of the germline configurations of the antigen-receptor gene loci for immunoglobulin heavy chain (IgH), immunoglobulin kappa (Igκ) and lambda (Igλ) light chains. Each gene is composed of several variable (V), joining (J), and constant (C) segments. Note that the IgH locus contains diversity (D) gene segments.

Molecular Genetic Basis for T-Cell Receptor Gene Rearrangements

A process similar to that described for the Ig genes occurs in the TCR genes (Figure 13-3), with the notable exception that somatic hypermutation is absent in TCR gene rearrangements. The developmental hierarchy of TCR genes is such that the TCRδ gene is the first to rearrange, followed by the TCRγ, TCRβ, and then the TCRα genes. The TCRδ gene is located on chromosome 14q11 and contains six or fewer Vδ (variable) segments, only two or three Dδ (diverse) segments, and three Jδ (joining) segments. The TCRα gene (Figure 13-3) is located on band 14q11 and flanks the TCRδ gene on either side.

Rearrangements may occur within or between gene segments (e.g., Vβ1 to Jβ1 or Vβ2 to Jβ1). There is extensive sequence homology between the constant Cβ1 and Cβ2 seg-

ments. This phenomenon is exploited in the utilization of a consensus Cβ probe in the Southern blot–based clonality assessment of the TCR genes. The TCRγ gene is located on chromosome 7 and contains about 11 Vγ segments and two Jγ genes. The simple structure and limited number of gene segments of the TCRγ loci favor its use as a target for TCR PCR. In TCR PCR, consensus primers are designed to recognize all of the relatively few Vγ and the Jγ gene segments.

Southern Blot Hybridization Analysis for Antigen-Receptor Gene Rearrangements

In this procedure, high-quality total cellular DNA extracted from a fresh or flash-frozen specimen is subjected to digestion using different bacterial restriction endonucleases, which produce DNA fragments of different sizes encompassing the Ig or TCR gene region segments to be interrogated (Figures 13-4 and 13-5). The enzyme-digested fragments of DNA are subjected to gel electrophoresis and transferred by blotting and immobilized on a membrane. A labeled probe complementary to the Ig J region segment is hybridized to the membrane. Clonal rearrangements are recognized by the identification of one or two novel rearranged bands that are distinct from the germ-line pattern obtained with placental DNA. One or two novel rearranged (nongermline) bands may be identifiable depending on whether there is a clonal monoallelic or biallelic rearrangement (Figure 13-6).

Material suitable for Southern blot analysis includes fresh tissue or aspiration biopsy material, as long as sufficient cellular material can be obtained from the specimen of interest. Ethanol-fixed tissue can also be used. However, formalin-fixed tissue produces chemical changes in DNA and yields DNA of insufficient quality to permit reliable Southern blotting. An SBH assay using three enzymes requires approximately 1.5×10^7 cells (approximately 15 µg of intact total cellular DNA). Hypothetically, all of the antigen-receptor genes could be used as potential targets for the assessment of clonality status. However, only the immunoglobulin heavy and light chain and the TCR beta chain loci have gained widespread use for clonality testing by Southern blot analysis. The TCRα locus is impractical because

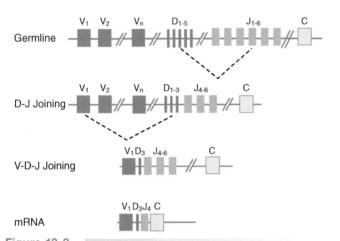

Figure 13-2
Schematic representation of antigen-receptor gene rearrangement mechanism using the IgH chain locus as a model. There is an initial D-to-J joining in a partial or incomplete recombination, followed by a V-D-J joining to complete the rearrangement. The C-regions are included at the mRNA level via RNA splicing to form a V(D)J-C transcript.

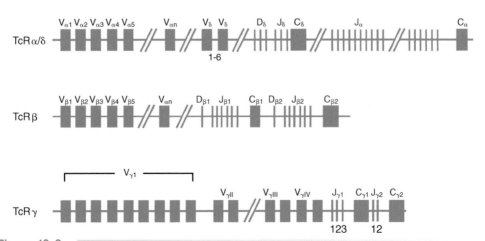

Figure 13-3
The T-cell-receptor locus contains α/δ-, β-, and γ-chain genes. The architectural configuration is similar to that of the Ig loci. Note that only β and δ contain diversity (D) regions.

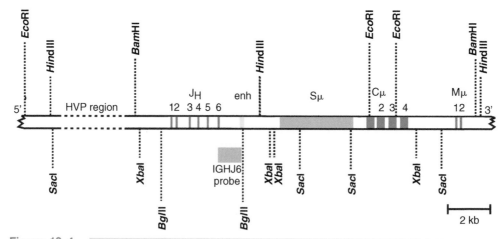

Figure 13-4

Restriction map of the Ig heavy locus. The sites of the enzyme restriction sites determine the sizes of the fragments that are visualized using the IgHJ6 probe as illustrated. The three restriction enzymes *Bam*HI, *Xba*I, and *Bgl*II yield fragments that are 16 kb, 6.2 kb, and 3.8 kb in length, respectively. Restriction patterns different from the germline patterns indicate a novel rearrangement event.

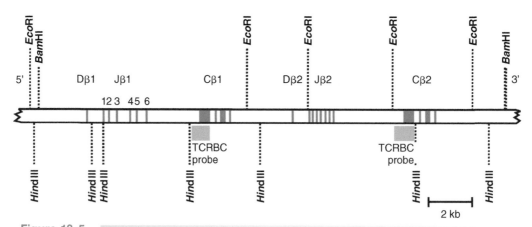

Figure 13-5

Restriction map of the TCRβ locus. The probe is complementary to the TCRβ constant region. There is extensive sequence homology between the Cβ1 and Cβ2 segments. Thus the Cβ probe hybridizes to both the Cβ1 and Cβ2 segments thereby resulting in two germline band signals for all enzymes depicted except *Bam*HI. The *Eco*RI site located between the Cβ1 and Jβ2 segments is notoriously resistant to digestion and may yield a partial digest with a band of 8.0 kb in size.

it contains several widely separated J segments; this would pose practical challenges in the optimization of assays for multiple probes. The TCRγ and TCRδ loci are also not favorable for Southern blot assays because they have only a limited number of V segments such that even reactive T-cell populations may yield confusing nongermline bands.

The presence of a clonal population is identified by the detection of one or two predominant nongermline rearranged bands on a gel (Figure 13-6). The presence of nongermline bands does not always indicate **monoclonality.** For example, perfectly normal alterations of single bases (often called single nucleotide polymorphisms or SNPs) may create or abolish restriction enzyme recognition sites, thus yielding novel bands on the gel following digestion of the DNA by the restriction enzymes. In this scenario, use of a different enzyme would yield a germline configuration. The potential of these SNPs to confound the interpretation of Southern blot studies justifies the

use of three or more enzymes for the unequivocal assignment of monoclonality. A second situation in which a nongermline band may occur and yet not indicate monoclonality is incomplete (partial) digestion by the restriction enzyme. This may be evident in the control sample (placental DNA) and if so invalidates the significance of any such band in the test sample. The placental DNA sample does not control for poor DNA extraction technique of the patient sample; poor extraction can reduce the efficiency of the restriction endonuclease (as would occur if the extracted DNA is contaminated by an inhibitor of the enzyme) and cause a novel DNA digestion pattern for the patient sample but not for the control.

Use of Clonal Rearrangements
to Determine Lineage

Clonal rearrangements of either the Ig or TCR genes have also been used to ascertain the lineage of hematological neoplasms

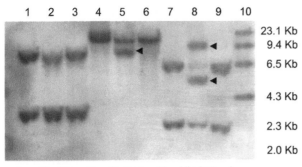

Figure 13-6
SBH analysis for clonal rearrangements of the TCRβ chain locus. DNA samples extracted from two different patients with a suspected diagnosis of T-cell lymphoma are assessed. Lanes 1 to 3 represent the *Eco*RI digests. Lanes 4 to 6 show the *Bam*HI digests, and lanes 7 to 9 demonstrate the *Hind*III digests from both samples run side by side. Lane 10 shows the DNA size marker. Lanes 1, 4, and 7 show the restriction patterns in the germline control (placenta) using the *Eco*RI, *Bam*HI, and *Hind*III enzymes, respectively. DNA from patient 1 (Lanes 2, 5, and 8) shows a germline pattern using *Eco*RI, but novel rearrangements *(arrowheads)* using *Bam*HI and *Hind*III. Patient 2 (lanes 3, 6, and 9) shows a germline pattern in all three enzyme digests. Accordingly, sample 1 is scored as showing evidence for a monoclonal T-cell population, and sample 2 is scored as showing evidence of a polyclonal T-cell population.

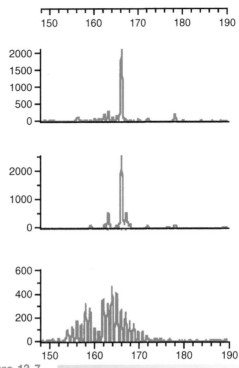

Figure 13-7
Polymerase chain reaction (PCR) analysis for clonal rearrangements of the antigen-receptor gene loci. PCR analysis of the TRC γ-chain locus is shown. The upper and middle panels show duplicate assays with monoclonal capillary electrohoretic peaks of identical size (~166 bp) in both replicates. The bottom panel shows a polyclonal pattern.

that do not express B- or T-cell specific markers. Intuitively, clonal rearrangements of the Ig genes would indicate B-cell processes, and clonal rearrangements of the TCR genes would indicate T-cell processes. However, some malignant lymphomas and leukemias may demonstrate both Ig and TCR rearrangements. In particular, acute leukemias and lymphoblastic lymphomas may demonstrate both Ig and TCR gene rearrangements. Further, up to 20% of acute myeloid leukemias (AMLs) may demonstrate rearrangements of either the Ig or TCR genes. Hence, lineage is best assigned using a combination of immunophenotypic and molecular studies.

Polymerase Chain Reaction Analysis of Antigen-Receptor Gene Rearrangements

PCR-based assays have become the mainstay for the detection of rearrangements of the Ig and TCR genes in many molecular diagnostics laboratories. This is because SBH is labor-intensive and slow. Additionally, SBH requires a substantial quantity of intact DNA and hence is less amenable to specimens with suboptimal DNA quality (as is the case with fixed, paraffin-embedded tissue samples). PCR, on the other hand, is well suited for analysis of such specimens, which constitute the majority of samples analyzed in the clinical laboratory.

The application of PCR for the identification of clonality entails the utilization of consensus V-region and J-region primers, in vitro amplification of DNA across the V(D)J junction followed by evaluation of the PCR products by gel electrophoresis, or other methods for analysis of the uniformity of PCR-generated fragments. In the germline configuration, these V- and J-region segments are located several kilobases apart and would not be amplifiable. However, the V(D)J recombination brings the VDJ segments into close proximity and thereby permits amplification of products that are less 80 to 350 bases

depending on the primers used. For T-cell assays by PCR, TCRγ is the most informative.

In these assays, monoclonal populations yield one or two dominant bands or peaks (Figure 13-7). By contrast a polyclonal mixture of cells will not show this pattern because each cell carries a unique gene rearrangement, and thus PCR products of many sizes are produced; this collection of DNA molecules is seen as a large number of bands ("ladder") or, if the bands are not distinct, as a "smear."[19] Thus the marker of clonality in PCR differs from that in SBH analysis in which the marker is the configuration of the rearranged antigen-receptor genes.

Following PCR, the PCR products are analyzed by electrophoresis (Figure 13-7). The PCR products are most commonly visualized by ultraviolet illumination of ethidium bromide–stained gels. Agarose and polyacrylamide gels have been commonly used for resolution of PCR products; capillary gel electrophoresis is perhaps the most common approach. A successful PCR exhibits PCR products in the expected size range, appropriate results in the positive and negative controls, and absence of bands in the template-free (H_2O) control.

Most PCR-based clonality assays are less sensitive in detecting all of the possible clonal rearrangements than is SBH analysis, which approaches 100% detection if a sufficient number of restriction enzymes and a variety of probes are used. Depending on the assay and the lymphoid neoplasm tested, PCR-based clonality studies may show false-negative rates from 10% to 40% when compared with SBH. High rates of false-negative results occurred in early PCR methods that did not detect partial DJ rearrangements, wherein the V and J region genes are not approximated to one another and are too distant for conventional PCR to generate an amplification product. Newer methods overcome this and most of the difficulties of earlier methods by the utilization of multiple primer sets. In the event of a negative PCR result, SBH analysis may be performed if sufficient high-quality genomic DNA is available.

The ability of PCR to detect rare DNA species carrying a specific molecular aberration depends on the particular application. For antigen-receptor gene rearrangement studies, PCR can detect a monoclonal population in a background of 10^2 to 10^3 polyclonal cells of the same phenotype (B or T cells). By comparison, PCR can detect one cell harboring a chromosomal translocation within a background of 10^5 to 10^6 cells negative for the translocation.

COMMON ("RECURRENT") CHROMOSOMAL TRANSLOCATIONS IN MALIGNANT LYMPHOMA

The Ig gene rearrangement process is susceptible to abnormal *translocation* of genes from other parts of the genome into the Ig gene. The abnormally regulated expression (deregulation) of these "foreign" genes underlies the development of lymphoid neoplasia. A *translocation* typically involves the transfer of a piece of one chromosome to a different chromosome.

Certain specific (nonrandom) chromosomal translocations are frequently observed in hematological neoplasia and in many cases are characteristic of specific types of tumors. The translocations typically result in one of two genetic consequences:

(1) An oncogene is placed in close proximity to an antigen-receptor gene. This leads to dysregulated expression of the oncogene and increased expression of the structurally normal (active) oncoprotein. This mechanism is exemplified by the translocation that is characteristic of follicular lymphoma. This translocation brings together the gene for bcl-2 from chromosome 18 and the gene for the IgH from chromosome 14.[21] Because the Ig gene is expressed in B lymphocytes, the adjacent gene for bcl-2 is also highly expressed.

(2) Two genes are brought together to create a novel chimeric gene. The chimeric gene is partly from one gene and partly from the other gene. The chimeric gene codes for a chimeric protein that has oncogenic properties. This mechanism is most commonly observed in the leukemias, but it is also seen in malignant lymphomas. For example, the translocation seen in anaplastic large cell lymphoma creates an abnormal fusion gene (*NPM-ALK*) that is central to the pathogenesis of malignant lymphoma. Testing for the presence of such a chimeric fusion is most readily done by use of reverse-transcriptase polymerase chain reaction (RT-PCR) (Chapter 5) to amplify the mRNA for the chimeric protein. Such testing is becoming increasingly available, particularly in reference laboratories. As a reference source, Chapter 14 includes a table (Table 14-8) of the common chromosomal translocations, the participating genes, and the associated lymphomas.

Southern Blot Hybridization Analysis for the Detection of Chromosomal Translocations

SBH analysis is an excellent method for the detection of chromosomal translocations. A sequence-specific probe to the gene of interest is used for SBH analysis as described for the antigen-receptor genes. Detection of a pattern in which bands of different sizes than are seen in the germline configuration of the gene of interest would suggest the presence of a translocation. It should be noted that this method does not identify the translocation partner of the gene of interest. As with the antigen-receptor gene rearrangement studies by SBH, single base alterations (SNPs) in the DNA sequence at enzyme restriction sites may result in nongermline patterns that may be misinterpreted as translocations. Use of a different restriction enzyme will correctly show the gene locus to be of germline size. The labor-intensive nature of SBH and the requirement for high quality DNA have diminished its popularity for routine detection of chromosomal translocations in the clinical laboratory.

Polymerase Chain Reaction Analysis for Detection of Chromosomal Translocations

The PCR is very well suited to the analysis of chromosomal translocations, particularly when the translocation breakpoints are clustered and the sequences flanking the translocation breakpoints are well characterized.

Follicular Lymphoma

The translocation that is characteristic of follicular lymphoma exemplifies the utility of PCR in the detection of a chromosomal translocation. Follicular lymphoma is associated with a gene translocation that inhibits cell death. The translocation involves the *BCL2* gene (on chromosome 18) and the locus coding for the IgH (on chromosome 14). Such a translocation involving chromosomes 14 and 18 is abbreviated t(14;18). (See Box 13-2 for more on abbreviations.) The locations at which chromosome 18 is broken (*breakpoints*) to allow the translocations are preferentially located in certain regions of chromosome 18 near the *BCL2* gene. The breakpoints in the majority of t(14;18) are clustered in the *major* **breakpoint cluster region (BCR)** (Figure 13-8). The BCR is a 150-bp sequence located within the 3'-untranslated region of exon 3 of the *BCL2* gene and harbors approximately 60% of the breakpoints found in follicular lymphoma. Another 20% are located at the *minor cluster* region, which is located 30 kb farther 3' from the *BCL2* gene. An additional cluster of breakpoints is located at the *variant cluster region* located 5' upstream of the *BCL2* gene that harbors approximately 5% of the breakpoints found in follicular lymphoma (Figure 13-8). More recently an intermediate cluster region (ICR) has been described[1].

FISH analysis can be used to detect this translocation. In one approach, a DNA probe labeled with a red fluorescent dye hybridizes with the IgH locus, and a probe labeled with a green

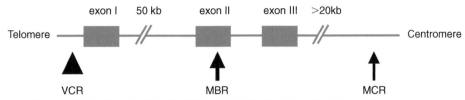

Figure 13-8
Schematic representation of the organization of the *BCL2* gene and most frequent breakpoints on chromosome 18q21 involved in t(14;18). The *BCL2* exons are represented as blue rectangles. MBR represents the major breakpoint cluster region where approximately 50% to 60% of the breakpoints occur. MCR represents the minor breakpoint cluster region where 20% to 25% of the breakpoints may be found. VCR represents the variant cluster region where 5% to 20% of the breakpoints may be found.

BOX 13-2

Shorthand Notation for Translocations

Translocations involve interchange of parts between different (nonhomologous) chromosomes, such as between a copy of chromosome 1 and a copy of chromosome 13. The shorthand notation for a translocation involving chromosomes 1 and 13 is t(1;13).

When the involved regions of the chromosomes are known, those regions also may be indicated in shorthand. For example, a t(1;13) translocation seen in a certain type of tumor places the *PAX7* gene of chromosome 1 next to the *FOXO1A* gene of chromosome 13. This t(1;13) translocation can be written as t(1;13)(p36;q14) because the *PAX7* gene is known to be located on the short arm (p) of chromosome 1 at band p36, and the *FOXO1A* gene is located on the long arm (q) of chromosome 13 at band 14 (q14).

As an exercise, what is the notation for a translocation of *PAX3* gene on chromosome 2 (2q35) to the *FOXO1A* gene on band 13q14?

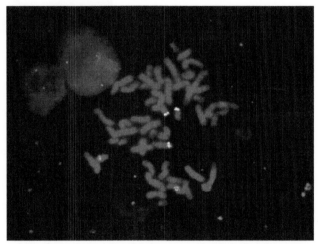

Figure 13-9
FISH for the t(14;18) anomaly on metaphase spreads from a case of follicular lymphoma. The IgH sequences on 14q32 *(red)* when juxtaposed to the *BCL2* sequences on 18q21 *(green)* yield a yellow fusion signal indicative of the presence of the t(14;18) (see Color Plate 9).

fluorescent dye hybridizes with sequences in or near the *BCL2* gene. In normal cells, the red and green signals appear on separate chromosomes. By contrast, when the two loci are together on the same chromosome, the red and green signals combine to produce a yellow signal. The image in Figure 13-9 shows this finding in cells from tissue with a translocation of DNA sequences involving chromosomes 14 and 18. Positive and negative controls must be used to establish the number of yellow translocation signals associated with the disease.

Mantle Cell Lymphoma

A different translocation is characteristic of mantle cell lymphoma, but rare in other types of malignant lymphoma. This translocation juxtaposes the *BCL1* locus on chromosome 11 with the IgH gene enhancer locus of chromosome 14. Multiple breakpoints have been seen on chromosome 11. The most frequently involved location is the major translocation cluster (MTC) region, which is located 110 kb 5′ of the *CCND1* (or *BCL1*) locus. Other breakpoints occurring within minor translocation cluster regions have also been described (Figure 13-10).

The *CCND1* gene encodes cyclin D1, and the translocations do not disrupt the coding region of the gene. Consequently the cyclin D1 produced is normal, but its expression is increased, leading to dysregulation of the cell cycle.

MOLECULAR GENETICS OF LEUKEMIAS

As indicated above, human leukemias are characterized by recurrent genetic abnormalities that can be used as genetic markers of the specific leukemia. The genetic abnormalities are most often chromosomal translocations that produce chimeric fusion proteins. These proteins may block cellular differentiation at a certain stage or increase cell proliferation.

The chronic leukemias of myeloid-derived cells are characterized by activation of tyrosine kinases. The kinases increase proliferation of cells and confer a survival advantage to the myelocytes. An example of this is the *BCR-ABL* chimeric fusion that is characteristic of chronic myeloid (or "myelogenous") leukemia (CML). Inhibition of the activated tyrosine kinase with imatinib mesylate (Gleevec) is a valuable treatment for CML[5].

In contrast to the chromosomal translocations in CML, the translocations in the AMLs typically result in loss-of-function aberrations. The translocations disrupt transcription factors and thereby lead to maturational arrest or differentiation blocks at early stages of myeloid development. These genetic changes appear to be insufficient to cause leukemia without

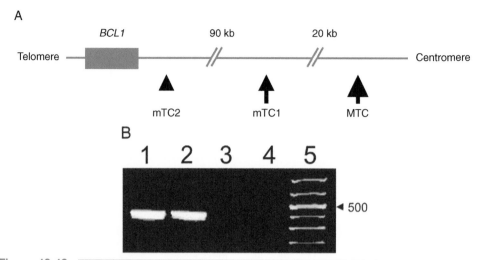

Figure 13-10

(**A**) Schematic representation of the organization of the *CCND1* (*BCL*) gene on chromosome 11q13 and the breakpoint regions associated with t(11;14). The *CCND1* (*BCL*) gene is represented as a blue rectangle. The relative locations of the MTC where up to 40% of the breakpoints are clustered and the minor translocation cluster regions (mTC1 and mTC2) are indicated. The size of the amplified PCR product may vary depending on the location of the breakpoints. (**B**) PCR analysis and agarose gel electrophoresis for the detection of t(11;14). The primers were directed against the MTC of *CCND1* (*BCL1*). Lane 1 represents a positive control with a band at ~450 bp. Lane 2 is the patient sample with a positive band also at ~450 bp. Lane 3 contains a negative control (reactive tonsil). Lane 4 represents a no-template (H₂O) control. Lane 5 shows the size marker.

concomitant mutations in *RAS* or in one of the tyrosine kinase genes, *FLT3* or *KIT* (formerly called *C-KIT*). Nonetheless, the translocations provide a target for disease detection, monitoring, and potential gene-specific therapy. A list of selected translocations occurring in human leukemias is provided for reference in Table 14-9 in Chapter 14.

The most frequently employed technique for the detection of the chimeric transcripts in the molecular laboratory is RT-PCR. The prevalence of specific genetic mutations often requires that screening for such mutations be performed in the diagnostic laboratory.

Acute Myeloid Leukemias

The translocations that occur in the AMLs target transcription factors or transcriptional coactivators. The transcription factors are involved in the differentiation of the myeloid cells, and disruption of their normal function by the translocation leads to developmental arrest and maturational block at immature stages of differentiation. The targeted transcription factors include the retinoic acid receptor alpha (RARα) (in acute promyelocytic leukemia [APL]) and several members of the core binding factor (CBF) complex. APL is characterized by translocations involving the *RARα* gene. These translocations result in a block of myeloid differentiation at the promyelocytic stage.

Acute Myeloid Leukemia

A translocation involving chromosomes 8 and 21 is found in approximately 7% of de novo AML and is more common in young individuals. The translocation is found in 20% to 40% of AMLs of the **FAB**-M2 subtype. It has also been reported infrequently in AML FAB M1, AML FAB M4, and rare cases of therapy-associated AML. The translocation leads to the fusion of the *RUNX1* and *RUNX1T1* genes. (*RUNX1* has been

called *AML1*, for AML 1 gene, and *RUNX1T* has been called *ETO*, for eight twenty one. The fusion is often called *AML1-ETO*. Other aliases and symbols for these genes can be found at the Web site of the HUGO Gene Nomenclature Committee that is discussed in Box 13-1.)

The translocation portends a good prognosis in cases of de novo AML, with a favorable response to treatment with cytosine arabinoside. The chimeric fusion is detectable by RT-PCR in the vast majority of AMLs with the translocation. The fusions join exon 5 of *RUNX1* (*AML1*) to exon 2 of *RUNX1T1* (*ETO*) (Figure 13-11), and the fusion transcript can also be detected in complex translocations in a significant proportion of cases in which the translocation is not found by conventional cytogenetic testing.[14] Specifically, RT-PCR has been reported to detect the fusion in 8% to 12% of AML. Interestingly, the fusion transcript may be detected using sensitive end-point PCR assays several years after chemotherapy or bone marrow transplant; this may limit its predictive value for relapse in affected patients. Quantitative studies using recently developed real-time PCR protocols (Figure 13-12) may provide a better indication of rising transcript copies and hence disease recurrence.

Acute Promyelocytic Leukemia

A translocation involving chromosomes 15 and 17 is the characteristic molecular abnormality in acute promyelocytic leukemia, which is classified as AML FAB M3. This abnormality is present in approximately 75% of cases of APL, which constitute 5% to 10% of all AMLs. The translocation results in juxtaposition of the putative transcription factor *PML* (promyelocytic leukemia) on chromosome 15 to the *RARA* gene (retinoic acid receptor α) on chromosome 17. The breakpoints on chromosome 17 are confined to a 15-kb fragment within intron 2 of

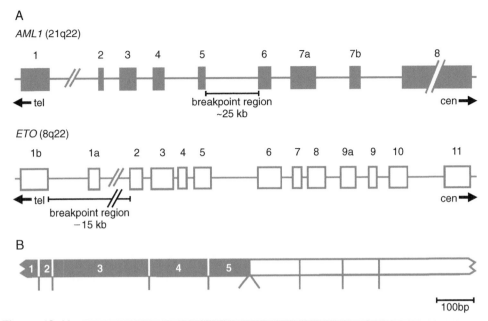

Figure 13-11
Schematic representation of the organization of the *RUNX1* (*AML1*) (21q22) and the *RUNX1T1* (*ETO*) genes (8q22) involved in the t(8;21) anomaly that is characteristic of FAB AML M2. The centromeric (c) and telomeric (tel) directions are indicated. In panel **A,** the exons of the *RUNX1* (*AML1*) gene are depicted in blue rectangles, whereas the exons of the *RUNX1T1* (*ETO*) gene are depicted in white rectangles. In panel **B,** the configuration of the *RUNX1-RUNX1T* (*AML1-ETO*) chimeric fusion is shown. The numbers below the fusion transcript indicate the position of the first nucleotide in the exon involved or the last nucleotide of the exon immediately 5′ to the fusion. The arrows depict the positions of oligonucleotide primers used for the PCR detection of the fusion transcript. The size of the amplified PCR product may vary depending on the location of the breakpoints.

the *RARA* locus. The breakpoints on chromosome 15 are more varied, with involvement of three or more distinct regions (Figure 13-13, panel A). The different breakpoints on *PML*, the alternatively spliced transcripts, and use of two different polyadenylation sites give rise to a great variety of fusion transcripts of different sizes (Figure 13-13, panel B). Recognition of these varied transcripts is important in the design of diagnostic RT-PCR assays that are capable of detecting the majority of these fusions (Figure 13-13, panel B). Most assays have been directed at the *PML-RARα* fusion since the reciprocal (*RARα-PML*) fusion is not detectable in some cases of APL.

The chimeric PML-RARα protein contributes to leukemogenesis by blocking the differentiation of myeloid cells at the level of promyelocytes. The persistent detection of fusion transcripts in treated patients is an ominous indication for a tendency for relapse. The recent availability of quantitative real-time protocols provides an opportunity for sensitive and specific monitoring of consecutive samples at appropriate intervals for the identification of patients with high relapse potential.

Chronic Leukemias of Myeloid/Monocytic Lineage

The chronic myeloid leukemias are characterized by translocations that lead to constitutive activation of tyrosine kinases. The most common of these is a translocation involving chromosomes 9 and 22 that results in the *BCR-ABL1* fusion that is characteristic of CML. Up to seven different chromosomal translocations are associated with the chronic leukemias of

myeloid and/or monocytic lineage, but all are characterized by the formation of a chimeric fusion with a tyrosine kinase domain and a motif that is important for activation of the tyrosine kinase. The increased kinase activity transforms the myeloid cells and confers growth potential.

Chronic Myeloid (or "Myelogenous") Leukemia
A translocation involving chromosomes 9 and 22, known as the Philadelphia chromosome, is the diagnostic hallmark of CML and is found in virtually 100% of cases. The translocation is also found in up to 20% to 50% of acute lymphocytic leukemias (ALLs) in adults and in 2% to 10% of childhood ALLs. The translocation juxtaposes 3′ sequences on the *ABL1* (also called *c-ABL*) tyrosine kinase proto-oncogene (chromosome 9) to the 5′ sequences of the breakpoint cluster region *BCR* gene (chromosome 22).[4] This forms two hybrid genes; *BCR-ABL* on the derivative chromosome 22 and *ABL-BCR* on the derivative chromosome 9. The *BCR-ABL* fusion encodes a chimeric protein with constitutively activated tyrosine kinase activity.

Whereas the breakpoints on chromosome 9 are relatively constant and 5′ to exon 2 of *c-ABL*, the breakpoints on chromosome 22 within the *BCR* gene are quite variable (Figure 13-14). Depending on the location of the breakpoint, the fusion protein resulting from the *BCR-ABL* fusion can vary in size from 190 to 230 kDa. Up to 95% of CMLs and 30% to 50% of adult t(9;22)-positive ALLs harbor breakpoints in the M-*BCR* region of the *BCR* gene.

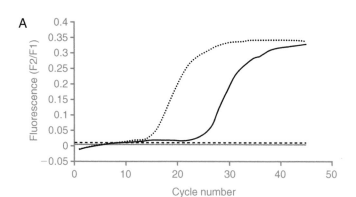

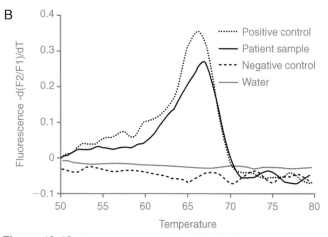

Figure 13-12

Real-time PCR detection of *RUNX1-RUNX1T1* (*AML1-ETO*) fusion transcript. Real-time PCR[24] detection was performed using a sequence-specific hybridization probe format with oligonucleotide probes labeled with fluorescein as the donor fluorophore and LCRed640 as the acceptor. Postamplification melting analysis was performed to provide confirmation of amplicon identity through the probe melting temperature. Panel **A** shows the fluorescence (F) versus cycle number (C) the LightCycler (Roche Diagnostics). The characteristic three-phase profiles of amplification curves are recognizable (i.e., initial lag, exponential or log/linear, and the final plateau phase). The dotted line represents the positive amplification signal for t(8;21) in the Kasumi cell line positive control. The heavy line represents the patient sample also showing the presence of the fusion. The dashed line represents a negative control (placental cDNA), and the light gray line is the no-template (H₂O) control. Panel **B** shows the derivative melting curves with positive melting peaks at ~65 °C in both the Kasumi cell line positive control and the patient sample. Both the negative and water controls show flat lines indicating the absence of the t(8;21) product (see Color Plate 10).

AC   The *BCR* breakpoints in virtually all of the CML cases occur in the 9.0-kb region between exons 13 and 15 (also known as b2 and b4, respectively). Fusion is to a breakpoint located in the large intron between exons 1b and 2 of the *ABL* gene (Figure 13-14). The resulting *BCR-ABL* transcript measures 8.5 kb and contains either *BCR* exon b2 or b3 and *ABL* exon 2 (exon a2). This transcript encodes the 210-kDa BCR-ABL chimeric protein (p210^{BCR/ABL}).

In rare cases of CML, the breakpoint in the *BCR* gene occurs at the ALL-associated m-*BCR*, which leads to the generation of the p190^{BCR/ABL} fusion protein.[18] p190^{BCR/ABL}-positive CML patients characteristically exhibit relative and absolute monocytosis in peripheral blood reminiscent of chronic myelomonocytic leukemia. Another distinct but rare fusion that has been described in t(9;22)-positive CML results in the formation of a large 230-kDa fusion protein as a consequence of a fusion between exon 19 (c3) of *BCR* and exon 2 (a2) of *ABL*. The *BCR* breakpoints for this fusion are located in the microbreakpoint cluster region (μ-*BCR*) located between exons 19 and 20 (Figure 13-14). The p230 fusion is characteristic of a peculiar form of CML with prominent neutrophilic proliferation. The clinical course of p230-positive CML is reportedly indolent in the majority of cases.

Up to 60% of t(9;22)-positive ALLs carry translocations in which the *BCR* breakpoints are located in a distinct region known as the "minor breakpoint cluster region" (m-*BCR*). m-*BCR* is located between the two alternative exons and exon 2 (Figure 13-14). The ABL breakpoints are located in the large intron between exon 1b and exon 2 of the ABL gene (Figure 13-14). The resulting e1-a2 fusion encodes a 190-kDa *BCR-ABL* chimeric protein that is expressed mostly in ALLs and rather infrequently as the exclusive *BCR-ABL* transcript in CML. On the other hand, the remaining 40% of t(9;22)-positive ALLs may express the p210 *BCR-ABL* fusion. A significant number of CML cases also express the low levels of e1-a2 transcripts in addition to the p210 via an alternative splicing mechanism.

Conventional **cytogenetics,** FISH, and RT-PCR have been reliably used for the laboratory detection of the t(9;22). RT-PCR detection is possible in up to 95% of cases and may detect up to 10% of cases missed by conventional cytogenetics and is an important modality for **minimal residual disease (MRD)** detection. Recently quantitative real-time PCR-based approaches have improved the ability to quantify *BCR-ABL* transcripts in CML patients[10] (Figure 13-15). The recent addition of the tyrosine kinase inhibitor imatinib mesylate[5] to the arsenal of therapeutic options for treatment of CML patients underscores the importance of methods for sensitive and specific identification and quantification of the *BCR-ABL* fusions. A t(9;22) translocation may also be seen in ALL. Its presence is an independent poor prognostic factor in ALL.

ONCOGENE AND TUMOR-SUPPRESSOR GENE MUTATIONS IN HEMATOPOIETIC MALIGNANCIES

The concomitant occurrence of additional genetic aberrations and chromosomal translocations is common in hematological malignancies. The *RAS* oncogene is one of the most frequently mutated genes in cancer[3] and is mutated in up to 25% to 44% of hematopoietic malignancies and myelodysplastic syndromes (MDS). The mutations are clustered in "hotspots" occurring at codons 12, 13, or 61, rendering them fairly easy to detect using different strategies for mutation detection, such as single-strand

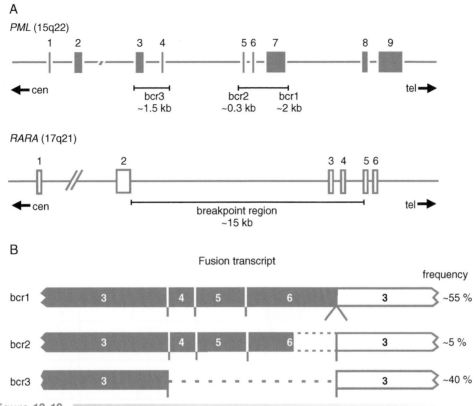

A

PML (15q22)

cen

bcr3
~1.5 kb

bcr2
~0.3 kb

bcr1
~2 kb

tel

RARA (17q21)

cen

breakpoint region
~15 kb

tel

B

Fusion transcript

frequency

bcr1   3   4   5   6   3   ~55 %

bcr2   3   4   5   6   3   ~5 %

bcr3   3   3   ~40 %

Figure 13-13

Schematic representation of the organization of the *PML* (15q22) and *RARA* (17q11) genes involved in the t(15;17) anomaly that is characteristic of FAB AML M3. The centromeric (c) and telomeric (tel) directions are indicated. In panel **A,** the exons of the *PML* gene are depicted in blue rectangles, and the exons of the *RARA* gene are depicted in white rectangles. In panel **B,** the configuration of the *PML-RARA* chimeric fusion is shown. The numbers below the fusion transcript indicate the position of the first nucleotide in the exon involved or the last nucleotide of the exon immediately 5′ to the fusion. The arrows depict the relative positions of commonly used primers employed for the PCR detection of the *PML-RARA* fusion transcript. The size of the amplified PCR product may vary depending on the location of the breakpoints.

conformation polymorphism analysis (SSCP) and denaturation gradient gel electrophoresis (DGGE) (see Chapter 5).

Mutations of another tyrosine kinase, *FLT3*, have been described in AMLs. The majority of these mutations are duplications (copies) of part of the DNA within the gene (internal tandem duplications or ITDs).[15] ITDs have been identified in *FLT3* in all FAB subtypes of AML, most frequently in APL (AML FAB M3). Figure 13-16, panel A shows an example of an ITD in *FLT3* that was detected by capillary electrophoresis of PCR products in a case of AML. The presence of the ITD was inferred from the presence of a PCR product for *FLT3* that was larger than the PCR product for wild-type *FLT3* (Figure 13-16, panel A). The duplication was confirmed by DNA sequencing of the gene. Additional mutations distinct from the ITDs occurring in *FLT3* have been described in a subset of AMLs. The most common of these is a base substitution occurring at the codon for aspartic acid residue 835. Such mutations have been identified in 7% of AML, 3% of MDS, and 3% of ALLs. *FLT3* may be the most frequently mutated gene in AML. Mutations in the activation loop of another receptor tyrosine kinase KIT (*C-KIT*) have been reported in mast cell proliferations and in a small proportion of AMLs.

The *p53* gene is the most commonly mutated tumor-suppressor gene in cancer.

Non–BCR-ABL Chronic Myeloproliferative Disorders: JAK2 Mutation in Polycythemia Vera, Essential Thrombocythemia, and Idiopathic Myelofibrosis

In several conditions, a common mutation (V617F) has been found in the *JAK2* gene (Janus kinase 2, a protein tyrosine kinase). This mutation has been identified in 60% to 90% of patients carrying a diagnosis of polycythemia vera (PV),[9] and in 30% to 50% of cases of essential thrombocythemia and approximately 30% of patients with idiopathic myelofibrosis. The mutation produces an activated JAK2 kinase, which makes the erythroid precursor cells grow without need for stimulation by erythropoietin (EPO). Mutations in the EPO receptor have been described in familial forms of PV and similarly lead to constitutive activation of the signaling pathway that includes the EPO receptor and the Janus kinase. However, the mutations in the EPO receptor are not identified in sporadic forms of the non–*BCR-ABL* chronic myeloproliferative disorders.

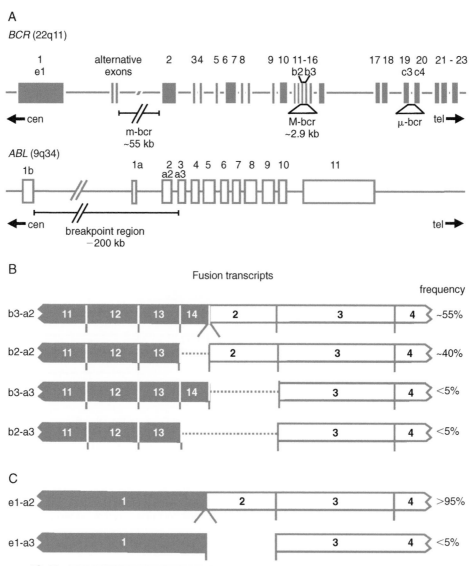

Figure 13-14

Schematic representation of the *BCR* (22q11) and *ABL* (9q34) genes involved in t(9;22) that is characteristic of all CMLs and a subset of ALLs. The centromeric (cam) and telomeric (tel) directions are indicated. The relative positions of the major breakpoint cluster (M-BCR), the minor breakpoint cluster (m-BCR), and the microbreakpoint cluster regions (μ-BCR) are shown. The previously used alternative nomenclature for the *BCR* and *ABL* exons is included where relevant. In panel **A,** the exons of the *BCR* genes are depicted in blue rectangles, and those of the *ABL* genes are depicted in white rectangles. In panel **B,** the configuration and varieties of the *BCR-ABL* chimeric fusions seen in CML are shown. In panel **C,** the configuration and varieties of the *BCR-ABL* fusions seen in ALL are shown. The numbers below the fusion transcript indicate the position of the first nucleotide in the exon involved or the last nucleotide of the exon immediately 5′ to the fusion. The e1-a2 transcript is most commonly detected in t(9;22)-positive ALL, whereas the b3-a2 and b2-a2 fusions are the most commonly detected in CML. The arrows depict the relative positions of commonly used primers employed for the PCR detection of the *BCR-ABL* fusion transcripts. The size of the amplified PCR product may vary depending on the location of the breakpoints.

The specific base change (V617F) in *JAK2* can be detected in the clinical laboratory by probe-based fluorescence real-time PCR with melting curve analysis, by allele-specific PCR, and by other techniques (see Chapter 5). DNA sequencing can be used for confirmation of the base change (Figure 13-16, panel B).

MINIMAL RESIDUAL DISEASE DETECTION AND MONITORING

Molecular techniques can detect small numbers of neoplastic cells that have characteristic genetic aberrations or the unique antigen-receptor gene rearrangement of a patient's lymphoid neoplasia. Detecting these cells can be useful clinically to

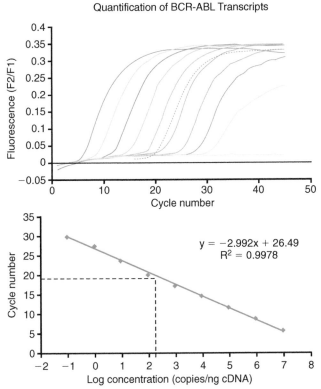

Quantification of BCR-ABL Transcripts

$$y = -2.992x + 26.49$$
$$R^2 = 0.9978$$

Figure 13-15

Real-time quantitative PCR of *BCR-ABL* transcripts with serial log dilutions of the plasmids containing the *BCR-ABL* sequence. Real-time PCR provides a remarkable dynamic range of quantification (10^9 to 10^0 template copies) in this example. The upper panel shows the amplification curves obtained using the *BCR–ABL*-containing plasmids and an unknown patient sample depicted as a dotted line. Note the regular ~3.3-cycle interval between log dilutions. The lower panel shows a calibration curve (linear regression of cycle number versus log template concentration). As indicated by the dotted line in the lower panel, the threshold cycle (Chapter 5) can be used to quantify the number of copies of the target sequence in the tested sample (see Color Plate 11).

detect MRD and to monitor therapy. Molecular techniques can detect one aberrant cell in a background of 10^3 to 10^6 normal cells and thus are superior to clinical or microscopic examination.

PCR-based methods have enjoyed the greatest utility for the detection of small numbers of cells with clonal antigen-receptor rearrangements and recurrent chromosomal translocations. Monitoring of MRD by use of antigen-receptor gene rearrangements requires previous identification of the specific gene rearrangement in the patient's tumor.

In patients with acute lymphoblastic leukemia or lymphoma, persistence of detectable cells with clonal rearrangements of the antigen-receptor genes at the end of induction therapy predicts a high likelihood of relapse. Moreover, persistent positivity for such cells in successive analyses is a strong predictor of future clinical relapse, and persistent negativity is indicative of a durable remission.

The implications of qualitative detection of cells with translocations vary with the translocation detected. For instance,

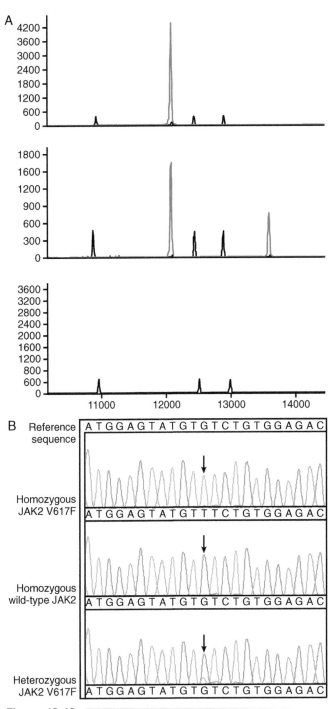

Figure 13-16

A, Detection of internal tandem duplications of the *FLT3* gene[15] by PCR and capillary gel electrophoresis of PCR products. Capillary electropherograms show clear resolution of PCR products. The *x*-axis represents the sizes of PCR products and the *y*-axis shows the fluorescence intensity, which correlates with the abundance of the PCR product. The upper panel shows a wild-type pattern (blue peak) and size markers (*black peaks*). The middle panel shows an additional peak of greater size (*blue peak on the right*) than the wild-type peak. This additional peak represents an *FLT3* internal tandem duplication. The lower panel shows the size markers (*black peaks*) also present in the upper and middle panels. **B,** Sequencing electropherogram showing the nucleotide substitution seen in PV (see Color Plate 12).

there is a very high risk of relapse associated with the detection of residual *PML-RARα* transcripts after therapy, but the t(8;21) *AML1-ETO* fusion may be detected in patients who have sustained remissions. The detection of the t(9;22) *BCR-ABL* fusion transcript strongly suggests relapse if conversion from negative to positive occurs within 6 to 12 months of treatment, whereas persistent molecular negativity for the transcript suggests a good response to therapy. In Ph-positive ALL, blood and marrow contain similar *BCR-ABL* transcript numbers, but some samples are discordant.[22] Marrow has been proposed as the preferred specimen type for residual disease studies.[22] Complicating the interpretation of results are reports that some fusion transcripts can be found in the peripheral blood of healthy individuals or in reactive lymphoid tissues without signs of malignancy.

Figure 13-15 shows a quantitative RT-PCR study for the *BCR-ABL* transcript that incorporated several calibrators.

MOLECULAR GENETICS OF SOLID TUMORS

The term *solid tumor* is generally used to describe nonhematopoietic tumors and includes the carcinomas (epithelial-derived cancers), and sarcomas (malignant tumors of connective tissue or tissues of mesenchymal origin). In comparison with the hematopoietic malignancies, fewer nonrandom chromosomal translocations have been described in association with carcinomas. By comparison, an increasing number of soft tissue sarcomas are associated with nonrandom chromosomal translocations. The solid tumors carrying recurrent chromosomal translocations include several that occur in the pediatric age group and the primitive neuroectodermal tumors (PNET). A brief discussion of the most characteristic molecular genetic abnormalities in a few well-characterized tumor entities is provided below. A table in Chapter 14 (Table 14-10) lists the common chromosomal translocations associated with soft tissue tumors. Determination of the unique fusion genes in a patient's tumor has become increasingly important for clinical management of tumors such as alveolar rhabdomyosarcoma, Ewing sarcoma/PNET, and synovial sarcoma.[17]

Rhabdomyosarcoma

Rhabdomyosarcoma is a malignant tumor with skeletal muscle differentiation. Rhabdomyosarcoma is the most common form of sarcoma occurring in pediatric patients and accounts for approximately 50% of cases. A number of distinct morphological subtypes with different behavior and prognostic significance are recognized. The alveolar and embryonal subtypes are most common. The sometimes difficult morphological distinction between the two subtypes has been facilitated by the presence of recurrent chromosomal translocations that are characteristic of alveolar rhabdomyosarcomas and distinguish them from the embryonal rhabdomyosarcoma. The distinction is important because alveolar rhabdomyosarcoma has an unfavorable prognosis, whereas embryonal rhabdomyosarcoma exhibits a more favorable prognosis. The two are distinguished by the finding of characteristic chromosomal rearrangements in the more aggressive alveolar form.

Alveolar Rhabdomyosarcoma

Alveolar rhabdomyosarcoma is molecularly characterized by a translocation that is detectable in approximately 75% of cases.[2]

The translocation leads to the juxtaposition of the *PAX3* gene on chromosome 2 (2q35) to the *FOXO1A* gene (forkhead box O1A [rhabdomyosarcoma]; previous symbol *FKHR*) on band 13q14, resulting in the formation of a chimeric fusion protein with aberrant transcription factor activity. Another translocation involving the *PAX7* gene on chromosome 1 (1p36) results in the formation of the chimeric *PAX7-FOXO1A* gene in the t(1;13)(p36;q14) and is observed in approximately 10% of cases. The PAX family of genes encodes transcription factors with paired homeobox domains. The PAX proteins are essential for normal embryonic development. The *PAX3* and *PAX7* genes demonstrate substantial sequence homology. They are both expressed in developing myotomes (embryological precursors of muscles), suggesting a mechanistic basis for the genetic deregulation of the genes that is thought to play a role in the pathogenesis of rhabdomyosarcoma. The forkhead box genes also encode transcription factors with important functions in embryogenesis.

Translocation fusions can be detected by a variety of molecular and cytogenetic techniques, such as RT-PCR[2] and FISH.

Embryonal Rhabdomyosarcoma

Unlike alveolar rhabdomyosarcoma, embryonal rhabdomyosarcoma does not exhibit characteristic nonrandom chromosomal translocations.

Primitive Neuroectodermal Tumor and Ewing Sarcoma

Primitive neuroectodermal tumor (PNET) refers to a group of tumors characterized histologically by a proliferation of "small round blue" cells that putatively represent an immature precursor cell of neuroectodermal origin. PNET is pathogenetically related to Ewing sarcoma, which is a malignant tumor of bone. The pathogenetic relatedness of the two tumors is supported by the fact that both are molecularly characterized by chromosomal translocations involving the Ewing sarcoma locus (often called EWS) at chromosome band 22q12. A common translocation is found in approximately 90% of cases of PNET and Ewing sarcoma and leads to the juxtaposition of the *EWSR1* gene at 22q12 to the *FLI1* gene at 11q24. This leads to the formation of a chimeric fusion protein EWS-FLI.[11] Deregulation of *FLI1* has been implicated in the pathogenesis of multiple neoplasias.

t(11;22) can be routinely detected by FISH in the diagnostic laboratory. Alternatively the EWS-FLI1 fusion can be detected by RT-PCR, but because of several different transcripts resulting from multiple breakpoints, RT-PCR detection may detect EWS-FLI-1 products of varying sizes. The EWS locus also partners with several other genes in many other chromosomal translocations that are found in PNET and Ewing sarcoma (listed in Chapter 14 for reference), and these may be detected by use of FISH or by analyses that use RT-PCR

In addition to the multiple translocation partners that are seen in PNET and Ewing's sarcoma, EWS is fused to several other genes in other soft tissue tumors. An example of these is fusion to the *ATF1* gene (activating transcription factor 1) in clear cell sarcoma.

Desmoplastic Small Round-Cell Tumor

Desmoplastic small round-cell tumor (DSCT) is another example of a small round blue cell tumor that has characteristic molecular genetic features that aid in its diagnosis. DSCT is characterized by t(11;22)(p13;q12). In this translocation, the Ewing sarcoma gene (EWSR1) on 22q12 is fused with the Wilm tumor-suppressor gene (WT1) on 11p13. The WT1 gene is normally expressed in developing kidney tissues, and its fusion with the EWSR1 gene generates a transcriptionally active chimeric protein that is involved in the pathogenesis of DSCT. As with the other EWSR1-fusion genes described earlier, the EWSR1-WT1 can be detected by FISH or RT-PCR to facilitate diagnosis.

Synovial Sarcoma

Synovial sarcoma is another rare soft tissue neoplasm with characteristic nonrandom chromosomal translocations. Synovial sarcoma is most frequently diagnosed in adolescents and younger adults. It is characterized by t(X;18)(p11;q11), which is detected in up to 95% of cases. The translocation can be detected by FISH and its resulting chimeric fusions by RT-PCR in the molecular diagnostic laboratory.

AC   Two histological subtypes of synovial sarcoma are recognized; monophasic and biphasic. The monophasic synovial sarcoma is composed exclusively of spindle-shaped tumor cells with mesenchymal morphology. The biphasic type displays both epithelial elements and mesenchymal elements. The t(X;18)(p11;q11) translocation most frequently leads to the fusion of the SS18 gene (18q11) to the SSX1 gene (Xp11). In other cases, the SS18 gene is fused to the SSX2 gene (Xp11.23-p11.22). Interestingly, synovial sarcomas with the SS18-SSX1 fusion exhibit a biphasic histology, whereas those with the SS18-SSX2 show a monophasic histology. The SS18-SSX fusion has been shown to be essential for the transformation of fibroblasts in culture, and it enhances cyclin D1 expression in synovial sarcoma cells.

Inflammatory Myofibroblastic Tumor

Inflammatory myofibroblastic tumor (IMT) is a rare soft tissue neoplasm putatively of indeterminate or low malignant potential that occurs predominantly in children and young adults. About 50% to 60% of tumors carrying a histological diagnosis of IMT show the presence of recurrent chromosomal translocations involving the anaplastic lymphoma kinase (ALK) gene on 2p23. Translocations involving the ALK gene[16] are readily detected by FISH and RT-PCR and are useful in the confirmation of a diagnosis of IMT.

AC   The most common translocation identified in IMT is t(1;2)(q22-23;p23) that fuses the nonmuscle tropomyosin gene 3 (TPM3) on 1q22-23 to the ALK gene on 2p23. The ALK gene product is a receptor tyrosine kinase, which is expressed preferentially in cells of neural derivation. Aberrant expression of the chimeric

ALK fusion leads to its constitutive activation and triggers diverse signaling events that underlie its role in oncogenesis.

As with the EWS (EWSR1) gene in PNET and Ewing's sarcoma, the ALK gene is fused to several different partners (see Table 14-10 in Chapter 14 for reference) in IMTs. Rearrangements involving the ALK gene are also characteristic of a subset of a type of non-Hodgkin's lymphoma known as anaplastic large cell lymphoma (ALCL). ALCL occurs in both the pediatric and adult age groups and is classified as a specific subtype of peripheral (postthymic) T-cell lymphoma. The most frequent translocation in ALCL is t(2;5)(p23;q35) and results in the chimeric fusion of the gene (NPM1) for nucleophosmin, a ubiquitously expressed nucleolar shuttling protein, to ALK. In addition to identification of the characteristic translocation in the molecular laboratory, immunohistochemical studies using an anti-ALK antibody reveal strong nuclear and cytoplasmic reactivity for ALK in cases of ALCL carrying the NPM1-ALK fusion. By contrast, the TPM3-ALK fusion protein found in both ALCL and IMT exhibits an exclusively cytoplasmic distribution. Indeed, all other non–NPM-ALK fusion proteins display a nonnuclear distribution.

Chromosomal Translocations in Prostatic Carcinoma

Prostatic carcinoma is a common cause of cancer morbidity and mortality in men. An estimated 200,000 men in the United States were diagnosed with prostate cancer in the year 2005, and more than 30,000 men succumbed to the disease, making it the second most common cause of cancer-related mortality in men. Recently, chromosomal translocations involving the ETS transcription factors ERG and ETV1 have been identified in up to 75% of prostate cancers.[20] An additional 2% of cases show translocations involving TMPRSS2 (21q22, transmembrane protease, serine 2) and ETV4 (17q21, ets variant gene 4; E1A enhancer binding protein, E1AF). This finding is important because of the relative paucity of recurrent chromosomal translocations in common epithelial malignancies. Translocations involving TMPRSS2 can be reliably detected using FISH and may be useful as an adjunct tool in the diagnosis of prostate cancer.

DETECTION OF VIRUSES INVOLVED IN THE PATHOGENESIS OF HUMAN CANCERS

Viruses thought to be involved in the pathogenesis of abnormal proliferations of hematopoietic cells include the human T-cell leukemia virus type I found in adult T-cell leukemia and lymphoma and Kaposi-sarcoma herpesvirus/human herpesvirus-8 (KSHV/HHV8) seen in primary effusion lymphoma and multicentric Castleman disease. In epithelial cancer, the human papillomavirus (HPV) is highly implicated in the pathogenesis of cervical carcinoma. Viral hepatitis is a precursor of liver cancer. All of these viruses can be detected using standard molecular biology techniques (Chapter 5; see also specific viruses, especially HPV, in Chapter 11).

The Epstein-Barr virus (EBV) is associated with nasopharyngeal carcinoma, although its role in the etiology of the cancer is less clear. EBV was identified in 1964 by Epstein, Achong, and Barr[6] in cultured cells obtained from a malignant lymphoma described by Denis Burkitt. EBV was subsequently identified by Werner Henle and colleagues[8] as the cause of infectious mononucleosis. EBV is a lymphotropic virus and has been associated with several conditions, including Burkitt lymphoma and posttransplant lymphoproliferative disorders. Figure 13-17 shows EBV signals seen by in situ hybridization in tissue from a case of posttransplant lymphoproliferative disease.

CONCLUSIONS AND ETHICAL CONSIDERATIONS

Human cancers are often associated with distinctive genetic aberrations that can be detected by the techniques used in the molecular diagnostics laboratory. In many cases, the identification of the molecular abnormality not only is useful for diagnosis but also carries important prognostic information and has implications for choice of treatment. The methodology chosen depends on the nature of the aberration being evaluated, the nature of the available samples, and the level of sensitivity afforded by the available methodologies. Technical issues aside, the clinical significance of each test has to be determined on an individualized basis. Most importantly, molecular tests should be used as adjunctive parameters in the evaluation of the patient and should never be used in isolation without consideration of clinical findings. Ideally the management of a patient incorporates the entire complement of clinical and diagnostic information pertinent to the individual and his or her disorder. In the setting of limited healthcare funding, molecular testing should be used only when it provides additional useful information and not when the diagnosis is clear.

Finally, the identification of germline genetic alterations that have strong associations with cancer raises important issues for society, some of which are raised for discussion in

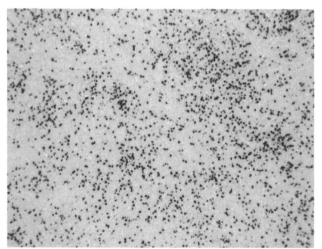

Figure 13-17
In situ hybridization (ISH) for the EBV. Numerous positive signals (*dark spots*) for EBV are visualized after hybridization of tissue with a fluorescently labeled DNA probe that is complementary to a region (EBER-1) of the EBV genome. The tissue sample was obtained from a solid-organ transplant patient who developed widespread nodal and extranodal masses. The positive reaction for EBV in this assay supports a diagnosis of posttransplant lymphoproliferative disease (see Color Plate 13).

ETHICS Box 13-1   Ethical Issues Associated With Breast Cancer–Related Genes *BRCA1* and *BRCA2*

It is now possible to estimate the likelihood that an individual who carries a mutation in *BRCA1*[13] or *BRCA2*[25] will develop breast and/or ovarian cancer. Should tests for these mutations be used only in families with a pattern of breast and/or ovarian cancer? (Many if not most breast cancer patients who have such mutations do not have strong family histories of the malignancy.) What should be done if an otherwise healthy individual is shown to carry a *BRCA* gene mutation? Carriers of a *BRCA1* gene mutation have an 85% risk of developing breast cancer and a 45% risk of developing ovarian cancer by the age of 85.[7] Should such patients have preventive surgeries, such as removal of the breasts (mastectomy) or ovaries (oophorectomy) or both? Should insurance companies and healthcare maintenance organizations be allowed to charge higher rates for carriers of *BRCA* mutations or even deny coverage completely? Is a daughter entitled to know the results of the test in her mother?

Identification of cancer risk has long been a goal of research. Now that it is possible, policies are needed on how best to use the tests and how to deal with the information.

Ethics Box 13-1. There is strong reason to argue that people with mutations in genes associated with cancer should not be segregated into higher premium categories for health insurance.

REFERENCES

1. Albinger-Hegyi A, Hochreutener B, Abdou MT, Hegyi I, Dours-Zimmermann MT, Kurrer MO, et al. High frequency of t(14;18)-translocation breakpoints outside of major breakpoint and minor cluster regions in follicular lymphomas: improved polymerase chain reaction protocols for their detection. Am J Pathol 2002;160:823-32.
2. Barr FG, Chatten J, D'Cruz CM, Wilson AE, Nauta LE, Nycum LM, et al. Molecular assays for chromosomal translocations in the diagnosis of pediatric soft tissue sarcomas. JAMA 1995;273:553-7.
3. Bos JL. ras oncogenes in human cancer: a review. Cancer Res 1989;49:4682-9.
4. de Klein A, van Kessel AG, Grosveld G, Bartram CR, Hagemeijer A, Bootsma D, et al. A cellular oncogene is translocated to the Philadelphia chromosome in chronic myelocytic leukaemia. Nature 1982;300:765-7.
5. Druker BJ, Talpaz M, Resta DJ, Peng B, Buchdunger E, Ford JM, et al. Efficacy and safety of a specific inhibitor of the BCR-ABL tyrosine kinase in chronic myeloid leukemia. N Engl J Med 2001;344:1031-7.
6. Epstein MA, Achong BG, Barr YM. Virus particles in cultured lymphoblasts from Burkitt lymphoma. Lancet 1964;1:702-3.
7. Ford D, Easton DF, Bishop DT, Narod SA, Goldgar DE. Risks of cancer in BRCA1-mutation carriers. Breast Cancer Linkage Consortium. Lancet 1994;343:692-5.
8. Henle G, Henle W, Diehl V. Relation of Burkitt tumor-associated herpes-type virus to infectious mononucleosis. Proc Natl Acad Sci U S A 1968;59:94-101.
9. James C, Ugo V, Casadevall N, Constantinescu SN, Vainchenker W. A JAK2 mutation in myeloproliferative disorders: pathogenesis and therapeutic and scientific prospects. Trends Mol Med 2005;11:546-54.
10. Kreuzer KA, Lass U, Bohn A, Landt O, Schmidt CA. LightCycler technology for the quantitation of bcr/abl fusion transcripts. Cancer Res 1999;59:3171-4.
11. Ladanyi M. EWS-FLI1 and Ewing's sarcoma: recent molecular data and new insights. Cancer Biol Ther 2002;1:330-6.
12. Medeiros LJ, Carr J. Overview of the role of molecular methods in the diagnosis of malignant lymphomas. Arch Pathol Lab Med 1999;123:1189-207.
13. Miki Y, Swensen J, Shattuck-Eidens D, Futreal PA, Harsham K, Tavtigian S, et al. A strong candidate for the breast and ovarian cancer susceptibility gene BRCA1. Science 1994;266:66-71.

14. Mitterbauer M, Kusec R, Schwarzinger I, Haas OA, Lechner K, Jaeger U. Comparison of karyotype analysis and RT-PCR for AML1/ETO in 204 unselected patients with AML. Ann Hematol 1998;76:139-43.
15. Nakao M, Yokota S, Iwai T, Kaneko H, Horiike S, Kashima K, et al. Internal tandem duplication of the flt3 gene found in acute myeloid leukemia. Leukemia 1996;10:1911-8.
16. Pulford K, Morris SW, Turturro F. Anaplastic lymphoma kinase proteins in growth control and cancer. J Cell Physiol 2004;199:330-58.
17. Qualman SJ, Morotti RA. Risk assignment in pediatric soft-tissue sarcomas: an evolving molecular classification. Curr Oncol Rep 2002:4:123-30.
18. Selleri L, von Lindern M, Hermans A, Meijer D, Torelli G, Grosveld G. Chronic myeloid leukemia may be associated with several bcr-abl transcripts including the acute lymphoid leukemia-type 7 kb transcript. Blood 1990;75:1146-53.
19. Sioutos N, Bagg A, Michaud GY, Irving SG, Hartmann DP, Siragy H, et al. Polymerase chain reaction versus Southern blot hybridization. Detection of immunoglobulin heavy-chain gene rearrangements. Diagn Mol Pathol 1995;4:8-13.
20. Tomlins SA, Rhodes DR, Perner S, Dhanasekaran SM, Mehra R, Sun XW, et al. Recurrent fusion of TMPRSS2 and ETS transcription factor genes in prostate cancer. Science 2005;310:644-8.
21. Tsujimoto Y, Gorham J, Cossman J, Jaffe E, Croce CM. The t(14;18) chromosome translocations involved in B-cell neoplasms result from mistakes in VDJ joining. Science 1985;229:1390-3.
22. van Rhee F, Marks DI, Lin F, Szydlo RM, Hochhaus A, Treleaven J, et al. Quantification of residual disease in Philadelphia-positive acute lymphoblastic leukemia: comparison of blood and bone marrow. Leukemia 1995;9:329-35.
23. Weinberg RA. The molecular basis of oncogenes and tumor suppressor genes. Ann N Y Acad Sci 1995;758:331-8.
24. Wittwer CT, Hermann MG, Moss AA, Rasmussen PP. Continuous fluorescence monitoring of rapid cycle DNA amplification. Biotechniques 1997;22:130-1, 4-8.
25. Wooster R, Neuhausen SL, Mangion J, Quirk Y, Ford D, Collins N, et al. Localization of a breast cancer susceptibility gene, BRCA2, to chromosome 13q12-13. Science 1994;265:2088-90.

REVIEW QUESTIONS

1. Cancer may result from
   A. deregulation of oncogenes.
   B. inactivation of tumor-suppressor genes.
   C. deregulation of genes involved in regulation of programmed cell death.
   D. all of the above.
   E. none of the above.

2. Malignant tumors arising in tissues of epithelial origin are known as
   A. sarcomas.
   B. odontomas.
   C. teratomas.
   D. ependymomas.
   E. carcinomas.

3. Immunoglobulin gene rearrangements are characteristic of
   A. CD4+ T cells.
   B. NK cells.
   C. mast cells.
   D. neutrophils.
   E. B cells.

4. All of the following are tumor-suppressor genes EXCEPT
   A. p53.
   B. Rb.
   C. p16/INK4A/CDKN2.
   D. k-ras.
   E. menin.

5. Follicular lymphoma is:
   A. a normal condition.
   B. an inflammatory condition.
   C. a form of lymphoid cancer.
   D. a tumor arising from epithelial cells.
   E. not malignant at all.

6. Clonal antigen receptor gene rearrangements:
   A. are characteristic of malignant lymphomas.
   B. can be detected by PCR.
   C. can be detected by Southern blot hybridization analysis.
   D. all of the above
   E. none of the above

7. Synovial sarcoma:
   A. is a rare soft tissue neoplasm.
   B. has characteristic translocations.
   C. is characterized by the t(X;18) aberration.
   D. has characteristic fusions that can be detected by RT-PCR.
   E. all of the above

8. Southern blot hybridization analysis
   A. involves analysis of RNA.
   B. is diagnostically useful in the identification of clonal lymphoid populations.
   C. involves the analysis of proteins.
   D. routinely uses nucleic acid extracted from fixed-paraffin embedded material.
   E. requires quantitatively less DNA than does PCR.

9. Structural abnormalities affecting genes encoding proteins involved in which of the following processes are frequently identified in human cancers?
   A. Receptor tyrosine kinases
   B. Transcription factors
   C. Antiapoptotic proteins
   D. None of the above
   E. All of the above (a, b, and c)

10. The Epstein-Barr virus is
    A. a retrovirus.
    B. involved in the pathogenesis of acute T-cell leukemia and lymphoma.
    C. frequently identified by in situ hybridization in cervical carcinoma.
    D. frequently identified in the tumor cells of endemic Burkitt lymphoma.
    E. also known as the human herpeslike virus type 8.

SECTION IV

APPENDIX

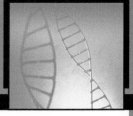

Chapter 14

Reference Information

Compiled by **David E. Bruns**, M.D.
Edward A. Ashwood, M.D.
Carl A. Burtis, Ph.D.

The reference information in this chapter was provided by the authors of the related chapters. The editors gratefully acknowledge the original contribution of the following works that were the sources for most of this material: Chapter 23, Tumor Markers, by Daniel W. Chan, Ronald A. Booth, and Eleftherios P. Diamandis; Chapter 39, Molecular Genetics and Diagnosis of Hematologic Malignancies, by Kojo S.J. Elenitoba-Johnson; Chapter 40, Inherited Disorders, by Cindy Vnencak-Jones; and Chapter 43, Pharmacogenetics, by Gwendolyn McMillin, all in Burtis CA, Ashwood ER, Bruns DE, editors: *Tietz Textbook of Clincal Chemistry and Molecular Diagnostics*, ed 4, St Louis, 2006, Saunders.

CONTENTS

TABLE 14-1	ACMG/ACOG Mutation Panel for Preconception and Prenatal CF Carrier Screening With Frequency of Each Mutation in Non-Hispanic CF Caucasian Alleles*		
Mutation	**Frequency (%)**	**Mutation**	**Frequency (%)**
ΔF508	72.42	7111G>T	0.43
G542X	2.28	R560T	0.38
G551D	2.25	3659delC	0.34
6211G>T	*1.57	A455E	0.34
W1282X	1.50	G85E	0.29
N1303K	1.27	R1162X	0.23
△I507	0.88	2184delA	0.17
R553X	0.87	18981G>A	0.16
R117H	0.70	R334W	0.14
384910kbC>T	0.58	I148T	0.09
27895G>A	0.48	31201G>A	0.08
1717–1G>A	0.48	1078delT	0.02
R347P	0.45	TOTAL	88.40

*ACMG, American College of Human Genetics; ACOG, American College of Obstetrics and Gynecology; panel as reported in Watson et al. Cystic fibrosis population carrier screening: 2004 revision of American College of Medical Genetics mutation panel. Genet Med 2004 Sep-Oct;6(5):387-91. Erratum in: Genet Med 2004 Nov-Dec;6(6):548. Genet Med 2005 Apr;7(4):286.

TABLE 14-2	FDA-Approved Molecular Tests for Bacterial Infections		
Test	**Manufacturer**	**Test Name**	**Method**
Chlamydia trachomatis detection (single organism)	Digene Corporation	HC2® CT ID	Hybrid Capture
	Gen-Probe, Inc.	APTIMA CT® Assay	TC, TMA, DKA
	Gen-Probe, Inc.	PACE® 2 CT	HPA
	Roche Molecular Diagnostics	COBAS AMPLICOR™ CT/NG Test	PCR
	Roche Molecular Diagnostics	COBAS AMPLICOR™ CT/NG Test	PCR
Neisseria gonorrhoeae detection (single organism)	Digene Corporation	HC2® GC ID	Hybrid Capture
	Gen-Probe, Inc.	APTIMA GC® Assay	TC, TMA, DKA
	Gen-Probe, Inc.	PACE® 2 GC Probe Competition Assay	HPA
	Roche Molecular Diagnostics	COBAS AMPLICOR™ CT/NG Test	PCR
	Roche Molecular Diagnostics	COBAS AMPLICOR™ CT/NG Test	PCR
Chlamydia trachomatis and Neisseria gonorrhoeae detection	Becton, Dickinson & Company	BD ProbeTec™ ET DNA Assay	SDA
	Digene Corporation	HC2® CT/GC Combo Test	Hybrid Capture
	Gen-Probe, Inc.	APTIMA Combo 2Ò Assay	TC, TMA, DKA
	Gen-Probe, Inc.	PACE® 2C CT/GC	HPA
	Roche Molecular Diagnostics	COBAS AMPLICOR™ CT/NG Test	PCR
	Roche Molecular Diagnostics	COBAS AMPLICOR™ CT/NG Test	PCR
Gardnerella, Trichomonas vaginalis, and Candida spp. detection	Becton, Dickinson & Company	BD Affirm™ VPIII Microbial Identification Test	Hybridization
Group A streptococci detection	Gen-Probe, Inc.	Group A Strep direct (GASD)	HPA
Group B streptococci detection	Gen-Probe, Inc.	Group B AccuProbe®	HPA
	GeneOhm Sciences, Inc.	IDI-Strep B™ Assay	Real Time PCR
	Cepheid	Xpert GBS	RT-PCR
Legionella pneumophila detection	Becton, Dickinson & Company	BD ProbeTec™ ET DNA Assay	SDA
MRSA for Staphylococcus aureus	GeneOhm Sciences, Inc.	IDI-MRSA™ Assay	Real Time PCR
Mycobacterium tuberculosis detection	Gen-Probe, Inc.	AMPLIFIED™ Direct Test (MTD)	TMA
	Roche Molecular Diagnostics	AMPLICOR™ M. tuberculosis Test	PCR
Mycobacteria spp., different fungi and bacteria culture confirmation	Gen-Probe, Inc.	AccuProbe® Culture Identification Tests	HPA

ASPE, Allele specific primer extension; bDNA, branched chain DNA signal amplification; DKA, dual kinetic assay; HPA, hybridization protection assay; NASBA, nucleic acid sequence based amplification; PCR, polymerase chain reaction; QC, quality control; RT-PCR, reverse-transcriptase PCR; SDA, strand displacement amplification; TC, target capture; TMA, transcription mediated amplification.

TABLE 14-3 **FDA-Approved Molecular Tests for Viral Infections**

Test	Manufacturer	Test Name	Method
Cytomegalovirus detection	Digene Corporation	HC1® CMV DNA Test	Hybrid Capture
	bioMerieux, Inc.	CMV pp67 mRNA	NASBA
HCV qualitative detection	Gen-Probe, Inc.	VERSANT® HCV RNA	TMA
	Roche Molecular Diagnostics	AMPLICOR™ HCV Test, version 2.0	PCR
	Roche Molecular Diagnostics	COBAS AMPLICOR™ HCV Test, version 2.0	PCR
HCV quantitation	Bayer HealthCare	VERSANT® HCV RNA 3.0 Assay	bDNA
HIV drug resistance testing	Celera Diagnostics	ViroSeq™ HIV-1 Genotyping System	Sequencing
	Bayer HealthCare	TruGene™ HIV-1 Genotyping and Open Gene DNA Sequencing System	Sequencing
HIV quantitation	Bayer HealthCare	VERSANT® HIV-1 RNA 3.0 Assay	bDNA
	bioMerieux, Inc.	NucliSens®HIV-1 QT	NASBA
	Roche Molecular Diagnostics	AMPLICOR HIV-1 MONITOR™	RT-PCR
HIV qualitative	Gen-Probe, Inc.	APTIMA HIV-1 Test, version 1.5	TMA
	Roche Molecular Diagnostics	COBAS AMPLICOR HIV-1 MONITOR™ Test, version 1.5	RT-PCR
HBV/HCV/HIV for blood donations	Gen-Probe, Inc.	Procleix™ HIV-1/HCV Assay	TMA
	Gen-Probe, Inc.	Chiron Procleix™ HIV-1/HCV Controls	QC controls
	Gen-Probe, Inc.	Chiron Procleix™ HIV/HCV Proficiency Panel	QC proficiency panel
	National Genetics Institute	UltraQual™ HCV RT-PCR Assay	RT-PCR
	National Genetics Institute	UltraQual™ HIV-1 RT-PCR Assay	RT-PCR
	Roche Molecular Diagnostics	COBAS AmpliScreen™ HBV Test	PCR
	Roche Molecular Diagnostics	COBAS AmpliScreen™ HCVTest, version 2.0	RT-PCR
	Roche Molecular Diagnostics	COBAS AmpliScreen™ HIV-1Test, version 1.5	RT-PCR
Human papillomavirus testing	Digene Corporation	HC2® HR and LR	Hybrid Capture
	Digene Corporation	HC2®HPV HR	Hybrid Capture
	Digene Corporation	HC2® DNA with Pap	Hybrid Capture

ASPE, Allele specific primer extension; bDNA, branched chain DNA signal amplification; DKA, dual kinetic assay; HPA, hybridization protection assay; NASBA, nucleic acid sequence based amplification; PCR, polymerase chain reaction; QC, quality control; RT-PCR, reverse-transcriptase PCR; SDA, strand displacement amplification; TC, target capture; TMA, transcription mediated amplification.

TABLE 14-4 **NAT Substrates**

Drugs	Potential Carcinogens or Toxicants
Aminoglutethimide	p-aminobenzoic acid (PABA)*
Amonafide	4-aminobiphenyl
Amrinone	2-aminodipyrido[1,2-a:3'2'd]-imidazole (Glu-P-2)
Caffeine	2-aminofluorene*
Clonazepam	2-amino-3,8-dimethylimidazo [4,5-f] quinoxaline (MeIQx)[†]
Dapsone	2-amino-3-methyl-imidazo [4,5-f] quinoline (IQ)[†]
Dipyrone	3-amino-1-methyl-5H-pyrido [4,3-b]indole (Trp-P-2)
Endralazine	p-aminosalicylic acid (PAS)*
Hydralazine	Benzidine
Isoniazid	3,4-dichloroaniline
Prizidilol	3,2'-dimethyl-4-aminobiphenyl
Prizidilol	B-naphthylamine
Procainamide[†]	p-phenetidine
Sulfonamides:[†]	
Sulfadiazine	o-toluidine[†]
Sulfadoxine	p-toluidine
Sulfamethazine	
Sulfamethoxazole	
Sulfapyridine	
Sulfasalazine	

Modified from Grant DM, Blum M, Beer M, Meyer UA. Monomorphic and polymorphic human arylamine N-acetyltransferases: a comparison of liver isozymes and expressed products of two cloned genes. Mol Pharmacol 1991;39:184-91; Grant DM, Goodfellow GH, Sugamori KS, Durette K. Pharmacogenetics of the human arylamine N-acetyltransferases. Pharmacol 2000;61:204-11; Hein DW, Doll MA, Rustan TD, Gray K, Feng Y, Ferguson RJ, et al. Metabolic activation and deactivation of arylamine carcinogens by recombinant human NAT1 and polymorphic NAT2 acetyltransferases. Carcinogenesis 1993;14:1633-8.
*Strong selectivity for NAT1 based on NAT1/NAT2 activity (nmol/min/U) ratio >300.
[†]Similar selectivity for NAT1 and NAT2 based on NAT1/NAT2 activity ratio <15.

TABLE 14-5	Common NAT1 and NAT2 Alleles Associated With a Slow Acetylator Phenotype				
Allele	**Nucleotide**	**Changes**			**Amino Acid Changes**
*NAT1*10*	1088T>A	1095C>A			None
*NAT2*5A*	341T>C	481C>T			I114T
*NAT2*5B*	341T>C	481C>T	803A>G		I114T, K268R
*NAT2*5C*	341T>C	803A>G			I114T, K268R
*NAT2*5D*	341T>C				I114T
*NAT2*5E*	341T>C	590G>A			I114T, R197Q
*NAT2*5F*	341T>C	481C>T	759C>A	803A>G	I114T, K268R
*NAT2*5G*	282C>T	341T>C	481C>T	803A>G	I114T, K268R
*NAT2*5H*	341T>C	481C>T	803A>G	859T>C	I114T, K268R, I287T
*NAT2*5I*	341T>C	411A>T	481C>T	803A>G	I114T, L137F, K268R
*NAT2*5J*	282C>T	341T>C	590G>A		I114T, R197Q
*NAT2*6A*	282C>T	590G>A	R197Q		
*NAT2*6B*	590G>A	R197Q			
*NAT2*6C*	282C>T	590G>A	803A>G		R197Q, K268R
*NAT2*6D*	111T>C	282C>T	590G>A		R197Q
*NAT2*6E*	481C>T	590G>A			R197Q
*NAT2*7A*	857G>A				G286E
*NAT2*7B*	282C>T	857G>A			G286E
*NAT2*14A*	191G>A				R64Q
*NAT2*14B*	191G>A	282C>T			R64Q
*NAT2*14C*	191G>A	341T>C	481C>T	803A>G	R64W, I114T, K268R
*NAT2*14D*	191G>A	282C>T	590G>A		R64Q, R197Q
*NAT2*14E*	191G>A	803A>G			R64W, K268R
*NAT2*14F*	191G>A	341T>C	803A>G		R64W, I114T, K268R
*NAT2*14G*	191G>A	282C>T	803A>G		R64W, K268R

TABLE 14-6	Additional Pharmacogenetic Targets	
Polymorphic Gene(s)	**Protein(s)**	**Drugs or Drug Classes Possibly Affected by Variants**
ACE	Angiotensin converting enzyme	ACE inhibitors
ABCB1	MDR1, p-glycoprotein	Immunosuppressants, antiretrovirals, anticonvulsants, cardiac glycosides
ADD1	Adducin 1 (α)	Diuretics
ADRB1 and 2	β-Adrenergic receptor	β-Agonists, β-blockers
AGT and AGTR1	Angiotensinogen and receptor	Antihypertensives
ALOX5	Arachidonate 5-lipoxygenase	Leukotriene receptors, 5-lipoxygenase inhibitors
APOE	Apolipoprotein E	Statins, acetylcholinesterase inhibitors (Alzheimer's therapeutics)
BCHE	Butyrylcholinesterase	Succinylcholine
BDKRB2	Bradykinin receptor B2	ACE inhibitors
CETP	Cholesteryl ester transfer protein	Statins
COMT	Catechol O-methyltransferase	Antipsychotics
CYP1A2, 2B6, 1E, 3A	Cytochrome P450 drug metabolizing enzymes	Several; <50% of all therapeutic drugs
DRD2, 3, and 4	Dopamine receptor	Antipsychotics
ERα	Estrogen receptor α	Hormone replacement therapy
FCGR3A	FcγRIIIa receptor	Rituximab
GNB3	Guanine nucleotide binding protein	Antipsychotics, antidepressants
GRIN2B	Glutamate receptor	Antipsychotics
HERG, KvLQT1, Mink, MiRP1	Ion channels involved in congenital long-QT syndrome	Antibiotics, quinidine
HLA-B	Major histocompatibility complex class I-B	Antiretrovirals
HTR2A	Serotonin (5-HTT) receptor	Antipsychotics, antidepressants
IL10	Interleukin 10	Prednisone and antivirals
LIPC	Hepatic lipase	Statins
SLC6A3	Dopamine transporter	Antipsychotics, antidepressants
SLC6A4	Serotonin transporter	Antipsychotics, antidepressants
TNF	Tissue necrosis factor	Immunosuppressants, carbamazepine
TPH1	Tryptophan hydroxylase 1	Antidepressants

Modified from Evans WE, McLeod HL. Pharmacogenomics—drug disposition, drug targets, and side effects. N Engl J Med 2003;348:538-49; Goldstein DB, Tate SK, Sisodiya SM. Pharmacogenetics goes genomic. Nat Rev Genet 2003;4:937-47.

BOX 14-1

Features of Selected Oncogenes

ras GENES

The *ras* genes were first identified as being responsible for the tumorigenic properties of the Harvey (H-*ras*) and Kirsten (K-*ras*) sarcoma viruses, which produce tumors in animals. Subsequent experiments with the human *ras* proto-oncogene provided the first evidence that alterations of normal human proto-oncogenes play a role in the development of human tumors. *Ras* mutations are among the most frequently identified aberrations in all of human cancer, but the presence of mutations in *ras* genes has little practical application in determination of prognosis.

The proteins encoded by the *ras* genes localize to the inner face of the plasma membrane. They bind to guanine nucleotides and function as molecular switches that regulate mitogenic signals from growth factors to the nucleus via signal transduction pathways. RAS proteins are activated in association with protein-tyrosine kinase receptors and are required for growth-factor proliferation or differentiation of a number of cell types.

The *NRAS* gene (for neuroblastoma ras) is a member of the ras family. It is found on the short arm of human chromosome 1. Changes in *NRAS* appear to be the critical step in carcinogenesis. The mutated *NRAS* gene is found in neuroblastomas and acute myeloid leukemia.

Mutated *KRAS* (the human counterpart of v-Ki-ras2 Kirsten rat sarcoma viral oncogene) is present in 95% of pancreatic cancers, 40% of colon cancer, 30% of lung and bladder cancers, and in lower percentages in other tumors. A single point mutation at the twelfth *KRAS* codon changes the coded amino acid from glycine to valine in the p21 protein. K-*ras* mutations appear to correlate with poor prognosis and shorter disease-free survival in patients with adenocarcinoma of the lung and endometrial carcinoma.

Activated *ras* is detected by expression of the gene product p21 in cancer tissue. By immunohistochemistry, p21 is found not only in about 40% of colon cancers, but also in colon polyps believed to be premalignant. The use of p21 as a tumor marker in tissue or serum is not well established. Mutations of *ras* oncogenes have been detected in the DNA in the stools of up to 60% of patients with curable colorectal tumors and thus have been considered as a target for screening for the presence of colon cancer.

c-myc GENE

The *MYC* gene (also called *c-Myc*) is the homolog of the v-myc oncogene of avian myelocytoma virus. The gene product p62 is a nuclear protein involved in transcriptional regulation, and levels of *MYC* correlate with the rate of cell division. Activation of the *MYC* is associated with B- and T-cell non-Hodgkin lymphomas, sarcomas, and endotheliomas. Genetic translocations and overexpression of *MYC* are studied by cytogenetics or immunohistochemistry.

In a specific subtype of acute lymphoblastic leukemias and Burkitt lymphomas, *MYC* (8q24) is involved in translocations with either the immunoglobulin heavy (14q32) or kappa light chain (2p12) or lambda chain (22q11) loci. In acute T-cell leukemias, there is an (8:14) (q24:q11) translocation that results in activation of the gene, and activation of the gene is associated with a poor prognosis. A decrease in expression of *MYC* after initiation of chemotherapy suggests a favorable response. Overexpression of p62 may be seen in 70% to 100% of primary breast cancers using immunohistochemistry, and the intensity of staining is greater with the increasing stage of the tumor. Amplification in lung carcinomas and gliomas correlates with increased clinical aggressiveness. There may be a fivefold to fortyfold higher expression of *MYC* in colon cancers when compared with normal mucosa, but the level of expression does not correlate with

progression. A similar relationship has been found for cervical, gastric, liver, and other cancers.

HER-2/neu

The HER-2/*neu* gene (also known as c-erbB-2, thus its symbol *ERBB2*) is named for its association with neural tumors (*neu*). The HER-2/*neu* gene encodes a 185-kDa transmembrane protein expressed on epithelial cells and belongs to the EGF family of tyrosine kinase receptors that is involved in cell proliferation, differentiation, and survival. The EGF family includes four members, the EGF receptor (*EGFR;* also known as ErbB1/HER-1), ErbB2/HER-2/*neu*, Erb3/HER-3, and ErbB4/HER-4. Members of the EGF family of receptors have similar protein structure. The extracellular portion of the protein can be split off (by metalloproteases), releasing a protein known as p105 into the blood where it can be detected. HER-2/*neu* protein is normally expressed on the epithelia of numerous organs, including lung, bladder, pancreas, breast, and prostate, and has been found to be elevated in cancer cells.

The HER-2/*neu* gene is amplified in breast, ovarian, and gastrointestinal tumors. Amplification of the gene in breast cancer tissue indicates a poor prognosis. Increased concentrations of HER-2/*neu* antigen in serum correlate with decreased response to hormone therapy of breast cancer. Because the breast cancer drug Herceptin is targeted at this gene, the drug is used for patients with amplification of the gene. Of the three oncogenes—HER-2/*neu*, *ras*, and c-*myc*—HER-2/*neu* has the strongest prognostic value in breast cancer. Serum levels of p105 are most useful in breast cancer, with some use in ovarian cancer patients. p105 levels in breast cancer correlate with a worse prognosis and a shorter disease-free state. Analyses of the EGF family for clinical purposes are performed by immunochemical and cytological techniques.

RET

The RET tyrosine kinase receptor, like other tyrosine kinase receptors, activates downstream growth pathways, and with uncontrolled signaling, cancer can result. RET is inappropriately activated in (1) papillary thyroid cancer, (2) multiple endocrine neoplasia type 2 (MEN2), and (3) familial medullary thyroid carcinoma (FMTC). In papillary thyroid cancer, a genetic event creates a fusion between the RET tyrosine kinase domain and a dimerization domain that can be donated by a number of genes. In MEN2A and FMTC, point mutations induce disulfide linkages between receptors. In MEN2B a point mutation in the kinase domain appears to alter the substrate specificity of the tyrosine kinase and presumably leads to inappropriate activation of downstream growth pathways.

Mutations in RET are identified in patients by testing in the molecular diagnostics laboratory. Testing of family members is important because it frees those family members who lack the family's characteristic mutation from undergoing the frequent traditional tests that are required to search for cancers before they are advanced.

EPIDERMAL GROWTH FACTOR RECEPTOR

The epidermal growth factor receptor (EGFR) is a prototype of a family of tyrosine kinase receptors. The natural ligands for the EGFR are epidermal growth factor (EGF) and transforming growth factor (TGF)-α, both of which can promote tumor growth. Overexpression of EGFR has prognostic value in a number of cancers. A number of anticancer compounds have been developed that inhibit EGFR.

Continued

BOX 14-1

Features of Selected Oncogenes—cont'd

bcl-2

The protein product of the *bcl*-2 oncogene is found primarily in the mitochondrial and other cellular membranes. The *bcl*-2 gene (symbol *BCL2*) is an oncogene with a mechanism different from that of the classical oncogenes *ras* and *myc*. The BCL2 protein inhibits apoptosis (programmed cell death) and contributes to survival of cancer cells, especially lymphoma and leukemic cells. The *bcl*-2 proto-oncogene was identified in follicular lymphomas wherein a 14 : 18 translocation (i.e., a translocation of pieces of chromosomes 14 and 18) results in formation of a fusion of the genes for *bcl*-2 and the immunoglobulin heavy chain. Activation of

the *bcl*-2 gene through the immunoglobulin promoter results in production of high levels of bcl-2 protein.

The *bcl*-2 oncogene is highly expressed in a variety of hematological malignancies, including lymphomas, myelomas, and chronic leukemias (malignancies characterized by prolonged cell survival). Abnormal expression of the *bcl*-2 gene appears to be an early event in colorectal carcinogenesis. In addition, overexpression of the *bcl*-2 gene is associated with development of resistance to cytotoxic cancer chemotherapy in a variety of tumors, including epithelial tumors and lymphomas. Thus detection of the *bcl*-2-gene product in tumors is an indication of progression.

BOX 14-2

Features of Selected Tumor-Suppressor Genes

RETINOBLASTOMA GENE

Retinoblastoma (RB) is a rare tumor of children that occurs both in families and sporadically. The work of Knudson on the familial-specific incidence of RB led to the two-hit hypothesis. He reasoned that in the *inherited* form of the tumor, one mutation was inherited in the germline (e.g., from the mother's egg) and was present in all cells of the patient's body. He hypothesized that the other mutational event (the second "hit") occurred somatically (not in the germline) in one of the cells of the developing retina. He hypothesized that, in the *sporadic* form of RB, both mutations occurred somatically in the same developing retinoblast, a relatively rare event. The two-hit hypothesis has served as a model for other tumor-suppressor genes.

The RB gene (symbol *RB1*) has been localized to a region of chromosome 13 by the finding of loss of a region of that chromosome in lymphocytes of patients with the familial form of RB. The finding has been confirmed by molecular studies of patients with RB. The same gene is affected in some patients with osteosarcomas. Most tumors do not have gross deletions, but point mutations or small insertions and deletions that result in a shortened protein product.

The protein product of the *RB1* gene is a nuclear phosphoprotein with a molecular mass of about 105 kDa (p105-RB).

This protein binds to a product of a DNA tumor virus, including the E1A protein of murine tumor virus and the E7 protein of human papillomavirus. When p105-RB is hypophosphorylated, it complexes with transcription factors, such as E2F, and blocks transcription of genes in S-phase cells. E2F dimerizes with a DP protein and regulates the transcription of several genes involved in DNA synthesis.

Inactivation or loss of p105-RB deregulates DNA syntheses and increases cellular proliferation. Thus RB is a tumor-suppressor gene because it suppresses DNA synthesis. Detection of mutations in RB is useful in determining the susceptibility of an individual to development of RB in the familial form, but it is not used as a tumor marker.

p53 GENE

The tumor protein p53 gene *TP53* is a tumor suppressor gene that encodes a nuclear phosphoprotein/transcription factor that regulates diverse cellular processes, including DNA repair, cell cycle arrest, and apoptosis. Wild-type p53 is believed to control cell division. This controlling effect of p53 protein may be lost by deletion of the gene or production of a competing mutant protein. The *TP53* gene is the most commonly mutated tumor-suppressor gene in cancer. *TP53* mutations

are commonly present in a variety of hematological disorders, including blast crisis in CML, AML, MDS, and adult T-cell leukemia and lymphoma. *TP53* mutations are also implicated in the histological transformation of follicular lymphoma into diffuse large B-cell lymphoma and have been described in a small subset of cases of Hodgkin disease. *TP53* mutations correlate with resistance to chemotherapy and portend a worse prognosis.

The *TP53* mutations are localized mainly to mutational "hot spots" in exons 5 to 8 and may be single-base substitutions, deletions, or insertions. Selective guanine to thymine mutations are found at codon 249 in human hepatocellular carcinomas taken from patients in high-incidence areas of Africa and Asia associated with aflatoxin exposure.

Mutations at codons 245 and 258 are found in Li-Fraumeni syndrome, a rare autosomal dominant syndrome characterized by diverse neoplasms at many different sites in the body. Inactivation of critical p53 protein function can be achieved by a mutation on one allele since the mutated protein can bind the wild-type protein and impair its function. In 75% to 80% of colon carcinomas, one p53 allele is deleted and the other contains a point mutation so that no wild-type p53 protein is present. Allelic deletion of p53 occurs only rarely in benign colon tumors, suggesting that p53 inactivation is a relatively late event in the development of colon carcinoma. Up to 70% of breast cancers also have deleted p53.

Mutations in *TP53* produce proteins that inactivate the wild type of p53 protein and allow cells to move through the cell cycle and contribute to the autonomous growth of cancer. Monoclonal antibodies to mutated p53 proteins have been developed. Wild-type p53 exhibits a short half-life and is normally not detected by immunohistochemistry. By contrast, the mutant protein accumulates to easily detectable levels.

Overexpression of mutant p53 proteins has been detected in up to 70% of primary colorectal cancers. Overexpression of p53 in breast cancers is associated with poor prognosis, but this association is not as strong as is the association of poor prognosis with c-*erb*B-2. Up to 75% of small cell lung carcinomas appear to overexpress a mutant protein.

Denaturing gradient gel electrophoresis, (DGGE), constant gradient gel electrophoresis (CGGE), and single-strand conformation polymorphism analysis (SSCP) have been used with great success for the detection of p53 mutations and can serve as effective tools in the molecular laboratory.

Features of Selected Tumor-Suppressor Genes—cont'd

p21 *(WAF1)*

The wild-type p53 protein activates transcription of a number of genes, including the *WAF1/CIP1* gene, the p21 protein product of the p21*WAF1* gene. The approved gene symbol *CDKN1A* refers to the fact that it is a cyclin-dependent protein kinase (cdk) inhibitor. The cell-cycle arrest function of p53 in response to DNA damage is mediated by p21.

One of the first events in the putative steps of progression of precursor lesions to colon cancer is loss of the adenomatous polyposis coli (symbol *APC*) gene in premalignant polyps. The *APC* gene encodes a large 300-kDa protein that may be truncated in cancer cells. The APC protein interacts with proteins that are involved in cell-cell interactions in epithelial cells. This gene is mutated in hereditary colorectal cancer syndromes, both polyposis and nonpolyposis types (see Chapter 9). The *APC* gene was detected by an interstitial deletion on chromosome 5q in a patient with hundreds of polyps. More than 80% of individuals with hereditary colorectal cancer have germline mutations in one of the *APC* alleles. The hereditary forms of colorectal cancer are relatively uncommon, but somatic mutations appear to be of great importance in the development of nonhereditary colorectal cancers. More than 70% of colorectal tumors have a specific mutation in one of the two APC alleles in the tumor tissue. APC mutations have also been described in other types of tumors, including breast, esophageal, and brain cancers.

For further discussion of familial colon cancer, including the role of testing for *APC* mutations, see Chapter 9.

NEUROFIBROMATOSIS TYPE 1

Neurofibromatosis type 1 (NF1), or von Recklinghausen disease, is a dominantly inherited syndrome manifested mainly by multiple benign tumors that develop along nerves (neurofibromas), brown ("café au lait") spots on the skin, and a type of nodule of the iris. Bones may also be affected, and learning difficulties are common. Mutations in the *NF1* gene have been found in about 20% of NF1 patients. Inactivating mutations of *NF1* have also been found in colorectal cancer, melanoma, and neuroblastoma.

The *NF1* gene has been localized to the pericentromeric region of chromosome 17q, band 11. It is a large gene coding for a 300-kDa protein, called neurofibromin. This protein has a high degree of similarity to GTPase-activating proteins. Although the exact mechanism of action of the protein is not known, it appears likely that loss or inactivation of neurofibromin function leads to alterations in signal transduction pathways regulated by small *ras*like G proteins, resulting in continuous "on" signals for cell activation.

WILMS TUMOR, *WT1*

The Wilms tumor-suppressor gene, *WT1,* located on chromosome 11p13, codes for a (45-kDa) protein that suppresses the expression of growth-inducing genes. Other chromosomal changes in Wilms tumors indicate that mutations of *WT1* may be only one step in the process of carcinogenesis. Thus identification and understanding of one tumor-suppressor gene in a given cancer may only provide a part of the information eventually required to understand the carcinogenic process.

BRCA1 AND BRCA2

A subset of breast cancer patients have been shown to have an autosomal dominant predisposition to developing breast and ovarian cancer. Two genetic loci have been identified: *BRCA1* on chromosome 17q and *BRCA2,* which localizes to 13q12-13. *BRCA1* encodes for an 1863-amino acid protein that may act as a transcription factor. The ability to detect mutations in *BRCA1* and *BRCA2* in somatic cells permits the identification of susceptible individuals in breast cancer families. As many as 1 in 200 women in the United States may have a germline mutation in the *BRCA1* gene. This has created an ethical dilemma for physicians, patients and their families, insurance companies, and health maintenance organizations. With further understanding of how the mutated gene products act, it may be possible to understand the molecular events in development of some breast and ovarian cancers.

For discussion of hereditary breast cancer, including the role of testing for *BRCA1* and *BRCA2*, see Chapter 9.

PTEN

PTEN stands for phosphatase and tensin homologue deleted on chromosome 10. The gene is also known by the acronym MMAC (mutated in multiple advanced cancers). The PTEN tumor-suppressor gene is mutated in numerous cancers.

PTEN functions as a phosphatase that negatively regulates phosphoinositide 3-kinase (PI 3-K) signaling by dephosphorylating the D3 position of phosphatidylinositol (3,4,5)-triphosphate [PtdIns$(3,4,5)P_3$]. PI 3-kinase and its product PtdIns$(3,4,5)P_3$ are involved in activation of signaling pathways leading to inhibition of apoptosis, cell migration, cell size, and chemotaxis. Mutation or inactivation of PTEN allows uncontrolled activation of the downstream pathways, which contribute to tumorigenesis.

Germline mutations in PTEN cause several autosomal dominantly inherited syndromes (Cowden, Lhermitte-Duclos, Bannayan-Zonana, and Proteus syndromes). The syndromes are characterized by development of benign tumors called hamartomas and by an increased likelihood of development of malignancies along with other growth-related symptoms. In various cancers, including breast, hepatocellular, endometrial, and cervical cancers, PTEN mutation and/or loss of expression is generally associated with a more advanced stage and is a poor prognostic indicator.

TABLE 14-7 — Detection Frequency of Antigen-Receptor Gene Rearrangements by Southern Blot Analysis

	CASES WITH ANTIGEN-RECEPTOR GENE REARRANGEMENT (%)					
	IMMUNOGLOBULIN GENES			T-CELL RECEPTOR GENES		
	IgH	Igκ	Igλ	TCRβ	TCRγ	TCRδ
B-CELL NEOPLASMS						
Precursor B-cell acute lymphoblastic leukemia/lymphoma	100	40-50	20-25	20-30	50-60	70-80
Chronic lymphocytic leukemia/small lymphocytic lymphoma	10	100	30	<10	<10	<10
Prolymphocytic leukemia	100	100	30	Rare	Rare	NA
Hairy cell leukemia/variant	100	100	30-50	Rare	NA	NA
Lymphoplasmacytic lymphoma/immunocytoma	100	100	30	Rare	NA	NA
Marginal zone B-cell lymphoma						
Low-grade, B-cell lymphoma of mucosa-associated lymphoid tissue	100	100	30	<10	Rare	NA
Splenic marginal zone lymphoma	100	100	30	0	NA	NA
Mantle-cell lymphoma	100	100	50	Rare	NA	NA
Follicular lymphoma	100	100	30	<10	<10	<10
Diffuse large B-cell lymphoma	100	100	30	<10	<10	NA
Burkitt lymphoma	100	100	30-40	Rare	Rare	NA
Plasma-cell myeloma	90	90	30	10	10	NA
T-CELL NEOPLASMS						
Precursor T-cell acute lymphoblastic leukemia/lymphoma	20	Rare	Rare	90-95	90-95	>95
Chronic lymphocytic leukemia/prolymphocytic leukemia	<10	0	0	100	100	>90
Large granular lymphocytic leukemia						
T cell	Rare	0	0	>90	>90	>90
Natural-killer cell	0	0	0	0	0	0
Peripheral T-cell lymphoma, unspecified	<10	Rare	0	>90	>90	>90
Peripheral T-cell lymphoma, specific variants						
Adult T-cell leukemia/lymphoma	<10	0	0	100	>90	>90
Nasal-T/NK lymphoma	0	0	0	<10	0	Rare
Angioimmunoblastic T-cell lymphoma	20	10-20	10-20	90	90	90
Intestinal T-cell lymphoma	0	0	0	100	NA	NA
Anaplastic large cell lymphoma	10	Rare	0	60-70	60-70	90
Hepatosplenic T-cell lymphoma	0	0	0	70-80	70-80	80-90
Subcutaneous panniculitis-like T-cell lymphoma	0	0	0	>90	>90	50
Mycosis fungoides/Sézary syndrome	0	0	0	70-80	70-80	>90

TABLE 14-8 — Common Recurrent Chromosomal Aberrations in Human Malignant Lymphoma

Cytogenetic Abnormality	Genes or Loci (@) Involved	Disease	Clinical Features	Frequency of Aberration (%)
t(14;18)(q32;q21)	BCL2/IGH@	FL	Indolent	~90
t(2;18)(p12;q21)	IGK@/BCL2	FL	Indolent	<5
t(3;14)(q27;q32)	BCL6/IGH@	FL	Indolent	~10
t(11;14)(q13;q32)	BCL1/IGH@	MCL	Aggressive	>90
Trisomy 3	Unknown	MZBCL-MALT	Indolent	Variable
t(11;18)(p21;q21)	API2/MLT	MZBCL	Indolent	50
t(1;14)(p22;q32)	BCL10/IGH@	MZBCL	Indolent	*
t(9;14)(p13;q32)	PAX-5/IGH@	LPL	Indolent-aggressive	*
t(8;14)(q24;q32)	MYC/IGH@	Burkitt lymphoma	Highly aggressive	75
t(2;8)(p12;q24)	MYC/IGK@	Burkitt lymphoma	Highly aggressive	15
t(8;22)(q24;q11)	MYC/IGL@	Burkitt lymphoma	Highly aggressive	10
t(3;14)(q27;q32)	BCL6/IGH@	DLBCL	Aggressive	~30
t(14;18)(q32;q21)	BCL2/IGH@	DLBCL	Aggressive	30
Amplification 9p	REL	PMLBCL	Aggressive	*
Del 13q14	Unknown	B-CLL	Indolent	25-50
Trisomy 12	Unknown	B-CLL	Indolent	30
t(11;14)(q13;q32)	BCL1/IGH@	B-PLL	Aggressive	*
t(2;5)(p23;q35)	NPM/ALK	ALCL,T/NK	Aggressive	~40
Inv 14(q11;q32) or complex translocations involving both chromosomes 14	Unknown	T-PLL	Aggressive	75
Isochromosome 7q	Unknown	Hepatosplenic γ/δ	Aggressive	*
Trisomy 8	Unknown	Hepatosplenic γ/δ	Aggressive	*

Note that IGK and IGL are symbols for genes Igκ and Igλ, respectively.

FL, Follicular lymphoma; MCL, Mantle-cell lymphoma; MZBCL, marginal-zone B-cell lymphoma; MALT, mucosa-associated lymphoid tissue; LPL, lymphoplasmacytic lymphoma; DLBCL, diffuse large B-cell lymphoma; PMLBCL, primary mediastinal large B-cell lymphoma; B-CLL, B-chronic lymphocytic leukemia; PLL, prolymphocytic leukemia; ALL, acute lymphoblastic leukemia; ALCL, anaplastic large cell lymphoma; NK, natural killer.

*An insufficient number of patients were studied to permit accurate assessment of percentage of tumors with the cytogenetic aberration indicated.

| TABLE 14-9 | Common Recurrent Chromosomal Aberrations in Human Leukemia |

Chromosomal Abnormalities	Frequency of Genes or Loci (@) Involved	Disease	Clinical Features	Genetic Alteration (%)
t(9;22)(q34;q11)	BCR/ABL (p210)	CML	Good prognosis	95
t(12;21) cryptic	TEL/AML1	Precursor B-cell ALL	Good prognosis	20-25
t(9;22)(q34;q11)	BCR/ABL (p190)	Precursor B-cell ALL	Poor prognosis	5-20
t(1;19)(q23;p13)	E2A/PBX	Precursor B-cell ALL	Pre-B phenotype (cytoplasmic μ), poor response to antimetabolites	3-6
t(4;11)(q21;q23)	MLL/AF4	Precursor B-cell ALL	Mixed lineage, infants, poor prognosis leukocytosis	3
t(11;19)(q23;p13)	MLL/ENL	Precursor B-cell ALL	Leukocytosis	<1
t(8;14)(q24;q32)	MYC/IGH@	B-ALL	FAB L3, mature B-cell phenotype extramedullary disease	85
t(2;8)(p12;q24)	MYC/IGK@	B-ALL	FAB L3, mature B-cell phenotype extramedullary disease	10
t(8;22)(q24;q11)	MYC/IGL@	B-ALL	FAB L3, mature B-cell phenotype extramedullary disease	5
None	TAL1 deletion	Precursor T-cell ALL	Extramedullary disease, CD2, CD10−	25
t(1;14)(p32;q11)	TRD@/TAL1	Precursor T-cell ALL	Extramedullary disease, CD2, CD10−	3
t(1;7)(p32;q35)	TRB@/TAL1	Precursor T-cell ALL	Extramedullary disease, CD2, CD10−	<1
t(8;14)(q24;q11)	TRA@/MYC	Precursor T-cell ALL	Extramedullary disease	2
t(11;14)(p15;q11)	TRD@/RBTN1	Precursor T-cell ALL	Extramedullary disease	<1
t(11;14)(p13;q11)	TRD@/RBTN2	Precursor T-cell ALL	Extramedullary disease	7
t(10;14)(q24;q11)	TRD@/HOX11	Precursor T-cell ALL	Extramedullary disease	4
t(1;7)(p34;q34)	TRB@/LCK	Precursor T-cell ALL	Extramedullary disease	1
t(8;13)(p11;q11-12)	FGFRI/ZNF198	Precursor T-cell ALL	Eosinophilia	<1
t(8;21)(q22;q22)	AML1/ETO	AML	AML-FAB M2	10-15 (30% of AML M2)
inv(16)(p13;q22)	CBFβ/MYH11	AML	FAB M4EO	10
t(6;9)(p23;q34)	DEK/CAN	AML	Basophilia	2
t(9;11)(p22;q23)	MLL/AF9	AML	FAB M4-M5, infants	5
t(8;16)(p11;p13)	MOZ/CBP	AML	FAB M4, M5	<1
t(7;11)(p15;p15)	NUP98/HOXA9	AML	FAB M2, M4	1
t(3;5)(q25;q34)	NPM/MLF 1	AML	Myelodysplastic syndrome	1
t(15;17)(q22;q21)	PML/RARA	AML	FAB M3, coagulopathy, good retinoic acid response	7 (75% of AML M3)
t(11;17)(q23;q21)	PLZF/RARA	AML	FAB M3, coagulopathy, poor retinoic acid response	<1
t(5;17)(q32;q21)	NPM/RARA	AML	FAB M3, coagulopathy, poor retinoic acid response	<1

CML, Chronic myelogenous leukemia; ALL, acute lymphoblastic leukemia; AML, acute myelogenous leukemia; p210 and p190, chimeric proteins (see text); FAB (with L3, M3, M4EO, etc), French-American-British classifications; TRB@, TRD@, T-cell receptor β and δ loci.
*Estimated frequency per clinical disease category.

TABLE 14-10 Chromosomal Aberrations in Soft Tissue Neoplasms

Type of Tumor	Chromosomal Aberration	Involved Genes	Prevalence
Rhabdomyosarcoma			
Alveolar	t(2;13)(q35;q14);	PAX3-FKHR	75%
	t(1;13)(p36;q14)	PAX7-FKHR	10%
Embryonal	Gains of 2, 7, 8, 12, 13	IGF2, GOK, PTCH TP53	NA
	Losses of 1, 6, 9, 14, and 17[50]		NA
Spindle cell	NA	NA	NA
Undifferentiated	NA	NA	NA
EWS/PNET	t(11;22)(q24;q12)	EWS-FLI-1	85%-95%
	t(21;22)(p22;q12)	EWS-ERG	5%-10%
	t(7;22)(p22;q12)	EWS-ETV1	<1%
	t(17;22)(q21;q12)	EWS-E1AD	<1%
	t(2;22)(q33;q12)	EWS-FEV	<1%
	Inversion of q22	EWS-ZSG	<1%
DSRCT	t(11;22)(p13;q12)	EWS-WT1	>95%
Clear cell sarcoma	t(12;22)(q13;q12)	EWS-ATF1	90%
Extraskeletal myxoid chondrosarcoma	t(9;22)(q22-23;q11-12)	EWS-TEC	75%
	t(9;15)(q22;q21)	TCF12-TEC	NA
	t(9;17)(q22;q11)	TAF2N-TEC	25%
Extraskeletal mesenchymal chondrosarcoma	der(13;21)(q10;q10)	NA	NA
Synovial sarcoma	t(X;18)(p11;q11)	SYT-SSX1	65%
		SYT-SSX2	35%
		SYT-SSX4	Rare
Congenital/infantile fibrosarcoma	t(12;15)(p13;q25)	ETV6-NTRK3	80%
Inflammatory myofibroblastic tumor	t(1;2)(q25;p23)	TPM3-ALK	NA
	t(2;19)(p23;q13)	TPM4-ALK	NA
	t(2;17)(p23;q23)	CLTC-ALK	NA
	t(2;11;2)(p23;p15;q31)	CARS-ALK	NA
Myxoid/round cell liposarcoma	t(12;16)(q13;p11)	TLS-CHOP	~95%
	t(12;22)(q13;q12)	EWS-CHOP	Rare
Tenosynovial giant cell tumor	t(1;2)(p11;q35-37)	CSF-COL6A3	40%
	t(1;5)(p11;q22-31)		10%
	t(1;11)(p11;q11-12)		10%
	t(1;8)(p11;q21-22)		10%
Lipoblastoma	Rearrangement of 8q12	PLAG1	70%
DFSP	Ring chromosome with sequences from chromosomes 17 and 22		
	t(17;22)(q22;q13)		
Giant cell fibroblastoma (juvenile form of DFSP)	t(17;22)(q22;q13)	COL1A1-PDGFB	NA
Desmoid tumor	+8, +20,	NA	NA
	Deletion (5)(q21-22)	NA	NA
Alveolar soft part sarcoma	t(X;17)(p11;q25)	ASPL-TFE3	>90%

NA, *Unknown;* EWS, *Ewing sarcoma;* PNET, *primitive neuroectodermal tumor;* DSCRT, *desmoplastic small round blue cell tumor;* Der, *derivative;* DFSP, *dermatofibrosarcoma protuberans.*

Answers to Review Questions

CHAPTER 1

1. D
2. E
3. D
4. C
5. D
6. B
7. E
8. C
9. A

CHAPTER 2

1. A
2. C
3. A
4. E
5. E

CHAPTER 3

1. E
2. A
3. D
4. B
5. A
6. C
7. B
8. A

CHAPTER 4

1. B
2. D
3. C
4. D
5. E
6. E
7. D

CHAPTER 5

1. E
2. A
3. E
4. C
5. B

CHAPTER 6

1. E
2. B
3. E
4. B
5. E

CHAPTER 7

1. A
2. D
3. E
4. B
5. C

CHAPTER 8

1. B
2. E
3. E
4. D
5. B
6. E
7. E
8. E
9. B
10. C
11. E
12. E
13. B
14. E
15. E
16. E

CHAPTER 9

1. A
2. D
3. D
4. B
5. E
6. C
7. A
8. C
9. B
10. C

CHAPTER 10
1. C
2. A
3. C
4. D
5. C
6. E
7. A
8. D
9. C
10. A

CHAPTER 11
1. C
2. D
3. D
4. D
5. B
6. D
7. E
8. D
9. A

CHAPTER 12
1. A
2. C
3. B
4. E
5. B

CHAPTER 13
1. D
2. E
3. E
4. D
5. C
6. D
7. E
8. B
9. E
10. D

Glossary

Absorbance The measurement of radiant energy absorbed by a solution (or a substance in a solution); this measurement can be related to the concentration of a substance, such as *DNA* or *RNA*, in that solution.

Adverse Drug Reaction (ADR) Any undesirable side effect or toxic reaction that is caused by the administration of a drug; ADRs are a leading cause of morbidity and mortality in the United States.

Allele A form of a *gene* found at a specific location on a *chromosome*; one of a number of alternative forms of the same gene at a given *locus* (position) on a chromosome; except for X chromosome genes in males, each person inherits two alleles for each gene, one allele from each parent; these alleles may be the same or may be different from one another; alleles may contain *sequence* variations (differences in the *sequences* of *base pairs*) that alter its expression or the functional characteristics of the corresponding protein.

Alteration A variation or change in *DNA sequence*; it may be benign or cause disease.

Amelogenin A low molecular weight protein found in tooth enamel; the amelogenin *gene* is used for sex identification because the male version is longer than the female version.

Amniocentesis Removal of amniotic fluid from the amniotic sac, normally through the mother's abdominal wall.

Amplicon The product of an amplification reaction, such as *PCR*; the amplified pieces of *nucleic acid* may contaminate reagents or samples in the laboratory.

Amplification Methods Techniques to amplify the amount of target (*DNA or RNA*), signal, or *probe* so that a detectable signal is produced from samples that contain the target or so that *sequence* alterations in the DNA or RNA can be readily observed.

Analyte-Specific Reagent Reagents that are used in the assessment of biochemical substances in biological specimens; the reagent(s), usually purchased, are used in laboratory-developed tests and confer specificity for detecting a particular analyte; ASRs include antibodies, specific receptor proteins, ligands, and *oligonucleotides*; in genetic testing, an ASR often is the key ingredient of a specially designed *in-house assay*.

Aneuploidy An abnormal number of *chromosomes*.

Anticipation A progressive increase in severity and/or age of onset of a genetic disorder in subsequent generations of a family; associated with trinucleotide repeat disorders (discussed in Chapter 9).

Anticoagulant Any substance that prevents blood clotting.

Apoptosis A specialized form of cell death known as programmed cell death; it involves the activation of a specific group of proteins known as caspases, with eventual nuclear fragmentation and formation of a characteristic ladder pattern on gel electrophoresis of the partially degraded DNA from the apoptotic cells.

Array A set of items that are randomly accessible by numeric index; an orthogonal pattern of parameters used to distinguish different assays; usually the parameters are spatial, as in linear, two-dimensional, or three-dimensional arrays.

Arthrocentesis Withdrawal of joint fluid.

Assay Controls Samples or specimens that test *preanalytical*, analytical, and postanalytical processes and components of assays.

Autosomal Dominant An autosomal dominant *gene* is one that is located on an *autosome* and that causes a specific *phenotype* even if only one copy of that gene is present and the copy on the other chromosome is different (a *heterozygous* state); an autosomal dominant disorder is one that is caused by an autosomal dominant disease gene and will be expressed in 50% of offspring if one parent is heterozygous for the gene; use of the word "dominant" typically refers to a *phenotype*.

Autosomal Recessive An autosomal recessive *gene* is one that is located on an *autosome* and that causes a specific phenotype to be expressed only if it is *homozygous*; an autosomal recessive disorder is one that is caused by two copies of a recessive gene and will be expressed in 25% of offspring if each parent carries one copy of the recessive gene; "recessive" typically refers to a phenotype.

Autosome A nonsex *chromosome*; there are 22 pairs of autosomes in the human *genome*.

B lymphocyte (B Cell) B lymphocytes are cells that are involved with the production of antibodies in the humoral immune response; the "B" in B cell represents the bursa of Fabricius, which is the organ where B cells mature in birds.

Base (in DNA or RNA) Bases are the *purines* and *pyrimidines* in a nucleic acid that define the *sequence* of the *nucleic acid*.

Base Pair A *purine* and a *pyrimidine nucleotide* bound by hydrogen bonds; in DNA base pairing, adenine (A) binds to thymine (T), and guanine (G) pairs with cytosine (C); in RNA base pairing, uracil replaces thymine.

Bias Systematic error that occurs when there is consistent overestimation or underestimation of a measured value, as opposed to random error, which is unpredictable.

Bioterrorism The use of pathogenic organisms or biological toxins to produce death and disease in humans for the purpose of spreading fear and terror in the community.

Breakpoint Cluster Region (BCR) The BCR refers to a region of *chromosome* 22 that is a partner in a large proportion of chromosomal *translocations* involving the *ABL1* (also called *ABL*) gene on chromosome 9; the breakpoints in this chromosome are clustered within this BCR region, hence its name; the *BCR-ABL* fusion occurs as a consequence of the translocation involving chromosomes 9 and 22 and is characteristic of chronic myeloid (or "myelogenous") leukemia; see also *Gene Rearrangement*.

Buccal Cells Epithelial cells from the inside of the mouth (cheek).

Carcinoma Malignant new growth (*neoplasm*) of cells that arises from epithelium; found in skin or the lining of body organs, such as in breast, prostate, lung, stomach, or bowel; tend to infiltrate into adjacent tissue and to spread to distant organs.

Centralization In regard to molecular diagnostics laboratory design, the sharing of equipment, reagents, personnel, and space for various disciplines, such as infectious disease (clinical microbiology) and inherited disease (genetics) testing.

Centromere A primary constriction in a *chromosome*; centromeres play an important role in directing the movement of chromosomes between daughter cells during cell division.

Chain of Custody A concept in jurisprudence that applies to the handling of evidence (such as a blood specimen) and its integrity; a process that tracks the movement of evidence through its collection, safeguarding, and analysis by documenting each person who handled the evidence, the date and time it was collected or transferred, and the purpose for the transfer.

Chimera An individual who has two genetically distinct types of cells, often the result of a bone marrow transplantation.

Chimerism The presence of more than one genetically distinct muscle *genome* in a single individual.

Chromatin Nuclear *DNA* and its associated structural proteins; chromatin is arranged and organized in a hierarchical fashion where the degree of its condensation increases with higher levels of structural organization.

Chromosome A highly ordered structure of a single double-stranded *DNA* molecule, compacted many times with the aid of structural *DNA-binding proteins*.

Terms in italic font within definitions are defined elsewhere in the Glossary.

Clinical Audit The review of case histories of patients against the benchmark of current best practice; used as a tool to improve clinical practice.

Clinical Practice Guidelines Systematically developed statements to assist practitioner and patient decisions about appropriate healthcare for specific clinical circumstances; in the laboratory, guidelines may include goals for accuracy, precision, and turnaround time of tests.

Clonal The term clonal refers to the origin of cells from a single progenitor (clone) that gives rise to progeny that are genetically identical to the original parental cell. The term is often used to encapsulate the concept that cancers arise from a single cancerous cell whose growth regulatory mechanisms have gone awry and that generates more tumor cells with cancerous growth characteristics.

Codon A three-nucleotide *sequence* that "codes" for an amino acid during translation; there are 64 possible codons in nuclear *DNA*.

College of American Pathologists An organization of board-certified pathologists that provides programs for proficiency testing and laboratory accreditation.

Crossover See *Recombination*.

Cytochrome P-450 (CYP) A large family of drug-metabolizing enzymes that are also important in metabolism of steroid hormones, fatty acids, and other substances; these isozymes are involved in metabolism of more than 50% of all drugs; many CYPs have *polymorphisms* (that is, their DNA sequences differ among individuals) and may account for variation among individuals in their response to drugs; *phenotypes* associated with *genotypes* range from poor to rapid metabolizers.

Cytogenetics The study of *chromosome* structure.

Decentralization The use of separate and distinct laboratory space, equipment, reagents, and personnel for each molecular laboratory discipline, such as infectious disease, inherited disease, and molecular oncology.

Deletion A *DNA sequence* that is missing in one sample compared with another. Deletions may be as small as one nucleotide or as large as an entire chromosome.

Detection Methods Techniques to identify *sequences* of *nucleic acids*, usually after purification and amplification.

Deoxyribonucleic Acid (DNA) A molecule that carries genetic information and is a double-stranded polymer of nucleotides.

Diagnostic Accuracy The closeness of agreement between a diagnostic test (index test) and the diagnosis made by use of a reference standard (gold standard) for a specific disease or condition; the agreement is expressed in a number of ways, including sensitivity and specificity, predictive values, likelihood ratios, diagnostic odds ratios, and areas under receiver operating characteristic (ROC) curves.

Diploid Having a full set of (paired) *chromosomes* (46 chromosomes in humans, half from each parent).

DNA-Binding Proteins Proteins that recognize and bind to specific *sequences* of *DNA*; some of these proteins are involved in the regulation of DNA *transcription*.

DNA Marker A *polymorphic locus* that is easily assayed, yielding reproducible results.

DNA Methylation The addition of a methyl residue to the 5 position of the pyrimidine ring of a cytosine base to form 5-methylcytosine and most often occurring at CpG *sequences* in *DNA*; DNA methylation can serve as a model of gene regulation by preventing gene transcription; this epigenetic process is implicated in growth and development of organisms.

DNase A *nuclease* that specifically degrades DNA.

dNTPs Deoxyribonucleotide triphosphates (usually dATP, dCTP, dGTP, and dTTP), the building blocks of DNA.

Downstream Located closer to the 3′ end of DNA molecule.

Drug Metabolism The process by which drugs are chemically modified in the body; most often metabolism involves one or more enzymes; although the primary purpose of drug metabolism is to promote inactivation and elimination of the drug, some drug metabolites possess pharmacological activity and may persist in the body longer than the parent drug.

Electrophoresis Movement caused by an electrical field, often through a gel matrix. Polyacrylamide and agarose are common matrices used to separate DNA molecules or RNA molecules in an electric field.

Endonuclease An enzyme that hydrolyzes an internal phosphodiester bond, splitting a *nucleic acid* into two or more parts.

Engraftment In *hematopoietic cell transplantation*, the process of infused donor stem cells homing to the bone marrow of the recipient and producing blood cells of all types.

Epigenetics Processes that alter gene function or its interpretation by mechanisms other than those that rely on changing the *sequence* of *bases* in *DNA*; these processes include *DNA methylation*, *genomic imprinting*, *histone* modification, *chromatin* remodeling, and others.

Euchromatin *Genomic* regions that are rich in genes; less intensely stained and less compactly organized (during interphase) than is *heterochromatin*.

Evidence-Based Laboratory Medicine The application of principles and techniques of evidence-based medicine to laboratory medicine; the conscientious, judicious, and explicit use of best evidence in the use of laboratory medicine investigations for assisting in decision making about the care of individual patients.

Evidence-Based Medicine The conscientious, judicious, and explicit use of the best evidence in making decisions about the care of individual patients.

Exclusion Results of an identity test that indicate that the tested individual was not the contributor of a tested sample.

Exon Part of the coding region of a gene that codes for a *gene* product; region that specifies the amino acid *sequence* of a polypeptide during *translation*; the coding region of a gene that will be expressed as protein following translation.

Exonuclease An enzyme that removes terminal *nucleotides* from a polynucleotide, nucleases release one nucleotide at a time (serially) beginning at one end of a *nucleic acid*; exonuclease activity excises incorrectly paired nucleotides during replication.

External Validity The degree to which the results of a study can be generalized to other patients.

Extraction The technique of removing a substance (in this case *DNA* or *RNA*) from surrounding material.

FAB French-American-British classification system for certain types of *leukemia*.

Fluorescence A physical property of some molecules that emit light at a longer wavelength when excited at a shorter wavelength.

Forensics A branch of science that deals with legal issues or criminalistics.

Formalin-Fixed, Paraffin-Embedded Tissue (FFPE) Tissue that has been permanently fixed with formalin and then embedded in paraffin before the preparation of microscopy slides.

Gene A unit of *DNA* that specifies production of RNA molecules (*transcription*), which then are *translated* to make the proteins that are required for cellular function.

Gene Deletion A circumstance in which all or part of a *gene* is lost.

Gene Dosage The number of copies of a particular *gene*; in most cases, there are two copies of each gene; in situations in which more or fewer copies of the gene are present, an increase or decrease in production of the protein product may occur.

Gene Duplication A condition in which all or part of a *gene* is repeated.

Gene Inversion A rearrangement of the *gene* or part of the gene causing the orientation of the *sequence* (order of *base pairs*) of *DNA* in the gene to be reversed in relation to the flanking *chromosomal DNA sequences*.

Gene Rearrangement Relocation of a segment of *DNA* within a *gene*.

Genetic Code The complete list of *nucleotide codons* and the amino acids or actions for which they "code."

Genome; Genomic The complete set of *chromosomes*; the total complement of hereditary information; the human genome contains two copies, termed *alleles*, of each *autosomal gene*.

Genotype The primary *nucleotide sequences* of the two *gene alleles*.

Genotyping Detection of specific genetic variants; some correlate with drug-response and other *phenotypes*.

Haploid Having a single set of *chromosomes*, as in gametes (eggs and sperm) (i.e., half the number of chromosomes present in a mature somatic cell).

Haploinsufficiency A situation in which an individual is clinically affected because of absence of one of the two copies of a *gene*; the remaining single copy of the normal gene is incapable of providing sufficient gene product (usually a protein) to assure normal function.

Haplotype The association of specific *alleles* at multiple loci on one *chromosome* strand; the genetic makeup of a single *chromosome*; shortened from "haploid genotype."

Hematopoietic Cell Transplantation (HCT) Transplantation of hematopoietic stem cells, usually from bone marrow, employed to treat some patients with disorders including *leukemias* and hereditary immune deficiencies.

Hemolysis Disruption of the membranes of blood cells causing release of hemoglobin and other components of the cells.

Heterochromatin Genomic regions that are *gene* poor or span transcriptionally silent genes and are more densely packed during interphase.

Heteroduplex A *sequence* of double-stranded *DNA* (DNA duplex) with internal mismatches of *bases* between the two strands.

Heteroplasmy The presence of more than one population of mitochondrial *DNA sequences* in a cell; a genetic state in which different *alleles* can be present in a continuously variable ratio.

Heterozygous The presence of different *alleles* at the same *locus* on the two copies of a *chromosome*; for example, one copy of the *gene* may be the usual (wild-type) gene, and the other copy may contain a disease-causing change in the *DNA*.

Histone A structural protein involved in the three-dimensional organization and function of nuclear *DNA*.

Homoduplex A perfectly matched *DNA* duplex (pair of strands) in double-stranded DNA or in a DNA-RNA hybrid.

Homologous Sequences *DNA sequences* that share a similar order of DNA *bases*; the term "homology" has other uses in biology; when quantifying the similarity of two DNA sequences, it is preferable to refer to "% sequence identity" rather than to "% sequence homology."

Homoplasmy The presence of a homogeneous population of *mitochondrial genomes* in a cell.

Homozygous Presence of the same *allele* on both *chromosomes*.

Human Genome Project A project undertaken by the International Human Genome Sequencing Consortium to decipher the three billion *base pairs* in the human *genome*; the project was completed in 2003.

Human Leukocyte Antigen (HLA) Classes of *polymorphic genes* located on *chromosome* 6p within the major histocompatibility complex that encode for the classic transplantation antigens found on the surface of nucleated cells; *alleles* of these *genes* are used for testing in transplantations of solid organs and bone marrow, in forensics and parentage investigations, and in documentation of *chimerism*.

Hybridization The binding (annealing, pairing) of two (complementary) *DNA* strands by *base pairing*.

Immunoglobulin Heavy and Light Chains Immunoglobulins are proteins composed of two light chains and two heavy chains; there are two types of light chains, kappa (κ) and lambda (λ); the heavy chains in an immunoglobulin may be gamma (γ), alpha (α), mu (μ), delta (δ), or epsilon (ε) to produce, respectively, immunoglobulins G, A, M, D, and E; an immunoglobulin molecule contains only κ or λ light chains and only one type of heavy chain.

Immunoglobulins Antibody molecules produced by mature B cells or plasma cells.

Imprinting (parental) Process that leads to differential expression of a *gene* in an offspring, depending on whether the gene was inherited from the mother or the father.

Inclusion A result of an identity test that indicates that the tested individual may be the contributor of the tested sample; often accompanied by the probability that the tested individual contributed the tested sample; contrast with *exclusion*.

Indel A *sequence* variant arising from both an *insertion* and a *deletion*.

Index Test In studies of diagnostic accuracy, the "new" test or the test of interest that is being studied.

Inheritance The biological process through which an offspring acquires characteristics of its parents.

Inhibition (of PCR) Failure to form the expected amount of products of the *PCR* reaction; produced by substances such as hemoglobin that inhibit the polymerase enzyme in PCR that catalyzes the production of copies of DNA (called amplifying the DNA); in many assays, a DNA that will always be amplified is added to the sample to determine whether an interfering substance is present.

In-House Assay A laboratory assay that is developed within a laboratory using ASRs and reagents made in the laboratory, and designed to respond to a need for a specific laboratory diagnosis; see also *Laboratory-Developed Test*.

Insertion An extra *DNA sequence* that is present in one sample compared with a reference *sequence*.

Intergenic Referring to regions of *chromosomes* that are located between *genes*.

Internal Validity The degree to which the results of a study can be trusted for the population of patients in the study; depends on the experimental design, research design, instruments used, calibration, etc.

Intron The noncoding region of a *gene* that will not be translated into protein; this *DNA sequence* is spliced out during mRNA processing; also called intervening sequence or IVS.

Isolation The separation of a substance from its surrounding material.

Label A molecule that is associated with an analyte that renders it easier to observe.

Laboratory-Developed Test (LDT) An *in-house assay* developed by a laboratory; in molecular diagnostics, this usually refers to a test for which no alternative is commercially available.

Leukemia Leukemias are *neoplastic* proliferations of hematopoietic cells and are characteristically based in the bone marrow and peripheral blood, but may be found elsewhere.

Ligase An enzyme that covalently joins two *DNA* strands.

Linkage Studies A method using *DNA* markers physically adjacent (i.e., linked) to a disease gene; this indirect analysis allows the disease gene to be tracked through a family; in this way, the genetic status of at-risk individuals can be determined even when the identity of the disease-causing DNA *sequence* variant is unknown.

Locus The location of a *gene* on a *chromosome*; a locus is said to be *polymorphic* when the least common allele has a population frequency of at least 1 in 100.

Lymphoma Lymphoma refers to malignant neoplasms that originate from lymphocytes in lymphatic tissues, such as lymph nodes, spleen, or tonsillar tissue; lymphomas are generally classified into Hodgkin or non-Hodgkin lymphoma; Hodgkin lymphoma is a specific category first described by Thomas Hodgkin in 1832 and characterized by the presence of the Reed-Sternberg cell, which accounts for only a small proportion of the cellular infiltrate;

non-Hodgkin lymphomas include all other types of lymphomas and may be of B-cell, T-cell, or natural killer (NK)-cell origin.

Lymphostasis Blockade of the normal flow of lymph.

Lyonization Random inactivation of one X *chromosome* in each cell of a female to circumvent excess protein product formation; named for Mary Lyon who first put forth the hypothesis.

Major Histocompatibility Complex (MHC) A large complex of *genes* located on *chromosome* 6p that contains the human leukocyte antigen region.

Malignant (Tumor or Cell) Having the potential to invade and destroy surrounding tissues and to spread to distant parts of the body.

Meiosis The two-step process of cell division that produces gametes (ova in females and sperm in males) with one half the number of *chromosomes* of the parent cell; contrast with *mitosis*.

Mendelian Inheritance Patterns of heredity that abide by a set of laws relating to transmission of inherited characteristics and assortment of *alleles*.

Metabolizer A description of the drug metabolism *phenotype*; specifically an individual's rate of metabolism as it relates to a specific therapeutic drug; poor metabolizers metabolize a drug slowly if at all, whereas an ultrarapid metabolizer converts a drug to its metabolite(s) very quickly, as compared with the usual (normal) so-called extensive metabolizer.

Microarray A small piece of silicon, plastic, or glass onto whose surface has been fabricated a structured, two-dimensional array of compartments that are accessed by their position in the *array*.

Microfabrication The collective term for the technologies used to fabricate components on a micrometer-sized scale.

Microfluidics A multidisciplinary field comprising physics, chemistry, engineering, and biotechnology that studies the behavior of fluids at the microscale and mesoscale; the term also encompasses the design of systems in which such small volumes of fluids are used.

MicroRNAs Short noncoding *RNA* molecules, about 22 nucleotides in length that play a role in regulation of *gene expression* by interfering with effective *translation* of mRNA to proteins.

Microsatellite Locus (Plural: Loci) A locus with a *short tandem repeat sequence (STR)* of DNA of, typically, 2-7 base pairs; usually the short sequences (e.g., AATG) are repeated 10 to 100 times (e.g., AATGAATGAATGAAT GAATGAATGAATGAATGAATGAA TGAATGAATG).

Microsatellite Repeat Markers Highly *polymorphic DNA sequences* of short repeats generally comprising <6 bases; these repeats are widely prevalent in the human *genome*.

Microsatellites Short segments of *DNA* (1 to 13 bases long) that are repeated end to end, also known as *short tandem repeats* (STRs).

Microtechnology Technology with features near one micrometer (one millionth of a meter, or 10^{-6} meter, or 1 μm).

Minimal Residual Disease (MRD) When used in relation to cancer, MRD refers to low-level residual disease after treatment, particularly after chemotherapy; especially in the hematological malignancies, molecular markers have been used to identify very low remaining tumor burden to establish disease persistence or relapse.

Minimum Feature Size The dimension of the smallest feature actually constructed in the manufacturing process of a chip.

Minisatellite Locus (Plural: Loci) Locus containing a *variable number of tandem repeats* of *DNA sequences* as short as 8 to 10 *base pairs* or as long as 50 to 100 base pairs.

Minisatellites Repeated segments of *DNA* that are 14 to 500 bases long, also known as *variable number of tandem repeats* or VNTRs.

Missense A *nucleotide* substitution that codes for a different amino acid; these *sequence* changes are commonly referred to as missense mutations.

Mitochondrial DNA The circular *DNA* within a mitochondrial organelle that codes for polypeptides involved in the oxidative phosphorylation pathway; this DNA is typically transmitted across generations by maternal *inheritance*.

Mitosis Process of cell division that produces daughter cells with the same number of *chromosomes* as the parent cell; contrast with *meiosis*.

Molecular Diagnostics A field of laboratory medicine that uses principles and techniques of molecular biology.

Molecular Test Tests or assays involving the extraction, purification, and processing of *DNA* or *RNA* (*nucleic acids*) in various ways to obtain specific information in the investigation of a given condition; often used for the diagnosis of an infectious disease.

Monoclonal Characterized by a single clone of cells; see *Clonal*.

Mosaicism The presence of two populations of cells in one individual, each with a different *genotype*.

Multiplex Assay The use of different *probes*, chromogens, *PCR* primers, etc. in a single assay to detect or quantify more than one target; in molecular microbiology, the targets are portions of the DNA or RNA of several infectious agents; in molecular genetics and molecular oncology, they often are several different DNA *sequences* of one or more *genes*.

Mutation A *sequence* alteration or, in some contexts (as in Chapter 9, Inherited Diseases), a sequence alteration that causes disease.

N-Acetyltransferase (NAT) A family of metabolic enzymes that acetylate drugs, such as procainamide (cardiac medication) and sulfonamides (antibiotics), in addition to a number of environmental toxins; slow and fast acetylator *phenotypes* are well characterized in several populations.

Nanotechnology Technology that "involves research and technology development at the atomic, molecular, or macromolecular levels in the dimension range of approximately 1-100 nanometers; nanotechnology research and development includes control at the nanoscale and integration of nanoscale structures into larger material components, systems, and architectures; within these larger scale assemblies, the control and construction of their structures and components remains at the nanometer scale." (http://www.becon2.nih.gov/nstc_def_nano.htm).

Neoplasia and Neoplasm; Neoplastic Neoplasia (in Latin, new growth) is used to refer to tumors and encompasses benign and malignant tumors, or *neoplasms*.

Nondisjunction Failure of *chromosomes* to separate during cell division.

Nonsense A *nucleotide* substitution that results in a stop *codon*, prematurely terminating *transcription*; may result in production of a shortened protein or no protein.

Northern Blot A method for detecting specific *RNA sequences* with labeled *probes* after they have been separated by size using *electrophoresis*.

Nuclease An enzyme that cleaves the (phosphodiester) bonds between the (nucleotide) subunits of a *nucleic acid* molecule (*DNA* or *RNA*); these enzymes catalyze the hydrolysis of *nucleic acid* by cleaving chains of *nucleotides* into smaller units; thus they are enzymes that degrade *nucleic acids*.

Nucleic Acid A polymer made of *nucleotide* monomers (a sugar moiety, a phosphoric acid, and a purine or pyrimidine base); examples are deoxyribonucleic acid (*DNA*) and ribonucleic acid (*RNA*).

Nucleosome A unit of *chromatin* consisting of nucleosome core particles (146 base pairs of double-stranded DNA) and linker DNA wound around an octamer of *histone* proteins.

Nucleotide A unit of *DNA* or *RNA*, consisting of one chemical base (purine or pyrimidine) plus a phosphate molecule and a sugar molecule (deoxyribose or ribose).

Oligonucleotide A short single-stranded polymer of *nucleic acid*.

Oncogene A deregulated *gene* that leads to uncontrolled cell growth and tumor formation; the normal cellular equivalent of the oncogene is known as a *proto-oncogene*.

Oncogenesis The progression of genetic and cellular changes that lead to formation of a malignant tumor.

Optimal Cutting Temperature Compound (OCT) A water-soluble compound composed of polyvinyl alcohol and polyethylene glycol that surrounds but does not infiltrate tissue.

Outcomes Results related to the quality or quantity of life of patients; examples include mortality, functional status, length of stay in a hospital, and costs.

Outcomes Studies Studies performed to determine if a medical intervention (such as a drug or a specific laboratory test) will improve patient *outcome*.

Pathogen An infectious agent that causes a disease in a patient.

PCR See *Polymerase Chain Reaction*.

Penetrance The percentage of individuals with the disease *genotype* who develop symptoms of the disease; complete penetrance implies that all individuals who possess the abnormal genotype will develop the disease, whereas incomplete or reduced penetrance indicates that not all individuals who have the disease genotype will become symptomatic; incomplete penetrance of a disease suggests that other genetic *loci* and/or environmental factors influence or modify the development of the disease.

Pharmacogenetics The variations in a single *gene* or small group of related genes that affect the pharmacology of a drug; the study of human genetic variation as revealed by various reactions to a drug.

Pharmacogenomics The variations in several *genes*, or the *genome*, that influence drug handling; the use of human genetic information for the design of new pharmaceuticals.

Phenotype The observable characteristics of an organism; includes visible features (eye color, height) and chemical and behavioral characteristics; reflects interaction of *genes* and environment.

Phenotyping In pharmacogenetics, the observable reaction or response of an individual (such as to a specific drug); the phenotype is based upon that individual's *genes*, but is influenced by other factors such as concomitant medications, liver function, and renal function.

Phlebotomist One who practices phlebotomy; the individual who withdraws blood from a patient.

Phlebotomy The puncture of a vein to collect blood.

Photolithography A process used to transfer a pattern from a photomask to the surface of a substrate, such as silicon, glass, plastic, sapphire, or metal.

Plasma The fluid portion of the blood in which the cells are suspended; differs from *serum* in that it contains fibrinogen and related proteins that are removed from blood when it clots and the specimen is centrifuged to obtain serum.

Polymerase An enzyme that sequentially adds *nucleotides* onto a growing polynucleotide, usually requiring a *primer* and a template (a nucleic acid strand whose base *sequence* serves as a pattern for the *sequence* of the new polynucleotide); polymerases are involved in DNA *replication* and *transcription*; DNA polymerase III reads a parent DNA template and attaches nucleotides to a growing daughter strand according to the *base-pairing* rules of double-stranded DNA; RNA polymerase II binds to a promoter region of a DNA strand to initiate transcription.

Polymerase Chain Reaction (PCR) An in vitro method for exponentially amplifying *DNA* (Chapter 5).

Polymorphism; Polymorphic A variation in the *sequence* of DNA; referring to differences in *nucleotide* sequences between two *chromosomes* at the same locus.

Preanalytical Variables Factors that affect specimens before analytical testing begins.

Preemptive Therapy Therapy administered to an identified high-risk group before development of symptoms in an attempt to prevent the development of active disease; genetic testing is used to identify individuals at high risk of disease; contrast with *Prophylactic Therapy*.

Preimplantation Genetic Testing Determining the *genotype* of an embryo relative to a specific genetic disease before choosing to implant the embryo in the womb.

Premutation Allele An *allele* with more copies of a trinucleotide (group of three nucleotides) than are present in a normal allele; for example, if the trinucleotide CAG is normally repeated four times (CAG CAG CAG CAG) in a certain gene, in a premutation allele of that gene it might be repeated 20 times; a premutation allele is at risk for expansion to a "full-mutation" allele (i.e., to gain even more copies of the trinucleotide) and thus cause disease; some premutation alleles produce clinical symptoms that are different from the clinical symptoms associated with a full-mutation allele in the same gene.

Primer   An *oligonucleotide* that serves to initiate *polymerase*-catalyzed addition of *dNTPs* by annealing to a template strand.

Probe   A *nucleic acid* used to identify a target by *hybridization*.

Prodrug   An inactive or less active drug that must first be metabolized to the active form of the drug to elicit the desired therapeutic effect.

Proficiency Testing   The process by which the same samples are analyzed by many laboratories with the results from each laboratory evaluated to determine the quality of laboratory performance; all steps in the testing process should be assessed.

Promoter   A regulatory region of *DNA* that serves to bind RNA *polymerase* II, which in turns binds other substances that will lead to initiation of *transcription*; promoters control the rate and timing of mRNA production and thus influence the rate of production of the corresponding protein.

Prophylactic Therapy   An approach to therapy in which all patients in a group of individuals are treated without further stratification of risk (as, for example, by genetic testing), thus involving treatment of a greater number of patients than in *preemptive therapy*.

Proto-oncogenes   Normal cellular genes that code for proteins that regulate cellular growth and differentiation; proto-oncogenes become *oncogenes* when they have been altered by dominant *mutations* or *chromosomal translocations*.

Pseudogene   A genetic element that does not result in a functional *gene* product, usually because of accumulated *mutations*.

Purine   A base containing two carbon-nitrogen rings; adenine and guanine are purines.

Pyrimidine   A base containing one carbon-nitrogen ring; cytosine, thymine, and uracil are pyrimidines.

Quality Assurance   The practice that encompasses all endeavors, procedures, formats, and activities directed toward ensuring that a specified quality is achieved and maintained.

Quality Control   The assessment of laboratory performance by testing assay controls and the statistical analysis of assay control values.

Quality Improvement   A process that uses a structured procedure to identify the causes of problems and to recommend appropriate remedies.

Randomized Controlled Trial   An experimental study in which study participants are randomly allocated to an intervention (treatment) group or an alternative treatment (control) group.

Real-Time PCR   A form of PCR in which the progress of amplification is observed at least once each cycle.

Recombination   Crossing over between DNA *sequences* resulting in the exchange of information between two *alleles*; this process occurs in *meiosis* between *homologous chromosomes* and during *mitosis* between sister chromatids; homologous recombination refers to this process when it occurs between similar sequences in corresponding regions; crossing over between misaligned yet similar sequences is called unequal homologous recombination; it is a mechanism to produce a duplication of the involved DNA segment on one chromosome and loss of the corresponding DNA (reciprocal deletion) on the other copy of that chromosome.

Reference Standard   The best available method for establishing the presence or absence of the target disease or condition; this could be a single test or a combination of methods and techniques.

Replication   The faithful reproduction of the *DNA* content from parent to daughter cells during cell division.

Resistance Testing   In molecular microbiology, genotypic assays that identify specific *mutations* or nucleotide changes that are associated with an increased *resistance* to an antiviral drug.

Resistance   The lack of response of an infectious agent to a therapy, such as an antibiotic, antiviral agent, or other therapeutic drug.

Restriction Endonuclease   An *endonuclease*, usually from bacteria, that cuts *nucleic acid* in a *sequence*-specific manner.

Restriction Fragment Length Polymorphisms (RFLP—"rif-lip")   *DNA polymorphisms* that are characterized by the ability of restriction enzyme digestion to generate fragments of different sizes; the fragment sizes are typically determined by electrophoresis; RFLPs thus include a subset of *single nucleotide polymorphisms (SNPs)* that are identified based on the ability of restriction endonucleases to digest double-stranded DNA at the sites of the variations in *sequence*.

Reverse Transcriptase   A polymerase that catalyzes synthesis of DNA from an RNA template.

Ribonucleic acid (RNA)   A molecule similar to *DNA* with the exceptions of being single stranded, containing ribose as the sugar moiety, having an extra hydroxyl group, and containing uracil instead of thymine; there are different functional types of RNA including messenger RNA (mRNA), ribosomal RNA (rRNA), and transfer RNA (tRNA).

RNase   A ubiquitous nuclease that specifically degrades RNA.

Sample   Part of a whole; a plasma sample is obtained from a blood specimen; a portion of a urine specimen that is taken for testing is a **sample** of the urine specimen; a blood specimen is also a sample of all the blood of the person being tested; and a liver biopsy is a sample of the patient's liver tissue; see also *specimen*.

Sarcoma   A malignant tumor of tissues of mesodermal origin, such as bone and muscle.

Sensitivity: Analytical Sensitivity   The change in the assay signal for a specific change in the quantity (or concentration) of a substance; the high sensitivity of PCR assays for pathogens is achieved through the several million-fold amplification of the pathogens' *nucleic acid*; "sensitivity" is often misused to mean the lowest concentration of an analyte that can be detected; **clinical sensitivity** (Chapter 2) of a test is the proportion of individuals with a specific disease whose test results are positive.

Sequence   Order of *bases* in a DNA or RNA molecule; a portion of a DNA molecule with a specific sequence.

Sequencing   Any method that determines the identity and exact order (*sequence*) of bases in a *DNA* molecule (or of amino acids in a protein).

Serum   The clear liquid that separates from blood on clotting; contrast with *plasma*.

Short Tandem Repeat (STR)   A nucleotide sequence, typically of 2 to 7 *base pairs*, that is repeated end to end; for example, in the sequence GATAGATAGATA, the tetranucleotide *GATA* (with 4 base pairs) is repeated three times; STRs are useful because the number of repeats (copies) of the STR varies among individuals and thus is useful in identifying the origin of DNA and in studying heredity; a region of a chromosome that contains the repeated nucleotide sequences is called a *microsatellite*.

Signal Amplification   Any method that increases the signal resulting from a molecular interaction that does not involve target amplification or *probe* amplification.

Single Nucleotide Polymorphism (SNP)   A single nucleotide variant that occurs in the population at a frequency of at least 1%; SNPs may be benign or cause disease.

Skewed X-Inactivation   A process by which inactivation of the X chromosome (lyonization) is not random.

Skin Puncture   Collection of capillary blood usually from a pediatric patient by making a thin cut in the skin, usually the heel of the foot.

Southern Blot   A method for detecting DNA *sequence* variants after restriction enzyme digestion and size separation by electrophoresis; hybridization with a labeled *probe* reveals *sequence* variants that result in a change in distance between restriction sites; detected variants include large insertions, deletions, and rearrangements.

Specificity: Analytical Specificity   The extent to which a method can identify or measure an analyte in a complex mixture without interference from other components in the mixture; the preferred term is selectivity; in molecular microbiology, specificity often refers to the ability of an assay to amplify and/or detect only the unique regions of the pathogen's genome without cross-reactivity with related species; specificity is sometimes used loosely to refer also to freedom from any interference; **Clinical Specificity** (Chapter 2) of a test is the proportion of individuals free of the target condition whose test results are negative.

Specimen   Tissue, fluid, or other material taken for testing; contrast with *sample*.

STARD   Standards for Reporting of Diagnostic Accuracy; a project designed to improve the quality of reporting of the results of studies of diagnostic accuracy of tests.

Systematic Review   A methodical and comprehensive review of all published and unpublished information about a specific topic to answer a precisely defined clinical question.

T Lymphocyte (T Cell)   T lymphocytes are a type of cells that are involved in the immune response; types of T lymphocytes include cytotoxic T cells, helper T cells, and regulatory T cells (also called suppressor T cells); the "T" in T cell represents thymus.

Target Amplification   Any method for increasing the amount of target *nucleic acid*; the "target" is the *nucleic acid* or nucleic acid *sequence* of interest.

T-Cell Receptor   These proteins are similar to immunoglobulins, but are found only on the surface of mature T lymphocytes; the T-cell receptors bind specific antigens.

Telomere   The DNA *sequences* at the end of a *chromosome*; telomeres contain repetitive nucleotide *sequences* that protect the ends of chromosomes from *recombination* with other chromosomes.

Thiopurine S-Methyltransferase (TPMT)   A metabolic enzyme that methylates and thereby inactivates 6-mercaptopurine (6-MP) and azathioprine, drugs used to treat several conditions, such as cancer and immune-mediated disease; individuals either lacking this enzyme or possessing enzyme with compromised function may require lower doses of the drugs to prevent toxicity.

Throughput   A term that describes analytical productivity; a process with high throughput is one in which a large number of *samples* are analyzed per hour or other appropriate time period.

Transcription   The process of transferring *sequence* information from the *gene* regions of DNA to an *RNA* message.

Translation   The process whereby an mRNA *sequence* forms an amino acid *sequence* with the help of tRNA and eventual enzymatic peptide bond formation between amino acids to synthesize polypeptides; translation occurs on cytoplasmic ribosomes.

Translocation, Chromosomal   A chromosomal translocation occurs when a piece of a *chromosome* breaks off and fuses to another chromosome; this added piece of chromosomal material can produce specific disorders, such as chronic myeloid leukemia (CML).

Transposon   A mobile genetic element that can delete and insert itself variably into the *genome*.

Tumor-Suppressor Gene   A *gene* that reduces the propensity of a cell to become malignant; thus loss of the proteins encoded by the tumor suppressor gene favors the formation of a *carcinoma*, *sarcoma*, *leukemia*, or *lymphoma*, depending on the cell in which the loss occurs.

UDP-Glucuronosyltransferase (UGT)   A family of metabolic enzymes that glucuronidate, and thereby inactivate, drugs, such as irinotecan (cancer therapeutic); genetic variants of *UGT1A1*, such as those with changes in its promoter region, are associated with *phenotypes* that have a higher risk of toxicity at usual doses of drugs; a lower dose is often appropriate for such individuals.

Uniparental Disomy   The inheritance of two copies of a *gene* from one parent and no gene from the other parent.

Upstream   Located closer to the 5′ end of DNA molecule.

Validity   (In research) the degree to which a measure is measuring what it is supposed to measure or the degree to which the study is able to answer the study question.

Variable Number of Tandem Repeats (VNTR) Locus   A locus with tandemly repeated segments of DNA (segments repeated end-to-end) that are typically more than 10 base pairs long and often more than 80 base pairs long; also known as a minisatellite locus; VNTRs can be used to identify individuals and their offspring; contrast with *STR* and *microsatellite*.

Venipuncture   The process of obtaining a blood *specimen* from a vein.

Venous Occlusion   Temporary blockage of return blood flow to the heart through the application of pressure, usually using a tourniquet.

Viral-Load Testing   Quantification of the concentration of genomic viral *nucleic acid* in blood (e.g., copies per liter of plasma); testing is done to determine when to initiate antiretroviral therapy, to monitor response to therapy, and to predict time to progression to AIDS.

X-linked Gene   An X-linked *gene* is one that is present only on an X chromosome; an X-linked disorder is a phenotype for which expression is dependent on the sex of an individual; in an X-linked *recessive* disorder, females are carriers of an X-linked gene when one of their (two) X chromosomes carries the gene variant, and are affected only when the variant is present on both copies; by contrast, males will exhibit the phenotype whenever they inherit the gene variant on their (single) X chromosome.

Index

Note: Page numbers followed by "f" refer to illustrations; page numbers followed by "t" refer to tables; page numbers followed by "b" refer to boxes.

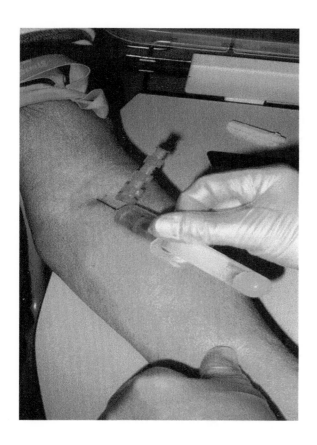

Venipuncture. (Courtesy Mayo Clinic, Rochester, Minn.) (See Figure 3-2.)

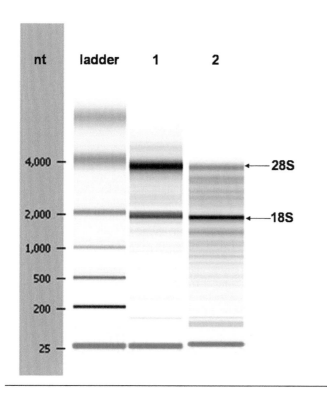

Assessment of total RNA quality by gel electrophoresis and densitometry. Total RNA extracted from whole blood specimens was analyzed by the Agilent 2100 bioanalyzer using the RNA 6000 Nano LabChip (Agilent Technologies). The gel electrophoretogram (shown here) is a simulated image based on the densitometry results. Extracted total RNA (lanes 1 and 2) appears as a smear with two prominent bands corresponding to the 18S and 28S rRNA, respectively. High-quality total RNA extractions (lane 1) are associated with high 28S/18S rRNA ratios with broad size distribution of the other RNA species. With RNase degradation as shown in lane 2, there is a reduction in the 28S/18S rRNA ratio and the overall RNA signal. There is also a shift towards shorter fragments of RNA. *nt*, Nucleotides. (See Figure 4-2, C.)

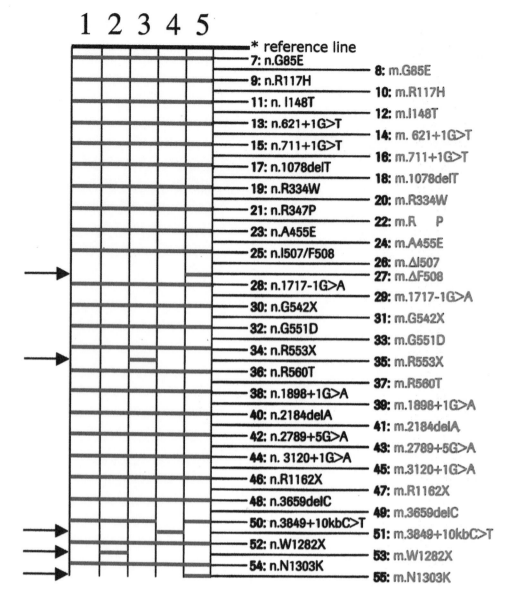

1 2 3 4 5

* reference line
7: n.G85E
8: m.G85E
9: n.R117H
10: m.R117H
11: n. I148T
12: m.I148T
13: n.621+1G>T
14: m. 621+1G>T
15: n.711+1G>T
16: m.711+1G>T
17: n.1078delT
18: m.1078delT
19: n.R334W
20: m.R334W
21: n.R347P
22: m.R   P
23: n.A455E
24: m.A455E
25: n.I507/F508
26: m.ΔI507
27: m.ΔF508
28: n.1717-1G>A
29: m.1717-1G>A
30: n.G542X
31: m.G542X
32: n.G551D
33: m.G551D
34: n.R553X
35: m.R553X
36: n.R560T
37: m.R560T
38: n.1898+1G>A
39: m.1898+1G>A
40: n.2184delA
41: m.2184delA
42: n.2789+5G>A
43: m.2789+5G>A
44: n. 3120+1G>A
45: m.3120+1G>A
46: n.R1162X
47: m.R1162X
48: n.3659delC
49: m.3659delC
50: n.3849+10kbC>T
51: m.3849+10kbC>T
52: n.W1282X
53: m.W1282X
54: n.N1303K
55: m.N1303K

Color Plate 3

CF mutation-detection assay CF Gold 1.0 developed by Roche Diagnostics Corp. Thirty to 45 ng of patient DNA is amplified in a multiplex amplification reaction. Amplicons are denatured and hybridized to membrane-bound oligonucleotide probes specific for 25 normal (n) and corresponding mutant (m) alleles. Lane 1 represents the pattern obtained from patient DNA in which none of the 25 common mutations is present; bands detected correspond only to normal alleles. Lane 2 represents the pattern obtained from patient DNA in which mutation W1282X is present in one allele, since bands corresponding to both nW1282X and mW1282X are present. In lane 3, mutation R553X is present in one allele since bands corresponding to mR553X and nR553X are present. Lanes 2 and 3 could represent CF carriers or could represent DNA from patients with CF for whom only one of their two mutations is identified. In the latter case, the second disease-causing mutation must be a mutation other than one of the 25 represented in this panel. Conversely, lane 4 represents patient DNA in which two copies of mutation 384910kbC>T are detected. Note that no band corresponding to n384910kbC>T is present. Lane 5 represents DNA from a CF patient who is a compound heterozygote with mutation delta F508 present on one allele and mutation N1303K present on the second mutant allele. Detection of 5, 7, or 9 T polymorphism in intron 8 has not been determined in these patients but can be performed by this assay. The strip contains oligonucleotide probes for the determination of this polymorphism in patient DNA above the reference line. However, before testing, this part of the strip is removed and is only performed as a reflex test if mutation R117H is detected. (See Figure 9-2.)

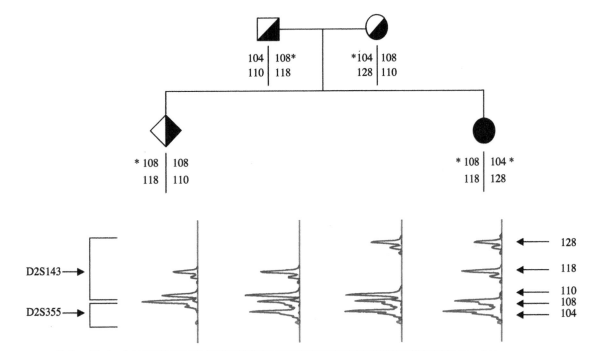

Color Plate 4

Electropherograms illustrating prenatal DNA-linkage studies on a family with CPSI deficiency. D2S355 (*blue*) and D2S143 (*green*) represent dinucleotide markers 4 centimorgans 5′ (D2S355) and 3 centimorgans 3′ (D2S143) to the *CPSI* gene, respectively. DNA samples from the affected child (*dark circle*), parents, and fetus are amplified by PCR using oligonucleotide primer pairs specific for each marker, with one primer of each pair labeled with a fluorescent dye. Amplicons are subjected to electrophoresis on a 5% denaturing polyacrylamide gel on an ABI 377 DNA sequencer and analyzed using GeneScan software 3.1 b3. The maternal haplotype donated to the affected child is 104,128, indicating that the mother's 108,110 allele is not linked to an abnormal *CPSI* gene. The paternal allele donated to the affected child is 108,118, indicating that the father's 104,110 allele is in repulsion with CPSI deficiency. The maternal allele donated to the fetus is 108,110. This allele is not linked to an abnormal *CPSI* gene. The paternal allele donated to the fetus is 108,118. This allele is linked to an abnormal *CPSI* gene. These results indicate that the fetus is a carrier of CPSI deficiency but is not affected. (See Figure 9-4.)

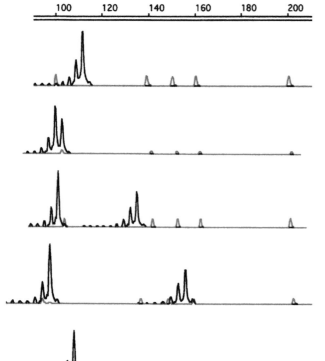

Color Plate 5

Electropherograms representing various patterns observed in patients referred for HD testing. The polyglutamine-encoding CAG repeat in exon 1 is amplified by PCR using flanking oligonucleotide primers, one of which is labeled with a fluorescent dye. Amplicons are subjected to electrophoresis on a 5% denaturing polyacrylamide gel on an ABI 377 DNA sequencer and analyzed using GeneScan software 3.1 b3. Amplicons 100 bp in length contain 18 CAG repeats and flanking DNA. Patient one (*row 1, top*) has amplicons 112 bp in length and has 22 CAG repeats on both HD alleles. Patient two (*row 2*) has 97 bp and 100 bp amplicons, corresponding to CAG repeats of 17 and 18. The diagnosis of HD can be ruled out in these two patients. Patient three (*row 3*) has 97 bp and 133 bp amplicons corresponding to CAG repeats of 17 and 29. The results would not support a diagnosis of HD. However, a CAG repeat of 29 is mutable and can undergo meiotic expansion to an HD allele. Patient four (*row 4*) has CAG repeats of 19 and 38 as depicted by amplicons 103 bp and 160 bp in length. In the symptomatic patient, these results would support the diagnosis of HD. However, in the presymptomatic patient, the phenotype of this HD allele with reduced penetrance cannot be predicted with certainty. Patient five (*row 5*) has CAG repeats of 21 and 44 since amplicons 109 bp and 178 bp in length were detected. These results would confirm the diagnosis of HD. Genetic counseling regarding the implications of the DNA findings in patients three, four, and five is indicated. (See Figure 9-7.)

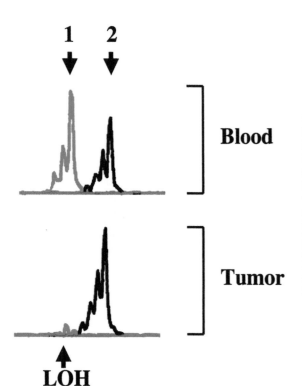

Blood

Tumor

LOH

Color Plate 6

Electropherograms illustrating loss of heterozygosity (LOH) in tumor DNA. Patient DNA is extracted from the peripheral blood and tumor tissue and amplified by PCR using an oligonucleotide primer pair specific for a polymorphic, microsatellite repeat locus contained within the chromosomal region thought to be deleted during tumorigenesis. One of the primers within the pair is labeled with a fluorescent dye. Amplicons are subjected to electrophoresis on a 5% denaturing polyacrylamide gel in an ABI DNA sequencer and analyzed using GeneScan software 3.1 b3. Constitutive DNA from the patient's blood illustrates heterozygosity for this marker with amplicons represented by alleles 1 and 2. In DNA from the tumor, a single peak representing a typical homozygous pattern is observed. Thus there is LOH in tumor DNA. This loss signifies the loss of the second allele and also indicates the loss of this region on the chromosome. (See Figure 9-14.)

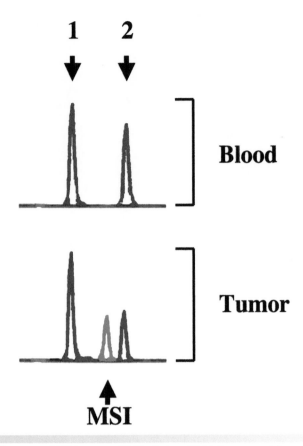

1 **2**

Blood

Tumor

MSI

Electropherograms illustrating MSI in tumor DNA. Patient DNA is extracted from the peripheral blood and tumor tissue and amplified by PCR using an oligonucleotide primer pair specific for a microsatellite repeat locus. One of the primers within the pair is labeled with a fluorescent dye. Amplicons are subjected to electrophoresis on a 5% denaturing polyacrylamide gel in an ABI DNA sequencer and analyzed by GeneScan software 3.1 b3. Constitutive DNA from the patient's blood illustrates heterozygosity for this marker with amplicons represented by alleles 1 and 2. In DNA from the tumor, in addition to constitutive alleles 1 and 2, amplicons representing DNA fragments of a different size are present; these indicate a change in repeat number for one of the alleles. Because of dysfunctional MMR enzymes, mistakes occurring during the replication of microsatellite repeat sequences resulting in expansions or contractions of the repeat number remain unrepaired. In this case, a contraction in the repeat number of allele 2 has occurred. (See Figure 9-15.)

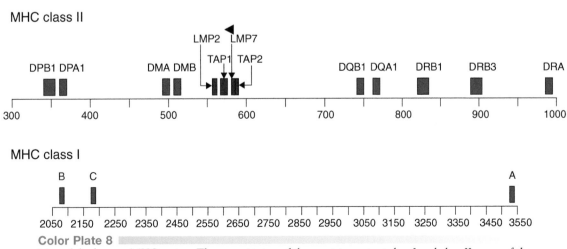

MHC class II

LMP2 LMP7

DPB1 DPA1   DMA DMB   TAP1 TAP2   DQB1 DQA1   DRB1   DRB3   DRA

300   400   500   600   700   800   900   1000

MHC class I

B   C   A

2050 2150 2250 2350 2450 2550 2650 2750 2850 2950 3050 3150 3250 3350 3450 3550

Map of the human MHC region. The organization of the most important class I and class II genes of the MHC is shown, with approximate genetic distances given in thousands of base pairs (kb). Genes are ordered from telomere to centromere. Not shown are MHC class III genes, which map between class I and class II genes. (See Figure 10-2.)

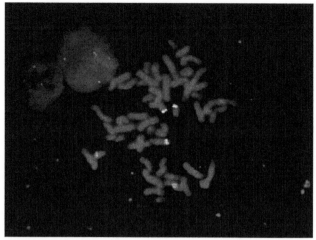

Fluorescence in situ hybridization for the t(14;18) anomaly on metaphase spreads from a case of follicular lymphoma. The immunoglobulin heavy chain sequences on 14q32 *(red)* when juxtaposed to the *BCL2* sequences on 18q21 *(green)* yield a yellow fusion signal indicative of the presence of the t(14;18). (See Figure 13-9.)

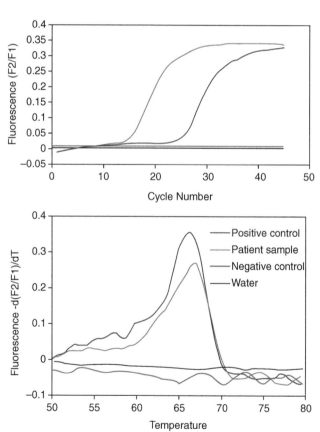

Real-time PCR detection of *RUNX1-RUNX1T1 (AML1-ETO)* fusion transcript. Real-time PCR detection was performed using a sequence-specific hybridization probe format with oligonucleotide probes labeled with fluorescein as the donor fluorophore and LCRed640 as the acceptor. Post-amplification melting analysis was performed to provide confirmation of amplicon identity through the probe melting temperature. The upper panel shows the fluorescence (F) versus cycle number (C) the LightCycler™ (Roche Diagnostics). The characteristic three-phase profiles of amplification curves are recognizable; i.e., initial lag, exponential or log/linear, and the final plateau phase. The red curve represents the positive amplification signal for the t(8;21) in the Kasumi cell line positive control. The blue curve represents the patient sample also showing the presence of the fusion. The green line represents a negative control (placental cDNA), and the black line is the no-template (H$_2$O) control. The lower panel shows the derivative melting curves with positive melting peaks at ~65°C, in both the Kasumi cell line positive control and the patient sample. Both the negative and water controls show flat lines indicating the absence of the t(8;21) product. (See Figure 13-12.)

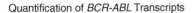

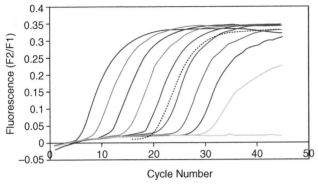

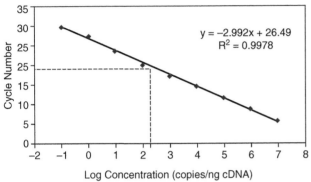

Real-time quantitative PCR of *BCR-ABL* transcripts with serial log dilutions of the plasmids (*colored curves*) containing the *BCR-ABL* sequence. Real-time PCR provides a remarkable dynamic range of quantification (10^9-10^0 template copies) in this example. The upper panel shows the amplification curves obtained using the *BCR-ABL*-containing plasmids, and an unknown patient sample depicted as a dotted line. Note the regular ~3.3-cycle interval between log dilutions. The lower panel shows a calibration curve (linear regression of cycle number versus log template concentration). As indicated by the dotted line in the lower panel, the threshold cycle (Chapter 5) can be used to quantify the number of copies of the target sequence in the tested sample. (See Figure 13-15.)

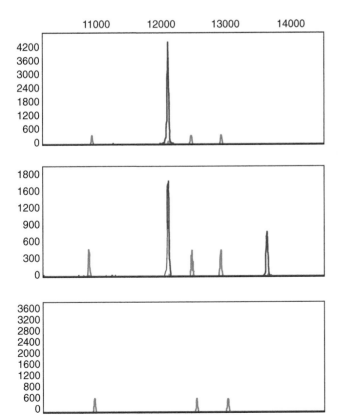

A, Detection of internal tandem duplications of the *FLT3* gene by PCR and capillary gel electrophoresis of PCR products. Capillary electropherograms show clear resolution of PCR products. The *x*-axis represents the sizes of PCR products and the *y*-axis shows the fluorescence intensity, which correlates with the abundance of the PCR product. The upper panel shows a wild-type pattern (*blue peak*) and size markers (*red peaks*). The middle panel shows an additional peak of greater size (*blue peak on the right*) than the wild-type peak. This additional peak represents an *FLT3* internal tandem duplication. The lower panel shows the size markers (*red peaks*), also present in the upper and middle panels. (See Figure 13-16, A.)

A

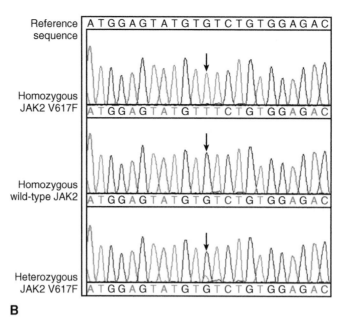

Reference sequence
`A T G G A G T A T G T G T C T G T G G A G A C`

Homozygous JAK2 V617F
`A T G G A G T A T G T T T C T G T G G A G A C`

Homozygous wild-type JAK2
`A T G G A G T A T G T G T C T G T G G A G A C`

Heterozygous JAK2 V617F
`A T G G A G T A T G T G T C T G T G G A G A C`

B

Color Plate 12

B, Sequencing electropherogram showing the 2343G>T nucleotide substitution seen in polycythemia vera. (See Figure 13-16, *B.*)

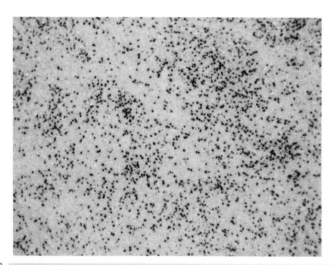

Color Plate 13

In situ hybridization (ISH) for the Epstein-Barr virus (EBV). Numerous positive signals (*dark-blue spots*) for EBV are visualized after hybridization of tissue with a fluorescently-labeled DNA probe that is complementary to a region (EBER-1) of the EBV genome. The tissue sample was obtained from a solid-organ transplant patient who developed widespread nodal and extranodal masses. The positive reaction for EBV in this assay supports a diagnosis of post-transplant lymphoproliferative disease. (See Figure 13-17.)